TEXTBOOK OF MEDICAL-SURGICAL NURSING

VOLUME 1: FOUNDATIONS OF ADULT HEALTH AND PROFESSIONAL PRACTICE

Michele McCarthy

ALLIED HEALTH PRESS

Textbook of Medical-Surgical Nursing

Volume 1: Foundations of Adult Health and Professional Practice

Author: **Michele McCarthy**

Allied Health Press
4164 Lakeshore Road
Burlington ON L7L 1A4
Canada
www.alliedhealthpress.com
Email: orders@arclereducation.com

ISBN: 978-1-77956-819-9

ABOUT THE AUTHOR

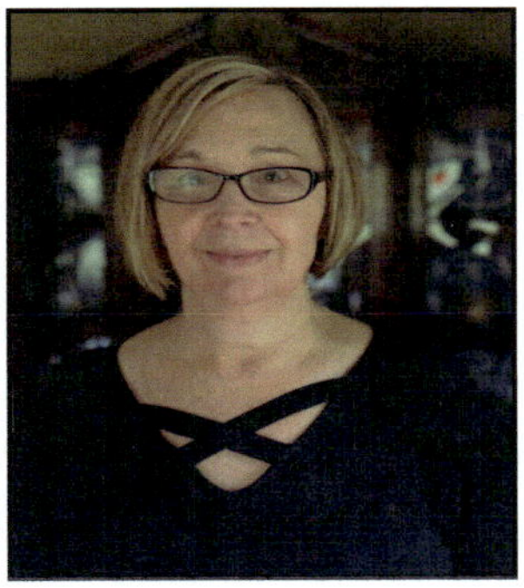

Michele is a registered nurse with over 25 years of clinical experience and a decade of service as a nurse educator. She holds national certifications as a Certified Nurse Educator (CNE) and Certified Healthcare Simulation Educator (CHSE), reflecting her commitment to excellence in teaching and experiential learning. Michele is passionate about advancing nursing education through learner-centered design, curriculum innovation, and the integration of simulation-based strategies.

Brief Table of Contents

Getting Started with This Book

Chapter Openers

A list of Chapter Outline is presented providing a brief Introduction to what will be covered in the chapter.

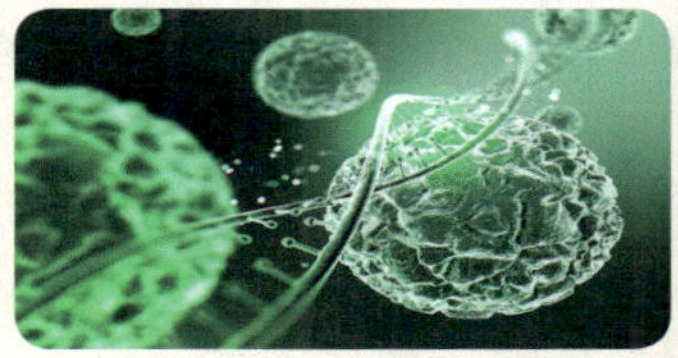

LEARNING OBJECTIVES

After studying this chapter, you will be able to:

1. Discuss the scientific method in biology;
2. Explain the cell theory;
3. Discuss the genetics and heredity;
4. Evolution and natural selection;
5. Focus on ecology and ecosystems;
6. Learn about human biology;
7. Evaluate the plant biology;
8. Explain the microbiology;
9. Focus on current trends in biology.

Introduction

Often referred to as the science of life, biology is a broad field of study aimed at comprehending the several kinds of life on Earth, from tiny creatures to sophisticated multicellular entities. Comprising several subfields, including molecular biology, ecology, and evolutionary biology, each of which advances our knowledge of living systems, this field clarifies the mechanisms controlling life events, including development, reproduction, and interaction with the surroundings, which is the central goal of biology. Moreover, biology fills in the void between the natural sciences and medicine by offering a necessary understanding of health, illness, and the interactions between organisms and their environments. Dealing with urgent global issues such as climate change, biodiversity loss, and new diseases depends on an awareness of these complex biological interactions, therefore highlighting the critical part biology plays in modern civilization. Fundamentally, biology explores and tests ideas about the living world using the scientific method. Through methodical observation and experimentation,

1.1. The Scientific Method in Biology

Learning Outcome

1. Describe the steps of the scientific method;
2. Focus on hypothesis formation;
3. Learn about experimental design.

Learning Outcomes

The beginning of each section of every chapter contains a set of Learning Outcomes that inform students of concepts they should understand. These outcomes help students understand what they should be able to do if they have mastered the material in that section.

Test Your Knowledge

Throughout each chapter, Test Your Knowledge cues you to note which topics have been covered and to self-test your understanding of the material presented.

Test Your Knowledge

1. Explain why correlation does not imply causation in scientific experiments.
2. How does the scientific method help reduce the influence of personal opinions in research?

Chapter Summary

The Summary Section appear at the end of each chapter and summarize main concepts covered throughout the chapter. These points provide key concepts in an engaging and meaningful way.

Summary

The investigation of biological principles highlights the importance of a comprehensive view of life by reflecting the intricate interactions that occur within living systems. The complexity of biology goes beyond individual species or systems, as this essay highlights; it also includes the interactions that mold ecosystems and affect biodiversity. Researchers can conduct in-depth analyses of metabolomic data using sophisticated technologies like MetaboAnalyst, which offer insights into the molecular mechanisms underlying these interactions. As demonstrated by the developments in MetaboAnalyst, for example, the integration of diverse omics data promotes a thorough understanding of metabolic pathways and helps identify important biological markers necessary for research on development and disease (Chong et al., 2018). Additionally, the phenomenon of ecological invasions is a key component of biological research and a vital field of study. The introduction of non-native species into unfamiliar habitats has significant ramifications and calls for multidisciplinary management strategies. Examining the origins and effects of these biological incursions, invasion science has become a crucial field that highlights the need to comprehend ecological dynamics and community interactions. As interest in biological invasions increases, new findings are emerging that put conventional ecological theories and practices to the test. The importance of incorporating various scientific viewpoints is shown by this developing discipline, which also highlights how invasive species shape ecosystems and advances our knowledge of ecological resilience (David et al., 2013). When taken as a whole, these discoveries from invasion science and metabolomics highlight the value of multidisciplinary biology research. Fostering cross-disciplinary collaboration and utilizing technological breakthroughs to improve our comprehension of intricate biological interactions are crucial as we look to the future of biological research. In addition to deepening our understanding of the complexities of life, this method lays the groundwork for tackling urgent environmental issues. Future studies can ensure the continued relevance of biology in a world that is constantly changing by acknowledging the interconnection of biological systems and opening the door to creative solutions that support sustainability and biodiversity conservation. We might imagine a thorough comprehension of life that serves both academia and society at large through ongoing investigation and integration of scientific knowledge.

Knowledge Assessment

The chapter includes material designed to review and reinforce each content. It includes Critical Thinking Questions to help test of your understanding of information presented in the chapter and Short answer Questions to review your understanding of the key concepts presented in the chapter.

Critical Thinking Questions

1. **Who is known as the "Father of Modern Biology"?**
   a. Aristotle
   b. Charles Darwin
   c. Gregor Mendel
   d. Louis Pasteur
2. **What is the basic unit of life?**
   a. Atom
   b. Molecule
   c. Cell
   d. Organism
3. **Which branch of biology studies the interaction of organisms with their environment?**
   a. Genetics
   b. Ecology
   c. Physiology
   d. Botany
4. **Which macromolecule is the main source of energy for living organisms?**
   a. Proteins
   b. Lipids
   c. Carbohydrates
   d. Nucleic acids
5. **DNA is primarily responsible for which function in living organisms?**
   a. Energy production
   b. Protein synthesis
   c. Storing genetic information
   d. Regulating body temperature

Short Answer Questions

1. What is biology, and why is it important to study biology?
2. What are the three main domains of life, and how are they different from one another?
3. Define homeostasis and give an example of how it works in living organisms.
4. What is the cell theory, and why is it fundamental to biology?
5. How do autotrophs and heterotrophs differ in the way they obtain energy?
6. What is the scientific method, and how is it applied in biological research?
7. Discuss how biology helps address global challenges such as climate change, disease, and food security.
8. Explain the levels of biological organization from the smallest unit to the largest. Provide examples at each level.
9. Describe the relationship between structure and function in biology, giving specific examples from cells or organs.
10. How has the discovery of genetics shaped our understanding of inheritance and variation among organisms?

Supplementary Materials

Key Terms: A list of key terms is given for quick reference

KEY TERMS FROM THIS CHAPTER

Annotation enrichment analysis	Biological structure	Cell
Cell theory	Cellular structure	Ecology
Ecosystems	Genetics	Human biology
Microbiology	Natural selection	Organism
Plant biology		

Further Resources: Recommendations for additional readings, websites, and multimedia resources.

References

1. Argelaguet, R., Velten, B., Arnol, D., Dietrich, S., Zenz, T., Marioni, J. C., Buettner, F., et al. (2018). Multi-omics factor analysis—A framework for unsupervised integration of multi-omics data sets. *Molecular Systems Biology, 14*. https://doi.org/10.15252/msb.20178124.
2. Bacher, S., Blackburn, T. M., Essl, F., & Genovesi, P. (2017). *Socio-Economic Impact Classification of Alien Taxa (SEICAT)*. https://core.ac.uk/download/286567949.pdf (accessed on 8th March 2025).
3. Barnett, R., Brace, S., Cucchi, T., & Dobney, K. (2013). *Divergent Evolutionary Processes Associated with Colonization of Offshore Islands*. https://core.ac.uk/download/20664364.pdf (accessed on 8th March 2025).

Detailed Table of Contents

CHAPTER 7

Disability, Chronic Illness, and Long-Term Care 203

CHAPTER 8

Genetics and Genomics in Nursing Practice 237

CHAPTER 11

Shock, Sepsis, and Multiple Organ Dysfunction Syndrome in Nursing 337

CHAPTER 12

Cancer Nursing: Principles of Oncologic Management 369

LIST OF FIGURES

PREFACE

Medical-surgical nursing is likely the first truly integrated and dynamic area of professional healthcare. It requires nurses to integrate scientific knowledge and practical expertise, compassion and clinical precision, with individualized care and systemic understanding and sensitivity. The profession is founded on delivering the full spectrum of adult health needs, both acute and chronic, in any environment. As the healthcare setting continues to evolve—driven by shifts in population, technological advancements, and global public health concerns—the role of the medical-surgical nurse is increasingly at the center of delivering safe, effective, and person-centered care.

In this formidable environment, professional nurses are not only caregivers but also teachers, advocates, and team members. They collaborate with patients, families, and interprofessional teams to promote wellness, minimize complications, and enhance health outcomes. The need for clinical competence, evidence-based practice, and ethical professional decisions among nurses is paramount. From postoperative recovery to end-of-life care, the medical-surgical nurse must conduct herself with confidence, accuracy, and compassion in a diverse array of situations. Preparation for such care requires a firm theoretical basis, clinical expertise, and the ability to adapt to the physical, psychological, and social aspects of adult health.

Textbook of Medical-Surgical Nursing – Volume 1 is designed to serve as a core textbook for nursing students, novice practitioners, and faculty. It emphasizes the integration of theory and practice, enabling nurses to respond to clinical needs with skill and insight. In thorough, evidence-based chapters, the book builds systematic knowledge of adult medical-surgical patient care. It presents essential clinical concepts while validating the values and professional roles required in nursing. With a focus on competence, communication, and the whole-person care approach, this textbook enables learners to develop critical and practical skills for contemporary nursing practice.

Chapter 1 addresses an introduction to professional nursing practice in medical-surgical environments, focusing on ethical responsibilities, the law, evidence-based practice, and the evolving role of the nurse within healthcare systems.

Chapter 2 covers guiding principles and the scope of medical-surgical nursing, including patient safety, interprofessional practice, and the nurse's role in various care settings.

Chapter 3 presents health education and health promotion strategies, emphasizing the importance of patient involvement, behavioral change theories, and educational planning in fostering long-term health behaviors.

Chapter 4 discusses the comprehensive assessment of adult health, such as physical examination, nutrition screening, and cultural competence in communicating with patients. It attempts to foster clinical judgment through having a specific and thorough approach to gathering and interpreting data.

Chapter 5 outlines the physiological response of the body to stress and the inflammatory processes, enabling nurses to recognize early warning signs and take prompt interventions.

Chapter 6 addresses the theory of gerontological nursing, including the physical, cognitive, and emotional characteristics of aging, as well as methods of support for the independence, comfort, and safety of older patient populations.

Chapter 7 addresses patient care for individuals with disabilities and chronic illnesses, as well as the issues of long-term care. It demands continuous emphasis on quality of life, caregiver support, and interprofessional planning. Chapter 8 explores the increasing importance of genetics and genomics in nursing practice, particularly in patient assessment, risk assessment, and ethical decision-making during genetic counseling and individualized care. Chapter 9 addresses pain control, including assessment techniques, pharmacological and non-pharmacological management, and the importance of patient-centered approaches in pain management. Chapter 10 outlines the regulation and clinical use of fluid, electrolyte, and acid-base balance.

It enables readers to monitor, interpret, and intervene in physiological imbalances that can compromise patient stability.

Chapter 11 addresses shock, sepsis, and multiple organ dysfunction syndrome, providing a complete understanding of pathophysiology, early recognition, and emergency priorities of care in life-threatening disease.

Finally, Chapter 12 discusses oncologic nursing management concepts, including cancer biology, treatments, symptom management, and emotional and psychosocial support for patients and families with cancer receiving care. This book is written for undergraduate nursing students, especially those in their clinical years, and a reliable reference for newly licensed nurses and nurse educators.

It is ideal for laboratory simulations, practice rotations, and classroom instruction. It is aligned with nursing curricula and practice standards to help learners apply academic knowledge to practice. Instructors may use it in lesson planning, exam creation, and discussions. Ultimately, the book is intended for anyone dedicated to establishing a solid, competent foundation in adult medical-surgical nursing, grounded in knowledge, compassion, and clinical excellence.

PROFESSIONAL NURSING PRACTICE IN MEDICAL-SURGICAL CARE

1

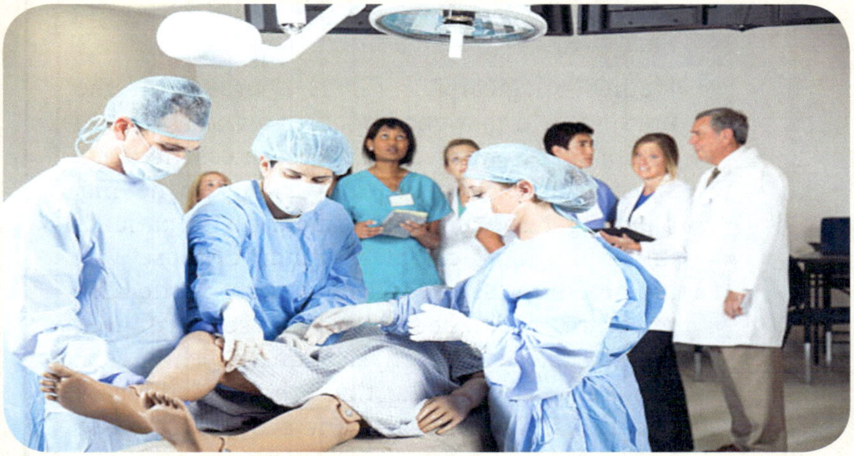

Introduction

Medical-surgical nursing is a vital specialty in delivering comprehensive care to patients across various clinical settings. Professional practice nursing as a specialty encompasses a wide range of competencies required in patient assessment, intervention, and education. With evolving healthcare, increased complexity of patient conditions requires, along with clinical competency, nurses to practice in collaboration with other health professionals. This integration ensures that patients receive comprehensive care tailored to their individual needs. The Foundation of Nursing Practice emphasizes evidence-based practice, and nurses should ensure they stay current with the latest research and developments in the healthcare industry to achieve optimal patient outcomes (Bonica et al., 2017). Advanced practice roles, such as nurse practitioners (NPs) and physician assistants (PAs), have focused on collaborative medical-surgical practice. These clinicians are valued additions to care teams, bridging gaps in healthcare

LEARNING OBJECTIVES

After studying this chapter, you will be able to:

1. Understand the evolution of medical-surgical nursing
2. Describe the central competencies in medical-surgical nursing
3. Discuss patient-centered care within medical-surgical environments
4. Identify medical-surgical nurses' challenges
5. Learn about practice innovations of nursing
6. Assess professional development and continuing education

delivery and enhancing patient interactions. The responsibilities and roles overlap, and communication and coordination with nurses, particularly in the operating room, require directness. Through close collaboration with residents and other healthcare professionals, PAs and NPs ensure an integrated environment that supports integrated care for patients.

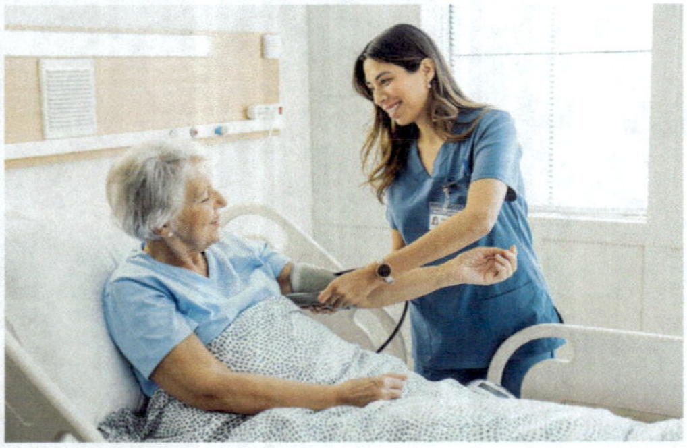

Figure 1.1. Medical-surgical nursing.

Source: https://external-content.duckduckgo.com/iu/?u=https%3A%2F%2Fassets-global.website-files.com%2F5babc11099f97ea5dbcf24d5%2F64de3ec56db3d89c7d78cab0_med-surg-nurse.jpg&f=1&nofb=1&ipt=6598dc00905997fdfa1a3d0e80222ec41d129b082860e0b38b2a9d509b1ec46e.

The transformation of care dynamics not only supports patient safety but also enables greater efficiency in care delivery, underscoring the indispensable role of professional practice nursing in medical-surgical care (Dunnington et al., 2018). With ongoing development in the healthcare setting, nurse roles in medical-surgical settings are increasingly considered to be the prescription for success of patient care initiatives. Advanced practice professionals introduced a reevaluation of the nursing role and an increased demand for more formal models of integration. This revision accommodates the needs of patients of different kinds in response to the problems of healthcare workforce shortages and growing service demands. In such a situation, nurses' education, as formal professional and mentoring programs, is the only solution to assist them with the complexity of patient care in modern times. This multifaceted plan is not only intended to promote patient outcomes but also to promote the sustained growth and job satisfaction of nursing professionals who work in a progressively dynamic healthcare landscape (Bonica et al., 2017) (Figure 1.1).

Definition of Medical-Surgical Nursing

Medical-surgical nursing is a branch of the nursing field that encompasses a wide range of complex patient care practices. In essence, this specialization involves assessing, diagnosing, planning, implementing, and caring for patients undergoing surgical interventions or those with medical illnesses requiring a therapeutic care program. Medical-surgical nurses are held accountable for the physical and psychological well-being of patients through extensive care programs. Such nurses can provide care for both pre- and post-operative phases, thereby ensuring continuity of care and addressing any complications that may arise. In contemporary healthcare systems, medical-surgical nursing is particularly critical due to the increased prevalence of chronic illness and the need for surgeries, and, consequently, the demand for competent nursing staff in delivering quality care daily. Emerging healthcare needs, specifically as systems struggle with workforce and resource issues, shape the practice of medical-surgical nursing. Healthcare environments are continually faced with the challenge of being timely while still ensuring patient quality and safety. For instance, as recognized by current scoping reviews, pre-scheduling semi-urgent surgical procedures involves intricacies in healthcare provision, wherein timely access to surgery is a central factor in achieving optimal patient outcomes (Coffey et al., 2024). All these nuances require successful healthcare systems interested in fulfilling patients' needs and promoting team-oriented methods among healthcare professionals. Medical-surgical nurses, in most instances, serve as patient advocates, resolving such system issues while delivering quality levels of care reflecting professional practice excellence in nursing. Interprofessional teamwork among healthcare teams is key to efficient medical-surgical nursing, supporting a model in which different professionals work together to advance patient-centered care. Initiatives such as the "Team Around the Patient" pilot programs in healthcare organizations aim at redefining the working roles of health providers, focusing on group innovation in addressing the varied needs of patients (Walsby et al., 2023). Through the integration of information from various stakeholders, including nursing, allied healthcare professionals, and administrators, this model aims to eradicate issues such as skill shortages and improve the delivery of patient care. Finally, the future of medical-surgical nursing depends on such interprofessional models that create interprofessional alliances and cultivate an adaptive workforce able to respond to issues in patient care in an increasingly changing healthcare setting.

Professional Nursing Practice Significance

Expert nursing practice is crucial to achieving the highest quality patient outcomes in medical-surgical settings. The severity of patient needs in such situations requires highly competent nursing practitioners to be readily available, ensuring high-quality care. Ideal nursing practice is based on clinical competence, which has a paramount influence on patient safety and the success of medical procedures. For example, studies have established a relationship between clinical competency and GPA scores for nursing students, where a higher GPA score is associated with better preparedness for practice (Khalafi et al., 2025). Thus, as medical-surgical practice becomes more complex, nursing education programs must prioritize the development of clinical competencies to professional standards. By fostering patient safety and clinical judgment skills, nursing education programs are crucial in equipping future practitioners to address the increasingly complex needs of healthcare. Communication and teamwork among healthcare providers are also critical components of professional nursing practice. The ability to perform effectively in diverse, multidisciplinary groups enhances interprofessional collaboration and, as a result, improves patient care outcomes. In medical-surgical settings, the introduction of Interprofessional Education (IPE) programs has been shown to enhance communication and teamwork among recently admitted medical doctors by a significant margin (Zhang et al., 2024). Through this education, nurses are equipped with the skills necessary to navigate the complexities of teamwork-oriented healthcare settings, thereby minimizing the likelihood of mistakes and enhancing the overall quality of service. Thus, an emphasis on teamwork in nursing school prepares an individual not only to work together but also instills a culture of teamwork and respect, fostering mutual accountability for patient outcomes. Constant professional development among medical-surgical nurses also ensures that high-quality care is consistently delivered in medical-surgical environments. Continuing education ensures that nurses are informed about the most recent advances in medical interventions, technology, and evidence-based practice. Ongoing learning is necessary to keep pace with the dynamic nature of healthcare environments, where treatment procedures and protocols are constantly evolving. Through the identification of gaps in communication and professional working by research that detects such gaps, closure of the gaps through direct training enhances nurses' ability and confidence (Khalafi et al., 2025). Besides, promoting professional practice standards among nursing professionals ensures that not just ethical standards but patient safety and best practices in integral care are enhanced among nurses. Ensuring professional development is the priority to ensure the nursing profession renews its fundamental purpose of promoting safe and effective practice in surgery and medicine (Figure 1.2).

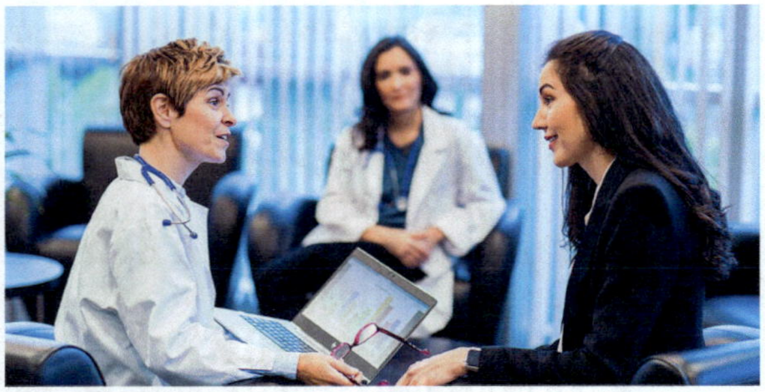

Figure 1.2. Professionalism in nursing.

Source: https://external-content.duckduckgo.com/iu/?u=https%3A%2F%2Fwww.usa.edu%2Fwp-content%2Fuploads%2F2020%2F06%2FMDP_2327.jpg%3Fis-pending-load%3D1&f=1&nofb=1&ipt=1363ec82adfb537c85f389c5d68c24cf7bad289dd41dbda49389c56b4bc403e4.

1.1. Historical Context of Medical-Surgical Nursing

Learning Outcome

1. Describe the evolution of nursing practice
2. Highlight milestones in medical-surgical nursing
3. Understand the influence of history on practice nursing

Medical-surgical nursing development is closely associated with advancements in medical technology and science, reflecting broader trends in healthcare as reflected in public opinion. In the late 19th century, the practice gradually became institutionalized, thanks primarily to the guidance of pathfinders such as Florence Nightingale, who focused on sanitation and public health, laying the groundwork for nursing practice. The establishment of schools of nursing, such as the Nightingale School of Nursing in 1860, continued to professionalize nursing roles and emphasized the importance of having competent staff within the operating room setting. Due to the development of the techniques of surgery, with the introduction of anesthesia and antisepsis care, specialized surgical nursing practice became an imperative, giving rise to a type of work focused on the pre-operative and post-operative management and instruction of the patient. This innovation set a pattern for medical-surgical nursing today, where comprehensive knowledge of patients' individualized requirements remains the primary focus. As the 20th century unfolded, medical-surgical nursing was compelled to adapt to significant transformations introduced by the increasing sophistication of operations and the growing demand for more complex patient care. Technological progress, including the use of imaging modalities and minimal access surgery techniques, transformed the science of surgery, necessitating changes in practice and education modalities for nurses. Studies conducted at this time revealed that appropriately trained nurses were able to perform procedures that had previously been performed by doctors safely, for example, the trial comparing pre-operative assessment by appropriately trained nurses (ATNs) and pre-registration house officers (PRHOs). The findings indicated comparative safety and quality when assessing patients, thereby maintaining nurses' positions in operating theaters (Alhameed et al., 2001). These innovations not only elevated the status of nurses in the operating rooms but also called for training programs capable of equipping nurses with suitable skills in a changing healthcare system. Higher responsibility, however, also introduced its own bag of challenges, including moral distress among nursing professionals. The research proposes that high-need surgical nurses indicate severe psychological distress around ethical judgment-making, and also care delivery (Aghaei et al., 2015). The observation highlights the need for emotional well-being awareness and effective nursing practice management. Amidst a transforming health environment, however, an urgent call remains for systematic evidence of moral distress and its influences on nursing practice in medical-surgical care. In the context of medical-surgical profession history, current practitioners can advocate for enhanced training, deliver high-quality care to patients, and develop coping skills to manage moral distress within the profession. In this regard, the history of the medical-surgical profession serves as a foundational pillar in addressing issues in current professional nursing practice (Figure 1.3).

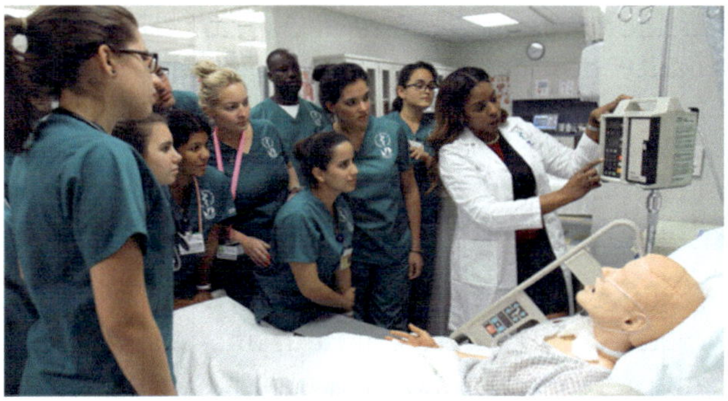

Figure 1.3. Appropriately trained nurses (ATNs).

Source: https://www.mdc.edu/nursing/img/featured-carousel-4.jpg.

1.1.1. Evolution of Nursing Practices

Throughout the decades, nursing practice has undergone significant changes, driven by historical advancements, evolving healthcare demands, and advancements in medical technology. The history of nursing dates back to the late 19th and early 20th centuries, characterized by the institutionalization of nursing education and the formation of professional nursing organizations. These facilities encouraged improved standards of training and the gravity of evidence-based practice in clinical settings. This set the pace for the future of nursing as a professionalized career and redefined nurses' interactions with patient care, especially in medical-surgical settings, where vast amounts of knowledge regarding patient needs are required. This context highlights the dynamic nature of nursing practice, which adapts to the nuances of delivering quality care. The nurse's role in medical-surgical care has emerged as a pivotal theme of today's healthcare. Nurses, while providing direct care to patients within these settings, act as patient safety champions, interact with interdisciplinary teams, and operate with advanced technologies to improve health outcomes. Over time, the establishment of evidence-based guidelines and standardized protocols has enhanced the quality of nursing care by emphasizing systematic interventions and assessments. Nurses are now better equipped with an integrated knowledge of pathophysiology, pharmacology, and evidence-based practice that allows them to act as caregivers as well as critical thinkers in today's healthcare setting. This evolution underscores the importance of continuing education and the adaptation of nursing practice to deliver optimal patient care within medical-surgical settings, where the complexity of patient presentations also necessitates advanced skills and knowledge. Furthermore, nursing practice changes are inextricably linked to broader societal trends, including the increasing use of technology and the rise in patient acuity within hospital settings. The integration of health information technologies has revolutionized nursing processes, making it simpler to document and communicate with one another among healthcare providers. For example, the use of electronic health records has ensured easy access to essential patient data to allow nurses to make decisions quickly and efficiently. Parallel to these advances in technology, the emphasis on patient-centered care has transformed nursing practice, with nurses now expected to be part of collaborative decision-making between patients and their families. This is yet another sign of a better understanding of holistic care in line with the dominant paradigms that emphasize the patient experience in medical-surgical care, and an indication of the profession's adaptability to address the needs of the healthcare environment and the patients being cared for (Figure 1.4).

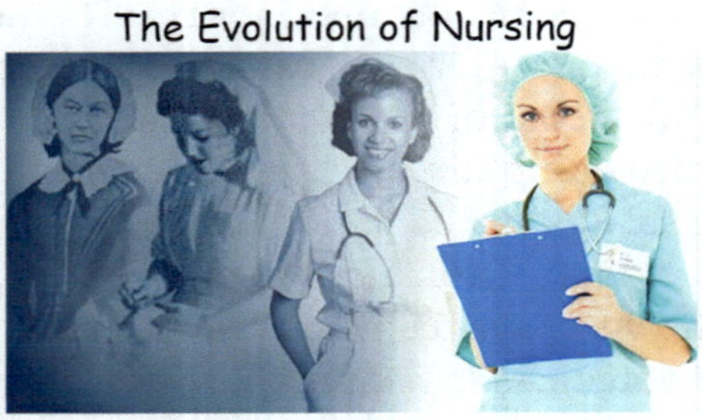

Figure 1.4. Evolution of nursing practices.

Source: https://external-content.duckduckgo.com/iu/?u=http%3A%2F%2F2.bp.blogspot.com%2F_uoJ_ksNzD2Y%2FS-gsczBMgHI%2FAAAAAAAAA5k%2FCt0A1NgXPkg%2Fs1600%2Fevolution%2Bof%2Bnursing.jpg&f=1&nofb=1&ipt=aac780210e15e7f8981da8ab17fc06aec8e84aa91e1ae87a446e34b7bc886ee9.

1.1.2. Key Milestones in Medical-Surgical Nursing

The history of medical-surgical nursing reflects significant developments with key milestones that have shaped the profession today. One of the most characteristic developments was the emergence of standardized care protocols, which seemed to respond to the increasing complexity of patient needs and the requirement for quality assurance. These standards provided the foundation for evidence-based practice, which enhances patient outcomes by enabling nurses to utilize current research and recommendations in their decision-making. Another milestone is the integration of technology and informatics in nursing, allowing for improved patient monitoring and data management. These technologies have enabled the medical-surgical nurse to deliver effective and efficient care, ultimately resulting in enhanced patient safety and quality outcomes. Greater interdisciplinary collaboration represents yet another significant advance in medical-surgical practice. Modern health care has recognized that total patient care is best delivered through an interdisciplinary team of physicians, pharmacists, and social workers. This collaborative approach facilitates a more comprehensive assessment of patient needs and enhances the coordination of care. For instance, the implementation of evidence-based infection prevention bundles, such as those for preventing central line-associated bloodstream infections (CLABSIs), underscores the importance of collaboration in achieving quality measures. There is evidence that unit work with a strong emphasis on workload management and prioritization of quality has resulted in higher adherence to CLABSI prevention guidelines, and that being collaborative to a certain degree is paramount in the pursuit of best patient safety and quality within med-surg settings (Lee et al., 2018).

Furthermore, the promotion of best practices by professional nursing associations cannot be overlooked as a turning point in this field. Nursing associations that aim to enhance nursing expertise have provided platforms for sharing innovative practices, thereby stimulating improved patient care. Quality improvement programs emphasize the importance of adopting evidence-based practices and a culture of continuous learning in health facilities. For example, initiatives that are integrated with organizational goals and include helpful tools for implementation promote not just adherence to clinical guidelines but also empower nurses to take an active role in quality improvement efforts. Through learning networks that maximize opportunities for learning, these types of organizations play a crucial role in the progressive evolution of medical-surgical nursing and its application to professional nursing practice in medical-surgical care (Stern et al., 2010) (Figure 1.5).

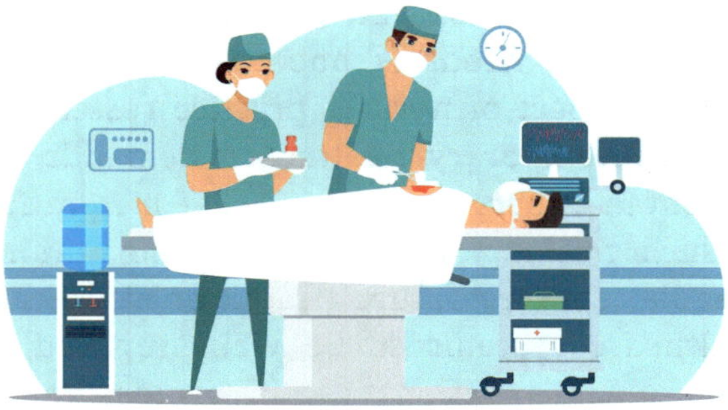

Figure 1.5. Surgical nurse.

Source: https://www.arizonacollege.edu/wp-content/uploads/2022/03/What-do-surgical-nurses-do.jpg.

1.1.3. The Impact of Historical Events on Nursing Roles

The profession of nursing has been significantly influenced by major historical events, such as wars, epidemics, and shifts in healthcare priorities. For instance, the role of nursing was not only expanded by nurses like Clara Barton during the Civil War, but also established nursing as a practical career for women. This period stressed the importance of educated care in chaotic times, ultimately leading to the institutionalization of nursing education. Nurses began to gain respect as important members of the healthcare team, resulting in significant improvements in nursing functions, particularly in areas such as triage and critical care administration, which are the cornerstones of medical-surgical nursing practice today. Past epidemics, such as the 1918 flu pandemic, also had an impact in shaping nursing roles by expanding public health advocacy and education. The enormous need for nurse care during the calamity led to increased nursing programs and a heavy emphasis on preventive care. When nurses took on more roles in community health, their roles included disease prevention and health promotion instruction. This shift marked a milestone in the nursing profession because it highlighted interdisciplinary solutions to public health problems, a concept as vital in the medical-surgical arena today. Recent developments in healthcare, particularly the expansion of advanced practice roles, are evidence of the evolution of nursing practice and a response to previous challenges. The development of physician assistants (PAs) and nurse practitioners (NPs) into care teams is evidence of a considerable shift towards team care models from the previous workforce deficit and the need for cost-cutting measures. Efforts to introduce programs supporting the expanded roles of advanced providers have fostered efficiency in patient care, thus justifying nursing's vital role in operating rooms. Through these focuses on integrating such providers into surgical teams, nursing continues to evolve, shaping professional practice according to the changing needs of patient care within complex medical-surgical environments (Adler et al., 2016; Dunnington et al., 2018).

Test Your Knowledge

1. What are the primary roles and responsibilities of a medical-surgical nurse who works in a hospital?
2. How is the nursing process applied in clinical decision-making within the medical-surgical practice?

1.2. Core Competencies in Medical-Surgical Nursing

Learning Outcome

1. Explain the clinical competencies and knowledge
2. Clarify the communication and interpersonal competencies

3.Explain the critical thinking and decision-making

With the evolving face of healthcare, key competencies in medical-surgical nursing are accountable for ensuring quality patient care. These include an in-depth knowledge base in patient assessment, care planning, and the application of evidence-based interventions. The medical-surgical nursing complexity requires practitioners to integrate clinical skills with evidence-based ability in research and quality improvement. As highlighted in Boaz et al. (2016), the clinical nurse specialist (CNS) demonstrates how engagement in evidence-based practice not only enhances direct patient care but also fosters a culture of inquiry among nurses.

By fostering these competencies, nursing professionals create an environment that values both clinical excellence and collaboration, emphasizing the importance of lifelong learning and adaptability in medical-surgical settings. Furthermore, core competencies extend beyond technical skills; they also encompass the ability to communicate effectively, think critically, and make informed ethical judgments. Nurses trained in medical-surgical care should also be capable of handling challenging patient scenarios that require immediate assessment and action. For instance, in the area of addressing health inequities with transgender and gender non-conforming (TGNC) patients, cultural competence and sensitivity competencies are essential. The educative module undertaken to raise awareness and competency around TGNC health needs is one that exhibits an integral aspect of nursing practice resonating with contemporary healthcare demands, as evident in Gilbert et al. (2016). The integration of such training programs into the nursing syllabus enables future practitioners within healthcare systems to be well-prepared to meet diverse patient needs professionally and compassionately. Lastly, constant working on core competencies is necessary to move medical-surgical nursing standards forward. To remain relevant to practice, continuous professional development and participation in research activities must be embedded in nursing education. The model of establishing an environment to foster professional growth, as presented in Boaz et al. (2016), includes collaboration between schools and clinical partners. Collaborations with organizations like these result in improved clinical outcomes and the advancement of best practices that target specific patient populations. A focus on increasing core competencies benefits immediate patient demand and positions nursing as a catalyst for future healthcare environments, ultimately leading to improved patient safety and quality care across various clinical settings (Figure 1.6).

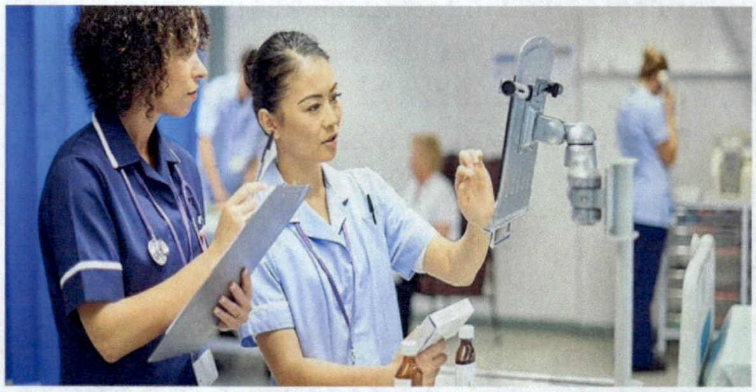

Figure 1.6. Clinical nurse specialist (CNS).

Source: https://external-content.duckduckgo.com/iu/?u=https%3A%2F%2Fnursinglicensemap.com%2Fwp-content%2Fuploads%2Fsites%2F62%2F2022%2F05%2FClinical-Nurse-

Specialist.jpg&f=1&nofb=1&ipt=fcfcc1c8dcdc5222fc25ba29dcf730ff02e4b47b9eca3e3f9bafc53fab77b239.

1.2.1. Clinical Skills and Knowledge

In medical-surgical nursing, clinical knowledge and competencies play a vital role in the delivery of efficient patient care. These competencies are a blend of practical skills and theoretical knowledge. From clinic to classroom, nursing students must be proficient in acquiring essential skills, such as vital sign monitoring, medication administration, and patient assessment. Besides, exposure to actual clinical scenarios enhances their ability to utilize evidence-based practices and the critical thinking attitude in patient management. Through a master's degree study of nursing students, it was established that, despite students holding positive attitudes toward evidence-based practice among nurses, their understanding of research terminology and its application in practice was significantly low (Abram et al., 2025). This gap highlights the need for a synthesis of intensive clinical training and research literacy, enabling future nurses to make informed, evidence-based decisions. The necessity for reflective learning in building clinical competencies cannot be overstated, particularly in the practice of medical-surgical nursing. Reflective practice allows nursing students to analyze their experience critically, gain from their errors, and apply the learned knowledge to subsequent patient experiences. This is essential to foster clinical judgment, professionalism, and communication skills—two of which are vital in handling multisided patient care cases. A quasi-experimental study found that a Blended Professional Holistic Reflective Learning course significantly increased professional competence among geriatric nursing interns (Mohajer et al., 2024). Such evidence supports the importance of systematic reflective practice in critical skill development in nursing, which requires that learning institutions emphasize this strategy in their curricula. The integration of clinical skills with a good understanding of evidence-based practice is crucial in advancing nursing competence in medical-surgical practice. While practice experience is vital, no less critical is having the ability to understand research and translate it into patient care. All attempts to enhance nursing education must bridge the gaps between research knowledge and practice (Abram et al., 2025). Increased standards in these areas will not only benefit nursing students during studies but also transfer into improved patient outcomes in practice settings. With the ever-evolving healthcare landscape, nursing curricula also need to adapt, preparing future professionals with the skills and knowledge to excel in various medical-surgical environments. This blended focus on clinical skills and knowledge will lead to a more competent and confident nursing staff (Figure 1.7).

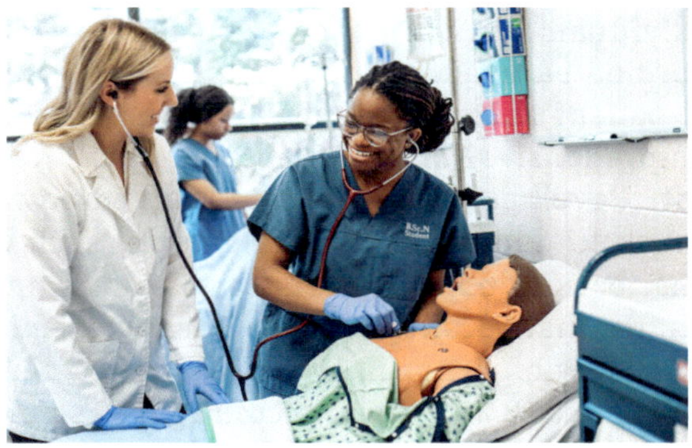

Figure 1.7. Clinical skills and knowledge.

Source: https://www.lakeheadu.ca/sites/default/files/uploads/86/photos/Copy%20of%20LU_Nursing-056.png.

1.2.2. Communication and Interpersonal Skills

Good interpersonal skills and communication are central to professional nursing practice, notably the medical-surgical setting. Nurses interact with diverse patient populations, healthcare professionals, and families, thus necessitating being able to convey information clearly and compassionately. Effective communication fosters rapport, enhances patient satisfaction, and promotes favorable health outcomes. For instance, research has highlighted that surgical residents who exemplify good professional behavior perform better in treating patients, irrespective of their socioeconomic status (Amoli et al., 2015). What it illustrates is that nurses who prioritize communication can create understanding gaps and offer respectful and individualized care that improves the patient's experience and reinforces the core nursing values. Interpersonal skills are also essential for conflict management and working in interdisciplinary teams. Nursing is about making fast decisions and building consensus among various healthcare workers, ranging from surgeons to pharmacists. These skills, therefore, such as maintaining open communication, listening actively, and appreciating other individuals' opinions, are crucial. A well-coordinated healthcare team is likely to meet the patient's needs more effectively and provide comprehensive, integrative care. Apart from that, developing these skills can empower nurses to address ethical dilemmas, such as conscientious objection-related dilemmas, in a manner that reconciles their moral principles with patients' rights and welfare (Dobrowolska et al., 2013). Thus, encouraging strong interpersonal skills helps nurses to advocate on behalf of their patients while establishing a collaborative environment. Of greater significance, integrating new communication techniques into nurse preparation can play a crucial role in facilitating the acquisition of these essential skills. Simulation training in domains such as active listening, empathy, and cultural competence prepares nurses to communicate more effectively with patients and their families. A curriculum incorporating simulation training enables nursing students to practice communication in real-life situations, thereby establishing confidence and competency. Effective communication, in the end, is not merely the passing of information; it is about understanding patients' needs, fears, and preferences, which is essential in medical-surgical practice. By prioritizing communication and interpersonal skills in professional nursing curricula, future nurses will be well-positioned to deliver quality care and contribute to favorable patient outcomes, aligning with the evolving demands of the healthcare setting (Figure 1.8).

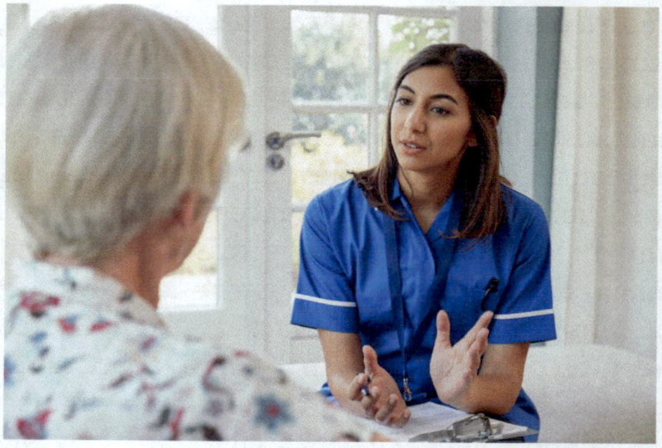

Figure 1.8. Effective nursing communication-skills.

Source: https://www.aiam.edu/wp-content/uploads/2023/01/Effective-Nursing-Communication-Skills.jpg.

1.2.3. Critical Thinking and Decision-Making

Critical thinking and decision-making are essential components of professional nursing practice, especially in medical-surgical care settings. Nurses are often expected to synthesize various forms of information to provide effective patient care, indicating the need to obtain and analyze multiple evidence sources. Research has shown that experienced nurses are more likely to rely on human information sources, such as clinical nurse specialists and experienced peers, than on text-based sources alone. This trend highlights the need to establish spaces for teamwork where nurses can interact freely with their colleagues to share information and enhance their decision-making capacity. By establishing such relationships, nurses can maximize the availability of vital information that determines patient outcomes, a step that aligns with the general goals of evidence-based practice, as highlighted in the existing literature (Cullum et al., 2001). Moreover, model building of nursing decision-making occurs as a consequence of the complicated clinical situations nurses encounter in medical-surgical practice. Older models, like information processing, have emphasized systematic thinking but have been criticized because they fail to incorporate intuitive judgment processes intrinsic to nursing. The introduction of the new multidimensional model, with its elements of patient-specific cues and pattern recognition, encapsulates the dynamic interaction between knowledge and experiential learning within clinical decision-making. The shift underscores the importance of nursing education incorporating these new models, enabling learners to develop the critical thinking skills necessary for effective nursing practice. As nurses practice with complex patient scenarios, an explicit understanding of these models can endow them with the skills to make informed decisions and promote patient-centered care (Aspiuynall et al., 2007). Finally, technology integration in nursing practice also enhances decision-making in medical-surgical practice. With greater access to online information, clinical decision-making is optimized through real-time access to evidence-based guidelines and literature. However, the reliance on technology must be weighed against the skills of critical evaluation, so that nurses can discern the quality of the information they are provided with. The latest research puts pressure on a strategic approach to ensure increased use of technological resources alongside traditional evidence to address problems nurses may encounter when seeking credible information. By developing critical thinking and decision-making abilities, nurses can significantly improve the quality of care for patients, demonstrating that quality nursing practice is largely a matter of resource allocation (Cullum et al., 2001).

Test Your Knowledge

1. What are the essential clinical competencies required for a medical-surgical nurse to deliver safe and effective patient care?
2. How does cultural competence enhance nursing care in a multicultural medical-surgical patient population?

1.3. Patient-Centered Care in Medical-Surgical Settings

Learning Outcome

1. Explain the importance of holistic approaches
2. Define successful patient engagement approaches
3. Describe the role of the family in patient care

Patient-centered care has evolved as a central aspect within medical-surgical settings, emphasizing the importance of individualized approaches tailored to meet the unique needs and preferences of each patient. This change in medical practices is founded upon the consideration that effective communication and interaction between patients and healthcare practitioners necessarily enhance patient outcomes. In medical-surgical units, nurses' work comes in the form of the implementation of patient-centered care, with the active participation of patients in the management of their own care and collaborative decision-making. Empowerment of patients, minimization of anxiety, and cooperation in their healthcare process come as a natural consequence of this, resulting in increased satisfaction and adherence to treatment plans. The integration of patient feedback into care provision demonstrates the transformative strength of this model, as it fosters trust and bonding between nurses and patients. Additionally, providing nursing students with adequate education in patient-centered care fundamentals is essential to enhance care provision in medical-surgical practice. There have been recent studies that have highlighted significant gaps in typical nursing curricula that may discourage students from learning the skills required for appropriate administration of medication and interaction with patients (Chorpenning et al., 2011). Students need additional training with simulated scenarios, communication skills, and conflict resolution channels to prepare them for the challenges faced in clinical practice. By embracing novel pedagogies based on experiential learning and peer-to-peer learning, nursing schools can educate a new generation of clinicians who are not only skilled in technical competency but also capable of designing patient-centered interactions. This integrated training is what is needed to graduate nurses capable of thriving in sophisticated healthcare environments. The NP role in medical-surgical practice also highlights the importance of patient-centered practice patterns. Evidence demonstrates that NPs dedicated to patient-centered care are associated with improved outcomes, thereby highlighting the unique contribution of nursing to quality care (Bandy et al., 2005).

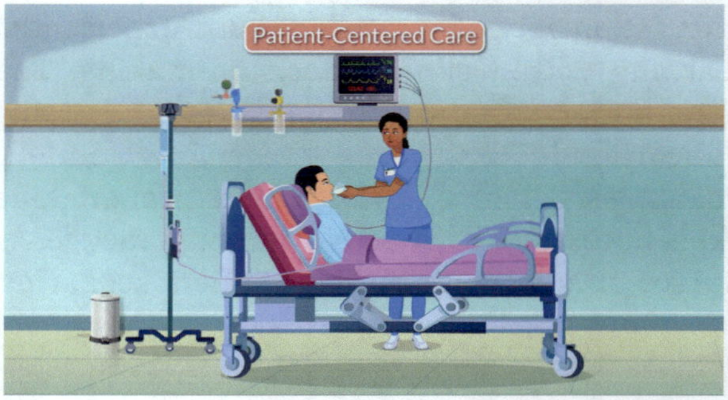

Figure 1.9. Patient-centered care in medical-surgical settings.

Source: https://cloudfront.jove.com/files/media/science-education/science-education-thumbs/13528.jpg.

As the widening scope of nurse practitioners increases, their contribution to individualized care becomes increasingly essential, ensuring that patients receive individualized interventions that are appropriate for their needs and health goals. In addition, placing emphasis on knowing the patient experience can bring about noteworthy positive changes in care quality, rates of adherence, and overall patient satisfaction. By consistently promoting and implementing patient-centered strategies, medical-surgical nursing practitioners can enhance the effectiveness of care delivery, ultimately achieving improved health outcomes for patients and upholding the core principles of professional nursing practice (Figure 1.9).

1.3.1. Importance of Holistic Approaches

Holistic strategies play a crucial role in the practice of medical-surgical nursing, offering comprehensive and effective patient care. The strategies not only incorporate the bodily aspects of health but also those of emotion, society, and spirit, as patients are holistic beings and not a collection of symptoms to be treated. By examining things holistically, nurses gain a deeper understanding of the complex interplay of factors that contribute to a patient's condition. This more holistic view enables more tailored care plans that resonate with patients' unique life history and values. This type of approach maximizes patient participation, enhances confidence, and promotes a culture of healing that is in harmony with the total mission of nursing: not only to treat the disease but also to care for the individual as an entire entity, which can significantly contribute to medical-surgical outcomes and patient satisfaction. Additionally, the worth of a holistic approach can be extended to promoting interdisciplinary practice among health practitioners. In implementing this model of holistic care, nurses are placing themselves as equal members of the healthcare team, working with physicians, therapists, and social workers to address the multifaceted needs of patients. Interdisciplinary practice facilitates communication, ensuring everyone is aligned on the patient's goals and needs. This collaborative practice enables the development of transdisciplinary care plans that are tailored to the unique circumstances of each individual patient. With nurses advocating for their patients within the team, they assist in cultivating a culture of integrated care that not only expands the scope of practice but also enhances the holistic health of patients as they navigate the process of medical-surgical interventions. Finally, holistic nursing practice is the key to bridging health disparities and promoting health equity among diverse patient populations. Holistic nurses are more attuned to the social determinants of health among their patients, such as socioeconomic status, culture, and access to resources. Such awareness enables nurses to advocate for healthcare delivery changes that are required and thus overcome the barriers that underrepresented groups face when trying to access quality care. Moreover, by integrating culture-informed practices into their care models, nurses can use interventions that appeal to patients' values and beliefs, ensuring greater compliance and improved health outcomes. According to Burton et al. (2021) and Glikson et al. (2021), effective nursing practice must be comprehensive and encompass multiple aspects of health, with the individual being dedicated to holistic care in bridging gaps and ensuring equitable care is provided to various communities (Figure 1.10).

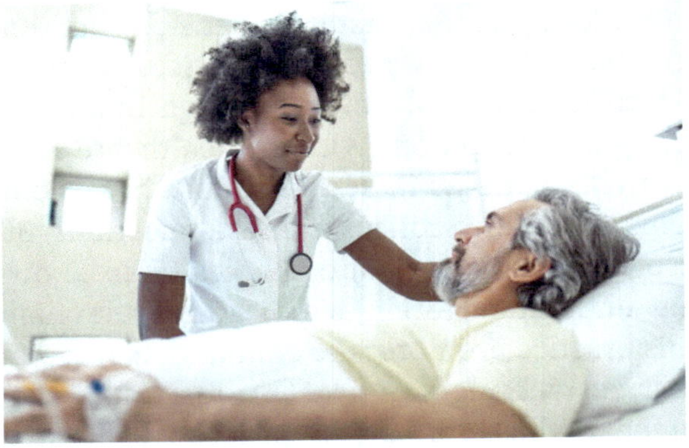

Figure 1.10. Holistic patient care.

Source: https://onlinenursing.cn.edu/sites/default/files/field/image/holistic-patient-care.jpg.

1.3.2. Strategies for Effective Patient Engagement

In practice, effective patient involvement is crucial in improving health outcomes and the overall healthcare setting. Active involvement of patients in their own care activities is one primary strategy that has the capacity to empower patients to make well-informed decisions about their health. The patient satisfaction not only improves, but treatment compliance also improves. Involving patients at various stages—ranging from the initial assessment to discharge planning—permits openness and trust in the nurse-patient relationship. Nurses can facilitate this involvement by employing communication strategies that focus on patient education and encouragement. Through the process of informing patients about procedures and related risks, nurses can ensure that patients appreciate and respect their care journey, thereby improving overall engagement in their health management. A second effective way to involve patients is through the use of formalized communication systems, such as the Team STEPPS model. The model targets teamwork and health communication practices in order to maximize interactions between medical teams and, therefore, create a harmonious environment for patient care. For instance, bedside rounding and bedside shift report practices enhance direct patient involvement through immediate care plan interactions with the healthcare team. Involving patients in such encounters not only helps them voice concerns or ask questions, but also empowers them and enables them to own and understand their health goals personally. This practice promotes the elimination of typical barriers among medical professionals and patients, which promotes a spirit of collaboration underpinning effective medical-surgical nursing practice (Beiler et al., 2019). Such collaborative practice ultimately improves both treatment outcomes and patient satisfaction. Additionally, nursing practice should incorporate constant feedback loops that accurately measure patients' levels of engagement. This can be achieved through use of tools such as patient interviews and questionnaires to quantify the quality of engagement practices. As shown by recent evidence, when nurses actively participate in critiquing their practice and incorporating patient feedback, both patient care quality and safety improve significantly (Lee-Riggins et al., 2014). Apart from that, systematic empowerment programs are also able to develop confidence among nurses in using innovative engagement strategies. As front-line nurses demonstrate an interest in participating in improvement activities, collaborative efforts not only enhance patient engagement but also promote professional development among nursing staff. Thus, a culture of continuous improvement and patient engagement is a platform for enhancing the quality of care offered in medical-surgical units (Figure 1.11).

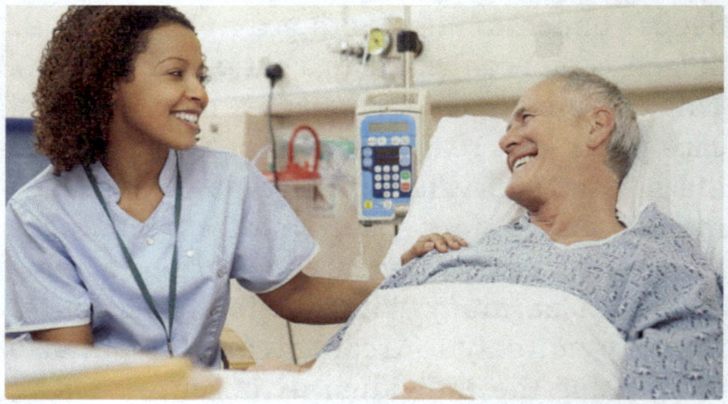

Figure 1.11. Keys to outstanding patient-education nurse patient relationships.

Source: https://get.goreact.com/wp-content/uploads/2019/08/5-Keys-to-Outstanding-Patient-Education-Nurse-Patient-Relationships-1024x591.png.

1.3.3. Role of Family in Patient Care

The involvement of family members in patient care is a crucial aspect of professional nursing practice, particularly in medical-surgical settings. Families are key emotional supporters and practical helpers that assist in removing patients' anxieties and promoting adherence to medical treatment. Moreover, family members can also serve as a link between the patient and the healthcare team, making it possible for them to effectively communicate the patient's needs and preferences. By engaging actively, not only do they enhance patient satisfaction, but they can also enhance better health outcomes. Through the active engagement of family members in care planning, nurses empower them to be active partners, a factor that leads to increased responsibility and advocacy for the patient. By involving family members in care, nurses create an integrated process that recognizes the vital role of the family as a unit in supporting recovery and health. Additionally, the extent of family involvement in patient care varies in relation to the nature of the medical condition and the complexities of the healthcare facility. In high-stakes settings such as critical care, where patients are likely to experience moral distress and ethical conflicts, having family members present can prove vital in providing moral support. Nurses may find themselves in situations where life-and-death choices result in ethical dilemmas not only for them but also for the family members who have to make difficult choices regarding their loved ones' care. Engaging families in discussions about such matters and more empathetic and informed decision-making can follow, ultimately reducing moral distress among nursing personnel. Such participative engagement highlights the nurse's role as a mediator and advocate who helps families understand healthcare practices and emotional needs associated with their loved ones' care, which can enhance the quality of care provided (Epstein et al., 2018). Training and education are essential for preparing nursing professionals to involve families meaningfully in patient care. Learning models should allow for the gaining of communication skills, empathy, and ethics decision-making so that nurses can handle the complexities of family processes. Workshops, seminars, and interdisciplinary collaboration may be utilized as platforms for sharing information, promoting best practices in family-centered care. The 3rd Java International Nursing Conference emphasized the importance of interprofessional collaboration in nursing, highlighting the value of shared knowledge and experience in enhancing patient outcomes (Nurmalia (Editor) et al., 2015). Successful collaboration modeling can also encourage families to be actively involved in medical decision-making. Lastly, championing a family-centered practice requires a concerted effort from nursing professionals, who must reconcile the technical components of care with the psychological and emotional requirements of patients and their families to effect holistic healing.

Test Your Knowledge

1. What is patient-centered care in the practice of medical-surgical nursing?
2. How can a nurse involve a patient and their family in care planning and decision-making?

1.4. Challenges Faced by Medical-Surgical Nurses

Learning Outcome

1. Define high patient-to-nurse ratios
2. Define emotional and physical stressors
3. Describe accessing complex healthcare systems

The medical-surgical nursing specialty presents an extensive range of challenges that exert significant impacts on the quality of patient care. One of the most emergent fields is the high patient-to-nurse ratio, which most likely leads to heavy workloads that can burden nursing staff. This state not only affects the physical load on nurses but also contributes to burnout, compromising patient outcomes and safety. With numerous patients at a time, nurses are more likely to make errors, which may lead to adverse effects. Additionally, low staffing levels limit nurses' ability to provide the empathetic care that underpins professional nursing practice, thereby weakening the fundamental principles of patient-centered care, which are essential in medical-surgical settings. Another problem that faces medical-surgical nurses is the complexity of patient care, which frequently requires specialized skills in various settings. The diverse nature of the medical conditions addressed requires nurses to be adaptable and competent in numerous practice areas. Therefore, continuing education and professional development become essential, as nurses must stay current with the latest medical advancements and evidence-based practices. However, inconsistency in training and availability of educational resources can hinder nurses ability to address these needs adequately. This kind of gap is particularly concerning in light of the evidence that overwhelming inequalities in the education and supervision of nurses, particularly in subspecialized tasks such as dermatological surgery, are bound to lead to variable quality of care across different healthcare facilities (Duffy et al., 2019). Moreover, the affective aspects of nursing present some serious challenges, particularly the moral distress experienced in intensive care units. Medical-surgical nurses are constantly faced with complex ethical issues of end-of-life choices, the boundaries of technology, and the broader effort of providing high-quality care. Instances of moral distress arise when nurses perceive that they cannot act consistently with their ethical values due to institutional barriers or conflict with physician orders. The psychological impact can lead to compromised care and decreased job satisfaction, with potential implications for patient outcomes (Epstein et al., 2018). Resolution of such emotional challenges through support interventions and encouragement of an environment conducive to ethical practice is necessary to continue providing effective and compassionate care within medical-surgical settings (Figure 1.12).

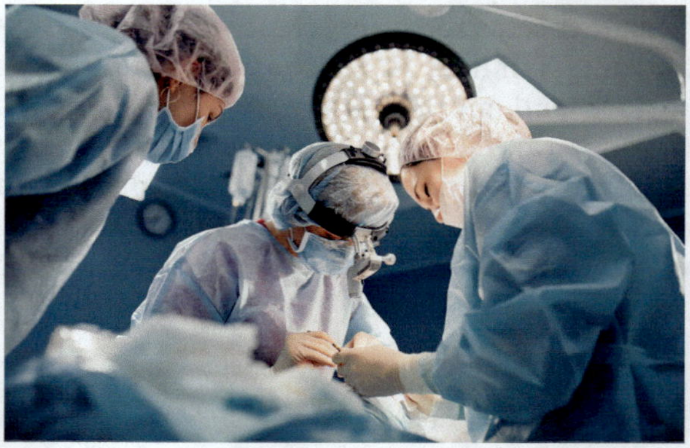

Figure 1.12. The challenges of working as an operating-room-nurse.

Source: https://everynurse.org/wp-content/uploads/2023/12/The-Challenges-of-Working-as-an-Operating-Room-Nurse.webp.

1.4.1. High Patient-to-Nurse Ratios

Large patient-to-nurse ratios are among the most formidable challenges in the field of medical-surgical care, with a direct impact on both patient outcomes and nursing staff health.

Repeatedly, studies have shown an extremely high correlation between large ratios and increased medical errors, patient complications, and adverse outcomes. A systematic review of various international studies emphasizes that reduced levels of nurse staffing have adverse effects that extend beyond hospital efficiency dimensions to permeate the very foundation of patient safety (Aiken et al., 2009). The nature of the problem lies in the inherent restrictions that stem from the allocation of inadequate nursing resources to manage the multifaceted needs of patient care, especially in high-acuity settings where prompt interventions are of critical importance. In addition, the effects of high patient-to-nurse ratios extend not only to patient care but also to extreme levels for nursing staff. They often lead to job dissatisfaction, burnout, and high nurse turnover, perpetuating a self-sustaining cycle that tends to exacerbate staffing shortages (Aleo et al., 2016). Evidence suggests that stressful work environments, characterized by inadequate staffing, are associated with reduced nurse retention and lower overall morale. Such conditions hinder professional practice of nursing by offering a limited scope for acquiring skills and negatively affecting cooperative practice, which is crucial for positive patient outcomes in med-surg settings. Therefore, nurse managers must position staffing adequacy in its rightful position as a prominent factor in ensuring a supportive work environment and maintaining nurse retention. Overcoming the problem of high patient-to-nurse ratios requires an integrated approach, including a systematic review of staffing policies and the incorporation of evidence-based practice into workforce planning. Policymakers and healthcare leaders must seek approaches that allow for maximum staffing levels in terms of nurse-patient ratios as well as intensity of care required (Aiken et al., 2009). Technology integration, enhanced training, and teamwork settings are most crucial in ensuring this. Additionally, fostering a culture of quality and safety improvement can encourage nursing professionals to take an active role in contributing to care solutions. As evidenced by the European RN4CAST study, strategic focus on the relationship between nurse staffing and quality of care can have extensive implications on patient safety outcomes (Aleo et al., 2016). The ongoing debate about staffing adequacy is thus also essential for advancing professional nursing practice in medical-surgical nursing (Figure 1.13).

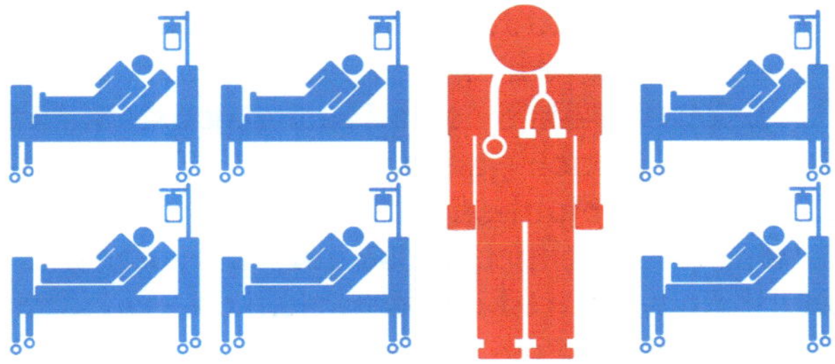

Figure 1.13. Nurse to patient ratio.

Source: https://theacademicinsights.com/wp-content/uploads/2020/10/staffing-slab3.png.

1.4.2. Emotional and Physical Stressors

In medical-surgical nursing practice, practitioners are exposed to numerous physical and emotional stressors that significantly impact their health and well-being. The stressful nature of the work compels practitioners into environments where they are forced to make extreme decisions under intense-pressure conditions, which impose significant stress on them due to the pressure to respond in a timely manner. This sudden stress can have a range of presentations, including anxiety symptoms, guilt, and lowered self-esteem, particularly following adverse occurrences or drug errors. Identification of phenomena such as the second victim syndrome highlights nurses' emotional distress from engaging in occurrences that affect patient outcomes. With research indicating that a large percentage of nurses do suffer from such emotional unrest, it is clear that prolonged pressure without relief can create long-term negative impacts on their working lives, necessitating specific interventions (Kuruvilla, 2025). Physical stressors exacerbate the challenges faced by nurses in medical-surgical care. With the physical demands of the job—like lifting and moving patients, working with heavy equipment, and standing for long periods of time—nurses are often exposed to developing musculoskeletal disorders or other disease. Physical demands are also supplemented by heavy workload and emotional stress of their work, which can lead to burnout, a condition marked by emotional exhaustion and depersonalization (Jain et al., 2024). This cross-dimensional, multi-stressor not only threatens patient care quality but also nurses' own mental well-being, as tired or overwhelmed providers can fall victim to making errors. Hence, creating healthy work environments that prioritize both physical safety and emotional resilience is essential to mitigate these stressors and enhance nursing practice in general within the medical-surgical setting. Nursing management of emotional and physical stressors entails a multi-level strategy that comprises organizational interventions and personal coping mechanisms. Health care organisations can play an active role by implementing a culture of support and free exchange of ideas on mental health. The implementation of mentorship programs or peer support schemes can enable nurses to overcome the emotional pressures associated with their profession, while also improving job satisfaction and reducing turnover (Kuruvilla, 2025). Additionally, individual nurses must develop self-care practices, such as mindfulness, exercise, and scheduled time away from work, to achieve a work-life balance. By understanding these stressors and taking deliberate steps to mitigate their impact, healthcare organizations and practitioners can contribute to overall improvements in the quality of patient care and a more stable nurse workforce, ultimately enhancing outcomes in the medical-surgical field (Figure 1.14).

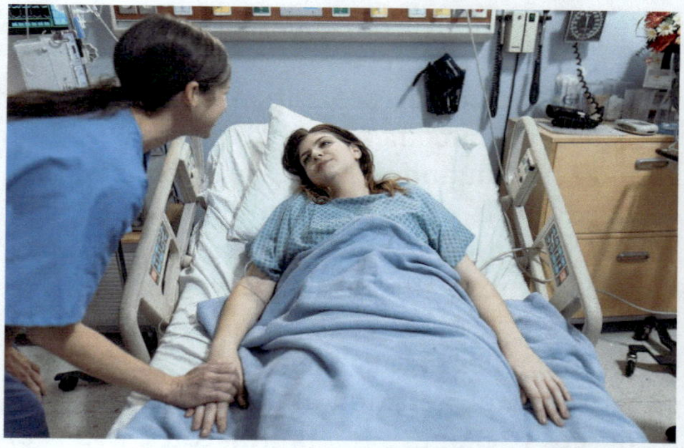

Figure 1.14. Emotional and physical stressors of medical-surgical nursing.

Source: https://images.pexels.com/photos/6129689/pexels-photo-6129689.jpeg.

1.4.3. Navigating Complex Healthcare Systems

Complexity in the healthcare system poses a significant challenge in the professional practice of nursing, particularly within medical-surgical care. Nurses in such environments are often faced with the challenge of managing complex patients' needs within multiple institutional processes and interprofessional teams. Understanding and utilizing these systems' resources is crucial for achieving maximum patient outcomes and providing quality care. Furthermore, the ever-more technological setting exacerbates these issues to such a degree that nurses find themselves confronted with moral dilemmas that compromise their capacity to provide empathetic care. Referring to such scenarios, as noted in the literature, highlights the imperative of creating a positive professional practice environment in which nurses can advocate effectively for their patients (Epstein et al., 2018). Effective communication dynamics are also essential for navigating complex healthcare systems. Not only is effective communication required to deliver quality patient care, but it is also required to facilitate collaboration among healthcare teams. In medical-surgical settings, nurses must clearly communicate vital information related to patients to other healthcare providers while ensuring that patients and families comprehend their treatment plan and goals. This dual obligation highlights the importance of communication skill building and building interpersonal relationships among the health care team in an effort to minimize errors and enhance patient safety. Secondarily, medication error and hospital-acquired infection data collection and reporting will enhance safety procedures and reduce adverse events across the health care system (Burke et al., 2008). Moreover, practice in advanced health systems necessitates ethical sensitivity towards the challenges of critical care settings. Moral distress, commonly experienced by healthcare professionals, is when providers perceive that they are being restricted from practicing as they should within their own ethics by institutional constraints or from beyond their own settings. While providing medical-surgical care, the practitioners are often confronted with end-of-life decisions and the implications of advanced medical technology, introducing conflict between professional duty and personal beliefs. Understanding the reasons for moral distress is crucial for maintaining integrity in nursing practice and maximizing patient care outcomes, as a lack of compassionate care would have catastrophic effects on both patients and caregivers (Epstein et al., 2018). Emphasizing the necessity of ongoing research into the impact of these ethical challenges is imperative for the future of medical-surgical nursing care and the operation of healthcare systems.

Test Your Knowledge

1. What are two problems that are commonly faced by medical-surgical nurses when managing patient workloads?
2. How do physical and emotional stress influence the performance of the role by medical-surgical nurses?

1.5. Technological Advancements in Nursing Practice

Learning Outcome

1. Describe the use of electronic health records (EHR)
2. Define telehealth and remote patient monitoring
3. Describe the advances in medical instruments and equipment

Incorporation of technological change into nursing practice has revolutionized the landscape of medical-surgical care. Through the use of tools such as electronic health records (EHRs), nurses are now equipped to capture, view, and share patient data in real-time, thereby fostering continuity of care. EHRs reduce paperwork, increase efficiency of processes, and decrease medical mistakes, which are central capabilities of exceptional value in hectic environments such as operating rooms. In addition, computer-based systems enable enhanced communication among nurses and other healthcare professionals, ensuring that everyone on the care team is up-to-date and engaged in patient care. As a result, this change not only optimizes the workflow but also optimizes patient outcomes, pointing to the key contribution of technology to the nursing profession. In addition, advances in technology, such as telehealth and remote monitoring, have become indispensable in elevating the level of patient care, particularly in medical-surgical practices. Telehealth facilitates consultations between nurses and patients who lack convenient access to healthcare facilities, enabling timely assessments and interventions. Additionally, remote monitoring devices can measure vital signs in real-time and alert nursing staff to any changes that require closer attention.

This is not only a more efficient response but also enables patients to be more involved in managing their own health. Evidence suggests that these technology tools are associated with improved patient satisfaction and adherence to treatment plans, both of which are significant components of successful nursing practice in the current medical-surgical environment. The value of continuous education in accessing these technological advancements cannot be stressed too much. Nurses should not only master new technologies but also be committed to ongoing education to keep pace with rapid advances. Educational institutions and healthcare organizations hold the fort in equipping nurses with the competencies to operate in such technological landscapes.

The provision of training programs in the effective use of EHRs, telemedicine, and remote monitoring enhances the competencies of nurses, equipping them to deliver high-quality services. Secondly, the development of a culture that encourages inquiry and adaptability to new technologies allows nurses to become change agents for their organizations. This commitment to lifelong learning will ultimately optimize technology integration in nursing practice, thereby improving the quality of medical-surgical care delivered to patients (Figure 1.15).

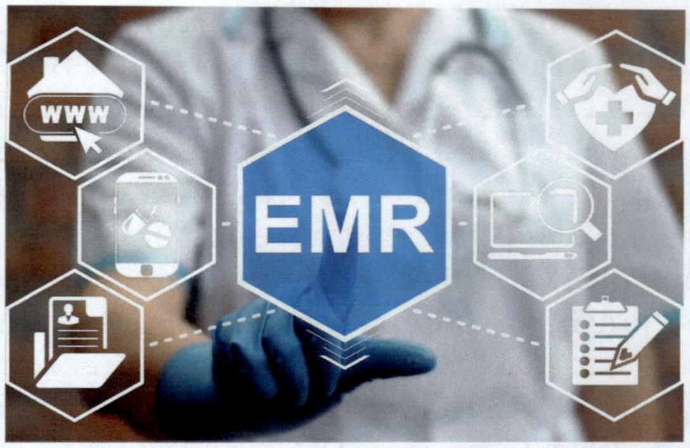

Figure 1.15. Electronic health records (EHRs).

Source: https://external-content.duckduckgo.com/iu/?u=https%3A%2F%2Fmedixonline.ca%2Fwp-content%2Fuploads%2F2020%2F06%2Femr.jpg&f=1&nofb=1&ipt=7e7de50806635f56bba25f5638a7cf4da38b4bf14d3eadecf6123a74462fc620.

1.5.1. Use of Electronic Health Records (EHR)

The utilization of EHRs has significantly transformed the face of professional nursing practice in medical-surgical care. EHRs support the streamlined documentation of patient data, greatly optimizing the efficiency of patient care delivery. EHRs enable nurses and other healthcare professionals to quickly access complete medical histories, allowing for informed decision-making that has a direct bearing on patient outcomes. With the ability to combine health data sources, EHRs support collaboration, allowing multiple discipline care teams to communicate more effectively. Interestingly, the transition from paper-based to electronic records is associated with a reduction in errors due to simpler communication and enhanced data management, proving highly useful in high-risk medical-surgical settings where accuracy is paramount. Additionally, the advantages of EHR systems extend beyond their direct clinical applications; they also support an evidence-based approach that influences healthcare policy and practice. The empirical data drawn from EHRs can be used to inform broader healthcare trends and policies, effectively serving as a database of knowledge that informs ongoing continuous quality improvement efforts. For instance, by reviewing the effectiveness of treatments using EHR information, healthcare organizations can identify best practices that improve patient safety and streamline workflows. Within this dynamic setting, nurses play a pivotal role, not only using EHRs as medical tools to treat patients but also being involved in policy reform discussions. According to industry analyses' quotes, understanding the interface between medical delivery systems and market forces is crucial for nurses in ensuring effective and efficient approaches to medical-surgical treatment (N/A, 2005).

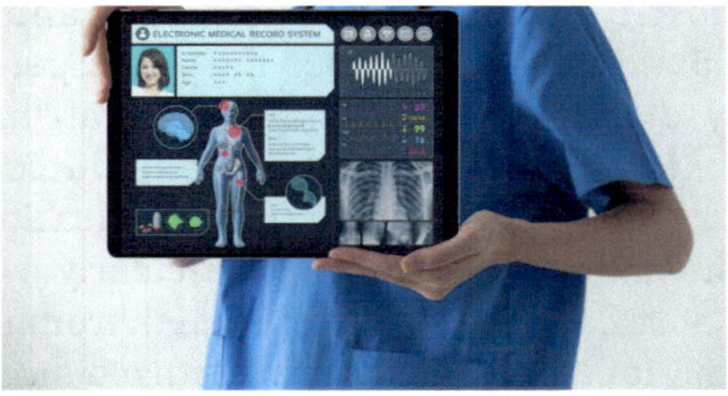

Figure 1.16. Use of electronic health records (EHR).

Source: https://www.aamc.org/sites/default/files/styles/scale_and_crop_1200_x_666/public/d/1/94-portable_ehr_story.jpg__992x558_q85_crop-smart_subsampling-2_upscale.jpg?itok=AhTchb2G.

The application of EHR systems also aligns with the specific needs of nurses, particularly in medical-surgical practice. Significant features like interoperability, real-time patient tracking, and access to drug processes enhance the nurse's ability to deliver quality care. As enshrined in recent studies, such technologies are central to ensuring that nurses are provided with the right equipment on hand to provide optimal patient safety, particularly in treating complex cases that involve the coordination of distinct specialist services. The ability to utilize hand-held devices also makes nurses more assertive by providing direct access to essential information at the point of care, as well as enhancing patient involvement and education. The integration of these cutting-edge technologies consequently leads to improved clinical outcomes and operating efficiencies, validating the crucial role of EHRs in current nursing practice (N/A, 2010) (Figure 1.16).

1.5.2. Telehealth and Remote Patient Monitoring

Telehealth and remote patient monitoring have transformed the landscape of professional nursing practice, particularly in medical-surgical care. As there is an increasing reliance on technology, nurses can now monitor, manage, and assess a patient's health from a distance. This not only makes care more accessible but also allows patients to receive timely interventions based on real-time data. For instance, programs like the Veterans Health Administration's (VHA) Care Coordination/Home Telehealth (CCHT) rely on remote monitoring technology to collect essential health information from individuals with chronic conditions, such as heart failure and diabetes. The use of such technologies has resulted in reduced hospitalizations and increased patient satisfaction, demonstrating the efficacy of telehealth in addressing complex healthcare needs within the nursing practice environment (Broderick, 2013). Furthermore, the pandemic has accelerated the adoption of telemedicine, bringing into focus its potential in ensuring quality nursing care for people from diverse backgrounds. The telemedicine framework improves patient-centered care as medical personnel can consult with patients remotely. It has been most beneficial in poor and rural areas, where access to healthcare is scarce. Telehealth has ensured ease in communication, reducing the expense of in-person visits, but without sacrificing high patient satisfaction levels. Remote monitoring technologies enable nurses to bridge critical gaps in healthcare delivery, effectively managing such ailments as hypertension and mental illness as well as safeguard against potential infections. Telehealth for nursing thus fulfills not only the immediate demands but also sets the stage for long-term healthcare solutions, delivering holistic care for patients (C V et al., 2025). Despite the numerous advantages telehealth has to offer, certain issues remain that require careful scrutiny by nursing practitioners. The installation of remote monitoring technologies into hospital infrastructures can be cumbersome and requires significant changes in workflows and processes. Nurses must ensure proper data entry, as well as accurately interpret remote biometric data, to make effective clinical decisions. Furthermore, maintaining the integrity of patient-nurse interactions remains a priority; the shift to virtual meetings calls for ongoing education and mentorship of healthcare practitioners to foster rapport and trust. As telehealth improves, it is essential that nursing practice evolves in tandem, capitalizing on its strengths and weaknesses to establish a robust and effective model of healthcare delivery that yields better patient outcomes (C V et al., 2025) (Figure 1.17).

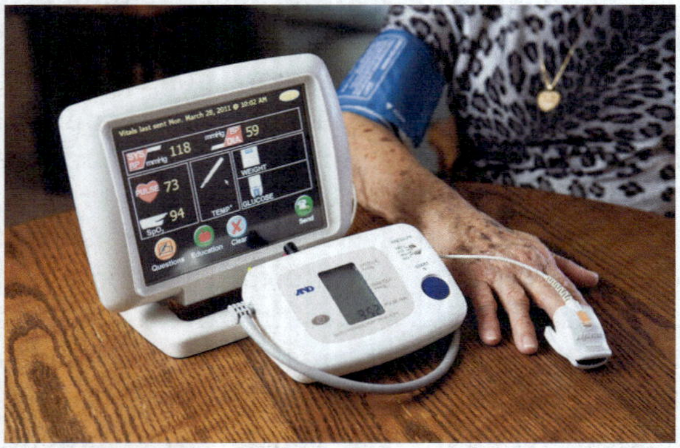

Figure 1.17. Care coordination/home telehealth (CCHT).

Source: https://i.pinimg.com/736x/0f/4e/ca/0f4ecaf764df5616aaacd9048157f334.jpg.

1.5.3. Innovations in Medical Equipment and Tools

The medical equipment and tools sector has changed significantly in the last few years, with the primary intention of enhancing safety and efficiency in healthcare. Technologies such as enhanced surgical tools, telehealth devices, and smart monitoring devices are key to improved patient care. One of the critical advances is the integration of robotic-assisted surgical systems, which provide greater precision for minimally invasive procedures. These systems not only minimize recovery times but also lower the risk of complications, thereby aligning with the overall objective of delivering higher-quality patient care in medical-surgical settings. Furthermore, the application of cutting-edge diagnostic technology, such as handheld ultrasound devices, enables nurses to perform timely diagnosis, which has a critical impact on clinical decisions and patient outcomes. In nursing practice, clear communication in patient handoff is crucial, particularly where life is at stake, such as in surgical environments. The implementation of standardized handoff safety checklists, based on research findings, has demonstrated significant improvement in the quality of communication among nursing staff (Rowe et al., 2015). Checklists aid in the prevention of sentinel events, such as retained foreign objects, that can cause irreparable damage to patients. This is done by offering a structured method for information transfer. By utilizing instruments like Rogers' diffusion of innovation theory and Donabedian's model, this approach not only adds to patient safety but also to nurse satisfaction through trust building and responsibility. Therefore, the ongoing evolution and utilization of these tools represent a revolutionary step towards best practices of nursing in medical-surgical care. Apart from that, the integration of information technology has also changed the management of patient information within medical-surgical environments, enhancing accessibility and accuracy. EHRs are technologies that allow for the sharing of real-time information among healthcare workers to improve collaborative work. The technology facilitates evidence-based nursing practice by providing immediate access to patient histories and treatment processes, thereby informing clinical decision-making. The emergence of telehealth platforms also illustrates how the technology is transforming the delivery of healthcare; these devices enable remote monitoring of patients, bridging the gap between home and hospital. These advances not only streamline work processes but also facilitate nurses in providing the best possible care, thereby reiterating their invaluable role in the medical-surgical setting.

Test Your Knowledge

1. In what ways has electronic health record (EHR) technology impacted nursing documentation and communication?
2. Recognize two emerging medical-surgical nursing technology tools and describe how they enhance patient outcomes.

1.6. Professional Development and Continuing Education

Learning Outcome

1. Describe the importance of lifelong learning
2. Define the options for certification and specialization
3. Identify the role of professional organizations in nursing

Professional development and continuous education are fundamental components of the medical-surgical practice, where the rapid evolution of healthcare requires practitioners to remain up-to-date on best practices as well as emerging trends. Continuous learning promotes not only individual proficiency but also enhances the overall quality of patient care on medical-surgical floors. Engaging in professional development activities helps nurses refine their abilities, integrate new information, and apply evidence-based practice effectively. By means of a culture of ongoing learning, healthcare organizations are able to provide nurses the capacity to manage complicated clinical environments effectively. A developmental focus directly facilitates the delivery of safe, quality care in a manner that enables nurses to meet the diverse needs of patients within a dynamic healthcare environment. Furthermore, highlighting the requirement to tackle work culture in professional development is the movement to prevent issues such as lateral violence among nursing staff. A pilot study in a small rural community hospital demonstrates how education programs specifically designed for registered nurses can foster a culture of civility, which is crucial for both staff morale and patient outcomes. The interventions employed in the study included a comprehensive review of organizational policies and a focused education retreat, providing an effective model for professional development that addresses not only clinical competencies but also interpersonal dynamics within medical-surgical settings. Such formative experiences have potent effects on the professional identity of nurses and result in greater collaboration, ultimately enhancing patient care through improved teamwork and communication among the staff (Lewis et al., 2017). Not all continuing professional development activities, however, are successful; it has been criticized that traditional CPD methods do not have a sufficiently significant impact to enhance the level of nursing practice. There is evidence that the more prevalent CPD methods, including lectures and conferences, are ineffective in significantly improving practitioner competence or impacting patient health outcomes. This challenges re-examination of the CPD approaches towards favoring active, reflective, and structured learning activities that capture nurses more effectively. For instance, CPD exercises that focus on practice skills, such as peer-to-peer communication or outcome-focused goals, are more likely to yield enhanced nursing performance and the standard of patient care. As the evolving nursing profession, stakeholders have to embrace innovative CPD models so that they can harness their maximum potential to enhance professional advancement (May et al., 2016) (Figure 1.18).

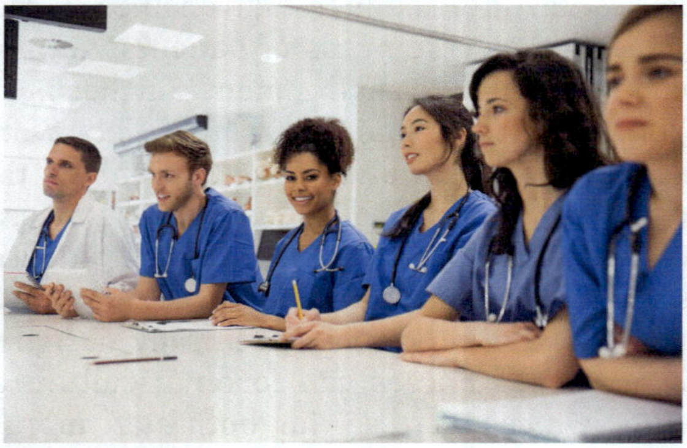

Figure 1.18. Professional development and continuing education in-nursing.

Source: https://nightingale.edu/_resources/images/blog/continuing-education-in-nursing.jpeg.

1.6.1. Importance of Lifelong Learning

The ever-evolving healthcare landscape necessitates that nursing practitioners engage in lifelong learning to remain effective practitioners, particularly in medical-surgical practice. As new modes of treatment and technology emerge, nurses must adapt their knowledge and skills to provide quality care. Critical thinking and flexibility are enhanced through lifelong learning, which enables nurses to handle complex patient cases, thereby improving patient outcomes. Continuing education, in the form of formal courses, workshops, and in-service training, allows nurses to receive the latest evidence-based practices. Continuing education also providesenables career advancement through specialized positions or a transition into management. Maintaining a commitment to lifelong learning ensures that nurses maintain their competence while fostering a culture of inquiry necessary in healthcare settings dedicated to improving patient care. Mentoring is a crucial process in promoting lifelong learning by nursing professionals, particularly in the delivery of medical-surgical care. Effective mentoring relationships can provide guidance and encouragement, helping nurses acquire the confidence and skills necessary to address the challenges of a changing healthcare system. According to recent findings, individuals who get engaged in mentoring have reported better problem-solving abilities and better career progress, particularly when transferring to higher levels of complexity (Dobrowolska et al., 2013). This highlights the importance of tailored support as a key component of a comprehensive professional development model. Apart from skill acquisition, mentoring can further facilitate vital professional relationships, allowing nurses to develop networks conducive to learning environments that foster collaboration. The integration of mentoring into nursing practice not only empowers individual nurses but also enhances the overall quality of patient care. The concept of lifelong learning encompasses not only knowledge acquisition but also ethical considerations that have a direct impact on nursing practice. Nurses frequently encounter dilemmas that require critical moral judgment, particularly in cases involving conscientious objection. There is a need to maintain a sense of ethical standards and legal expectations, particularly considering that nurses work with a multicultural patient population that has different needs and expectations (Dobrowolska et al., 2013). Lifelong learning as a practice enables nurses to address such ethical dilemmas, promoting patients' rights appropriately and remaining sensitive to their moral values. Through participation in ethical education and reflection, nursing practitioners are equipped to integrate their personal values with professional responsibilities. Ultimately, this integrated notion of lifelong learning contributes not only to individual improvement but also enhances the ethical climate of healthcare organizations, with patient care remaining at the forefront of practice (Figure 1.19).

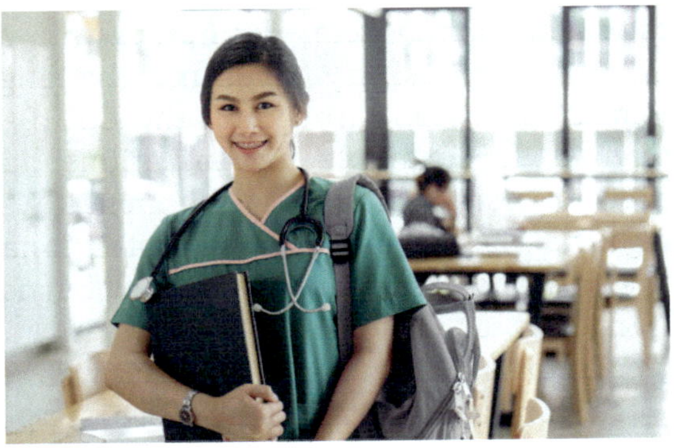

Figure 1.19. The-importance-of-lifelong-learning-in-nursing.

Source: https://www.sflhealthcareinstitute.com/wp-content/uploads/2024/04/the-importance-of-lifelong-learning-in-nursing.jpeg.

1.6.2. Certification and Specialization Opportunities

The professional nursing practice environment, particularly in medical-surgical care, is primarily influenced by certification and specialization. They provide the nurses with the potential to develop their skills and knowledge, which indirectly leads to improved patient outcomes and professional prestige. Certification provides a formal vehicle through which nurses can certify their competence in specific specialties in a bid to demonstrate that they meet high expectations in contemporary healthcare settings. As nursing roles evolve, particularly in response to the needs of medical-surgical units, becoming certified also leads to better work prospects and, in most cases, higher pay, highlighting the value of continuing education in a competitive job market. Additionally, specialization offers nurses the opportunity to focus on specific domains of patient care, such as pre-operative and post-operative management, chronic illness management, or specialized surgical interventions. Engagement in specialized education programs most commonly leads to advanced practice positions, e.g., NP or CNS, which are critical in managing complex patient populations within the medical-surgical environment. According to the stipulations in the present work, the National Nursing Research Unit of King's College London (Griffiths et al., 2007), an understanding of the regulatory framework in different countries can demonstrate how the same certifications are viewed around the world and can inspire a culture of excellence for nursing practice. Beyond enhancing individual career lives, specialization and certification enhance the overall quality of patient care in healthcare organizations. The more certified and specialized nurses an organization has, the higher its patient safety and satisfaction levels. In addition, these certifications can serve as evidence-based practice and leadership for nursing. The more that healthcare systems rely on educated nurses to manage complex patient cases, nursing incorporation becomes the focal point. Not only does it reflect a dedication to a nurse's own career advancement, but it also stays in step with the broader trends throughout healthcare that demand an ever more current skill set (Snyder et al., 1995) (Figure 1.20).

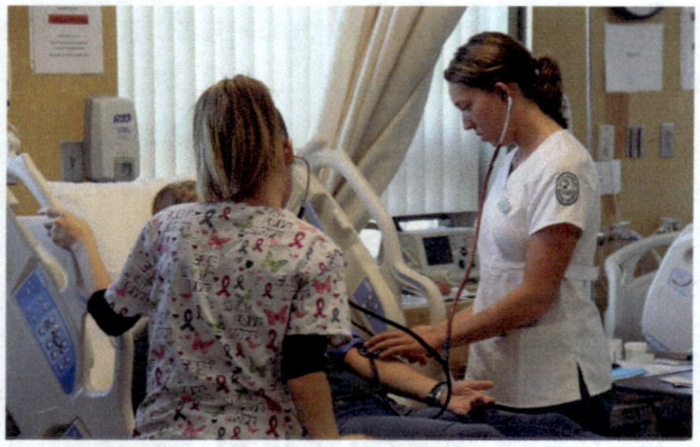

Figure 1.20. Nurse practitioner working.

Source: https://www.husson.edu/online/blog/2021/11/IMG_5655-min.JPG.

1.6.3. Role of Professional Organizations in Nursing

Professional nursing associations play a crucial role in shaping medical-surgical care, and their activities and functions encompass a wide range of initiatives that support professional activism and nurse development. Professional associations provide vital resources such as continuing education, certification, and evidence-based practice guidelines to keep nurses up-to-date in terms of evidence-based practice. By establishing standards of practice and supporting compliance with professional codes of ethics, nursing organizations ensure that members provide quality care, resulting in improved patient outcomes in medical-surgical settings. Nursing organizations also advocate for nurses at policy-making and legislative levels, thus influencing the healthcare environment in a manner that enhances nursing practice and workforce development more. In return, professional associations are networking sites that consolidate medical-surgical nursing experts from various medical-surgical settings. Through the bridge they create between nurses at stages of their careers, such professional associations offer mentorship and sharing of best practices. The dissemination of information and procedures through collaborative efforts helps share information and processes regarding common issues faced by patients during medical-surgical care, thereby enhancing the overall quality of patient service. Conference and seminar sessions organized by such professional associations provide excellent prospects for career development and knowledge sharing among registered nurses. As time passes, such associations forge a bond of fellowship and belonging among nursing fraternity members that helps balance burnout and alienation, especially during times of hardship, such as the COVID-19 pandemic. In times of crises, professional organizations are even more apparent because it is striving to establish effective support systems for nurses who are faced with increasingly mounting challenges in clinical practice. Throughout the COVID-19 pandemic, for example, organizations have opened to design content for the mental well-being and health of nursing professionals, giving tips and assistance to prevent burnout (Sasangohar et al., 2020). Leaders in such organizations have promoted clinician wellness through formal programs and peer support mechanisms (Dewey et al., 2020). Through lobbying for vital resources and nurse-friendly policies, professional groups enable practitioners to build resilience and sustain the nursing workforce, thereby delivering quality care in medical-surgical environments. With the continued advancement of nursing practice, these groups play a crucial role in building an effective and responsive healthcare system.

Test Your Knowledge

1. Why is continuing education so important to medical-surgical nurses?
2. Explain why continuous learning and continuous education are essential in achieving professional nursing practice, leadership, and patient safety in medical-surgical practice.

SUMMARY

Medical-surgical professional nursing practice, leadership, and patient safety require a thorough understanding of ethical responsibilities, as well as the nuances of patient care. Given the diversity of scenarios that nurses must navigate, including those involving conscientious objection, it is essential to balance personal beliefs with the ethical requirement to provide care. Nurses are confronted with such cases where moral belief conflicts with the requested medical interventions, particularly in reproductive health and end-of-life care. Such scenarios underscore the requirement for institutions to develop clear guidelines that enable both patients' rights to benefit from legal medical services and nurses' rights to uphold their moral integrity. Sustaining these dynamics not only perpetuates the ethical culture of nursing practice but also enhances patient-provider trust (Dobrowolska et al., 2013). Additionally, the emotional burden of moral distress on nurses cannot be overstated. As seen in existing literature, high-stakes situations and technological devices are among the factors that contribute to ethical dilemmas, particularly in critical care units. Failure to provide empathetic care due to moral distress significantly lowers the quality of care provided to patients, thereby impacting clinical outcomes. Results of research into moral distress indicate that poor communication and challenging work environments contribute to exacerbating this issue, highlighting the vital need for interventions to empower nurses in fulfilling these emotional demands. Therefore, it is essential to address moral distress in nursing practice, not only for the nurses' well-being but also for the overall quality of patient care (Epstein et al., 2018). Ultimately, these findings extend beyond individual practice to have implications for systemic change in healthcare organizations. Once it becomes apparent to health care system stakeholders that creating ethical environments supportive of professional nursing practice is essential, there must be balanced training and support systems set up. Active engagement in interprofessional discussion forums for ethical issues and policy development that protects nurses while enhancing patient rights is key to advancing healthcare service delivery. Through establishing a culture of moral strength and ethical reflection, the profession can improve its capacity to meet the evolving needs of patients in medical-surgical practice. In short, developing a culture of moral agency and high-quality care is of utmost importance for the future of professional nursing (Dobrowolska et al., 2013; Epstein et al., 2018).

In medical-surgical practice and nursing, obtaining valid and relevant information is crucial for effective clinical decision-making. In one study, it was hypothesized and demonstrated that nurses require access to credible evidence that will minimize uncertainty in the clinical environment. It explained that human sources of information, i.e., clinically experienced colleagues and clinical nurse specialists, are going to be perceived as being more accessible to the nurses than traditional text-based information. This application of human communication likely arises from the pragmatic issue of coping with outdated literature, coupled with the absence of evidence-based guidelines. It is therefore an issue of acute necessity for him to ensure maximum interfacings between technology and indigenous resources so that nurses can bridge the gap between clinical practice and research evidence, culminating in better patient outcomes (Cullum et al., 2001). Among these, one of the most pressing is the transfer of information among nursing staff. Scholarship has identified the nursing handoff as a uniquely at-risk site in which communication errors will have catastrophic consequences. In nursing simulations, for example, students have organized patient handoffs by employing collaborative documentation in the form of patient charts and personal notes to assure continuity of care. Observational studies emphasize the importance of quality text mediation in the situation of such handoffs, and it is inferred that with greater experience for nursing students, they talk more, leading to the passing on of clearer information about patients. Understanding the nature of such handoff experiences is fundamental to developing effective communication plans that strengthen the nurse-patient relationship and foster a culture of safety in the medical-surgical environment (Campbell et al., 2019). The incorporation of best practice into evidence-based nursing creates a culture of continuous improvement in medical-surgical care. The challenge lies in transforming theoretical gains into meaningful interventions for the dynamically changing clinical setting. By leveraging knowledge from experienced practitioners and creating facilitative environments for knowledge transfer, new interventions can be crafted to suit local conditions and enhance nursing practice. Above all, such projects that promote collaboration among the nursing staff, as well as make it easier to access life-altering information, empower nurses to adopt cutting-edge practices in patient care. Embracing education- and mentorship-supportive cultures positively impacts the quality of medical-surgical nursing care being delivered, leading the way towards improved patient outcomes and a more educated nursing profession, which is essential for meeting the needs of modern healthcare challenges (Cullum et al., 2001).

KEY TERMS FROM THIS CHAPTER

- Assessment
- Communication
- Critical Thinking
- Documentation
- Evidence-Based Practice
- Infection Control
- Leadership
- Nursing Process
- Patient-Centered Care
- Therapeutic Communication
- Clinical Judgment
- Continuity of Care
- Cultural Competence
- Ethical Practice
- Health Promotion
- Interprofessional Collaboration
- Nursing Interventions
- Patient Safety
- Quality Improvement
- Time Management

CRITICAL THINKING QUESTIONS

1. **Which of the following best defines the nurse's central role in caring for patients within a med-surg unit?**
   a. Writing patient prescriptions
   b. Diagnosis of disease and treatment planning
   c. Direct patient care and communication with the healthcare team
   d. Surgery
2. **Which of the following nursing interventions is most important during the postoperative phase?**
   a. Disease prevention education
   b. Infection and complication monitoring
   c. Renewing patient medications
   d. Ordering laboratory tests
3. **A nurse is practicing evidence-based practice with patients. What is that?**
   a. Staff-convenient routine following
   b. Habits of decision
   c. Incorporating the best available evidence, clinical judgment, and patient values
   d. Only the physician order follows
4. **Why is the nursing process implementation necessary in professional practice?**
   a. To limit patient contact
   b. To ensure the nurse follows hospital policy
   c. To provide a formal, patient-centered method of care
   d. To reduce documentation
5. **What ethical principle is demonstrated when a nurse upholds a patient's right to autonomy in decision-making regarding their healthcare?**
   a. Beneficence
   b. Nonmaleficence
   c. Justice
   d. Autonomy

Short Answer Questions

1. What is the nursing process, and what are its five steps?
2. What are two significant differences between medical and surgical nursing care?
3. What is the nurse's role in preparing the patient preoperatively?
4. What are two nurse roles for managing postoperative pain?
5. What is "evidence-based practice" in nursing?
6. Explain the importance of communication and cooperation for the medical-surgical nursing team. Provide examples.
7. Show how a nurse prioritizes and assesses care for a respiratory distress-admitted patient.
8. Apply the nursing process to patient care for a med-surg patient recovering from abdominal surgery.

Answers to Critical Thinking Questions

1. (c) 2. (b) 3. (c) 4. (c) 5. (d)

REFERENCES

1. Abram, B., Radzimska, O., Janiszewska, J., Świniarska, A., Papierkowska, R., Czapla, M., & Uchmanowicz, I. (2025). Evaluation of knowledge, attitudes, and skills in Evidence-Based Nursing Practice among Master's degree nursing students. *Nursing Reports, 15*(4), 117. https://doi.org/10.3390/nursrep15040117Adler, P. S., Balkundi, P., Barrow, J., Baxter, R., Bishop, M., Braun, B., et al. (2016). The case of veterinary interprofessional practice: From one health to a world of its own. https://core.ac.uk/download/45467950.pdf (accessed on 28th June 2025).
2. Aghaei, N., Esmaeili, R., Heidari, M. R., Saadatmehr, A., et al. (2015). Investigating the level of moral distress and its related factors among nurses in Mazandaran burn center. https://core.ac.uk/download/52205769.pdf (accessed on 28th June 2025).
3. Ahmadi Amoli, H., Aminian, A., Khashayar, P., Khashayar, J., et al. (2015). Using 360-degree multi-source feedback to evaluate professionalism in surgery departments: An Iranian perspective. https://core.ac.uk/download/55798643.pdf (accessed on 28th June 2025).
4. Aiken, L. H., Al-Kandari, F., Arthur, D., Audit Commission, Buchan, J., Budge, C., et al. (2009). Nurse staffing levels revisited: A consideration of key issues in nurse staffing levels and skill mix research. https://core.ac.uk/download/9632672.pdf (accessed on 28th June 2025).
5. Aleo, G., Bagnasco, A., Catania, G., Icardi, G., et al. (2016). The general results of the RN4CAST survey in Italy. https://core.ac.uk/download/151161294.pdf (accessed on 28th June 2025).
6. Alhameed, H., Czoski-Murray, C., Fernandez, N., George, S., et al. (2001). Extended scope of nursing practice: A multicenter randomized controlled trial of appropriately trained nurses and pre-registration house officers in pre-operative assessment in elective general surgery.
7. Ammenwerth, E., Berg, M., Bostrom, J., Bryman, A., Carlsson, M., Carlsson, M., Chiasson, M., et al. (2009). A quantitative analysis of the impact of a computerized information system on nurses' clinical practice using a realistic evaluation framework. https://core.ac.uk/download/50210.pdf (accessed on 28th June 2025).
8. Aspiuynall, M. J., Benner, P., Carnevali, D., Gerrity, P., Gordon, M., Harbison, J., et al. (2007). A review of clinical decision-making: Models and current research. https://core.ac.uk/download/334115.pdf (accessed on 28th June 2025).
9. Bandy, K. (2005). Practice patterns contributing to positive patient outcomes by nurse practitioners. https://core.ac.uk/download/223074284.pdf (accessed on 28th June 2025).
10. Beiler, J., Opper, K., & Weiss, M. E. (2019). Integrating research and quality improvement using TeamSTEPPS: A health team communication project to improve hospital discharge. https://core.ac.uk/download/286544062.pdf (accessed on 28th June 2025).
11. Boaz, L., Bull, M. J., Gettrust, L., Hagle, M. E., et al. (2016). Engaging nursing staff in research: The clinical nurse specialist role in an academic-clinical partnership. https://core.ac.uk/download/213076328.pdf (accessed on 28th June 2025).
12. Bonica, M., & Students of Health Management 721.01. (2017). *Healthcare Management Primer*. University of New Hampshire. https://core.ac.uk/download/215509297.pdf (accessed on 28th June 2025).
13. Broderick, A. (2013). The Veterans Health Administration: Taking home telehealth services to scale nationally. https://core.ac.uk/download/75777635.pdf (accessed on 28th June 2025).

14. Burke, J., Smith, L. N., Sveinsdóttir, H., Willman, A., et al. (2008). Patient safety in Europe: Medication errors and hospital-acquired infections. https://core.ac.uk/download/90014.pdf (accessed on 28th June 2025).
15. Burton, M. J., Ramke, J., Marques, A. P., Bourne, R., Congdon, N., Jones, I., Ah Tong, B. A. M., et al. (2021). The Lancet Global Health Commission on global eye health: Vision beyond 2020. *The Lancet Global Health, 9*, e489–e551. https://doi.org/10.1016/s2214-109x(20)30488-5 (accessed on 28th June 2025).
16. Buyanova, I., Chen, S., & Chen, W. (1967). Innovations and experiments in uses of health manpower—The effect of licensure laws. https://core.ac.uk/download/62555863.pdf (accessed on 28th June 2025).
17. Campbell, L. (2019). Textual mediation in simulated nursing handoffs: Examining how student writing coordinates action. https://core.ac.uk/download/223025148.pdf (accessed on 28th June 2025).
18. Chorpenning, L., Krautscheid, L. C., Orton, V. J., Ryerson, R., et al. (2011). Student nurse perceptions of effective medication administration education. https://core.ac.uk/download/232742004.pdf (accessed on 28th June 2025).
19. Coffey, E. K., Walker, R., Nicholson, P., & Gillespie, B. (2024). Prioritizing patients for semi-urgent surgery: A scoping review. *Journal of Clinical Nursing*. https://www.semanticscholar.org/paper/491b3dea03d678a55822c2ac8b63890b01b32142 (accessed on 28th June 2025).
20. Cullum, N., McCaughan, D., Mulhall, A., Sheldon, T., et al. (2001). The accessibility of research-based knowledge for nurses in United Kingdom acute care settings. https://core.ac.uk/download/60166.pdf (accessed on 28th June 2025).
21. Dewey, C. M., Hingle, S., Goelz, E., & Linzer, M. (2020). Supporting clinicians during the COVID-19 pandemic. *Annals of Internal Medicine, 172*, 752–753. https://doi.org/10.7326/m20-1033 (accessed on 28th June 2025).
22. Dobrowolska, B., Kane, R., Linsley, P., Pilewska-Kozak, A., et al. (2013). Conscientious objection–Does it also apply to nursing students? https://core.ac.uk/download/20320976.pdf (accessed on 28th June 2025).
23. Dobrowolska, B., Kane, R., Linsley, P., Pilewska-Kozak, A., et al. (2013). Academic careers: The value of individual mentorship on research career progression. https://core.ac.uk/download/20320977.pdf (accessed on 28th June 2025).
24. Duffy, R., & Eddy, L. (2019). A study of the skills, education and qualifications of nurses performing dermatological surgery in the United Kingdom. https://core.ac.uk/download/287613433.pdf (accessed on 28th June 2025).
25. Dunnington, G., Hockaday, M., Smith, C., Torbeck, L., et al. (2018). Optimizing the integration of advanced practitioners in a department of surgery: An operational improvement model. https://core.ac.uk/download/161229732.pdf (accessed on 28th June 2025).
26. Epstein, E. G., Falcó-Pegueroles, A., Jameton, A., Jameton, A., Leske, J., Schroeter, K., Meyers, L. S., et al. (2018). Moral distress in critical care nursing: The state of the science. https://core.ac.uk/download/213088610.pdf (accessed on 28th June 2025).
27. Fatkin, K. J. (2012). Using organization theory to explore the changing role of medical libraries. https://core.ac.uk/download/215412957.pdf (accessed on 28th June 2025).

28. Gilbert, C. L. (2016). Expanding hearts and minds: The impact of transgender and gender non-conforming educational interventions on nurse practitioner students' knowledge and comfort. https://core.ac.uk/download/79664893.pdf (accessed on 28th June 2025).

29. Glikson, M., Nielsen, J. C., Kronborg, M. B., Michowitz, Y., Auricchio, A., Barbash, I. M., Barrabés, J. A., et al. (2021). 2021 ESC guidelines on cardiac pacing and cardiac resynchronization therapy. *European Heart Journal, 42*, 3427–3520. https://doi.org/10.1093/eurheartj/ehab364 (accessed on 28th June 2025).

30. Gonzalez, E. L. F., & Seaton, H. J. (1995). *Internet Sources for Nursing and Allied Health*. https://core.ac.uk/download/187423840.pdf (accessed on 28th June 2025).

31. Griffiths, P., & Robinson, S. (2007). *Nursing Education and Regulation: International Profiles and Perspectives.*

32. Jain, M., Sakale, H., Sriramka, B., & Shyam, A. (2024). Surgeon burnout–Time to heal the healers. *Journal of Orthopedic Case Reports, 14*, 5–6. https://www.semanticscholar.org/paper/95da1e9e1730ee40c0ef922b7d2751c0326fc330 (accessed on 28th June 2025).

33. Johnstone, E. M. (2016). *Perioperative Orientation, Education, And Mentoring (POEM) Program*. https://core.ac.uk/download/147835250.pdf (accessed on 28th June 2025).

34. Khalafi, A., Choopani, S., & Sarvi Sarmeydani, N. (2025). Clinical competency in anesthesia nursing education: A descriptive cross-sectional study at Jundishapur University of Medical Sciences. *Archives of Anesthesia and Critical Care*. https://www.semanticscholar.org/paper/e768d8b03093af04baa5d425deb8af97e745059b (accessed on 28th June 2025).

35. Kuruvilla, J. (2025). Unveiling the hidden strain: Exploring second victim phenomenon among critical care nurses. *International Journal of Critical Care*. https://www.semanticscholar.org/paper/ff2d3ecfb0ac4096a5b324cd74f93448c60d435d (accessed on 28th June 2025).

36. Lee, Y. S. H., Nembhard, I. M., Pogorzelska-Maziarz, M., Stone, P. W., et al. (2018). Differences in work environment for staff as an explanation for variation in central line bundle compliance in intensive care units. https://core.ac.uk/download/213449746.pdf (accessed on 28th June 2025).

37. Lee-Riggins, A. M. (2014). Nurses' perceptions of structural empowerment: A practice review process pilot. https://core.ac.uk/download/70419786.pdf (accessed on 28th June 2025).

38. Lewis, N. M. (2017). Applying a multidimensional strategy to mitigate lateral violence in a small rural community hospital in Western New York. https://core.ac.uk/download/84856763.pdf (accessed on 28th June 2025).

39. May, S. A., & Wallace, S. (2016). Assessing and enhancing quality through outcomes-based continuing professional development (CPD): A review of current practice. https://core.ac.uk/download/76981001.pdf (accessed on 28th June 2025).

40. Mohajer, S., Bagheri, N., Chan, C. M., Danaee, M., Mazlum, S. R., Yoong, T. L., Lopez, V., et al. (2024). Effect of holistic reflective learning program on development of nursing students' professional competency in geriatric clinical practice: A quasi-experimental study. *BMC Medical Education, 24*. https://www.semanticscholar.org/paper/84d8ce77c0ed2e58620c98966dc4fcdfbcb248c9 (accessed on 28th June 2025).

41. N/A. (2005). Can this marriage be saved? https://core.ac.uk/download/71339012.pdf (accessed on 28th June 2025).

42. N/A. (2010). Technology target studies: Technology solutions to make patient care safer and more efficient. https://core.ac.uk/download/71355358.pdf (accessed on 28th June 2025).

43. Nurmalia, D., Padmasari, S., Rokhana, N., Utami, N., et al. (2015). *Proceeding: 3rd Java International Nursing Conference 2015 "Harmony of Caring and Healing Inquiry for Holistic Nursing Practice; Enhancing Quality of Care," Semarang, 20–21 August 2015*. https://core.ac.uk/download/76930906.pdf (accessed on 28th June 2025).

44. Prathiba, P. M., Umar, M., C. V., S., Rathore, M. I., Geetha, P. A., Karfe, K., Suhashini, S., & Deepa, N. R. (2025). Optimizing healthcare outcomes and broadening nursing capabilities in digital era: Telemedicine transformative impact. https://core.ac.uk/download/655504253.pdf (accessed on 28th June 2025).

45. Rowe, S. T. (2015). Improve intra-operative nurse-to-nurse communication using a safety checklist. https://core.ac.uk/download/70419776.pdf (accessed on 28th June 2025).

46. Sasangohar, F., Jones, S. L., Masud, F., Vahidy, F., & Kash, B. A. (2020). Provider burnout and fatigue during the COVID-19 pandemic: Lessons learned from a high-volume intensive care unit. *Anesthesia & Analgesia, 131*, 106–111. https://doi.org/10.1213/ane.0000000000004866 (accessed on 28th June 2025).

47. Snyder, M. (1995). Post-graduate nursing education in the United States. http://ir.library.osaka-u.ac.jp/dspace/bitstream/11094/56893/1/njou1_1_039.pdf (accessed on 28th June 2025).

48. Stern, A. F., Yuan, C. T., Bradley, E. H., Krumholz, H. M., Nembhard, I. M., & Brush, J. E., Jr. (2010). Blueprint for the dissemination of evidence-based practices in health care. https://core.ac.uk/download/71349600.pdf (accessed on 28th June 2025).

49. Walsby, A., Williams, S., & Best, S. (2023). Team around the patient: Multi-professional opportunities to support care delivery in hospitals. *International Journal of Integrated Care*. https://www.semanticscholar.org/paper/92cbcfb475d678e267265725c83580034f0b3066 (accessed on 28th June 2025).

50. Zhang, M., & Wang, W. (2024). Research on the application effect of inter-professional training program for newly enrolled medical staff in operating room based on digital information technology. *BMC Medical Education, 24*. https://www.semanticscholar.org/paper/e7e7727e601d931cf5b1b1fe3a68bb6ef01682b6 (accessed on 28th June 2025).

PRINCIPLES AND SCOPE OF MEDICAL-SURGICAL NURSING

2

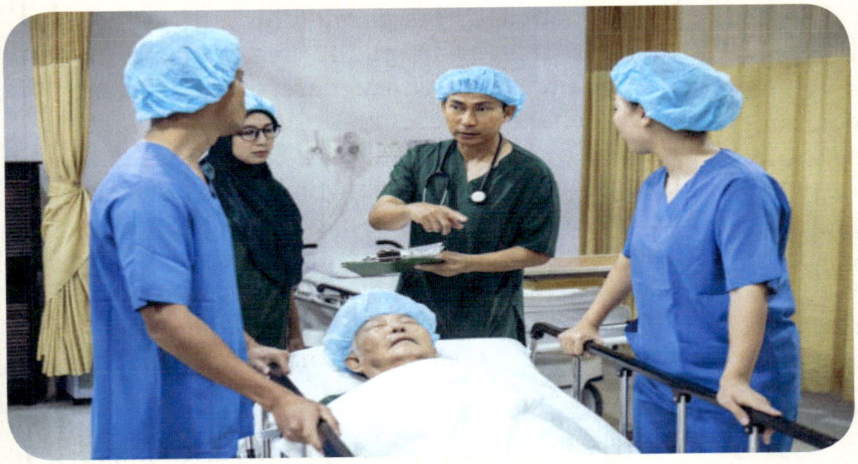

LEARNING OBJECTIVES

After studying this chapter, you will be able to:

1. Describe the history of medical-surgical nursing
2. Discuss the essential principles of medical-surgical nursing
3. Describe the practice scope of medical-surgical nursing
4. Prioritize management and assessment of patients
5. Learn the conditions of medical-surgery
6. List medical-surgical nursing challenges

Introduction

Medical-surgical nursing is the core of care, serving as a bridge between sophisticated medical knowledge and bedside patient care daily. As healthcare continues to become more refined, the demand for competent nurses who can provide holistic and quality care is at its peak. Medical-surgical nurses are tasked with delivering a range of patient health conditions, which is proof of clinical competence and providing supportive care. The principles in this specialty include thorough patient assessment and the application of evidence-based practice, which are essential for achieving favorable outcomes. Furthermore, this dynamic nursing specialty is at the core of patient education, empowering individuals to make informed decisions about their health. Understanding the scope and principles of medical-surgical nursing is essential for developing competent practitioners who can effectively address the complexities of modern healthcare. Through the discussion of medical-surgical nursing practices, it is evident that the practice is founded on safety, care, and effective communication. The integration of patient safety interventions into healthcare systems has helped reduce errors and enhance patient care. Recent studies highlight the importance of systematic practice and tool development, emphasizing accountability and goal setting in nursing practice (McCarthy et al., 2011). Such concepts not only define the clinical competencies that medical-surgical nurses are required to meet, but also confirm continuous improvement in the delivery of healthcare. Thus, nurses need to be skilled in a variety of areas, from technical skills to human interactions, in order to appropriately address the various needs of patients. The medical-surgical nursing practice is not confined to direct patient care but entails a wide range of strategies in handling healthcare. As highlighted in academia, e.g., programs offered by institutions with expertise in health management and policy, the role of the nurse often extends beyond organizational management, where patient care strategic plans are discussed (Bonica et al., 2017).

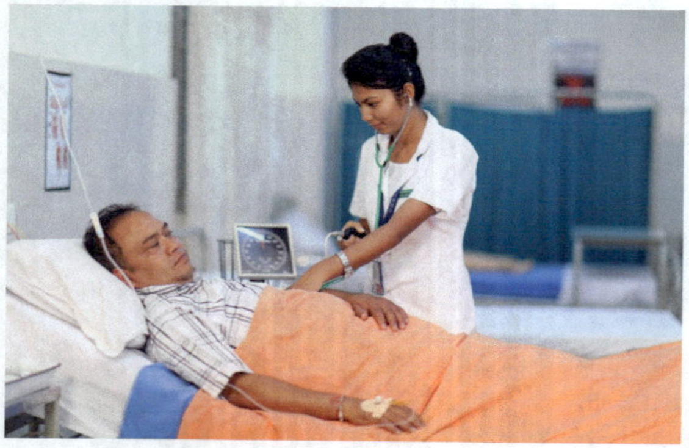

Figure 2.1. Principles and scope of medical-surgical nursing.

Source: https://lvtgnursing.com/wp-content/uploads/2016/03/Medical-Surgical-1.jpg.

This highlights how the medical-surgical nurse is engaged in interdisciplinary teams to address patients' needs, implement quality improvement interventions, and advocate for patients in the healthcare organization. By developing teamwork, clinical decision-making, and leadership competencies, medical-surgical nurses can enhance patient safety and improve health outcomes. In the end, the study of these principles and the depth of the scope of nursing is essential to people who want to master this vital area of healthcare (Figure 2.1).

Importance in the Healthcare System

The relevance of the healthcare system can be described by its three-fold contribution to improvement in public health, ensuring the quality of medical care, and efficient management of resources. Here, the role of medical-surgical nursing is a central one that bridges the gap between theoretical science and practical application in the care of patients. The professionals in this profession not only have the responsibility of direct care of surgical procedures but also of providing whole-patient care to patients suffering from complex health conditions.

Through the practice of interdisciplinary nursing, medical-surgical nurses facilitate the integrative assessment and care of patients, thereby enhancing the quality of care and improving health outcomes, which reinforces the overall integrity of the healthcare process (Bonica et al., 2017). Besides, safety guidelines and models of patient-centered care development have also highlighted the value that may be added to quality assurance by the healthcare system. As the medical environment continues to evolve, evidence-based care is becoming increasingly crucial in preventing medical mistakes and enhancing patient safety. Medical-surgical nursing complements this emphasis by employing formal training protocols and designing effective tools to reduce the risks associated with patient care. Through the implementation of goal-setting and responsibility systems, nurses promote a culture that prioritizes safety and quality.

Through evidence-based research examining the development of patient safety interventions by four healthcare systems over a five-year period, the study illustrates how system-wide interventions can significantly minimize errors and enhance the delivery of care (McCarthy et al., 2011). The healthcare system also highlights its importance through its capacity to adapt to new challenges and evolving healthcare demands.

The imperative call for innovation in medical-surgical nursing is essential, as the healthcare environment is changing due to social, technological, and epidemiological trends. Medical-surgical nurses spearhead the effort to implement these changes through their professional judgment, adapting practices to meet the needs of the patient. These adaptations not only improve the quality of care but also strengthen public health efforts and community health outcomes. Therefore, as the basic principles of medical-surgical nursing evolve, so does the ability of healthcare systems to cope with diverse and often changing needs and provide an enhanced level of care for all patient populations (Figure 2.2).

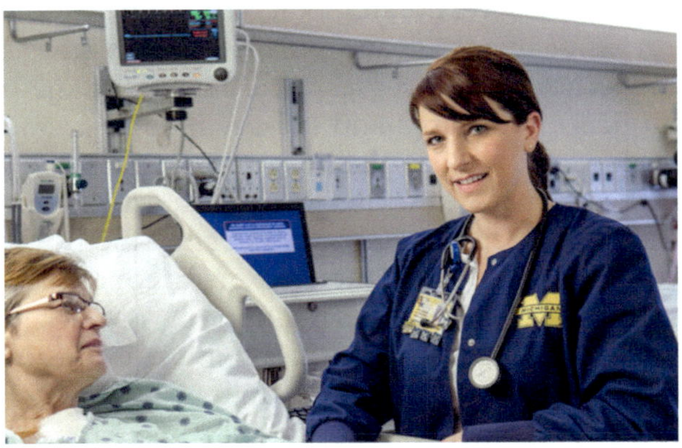

Figure 2.2. Importance in the healthcare system.

Source: https://cdn-static.findly.com/wp-content/uploads/sites/398/2015/10/BannerMedicalSurgical.jpg.

2.1. Historical Background

Learning Outcome

1. Explain the evolution of medical-surgical nursing
2. Emphasize the development of medical-surgical nursing
3. Learn nursing education and practice milestones

The history of medical-surgical nursing is deeply rooted in the revolutionary shifts in healthcare practices that occurred over the last century. The evolution of nursing as a profession accelerated during the late 19th and early 20th centuries, driven by the formation of institutions and the establishment of formalized school of nursing programs. It was early pioneers such as Florence Nightingale who established the foundation by emphasizing the importance of hygiene, patient care environments, and evidence-based practice. With the increased complexity in patient care resulting from advances in medical technology and surgery, the role of the nurse has expanded from uncomplicated care to critical decision-making and high-order patient management. This change also reflected a broadened vision for the healthcare setting and paved the way for the inclusion of advanced providers, such as physician assistants and nurse practitioners, in the operating room, thereby expanding the range of medical-surgical practice. The integration of advanced practice providers within surgical health teams has undergone significant evolution over this period, revolutionizing patient care paradigms. High-level practitioners, such as physician assistants (PAs) and nurse practitioners (NPs), have become integral to medical-surgical nursing, as they collaborate with physicians from various specialties. These practitioners fill several roles, from conducting pre-operative assessments to managing post-operative care. Studies have compared the effectiveness and cost-effectiveness of these practitioners, demonstrating that they can deliver quality care while alleviating some of the pressures on surgical teams. While data on the formal integration of advanced providers within surgery departments remains limited, existing studies suggest that formalized programs enhance teamwork and patient care. In this context, it highlights the need for cultivating multidisciplinary models to integrate such roles, addressing the operational and educational dimensions of surgical care (Dunnington et al., 2018). This is reinforced by the historical context of nursing jobs, particularly in military settings, which further illuminates the evolution of medical-surgical practice. The establishment of the Navy Nurse Corps in 1908 was a turning point in the professionalization of nurses in military settings. Navy nurses served in surgery and emergency care in World War II, frequently in hazardous circumstances, as they delivered badly needed services. Although accounts of the Army Nurse Corps typically overshadow naval nurses, Dora Cline Fechtmann's and Dorothy Still Danner's lives are typical of the commitment and resilience of nurses in stressful environments.

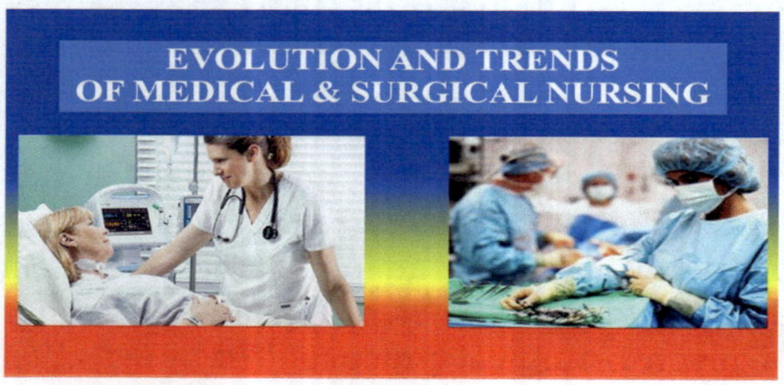

Figure 2.3. Evolution of medical-surgical nursing.

Source: https://i.ytimg.com/vi/hkaLSCXduTM/maxresdefault.jpg.

Their assignments not only made nursing history but also influenced the overall principles that regulate medical-surgical practice today. By gaining such an understanding of their past role, current practicing nurses can more fully grasp the foundation on which medical-surgical nursing rests, blending the heritage of the past into their current practice (Thibault et al., 2016) (Figure 2.3).

2.1.1. Evolution of Medical-Surgical Nursing

The evolution of medical-surgical nursing reflects broader societal and technological changes that have shaped healthcare practices over the centuries. Initially, nursing was primarily an extension of homemaking skills, emphasizing care and comfort for the ill. However, as the field advanced, particularly in the late 19th and early 20th centuries, nursing began to embrace a more scientific approach. Pathfinders such as Florence Nightingale established standards that included hygiene and sanitation, leading to changes in patient care over time. The change was a significant transition from intuitive care to evidence-based practice, influencing the core values of modern medical-surgical nursing. With the advancement of healthcare technology, nurses have taken on more tasks, including patient management and education, to address upgraded patient demands and develop critical thinking in practice. In the mid-20th century, medical-surgical nursing experienced significant expansion due to advances in medical knowledge and technological progress. The invention of new surgical procedures and life-saving operations necessitated a more qualified nursing personnel with extensive knowledge and expertise. Not only did medical-surgical nursing focus on postoperative care, but also on preoperative assessment and interdisciplinary coordination, allowing nurses to play a significant role in the operating team. This evolution also led to the development of specialized educational programs and certifications, acknowledging the unique skills required to function effectively in this field. Furthermore, the incorporation of nursing models and theory within the curriculum helped define professional roles and competencies, reaffirming the importance of medical-surgical nursing in the continuum of healthcare. The evolution of medical-surgical nursing is further enhanced as healthcare shifts in response to the dynamics of patient-centered care and the growing complexity of managing chronic conditions. Modern medical-surgical nurses are confronted with a paradigm of interprofessional practice, health reforms, and altered patterns in patient populations. As healthcare shifts toward a model with a vision for holistic practice, nurses serve as patient advocates while facilitating care across various settings. The ongoing debate of healthcare policy, particularly issues such as reproductive rights, makes it essential for nurses to remain current and engaged in the political environment that affects their practice. Therefore, as the profession evolves, medical-surgical nursing continues to develop, symbolizing values that emphasize comprehensive, humane, and effective patient care, consistent with the tradition of nursing, yet sensitive to the issues in healthcare today (Sheldon et al., 2015; Bonica et al., 2017).

2.1.2. Key Figures in the Development of the Field

The evolution of medical-surgical nursing has been significantly impacted by major players who introduced new practice patterns and educational frameworks. Virginia Henderson is a major contributor who has been highly praised as one of the founders of nursing theory. Henderson's perspective, which defines nursing as assisting individuals to perform activities that result in health and restoration, is the foundation for medical-surgical nursing. Her work emphasized the patient advocate role and care-giving of the nurse, advocating an integrated approach to patient care. Altered conceptions of patients as active participants in the healing process have impacted education programs and nursing practice, emphasizing caring and critical thinking as essential dimensions of the profession. As the profession continues to grow, Henderson's legacy remains within it, challenging today's nurses to merge technical skills with a human touch in their patient care. The other most significant development in the evolution of medical-surgical nursing is advanced practice, which has transformed patient care delivery in operating rooms. The PA and NP role has been central to improving the efficiency and effectiveness of surgical care. As discussed in recent literature, PAs and NPs not only expand the scope of practice for physicians but also improve patient outcomes through multidisciplinary models of care. Advanced practitioners play a significant role in governing a variety of healthcare practices, such as general surgery and subspecialties. Their contributions have informed the necessity for practice-based teams, wherein interdisciplinary practice leads to improved service provision and patient satisfaction. The role transformation of NPs and PAs reflects how the medical-surgical nursing profession evolves to meet the complexities of today's healthcare demands (Dunnington et al., 2018). Mentoring has also emerged as a core component in developing nursing careers, particularly in advancing clinical academic progression. As highlighted by the pertinent research, successful mentoring contacts provide incredibly beneficial support to novice and experienced nurses navigating their careers. Mentees report increased confidence and enhanced competency, leading to improved patient care in the operating room. These formal and informal mentoring experiences are crucial for developing the next generation of leaders and researchers in nursing, ultimately shaping the future of medical-surgical nursing. While the advantages are acknowledged, participation in formal mentoring programs is sporadic, which reflects the lack of support mechanisms necessary for professional and personal growth in this profession. A more comprehensive national strategy for mentoring would significantly enhance the career trajectory of nursing, thereby enriching the principles and practice of medical-surgical nursing (Dobrowolska et al., 2013) (Figure 2.4).

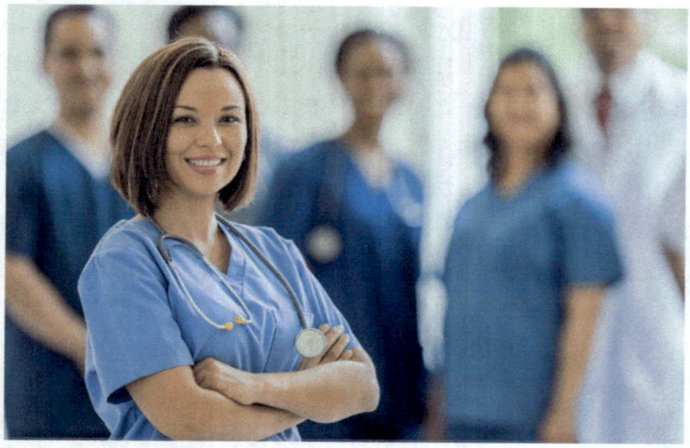

Figure 2.4. The evolving role of physician assistants (PAs) in healthcare.

Source: https://talhealthcare.com/wp-content/uploads/2024/10/Physician-Assistants-2.png.

2.1.3. Milestones in Nursing Education and Practice

The history of nursing education and practice has been marked by significant milestones that reflect broader societal trends and advancements in healthcare. Possibly the most significant landmark was the establishment of formal nursing education in the 19th century, as demonstrated by the activities of Florence Nightingale, which laid the groundwork for the establishment of nursing as a respected vocation. This initial phase initiated reforms in curriculum development, focusing on both theoretical knowledge and clinical practice. The move toward competency-based education has come to shape nursing education worldwide, promoting holistic training based on principles of holistic patient care. Also, the concordance of nursing curriculum to national standards, as demonstrated in most countries, confirms the global nature of nursing education and its commitment to preparing effective practitioners to meet the differing needs of community health, as presented through comparative studies on nursing programs in Brazil and Portugal, indicating similarities and divergence according to regional variance (Fonseca et al., 2014). The use of standardized accreditation processes and the incorporation of research into nursing curricula also transformed nursing education. Accreditation not only enhances the quality of educational programs but also ensures the public that nursing graduates are competent. The Bologna Process is a demonstration of this commitment to harmonizing the education system within Europe, aiming to achieve a recognized level of nursing qualifications and competencies that facilitate mobility among health professionals. In Brazil, for instance, nursing education is competency-based through specialist disciplines tailored to the nation's health reality, including mandatory subjects in geriatric care and research (Fonseca et al., 2014). These curricula are based on regional health requirements, developing nursing professionals who can effectively handle diverse patient populations. These innovations align with the fundamental principles of medical-surgical nursing, which emphasize holistic knowledge combined with practical skills in delivering optimal patient care. Finally, ongoing professional development of nurses is necessary to address the dynamic nature of healthcare practice and education. This is particularly necessary in midwifery education, which has faced numerous challenges in the past five decades in Jordan, as in nursing education. Education and training continuously, as well as employing trained graduates and faculty members, is required to maintain nursing and midwifery practice functionality and integrity. With regard to intricate issues like chronic diseases and aging, which healthcare systems are encountering, nursing education development has to keep pace with adaptation. By developing a learning environment conducive to ongoing learning, nurses can be assured of their ongoing capacity to deliver competent practice, which ultimately translates into improved patient outcomes and better quality of care within medical-surgical settings (Figure 2.5).

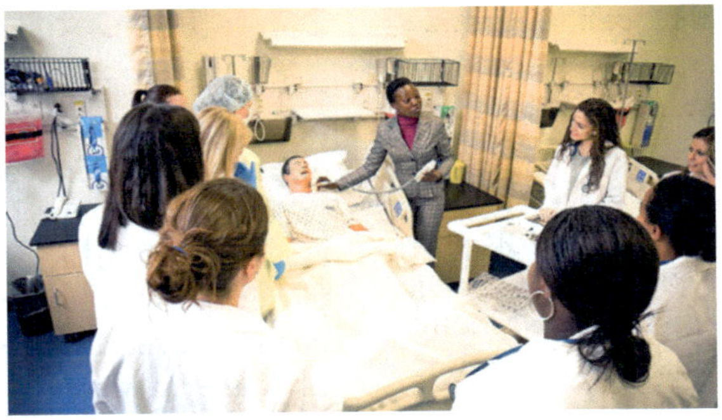

Figure 2.5. Nursing education and practice.

Source: https://external-content.duckduckgo.com/iu/?u=https%3A%2F%2Fmarymount.edu%2Fwp-content%2Fuploads%2F2024%2F08%2FFOR-WEB-2.jpg&f=1&nofb=1&ipt=b865b1edeb720e51f06f5e30ead8697cafeb9a190b4b7a96eeacb656610cbeba.

Test Your Knowledge

1. What are the primary functions of nurse practitioners (NPs) within surgical care settings?
2. In what ways do NPs improve the quality of care within surgical settings and contribute to improved patient outcomes?

2.2. Core Principles of Medical-Surgical Nursing

Learning Outcome

1. Explain the patient-centered care
2. Define the evidence-based practice (EBP) of medical-surgical nursing
3. Discuss the interprofessional collaboration of medical-surgical nursing

The underlying principles of medical-surgical nursing are founded on two pillars: patient safety and whole-person care. These principles form a foundation that guides nursing practice in the clinical setting through the imperatives of continuous assessment and evidence-based action. By integrating exhaustive analyses of patients' physical, emotional, and social needs, nurses are ideally suited to create personalized care plans that treat not only acute illness but also such lifestyle factors as may impact recovery. Improved patient outcomes rely heavily on this comprehensive process, which capitalizes on the therapeutic benefits of treating individuals, rather than just their symptoms. Thus, medical-surgical nurses are not just caregivers but also advocates of integrated health care management throughout the patient's course of care. Additionally, the integration of evidence-based practice into the protocol of medical-surgical nursing best practice enhances decision-making and enhances higher standards of care. This approach necessitates ongoing education and adherence to prevailing research to ensure care delivery conformance in response to the latest clinical guidelines. For instance, as noted in previous studies, healthcare organizations have increasingly focused on improving patient safety interventions through setting effective training processes and practical tools for error reduction, which are integral components of evidence-based practice. Through goal setting and being responsible, nurses can minimize risks and enhance patient safety outcomes in their practice environment. Therefore, incorporating evidence-based practices into regular nursing procedures on an ongoing basis not only improves the efficacy of care but also demonstrates the core principles of providing safe and effective patient-centered care. Finally, the core principles of medical-surgical nursing also encompass interdisciplinary collaboration, which is essential for maintaining comprehensive patient care. When health professionals, including physicians, pharmacists, and social workers, exchange information effectively, coordination of effort ensues, ultimately benefiting the patient. Practice models involving teamwork facilitate broader evaluations and enhanced understanding of various health conditions affecting the patients. For instance, strategic interventions through critical discourse among healthcare providers can lead to enhanced patient safety protocols and improved health literacy. As medical-surgical nursing evolves with the expanding science of healthcare, it will increasingly become more necessary for the implementation of interdisciplinary collaboration into the very core of medical-surgical nursing to address greater complexities of patient care and deliver holistic and effective care, and thereby establish the promise of the nursing profession to compassionate and personalized patient care (Figure 2.6).

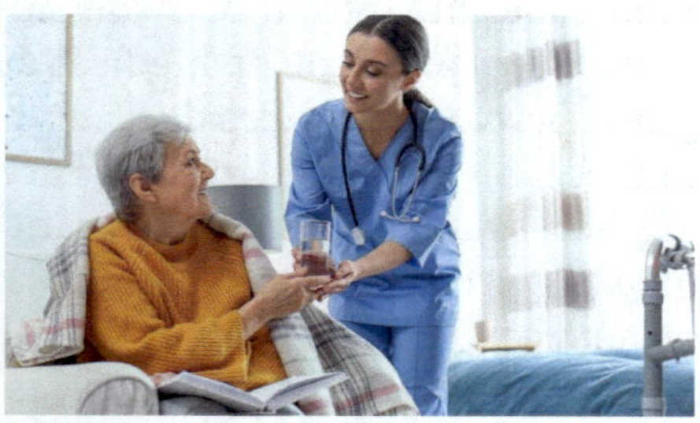

Figure 2.6. Benefits of holistic hospice care.

Source: https://www.wphealthcarenews.com/wp-content/ uploads/2022/05/ DTgZm2xQb YhJXEEv JfrCibBqYwGqOeRL 1650388965.jpg.

2.2.1. Patient-Centered Care

Patient-centered care in Medical-Surgical Nursing is a key practice philosophy that enables and enhances patient outcomes. Patient-centered care is concerned explicitly with enabling recognition of and respect for the individual patient's own needs, values, and preferences. Patient-centered care allows for the adaptability of care delivery to address the unique circumstances surrounding each patient through the development of a partnership between healthcare workers and patients. This paradigm shift not only improves patient satisfaction but has also been correlated with shorter hospital stays and decreased readmission rates. Building trust and communication in this model is crucial, as it facilitates the patient becoming an active participant in their healthcare decisions, which can vastly enhance their entire treatment experience and efficacy. At the core of patient-centered practice is effective communication between patients and healthcare professionals. Clear and accurate information shared enables the demystification of the medical-surgical process complexity, which ultimately provides a supportive environment that fosters the expression of concern and preference by patients. In addition, the development of an open line of communication enables the determination of patient-specific goals, with the potential for a tailored treatment strategy that respects individual values and cultural contexts. Education of medical professionals in the subtleties of empathetic communication is paramount, as it enables them to communicate with patients on a more sophisticated level. Hence, such a link is the foundation for establishing trust and collaborative decision-making, which play an essential role in achieving optimal health results in different patient groups. Moreover, the integration of patient safety interventions into healthcare systems plays a vital role in promoting patient-centered care programs. Over the last couple of years, several systems have adopted integrated approaches that aim to minimize errors by establishing an accountability culture and setting goals among health teams. These are key strategies that have been employed to develop effective training methods and high-quality tools to enhance patient safety, which is inextricably linked to the fundamental principles of patient-centered care. By placing equal value on safety and patient preference, healthcare providers can create an environment in which patients feel safe and empowered to manage their own health. Supported by a system of safety and valuing individual choice, patients are more likely to be fully engaged in their treatment plans, hence enhancing the overall effectiveness of medical-surgical nursing practice (Schenk et al., 1959; McCarthy et al., 2011) (Figure 2.7).

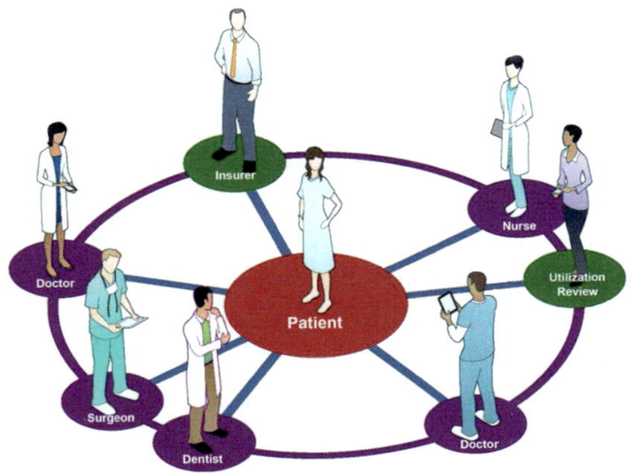

Figure 2.7. Patient centered care.

Source: https://medico.co.jp/wp-content/uploads/2020/08/patient-centered-care-4-768x603.jpg.

2.2.2. Evidence-Based Practice (EBP)

Introduction of EBP in medical-surgical nursing is a foundation for enhancing patient care quality and clinical outcomes. EBP provides a systematic approach that combines clinical expertise, patient values, and the best current research evidence to inform decision-making for nursing practice. This three-pronged approach is particularly crucial in medical-surgical settings, where healthcare practitioners frequently face an array of disorders requiring multifaceted interventions. With the aid of firm evidence, nurses can design and implement care plans that address both the short-term needs of patients and their long-term health trends. Such a framework enables a culture of inquiry in nursing, as health professionals continually seek ways to integrate recent research findings into their daily practice, foster discussion, and enhance the overall efficacy of nursing interventions. In addition, the evolving nature of healthcare requires ongoing efforts to ensure that nursing education remains aligned with current and future practice needs. As depicted by recent research, nursing curricula need to change to accommodate new and emerging standards, as well as contemporary health issues. For instance, the requirements for advanced practice nurses and nurse practitioners to manage complex ethical problems, such as abortion services, affirm the far-reaching undertones of EBP in advanced practice nursing education and practice. Findings indicated that, while most students in advanced practice nursing may not intend to provide abortion services, they realize the importance of being skilled and informed in referral when necessary. This emphasizes a key aspect of EBP: equipping nurses with the competencies and expertise to address ethical issues in practice while considering the values and needs of their patients and ensuring that care is patient-centered and evidence-based (Fehring et al., 2005). As the nursing environment changes in parallel with changes in the provision of care and patient populations, namely an aging population, the cornerstones of EBP must change similarly. Evidence suggests that future nursing practice will increasingly require competencies in gerontology, home care, and community health, necessitating a reassessment of nursing education programs. A focus on preparing nurse graduates for these evolving challenges can help ensure that they are equipped to meet the complexity of patient care across settings. By addressing these educational needs, nursing programs can strengthen the foundational elements of EBP, ultimately preparing nurses to deliver care in accordance with contemporary best practices. This alignment not only enhances the effectiveness of nursing interventions but also fosters a collaborative, interdisciplinary approach to healthcare that prioritizes patient wellness across diverse environments (O\u27Brien et al., 1989) (Figure 2.8).

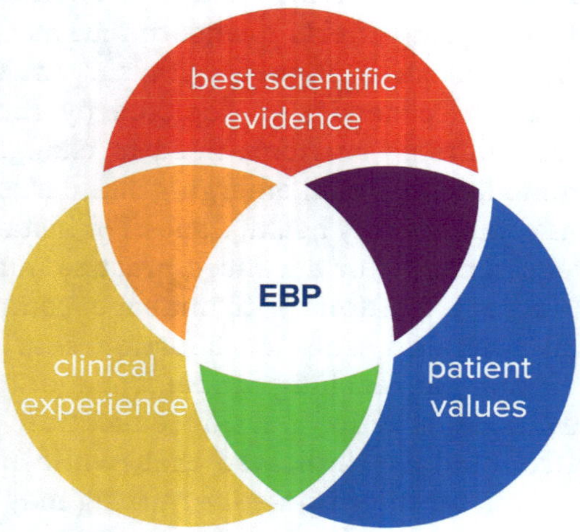

Figure 2.8. Evidence-based practice (EBP).

Source: https://pressbooks.umn.edu/app/uploads/sites/150/2022/08/EBP-venn-diagram-768x726.jpg.

2.2.3. Interprofessional Collaboration

Collaborative practice is vital in medical-surgical settings, and it is essential for enhancing patient care and outcomes. The collaborative process involves health professionals from various disciplines, including physicians, nurses, physician assistants, and pharmacists, working together to give integrated, holistic care. Effective communication among the members of the team improves a holistic understanding of the needs of the patients, and the services are therefore well-integrated. Through collective decision-making and diverse perspectives, interprofessional collaboration enhances problem-solving, which ultimately results in improved patient safety and satisfaction. Through combining the composite knowledge of different health professionals, this collaborative setting not only maximizes the care process but also reduces medical mistakes, which is a critical element under challenging settings prevalent in medical-surgical settings. The use of advanced practice providers, such as physician assistants and nurse practitioners, is a symbol of interprofessional practice in medical-surgical nursing. As these professionals take on increased tasks in patient care, they contribute immensely to the multidisciplinary team through their specialized skills and enhanced availability for interacting with patients. Recent initiatives described in the literature suggest that integrating advanced providers into surgical teams may potentially lead to operational efficiencies and improve surgical patient outcomes. One can clearly see that the findings reflect a demand for systematic approaches to facilitate such integration, so that teamwork works to continuously improve care (Dunnington et al., 2018). By recognizing the unique contributions of advanced practice providers, healthcare teams are better equipped to manage the complexities of patient care in surgical environments, resulting in improved quality of service. The literature also emphasizes the need for formally structured interprofessional interventions that focus on safe patient care practices. A narrative review illustrated several intervention approaches, including TeamSTEPPS, aimed at enhancing healthcare professionals' capacities through educational interventions. Not only do these interventions and improve communication skills, but also facilitate teamwork, significantly boosting attitudes towards collaborative practice among medical and nursing professionals (Clark et al., 2017). Still, the review also suggests a gap in evaluating the long-term impact of such interventions on patient outcomes and safety measures. As medical-surgical nursing increasingly emphasizes quality and safety, ongoing research on the effectiveness of interprofessional collaboration is crucial. Strengthening these alliances can facilitate the development of best practices that enhance patient care, thereby improving the culture of safety in healthcare institutions.

Test Your Knowledge

1. How does evidence-based practice (EBP) improve patient-centered care in medical-surgical nursing?
2. What are two steps in the EBP process that medical-surgical nurses commonly use to improve patient outcomes?

2.3. Scope of Practice

Learning Outcome

1. Explain the role and responsibility of medical-surgical nurses
2. Define settings of medical-surgical nursing practice
3. Describe the legal and ethical aspects of medical-surgical nursing

The concept of Scope of Practice is at the core of determining the duties and boundaries of medical-surgical nursing. It identifies the various roles and tasks nurses can perform safely, as per their education, skills, and legislation. With the advancement of healthcare delivery, especially in the development of medical technology, the scope is typically broadened to include complex procedures and tasks. However, adherence to such defined boundaries is paramount, as they not only ensure safety for the patient but also protect healthcare professionals from potential ethical and legal consequences. Delineating the scope in a concise manner enables nurses to practice comfortably within their field of expertise and fosters a conducive working environment in multidisciplinary healthcare facilities. Advanced practice nurses play a significant role in shaping the scope of practice, particularly in specific areas such as women's health. Recent studies indicate a rise in the acceptance of such practitioners to provide reproductive healthcare services, such as abortion, under existing ethical and personal constraints. For instance, one study found that while the majority of advanced practice nursing students refused to incorporate abortion into practice based on institutional policy and personal values, there existed much enthusiasm among them to refer patients for the same (Fehring et al., 2005). This duality reflects the multifaceted tension between personal belief and professional duty, ultimately impacting the changing face of medical-surgical nursing and its educational needs. Additionally, the ethical dimensions of the scope of practice highlight the necessity for ongoing professional education and development within the nursing profession. As health practices shift, so must the knowledge base of ethical principles governing patient care. Nurses are forced to encounter circumstances where their own faith may conflict with the medical needs of the patients, particularly where such controversial issues as abortion services (Nassar et al., 1950) are involved. It is vital to create a learning and discussion space for such issues between the students and practicing nurses. It facilitates a reflective approach to how their scope of practice may shift and still stay within ethical boundaries, ultimately driving holistic patient care in medical-surgical facilities (Figure 2.9).

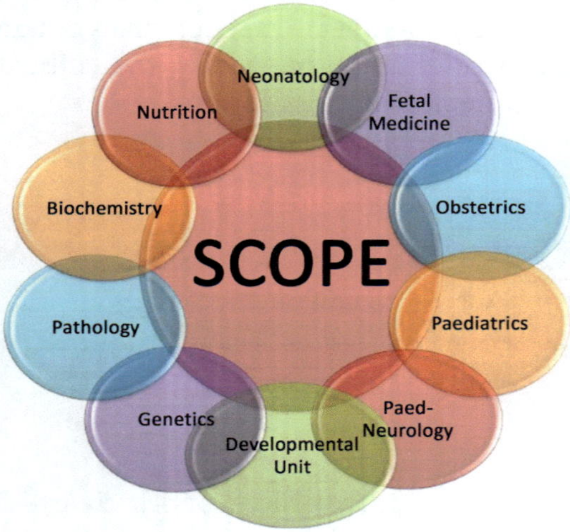

Figure 2.9. Scope of practice of nursing.

Source: https://www.sriramachandra.edu.in/university/update/research-webpage-sriher-27th-july-2019/scopeintro2.jpg.

2.3.1. Roles and Responsibilities of Medical-Surgical Nurses

In the ever-changing healthcare environment, the roles and responsibilities of medical-surgical nurses play a crucial role in delivering comprehensive patient care. These nurses serve as the primary carers of patients with a wide variety of medical and surgical illnesses, often coordinating intricate treatments and interventions. Medical-surgical nurses are tasked with constantly assessing patients' needs, using critical thinking skills to implement care plans derived from individual health profiles. In addition to their physical care activities, they also provide emotional support and education, which are essential components of the healing process. They coordinate extensive healthcare systems with the support of interdisciplinary teams, adhering to best practices and standards governing nursing care. Consequently, their work is no longer confined at the bedside, but they become an indispensable communication link between patients, families, and other healthcare professionals, hence optimizing overall care delivery (Bonica et al., 2017). As front-line care professionals, medical-surgical nurses are well-acquainted with the ideals of patient safety and quality nursing care. This involves the effective management of drug administration, taking vital essential signs, and detecting complications or a decline in a patient's status. They play a crucial role in infection control through the implementation of stringent measures that lower the risk of hospital-acquired infections. Besides, medical-surgical nurses also stand up for patients, thus their voices being heard during decision-making. The focus on evidence-based practices also more strongly establishes their mandates, requiring nurses to remain abreast and adjust to innovations in guidelines and technologies within care models. In upholding ongoing learning and professional growth, nurses foster a culture of safety and excellence in care, which has a direct impact on patient outcomes (Dunnington et al., 2018). Besides their clinical practice, medical-surgical nurses are teachers and managers in the healthcare environment. They also offer patient and family education by educating patients on their diagnoses, treatment, and post-discharge care, enabling them to play important roles in their own healing journeys. This process of education typically entails deconstructing complex medical terms to easier language for understanding by the patients to maintain compliance with regimens. Medical-surgical nurses are also capable of becoming leaders in their workplaces, promoting care delivery and patient experiences through the initiatives they initiate. These roles may involve precepting new nurses, developing care plans, or collaborating on quality improvement projects. With these types of programs, they not only assist with direct patient care but also advance nursing practice and the healthcare organization's culture as a whole (Dunnington et al., 2018) (Figure 2.10).

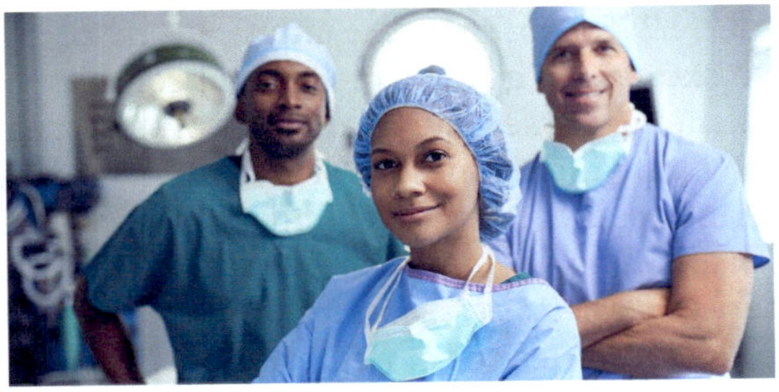

Figure 2.10. Roles and responsibilities of medical-surgical nurses.

Source: https://careers.eisenhowerhealth.org/wp-content/uploads/Surgical-Nurses-Standing-Together-in-Uniform.jpg.

2.3.2. Settings for Medical-Surgical Nursing Practice

In various clinical settings within medical-surgical nursing practice, different patient outcomes and nursing interventions are observed. They encompass acute care hospitals, outpatient surgical centers, among others, with various challenges and nursing interventions. The acute care setting, characterized by its active nature and fast patient turnover, requires nurses to possess a mix of clinical competence and effective time management. On the other hand, outpatient settings prioritize follow-up and education for patients, promoting individuals after discharge. Prioritizing the importance of flexibility, medical-surgical nurses thrive by adapting their styles to meet the specific demands of their settings, thereby advancing patients' optimal recovery and satisfaction. Another essential aspect of medical-surgical nursing practice is the implementation of evidence-based practices in various settings. Protocol-based care, according to the latest research, facilitates the coordination of treatment methods across various clinical environments, with the ultimate goal of enhancing patient care quality. Utilizing realistic evaluation methods, nursing staff can accurately identify the protocols most likely to produce the best outcomes based on specific contexts. Through this, not only is patients' safety improved but nurses are also encouraged to pursue ongoing professional development and maturation. Therefore, understanding the interplay between context and protocol implementation is crucial to nursing competence in achieving the overall goal of optimizing patient care in medical-surgical settings (Hunter et al., 2010). Furthermore, education and training of medical-surgical nurses play an essential role in preparing them for the complexity of their practice environments. Nursing schools are increasingly emphasizing experiential learning activities across a range of environments, allowing for the development of foundational skills that can be applied in both inpatient and outpatient settings. Through clinical rotations and simulations, future nurses become familiarized with diverse patient populations and acute health conditions. This exposure is crucial in developing critical thinking, problem-solving, and communication strategies that are essential for navigating the complexities of medical-surgical nursing. With the evolution of nursing curricula, the acquisition of interprofessional collaboration and patient-centered care concepts becomes imperative, ultimately broadening the scope of practice in nursing in this regard (Bonica et al., 2017) (Figure 2.11).

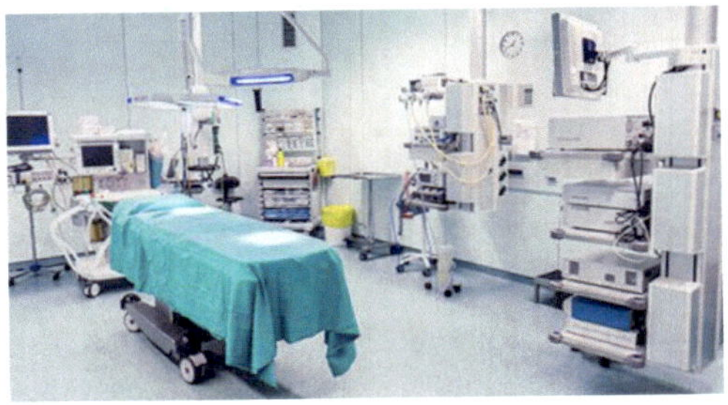

Figure 2.11. The surgical setting.

Source: https://external-content.duckduckgo.com/iu/?u=https%3A%2F%2Ftse4.mm.bing.net%2Fth%3Fid%3DOIP.aNLBjKSydF1_qONKYTMIOwHaEO%26pid%3DApi&f=1&ipt=e5e0523b2426e0eb0e24c7bf77aa17aa88ba9a2d5106d15d6f12efd93b701811.

2.3.3. Legal and Ethical Considerations

In the practice and decision-making of medical-surgical nursing, legal and ethical concerns intersect in a useful manner to inform practice and decision-making. Practitioners frequently encounter complex problems that involve a combination of legal statutes and ethical principles. For instance, the legal mandate of informed consent is a fundamental requirement that ensures patients are appropriately informed and consenting to the interventions and procedures they are to undergo. This legal mandate is interwoven with ethical demands that call on nurses to uphold patient autonomy while ensuring that patients have adequate comprehension to make informed decisions concerning their care. The balance between compliance with legal standards and upholding ethical practice is of significant interest to patient outcomes and the integrity of nursing practice. One of the major areas that is noteworthy both legally and ethically in medical-surgical nursing is the scenario where decisions are made about end-of-life care. The Airdale NHS Trust V Bland case vividly illustrates the contentious issues surrounding the withdrawal of life-sustaining treatment, particularly where patients remain in a persistent vegetative state (PVS). As Dobson et al. (1995) observe, the implications of this case extend far beyond mere legal compliance, challenging nurses and healthcare professionals to navigate the nuanced world of balancing the best interests of the patient with the ethical ideal of prolonging life. Implementation of the best interests test involves careful consideration of the patient's current state of health, prognosis, and previously expressed wishes, but ultimately rests with the nurses as champions of ethical decision-making in the context of competing agendas. Additionally, moral principles such as beneficence, non-maleficence, and justice must be embedded within nursing practice culture. Nurses are then faced with the challenge of doing good and not harm, particularly when resources are scarce or patient wishes do not align with medical recommendations. The Bolam test employed in Dobson et al. (1995) is a benchmark used to guide practice according to the reasonable standard adopted by professionals within similar situations. By integrating such ethical and legal concerns into practice, nurses can navigate the tightrope of adversity present in medical-surgical settings, with patient care that meets both legal requirements and ethical standards that promote professional integrity and caring.

Test Your Knowledge

1. What are three primary responsibilities of a medical-surgical nurse in patient care?
2. Explain the evolving roles of the medical-surgical nurses in varied clinical environments and explain how they facilitate interdisciplinary teamwork and patient outcomes.

2.4. Patient Assessment and Management

Learning Outcome

1. Identify the holistic patient assessment techniques
2. Define the development of nursing care plans
3. Describe the monitoring and evaluation of patient outcomes

Patient assessment and management in medical-surgical nursing are essential components that determine the type of care provided. This step-by-step procedure begins with a detailed patient assessment through physical examination, medical history, and psychosocial assessment. With a methodical process, nurses collect and synthesize data to identify current and potential health issues. Practical assessment not only aids in the development of a comparison baseline throughout the patient's hospitalization but also informs nursing diagnoses that guide individualized care plans. By utilizing evidence-based methods and tools, medical-surgical nurses facilitate the detection of slight differences in a patient's condition with expedience, consequently enabling timely intervention. For example, ongoing assessment facilitates monitoring for complications, enabling optimal inpatient outcomes and safety —a key target domain in patient management practice. Following assessment, the management phase entails the strategic use of interventions based on the determined needs. Prioritization of care based on urgency and impact is crucial in the high-pressure medical-surgical setting, where patient status can change rapidly. Nurses must collaborate to develop care plans, often through interdisciplinary teams, to manage the varied dimensions of a patient's health, physical recuperation, emotional status, and social support systems. Interdisciplinary approaches enhance the level of care while encouraging a patient-centered atmosphere. Furthermore, programmatic management methods, such as the implementation of patient engagement programs, have been shown to significantly reduce errors. Patient engagement programs create care plan discussions via active patient participation in recovery and adherence to the treatment regimen, thus improving health outcomes and satisfaction rates. Apart from direct patient management, the application of safety procedures and programmatic practices significantly contributes to improving patient outcomes in medical-surgical settings. Notable success stories of successful interventions are evident in the practices within healthcare organizations that focus on ensuring patient safety, such as those observed in the case of the Veterans Affairs (VA) system.

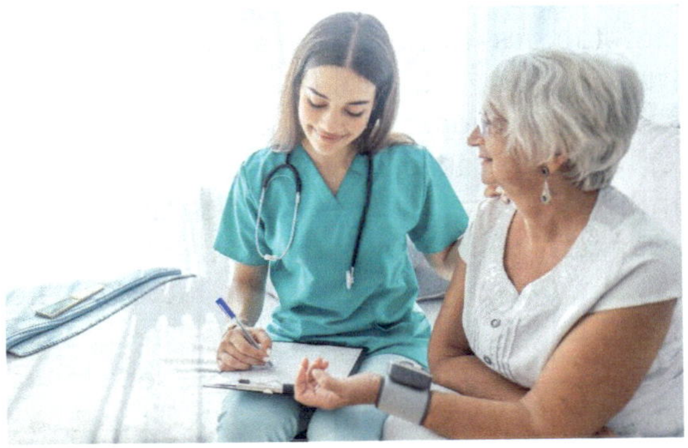

Figure 2.12. Patient assessment and management.

Source: https://s3.amazonaws.com/utep-uploads/wp-content/uploads/online-regis-college/2019/06/06095024/HEENT.jpg.

Through the creation of the National Center for Patient Safety, the VA has established a culture of safety, as well as implemented initiatives to enhance communication among personnel, including targeted training programs for operating room staff. Such strategies have also proven promising in terms of reducing surgical mortality and improving overall quality of care. In addition, leadership responsibility and organizational support for ongoing improvement efforts provide a platform that amplifies nursing practice, allowing for the effective identification and correction of safety events. As patient assessment and management principles are integrated into thorough strategies, they become a strong platform for high-quality medical-surgical nursing care, benefiting both patients and healthcare professionals equally (Chase et al., 2011; McCarthy et al., 2011) (Figure 2.12).

2.4.1. Comprehensive Patient Assessment Techniques

Comprehensive patient assessment techniques in the field of medical-surgical nursing are crucial for ensuring optimal patient outcomes. These approaches encompass a comprehensive strategy that involves physiological, psychological, and social factors influencing a patient's health status. Proper evaluation not only facilitates accurate diagnoses but also guides nursing interventions based on individual needs. With standardized assessment tools and models, nurses can interpret a patient's history, present symptoms, and potential risk factors. These systematic evaluations serve as the basis for effective communication among interdisciplinary teams, thereby enhancing teamwork in patient care. The increasing emphasis on patient safety within healthcare underscores the need for accurate evaluation, as evidenced by research that demonstrates how specific training methods can reduce errors and enhance overall care quality (McCarthy et al., 2011). Besides improving patient safety, medical-surgical nurses are encouraged to pursue ongoing education and training on assessment methods. The development of efficient tools for error reduction has benefited the use of assessment techniques in various healthcare settings. Goal setting and accountability in clinical practice become the focal points. Continuous professional development enables nurses to enhance their assessment skills, adapt to emerging healthcare technologies, and stay current with evolving assessment methods. Additionally, integrating patient feedback into assessment processes can provide valuable insights into patients' subjective experiences and thus complement the data gathered during assessments. Innovation and research-driven revolution of healthcare practices is crucial in instilling a safety culture, as uncovered in most case studies showing effective strategies implemented by health organizations (Blumenthal et al., 2006). Ultimately, comprehensive patient assessment is not only a daily practice but also the foundation of practical medical-surgical nursing. It helps nurses identify subtle indications of change in a patient's status early on, thereby enabling them to take timely interventions that have a major bearing on patient outcomes. The values that inform rigorous assessment practices align with the overall mission of medical-surgical nursing, which aims not only to treat disease but also to promote overall wellness. By incorporating rigorous assessment practices into practice, nurses play a key role in spearheading the enhancement of healthcare quality within the system as a whole, ultimately serving to improve patient experience and outcomes. The continued refinement of these evaluation techniques is a significant area of concern, reflecting the constantly evolving discipline of patient care within the medical community (Figure 2.13).

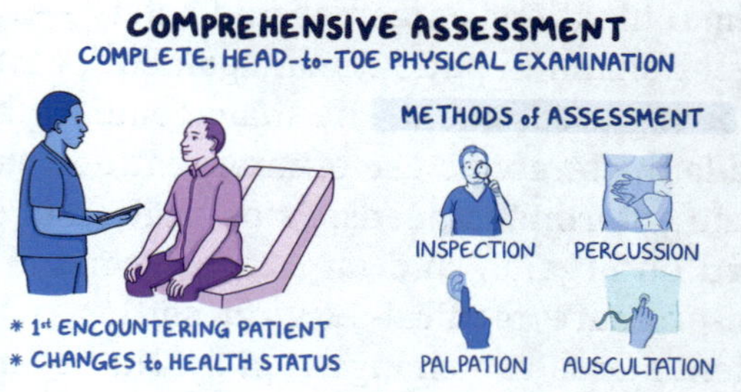

Figure 2.13. Comprehensive patient assessment techniques.

Source: https://osmose-it.s3.amazonaws.com/-vU9gnHSRYGWxR3bjI1iOC5OQ3yy7kC6/_.jpg.

2.4.2. Development of Nursing Care Plans

Development of the nursing care plan is essential component within the organization of medical-surgical nursing that guarantees the unique needs of each individual patient are addressed through systematic planning and assessment. To begin with, the nursing process begins through a thorough evaluation involving the gathering of complete information about a patient's health history, present health status, as well as psychosocial concerns. Everything forms the groundwork for constructing nursing diagnoses, which are essential in tailoring individualized care plans. Through recognizing the strengths and weaknesses faced by each patient, nurses can develop specifically tailored interventions. This personalized strategy not only facilitates better patient outcomes but also enhances the efficiency of health services. In this way, individualized care emphasizes the inherent principles of medical-surgical nursing, cementing its position in facilitating whole-person recovery. Following the assessment period, nursing care planning requires setting specific, measurable, achievable, relevant, and time-bound (SMART) goals and outcomes. This structure assists nursing professionals in tracing the patients' progress systematically. For instance, when creating a care plan for a patient who has just undergone surgery, interventions that address pain control, mobilization, and dressing are crucial. Following each objective are associated interventions that could be administered, such as medicine, post-operative education, and exercises. Incorporation of evidence-based practice at this point is necessary because it grounds nursing interventions in research and evidence of efficacy, thereby enhancing the overall quality of care. The motivation for excellence in nursing care planning eventually translates into the general objectives of medical-surgical nursing and healthcare delivery. Finally, continuing reassessment and revision of nursing care plans are necessary for them to work. This dynamic process ensures care is maintained in harmony with evolving patient needs and clinical evidence. While patient responses are being monitored, nurses must be prepared to adjust care strategies as necessary, in response to changes in patient conditions or feedback from members of the interdisciplinary team. Such flexibility is essential for resolving complex medical-surgical issues and achieving optimal health outcomes. Besides, integrating steps to enhance care processes, optimize staffing, and promote safe work habits can also boost the effectiveness of nursing care plans (Nassar et al., 1950; N/A, 2009). Thus, this ongoing development process embodies the medical-surgical nursing philosophy, ensuring that patients receive the best quality of care through highly customized, evidence-based interventions (Figure 2.14).

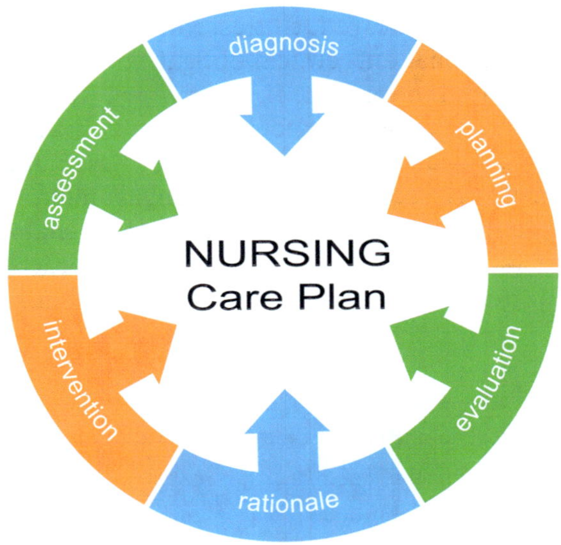

Figure 2.14. Nursing care plans.

Source: https://www.courtemanche-assocs.com/wp-content/uploads/2022/07/Aug-newsletter-care-plans-1.jpeg.

2.4.3. Monitoring and Evaluating Patient Outcomes

Monitoring and assessing patient outcomes is a crucial component of medical-surgical nursing, which can enhance the quality of care provided to patients. It's the systematic gathering and processing of patient data to determine the effectiveness of interventions, treatment, and patient recovery pathways. By applying evidence-based practice, nurses can identify which interventions yield the most favorable results in specific patient populations. The emphasis on standardizing care through guidelines and protocols in various clinical settings enables a more consistent approach to patient care. The adaptability in the process requires consideration of contextual determinants that influence patient outcomes, thereby optimizing the effectiveness and responsiveness of nursing interventions to address individualized needs (Hunter et al., 2010). Furthermore, the proactive engagement of nurses in ongoing monitoring and evaluation fosters a culture of quality and safety in healthcare facilities. Nurses have both a professional and ethical obligation to engage in evaluation processes that work towards enhancing patients' safety and the delivery of care, as set by the American Nurses Association (Lee-Riggins et al., 2014). Such engagement not only empowers frontline nurses but also enables a feedback loop that informs clinical practice and policy-making. The use of structured frameworks, such as nurse practice algorithms, enables nursing personnel to participate in the evaluation process actively. Research conducted at Fresno Heart & Surgical Hospital discovered nurses enjoyed the opportunity to engage in these improvement endeavors, indicating the effectiveness of such evaluations in promoting a proactive and cooperative culture in patient care (Lee-Riggins et al., 2014). Besides enhancing nursing practice, patient outcomes evaluation forms the foundation for accountability in healthcare. Tracking essential measures of success in patients, including recovery times, rates of complications, and satisfaction with treatment, is paramount to medical-surgical nurses. By standardized review of such information, clinicians to identify trends, inform clinical decisions, and prepare for improvement. Beyond that, this focus on outcomes facilitates interprofessional practice, enabling teams to collaborate and overcome challenges to deliver the best care and implement effective interventions. Lastly, continuous monitoring and evaluation of patient outcomes not only improve the quality of care but also reinforce a culture of excellence in medical-surgical nursing, ultimately improving health outcomes on a broader level (Hunter et al., 2010).

Test Your Knowledge

1. What are the four primary components of an in-depth patient assessment in medical-surgical nursing?
2. How does continuous assessment improve effective patient management in surgery?

2.5. Common Medical-Surgical Conditions

Learning Outcome

1. Describe the acute and chronic conditions
2. Operate and define the surgery and nursing interventions
3. Discuss post-operative complications and care

A good understanding of medical-surgical conditions is essential for nursing professionals, as these conditions frequently occur in healthcare facilities and have a significant impact on patient outcomes. The most prevalent conditions are cardiovascular diseases, which account for a substantial percentage of morbidity and mortality. Conditions such as hypertension and heart failure need close nursing observation to monitor their vital signs and detect the onset of signs of deterioration. Secondly, nursing interventions have to be tailored to address the multiple needs of these patients. These include medication management, lifestyle modification education, and psychosocial support. The medical-surgical nurse not only provides immediate care but also offers ongoing support to patients and their families through interaction, helping them understand their illness and treatment. Such holistic care aligns with patient-centered care nursing theories and conveys the concept that education plays a significant role in the effective management of diseases, as noted in Nassar et al. (1950). A Second set of common medical-surgical illnesses.is a respiratory illness, and examples for frequent diseases are COPD and pneumonia. These illnesses are frustrating in the inpatient setting, often requiring nursing to get patients on respiratory therapy and monitor for respiratory distress. Maintaining airway patency, maintaining optimal oxygenation, and instructing patients on the use of inhalers and lung function are key components of care. Nurses also need to recognize the psychosocial impact of such illnesses, including depression and anxiety, that interfere with recovery and compliance with treatment. Therefore, incorporating holistic assessment and team-oriented practice is essential in addressing the complexity arising from respiratory illnesses, meeting both the physical and emotional needs of the patient, a concept emphasized in Hall et al. (1959). Surgical conditions, including surgical complications and postoperative management, are another significant area of concern within the context of medical-surgical nursing.

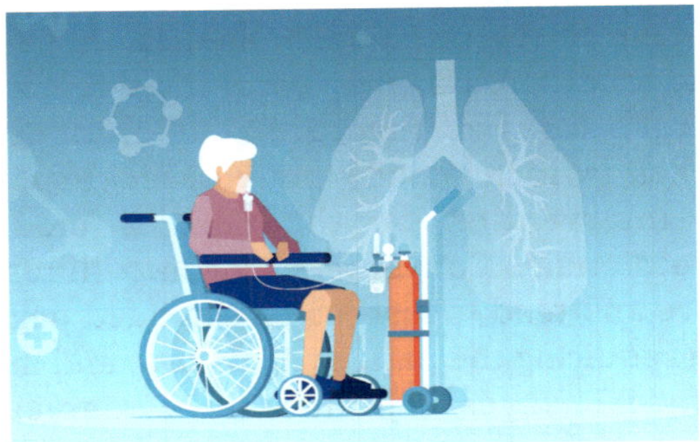

Figure 2.15. Chronic obstructive pulmonary disease (COPD).

Source: https://www.americaspharmacy.com/media/gy4a55bq/copd.jpg.

Surgical infection sites, pain management, and threat of thromboembolic complications are traditional areas of post-operative care that necessitate precise nursing interventions. Asepsis procedure and effective pain management are essential; nurses are at the forefront, employing measures that decrease complications and promote rapid recovery. Furthermore, patient education regarding post-operative care—encompassing wound care, activity restriction, and other relevant aspects—enhances recovery outcomes and reduces the rate of readmission. This role of education has a significant impact on patient empowerment in the recovery process, as it fosters a culture of knowledge and support.

Lastly, these types of programs illustrate the broad scope of medical-surgical nursing and its integral contribution to healthcare, aligned with best practices specified in existing nursing literature, as referenced by Hall et al. (1959) and Nassar et al. (1950) (Figure 2.15).

2.5.1. Overview of Acute and Chronic Conditions

Understanding acute and chronic conditions is at the heart of the principles and scope of medical-surgical nursing. Acute conditions are typically characterized by their fast development and tend to require a quick medical response. Acute conditions can manifest as life-threatening emergencies, like myocardial infarctions or strokes, which need immediate response and intervention on the part of medical professionals. Conversely, chronic illnesses evolve and tend to last for an extended period, even requiring the patient to manage and make lifestyle changes continuously. Examples of such conditions include diabetes, high blood pressure, and chronic obstructive pulmonary disease, which present particular challenges for patients and medical-surgical nurses alike. The nurses' work in resolving the intricacies of these conditions is crucial because they bridge the interface between acute and long-term care, emphasizing the importance of holistic and patient-centered nursing. In medical-surgical nursing, the successful management of acute and chronic conditions depends on the synthesis of best practices and evidence-based care. For example, in the case of acute care, emergency nursing protocols are imperative because the policies keep patients stable and prevent complications. Chronic diseases also usually require a holistic approach that includes education and self-management strategies. Nurses also need to enable their patients by sharing information regarding the diseases they have and encouraging adherence to treatment regimens. These strategies lead to improved health status and quality of life for patients. Moreover, addressing the social and psychological determinants of health is now a part of the action, with nurses ensuring that not only are patients cured of the diseases of their bodies, but also informed so that they are empowered in their overall health. Furthermore, achievement of low readmission rates for conditions such as heart attack, heart failure, and pneumonia is a benchmark for excellence in medical-surgical nursing. New models, such as the employment of advanced practice nurses, are central to enhanced patient care through the utilization of evidence-based criteria. Investing in these professionals ensures a maximum understanding of the intricacies that accompany acute and chronic conditions, which in turn creates favorable patient outcomes. Learning from implemented plans provides significant insights into the ongoing evolution of nursing practice, underscoring the importance of continuous education and adaptation. Medical-surgical nursing is grounded in a solid foundation that emphasizes interprofessional teamwork, critical thinking, and lifelong learning, reflecting its central position in the larger healthcare system (Nassar et al., 1950; Lashbrook et al., 2011) (Figure 2.16).

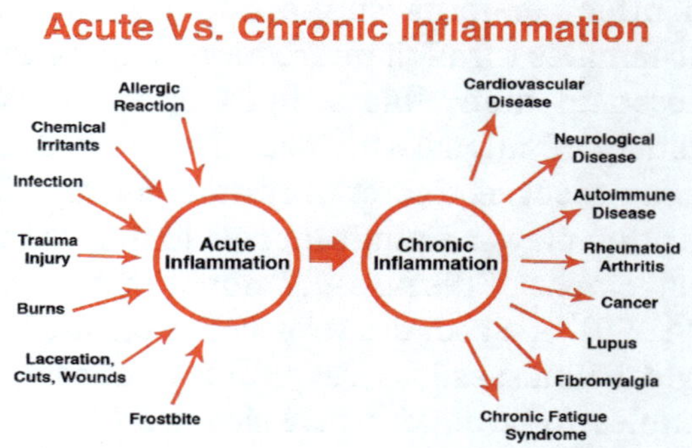

Figure 2.16. Acute and chronic conditions.

Source: https://img1.rapidleaks.com/2022/06/inflammation-types-1024x788.jpg.

2.5.2. Surgical Interventions and Nursing Care

In medical-surgical nursing, operating procedures are a critical part of patient care that requires a comprehensive understanding of the procedure itself and the subsequent post-procedure nursing care needs. Evolutions in surgical procedures, particularly day surgery, have necessitated nurses to be flexible enough to cope with the varying array of operating procedures. Effective nursing practice involves not only preparation for interventions of this kind but also post-surgery care to allow the patient's recuperation. One of the central aspects of this kind of care is the implementation of evidence-based procedures that optimize outcomes and ensure patient safety. As stipulated in recent research, the implementation of standardized care strategies, via protocols and guidelines, is imperative in overcoming the intricacies of modern-day surgical units and ensuring equal care within diverse clinical settings (Hunter et al., 2010). Nursing roles in operating rooms extend beyond traditional preparation to encompass thorough patient assessment and education. Nurses must be well-equipped to assess patients' pre-surgical conditions, identify what can go wrong, and modify their educational programs to accommodate. Research is revealing a disconcerting gap in nursing education regarding modern surgical practices, as most newly graduated staff nurses report minimal exposure to day surgery procedures during their training. This lack of preparation can overwhelm nursing contributions to the post-operative recovery process, provoking the imperative for nursing curriculum reform towards alignment with advances in surgical practice. The comparative neglect of contemporary surgical methods in pre-registration curricula highlights a principal challenge to nursing education (Mitchell et al., 2005); without rebalancing this disparity, opportunities for best practice among surgeons' unit nurses could be irretrievably lost. Furthermore, the increased demand for intricate surgical processes necessitates a robust multidisciplinary approach that engages nurses, surgeons, and other healthcare providers. The successful delivery of surgical care is contingent upon an integrative effort to construct up evidence-based protocols that are tailored to fit unique clinical contexts. An integrated approach not only enhances patient outcomes but also provides a learning system that is conducive to continuous improvement and modification. The emphasis on realistic evaluation in understanding the dynamics of surgical procedures—what works, for whom, and under what conditions—gives merit to the use of standardized care protocols. Using such a strategy, medical-surgical nursing can be revolutionized, where nurses are adequately trained and educated to attend to surgical patients properly, thereby influencing the way surgical care is delivered in the healthcare system (Hunter et al., 2010) (Figure 2.17).

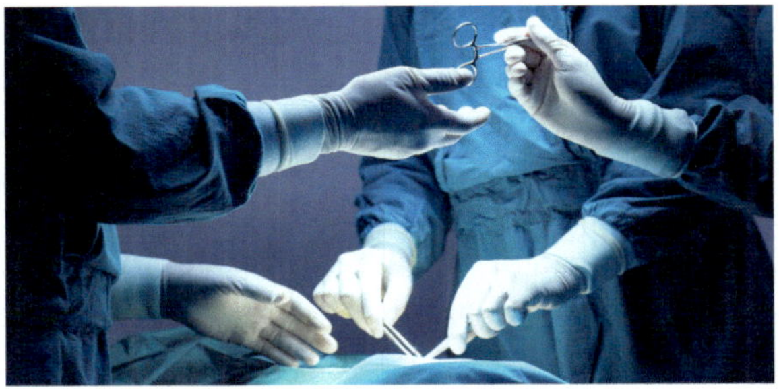

Figure 2.17. Surgical-intervention-superior-to-drugs-in-patients-with-atrial-fibrillation.

Source: https://www.healthindustryhub.com.au/wp-content/uploads/2023/09/Surgical-intervention-superior-to-drugs-in-patients-with-atrial-fibrillation.png.

2.5.3. Postoperative Care and Complications

Adequate postoperative care is a crucial factor in preventing complications that can arise after surgery. The postoperative period is characterized by the need for close observation of vital signs, wound integrity, and patient comfort, as any deviation can indicate possible complications, such as infection or hemorrhage. Nurses play a central role in this respect, using their assessment to identify evidence of abnormal healing or distress. A study found that patients who did not have their stoma site marked preoperatively had greater pouch leakage issues than those who were, highlighting the value of preoperative intervention in achieving better postoperative outcomes (Cantara et al., 2008). Lastly, evidence-based practice, paired with judicious postoperative care, meets patient needs both in the short and long term. Surgical complications have the ability to influence patient recovery significantly and must as such be tackled by a suitable strategy in multidisciplinary care. SSIs, venous thromboembolism, and anesthesia adverse reactions are only a few of many, and emphasize the necessity of active control. By implementing protocols that focus on prevention, such as prophylactic antibiotics and early mobilization, surgical teams can minimize these issues to a significant extent. Moreover, organizations like the Veterans Affairs have implemented training programs aimed at enhancing communication and teamwork in the operating room, which has led to fewer deaths and improved quality of care (Chase et al., 2011). This emphasis on cooperation and open communication fosters a safety culture essential in medical-surgical practice, ultimately leading to improved patient outcomes. Patient education is a vital component in the management of postoperative patients, empowering them to recognize signs of complications and adhere to recovery protocols. An informed patient is better equipped to engage in self-care interventions, monitor their health status, and communicate effectively with healthcare providers. Nurses must make an effort to give thorough and straightforward discharge instructions, emphasizing the necessity of follow-up visits and lifestyle changes that favor healing. Understanding psychosocial recovery is also essential, since emotional well-being can have a direct influence on physical health outcomes. As shown through evidence, interventions such as preoperative stoma site marking have been associated with a better patient experience and reduced complications, demonstrating the importance of an integrated care model that incorporates both physical and emotional support interventions (Cantara et al., 2008). In general, patient education emphasis is essential for postoperative complication prevention and a successful recovery course.

Test Your Knowledge

1. What are two common medical-surgical illnesses, and how are they typically managed in the hospital setting?
2. Describe the nurse's role in monitoring for complications in patients with chronic medical-surgical illnesses.

2.6. Challenges in Medical-Surgical Nursing

Learning Outcome

1. Describe the large patient-to-nurse ratios
2. Define the physical and emotional demands of the job
3. Identify the need to keep pace with advances in medical technology

The world of medical-surgical nursing is filled with numerous challenges that healthcare practitioners must overcome to deliver the best care. One of the most significant challenges is keeping pace with emerging medical technologies and surgical techniques. With technological innovations, nurses must acquire new skills and knowledge to keep patients safe and maintain the efficiency of care delivery. This necessity to continually learn can create anxiety and feelings of inadequacy in nursing staff, particularly if schools of nursing do not align their curricula with current practices. An imbalance between clinical needs and educational training can have adverse effects on nurses' confidence and competence, which are central components of delivering high-quality patient care (Bonica et al., 2017). Hence, the gap has to be filled with what nurses are exposed to in the medical-surgical environment. Moreover, the greater complexity and acuity of patients in medical-surgical units pose additional barriers to nursing practitioners. Nurses have to treat patients who have complicated health conditions requiring multi-management approaches, i.e., patients with chronic diseases and multiple comorbidities. This situation proves challenging for nursing personnel, who must set aside time for comprehensive assessments, coordinate care, and provide patient and family education while maintaining an efficient workload. Studies indicate that inadequate education on modern surgical practices is a contributing factor to this situation, as most nurses lack sufficient training to meet the demands of contemporary patient care (Mitchell et al., 2005). Thus, the practice must align with incorporating training that bridges these gaps, equipping nurses with the necessary tools to address complex patient situations effectively. Beyond educational deficiencies and increased patient acuity, system issues in healthcare settings complicate medical-surgical nursing practice. Staffing problems and turnover increase an unstable environment that not only impacts nurse morale but also affects patient outcomes. Understaffing, in turn, can lead to burnout, lower job satisfaction, and ultimately, a diminished effect on the quality of care delivered. Nurses themselves consistently complain of being stretched too thin, with challenges in maintaining individualized relationships that are essential for therapeutic interactions with patients. This fragmentation can interrupt the integrative attention ideally applied in medical-surgical nursing, which emphasizes whole-person care. The cause of these problems is a critical need for systemic changes, including more appropriate staffing ratios and greater assistance for ongoing education, to create a sustainable and effective nursing pool in the medical-surgical setting (Bonica et al., 2017).

2.6.1. High Patient-to-Nurse Ratios

High patient-to-nurse ratios are a significant concern in the practice of medical-surgical nursing, with effects that directly impact the outcomes of patient care and healthcare settings generally. If a single nurse has too many patients, the quality of care is compromised due to a high workload and reduced time per patient. This can lead to miscommunication, medication errors, and a reduction in attention to detailed assessments, all of which jeopardize patient safety. The principle of quality nursing requires that every patient be treated with respect and care; however, high patient-to-nurse ratios detract from this core principle, essentially establishing a system where nursing staff are likely to feel overwhelmed and unable to provide the individualized attention each patient needs. The relationship between high patient-to-nurse ratios and poor health outcomes has been substantiated through several studies that determined the increased risk of complications and mortality. In circumstances when nurses are overextended, patients are exposed to delays in essential interventions, thereby worsening their general health status and contributing to extended hospital stays. Not only does this affect the patient, but it also subjects nursing professionals to an excessive workload, leading to additional stress, burnout, and work dissatisfaction among staff. Additionally, excessive turnover can be caused by nurses seeking employment in less stressful environments, which further widens healthcare staffing gaps in institutions. Such dynamics call for the imperative of ensuring that healthcare management prioritizes productive staffing practices that balance patient needs and nurse workloads. Furthermore, a remedy for excessive patient-nurse ratios demands a holistic approach that brings together healthcare unions, management, and nursing staff. Innovations that enable transparent communication and cooperation among unions and healthcare institutions are capable of significantly improving work conditions. By engaging the expertise of frontline healthcare workers in practice, they contribute to designing the delivery of care that improves both clinical outcomes and worker satisfaction. Involvement through shared governance models not only and enhances the practice of nursing but also a healthier and stable health system as well. The emphasis on collective decision-making and openness can create healthier work environments where nurses are valued and feel connected, eventually decreasing the adverse effects of high patient-to-nurse ratios (Figueroa et al., 2012; Bonica et al., 2017) (Figure 2.18).

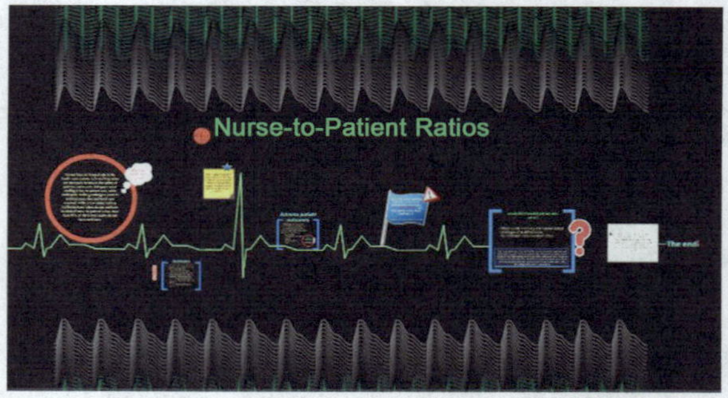

Figure 2.18. High patient-to-nurse ratios.

Source: https://0901.static.prezi.com/ preview/ v2/ght6u ymozbyfwxxpni7 eqchm 4p6jc3sa chvcdoaizecfr3dnitcq_3_0.png.

2.6.2. Emotional and Physical Demands of the Role

The medical-surgical nursing profession is characterized by its high physical and emotional demands, which impact practitioners in several ways. Nurses in this specialty are often subjected to high-stress scenarios that require instant decision-making and continuous monitoring of patients' needs. Emotional suffering derives from carrying the burden of handling varying patient conditions, witnessing patients enduring suffering and bereavement. The development of such experiences fosters powerful emotional connections between nurses and patients, making it necessary for nurses to implement self-care mechanisms to minimize the risk of burnout. Emotional labor deployed in the provision of empathetic care requires resilience as well as emotional intelligence, underscoring the inherent value of psychological support structures for nursing professionals (Hall et al., 1959). By understanding these dynamics, the scope of medical-surgical nursing is appreciated not only as a technical science but also as a foundation of deep emotional care. Beyond the emotional strain, medical-surgical nurses also have to withstand some physical burdens. The nature of the job often requires standing for long hours and performing activities that demand physical strength, dexterity, and coordination. Activities such as patient repositioning and lifting can potentially induce musculoskeletal trauma, and hence, proper ergonomics and equipment aids are a necessity within healthcare settings. Furthermore, nurses frequently execute life-saving maneuvers that require equal amounts of physical effort and mental focus, such as administering medications or assessing patients. This physical nature renders physical fitness and health promotion an essential element among nursing professionals. By meeting these physical needs, institutions can foster a healthier workforce that can sustain the intense responsibilities described in the principles of medical-surgical nursing (Genereux et al., 1963). Knowing the interplay between physical endurance and emotional resilience is critical in informing nursing practice and education. Adding training courses that deal with both can enhance nurses' readiness for the numerous problems they face.

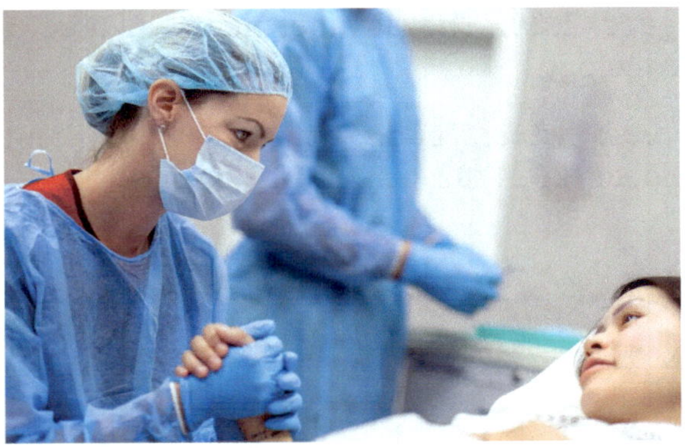

Figure 2.19. Emotional and physical demands of the role for nursing.

Source: https://www.baker.edu/wp-content/uploads/H1-Certified-Nurse-Midwife2x-1536x1016.jpg.

For instance, curriculum components that focus on stress management, coping skills, and physical health can expand the context of nursing education. Moreover, creating healthy work environments that prioritize well-being can act as buffers for the ill effects of the emotional and physical strains of work. Institutions that organize wellness programs and promote work-life balance benefit their staff while also contributing to better patient care, thereby strengthening the core philosophy of medical-surgical nursing. Ultimately, while nurses navigate the intricacies of the profession, developing their emotional and physical resilience becomes equally the responsibility of educators and healthcare organizations (Hall et al., 1959) (Figure 2.19).

2.6.3. Keeping Up with Advancements in Medical Technology

Medical technology advances have significantly influenced the trend of medical-surgical nursing, and this demands continuous education as well as flexibility on the part of nursing practitioners. New technologies, including robotic surgery and telemedicine services, are transforming conventional patient care paradigms, improving outcomes and streamlining delivery. As such technologies find their place in healthcare facilities, nurses need to stay current regarding their functions and use to enhance the delivery of care to patients. This requires formal education, as well as continuous professional development, and participation in multidisciplinary teams where technology plays an essential role. An understanding of the effects of these tools is critical not only for effective implementation but also to address any ethical problems and ensure the safety of the patients in different care environments. One of the most significant developments in the past few years has been the application of robotics to medicine, which provides a range of benefits that enhance the precision of surgery and reduce the period of recovery for patients. For instance, the use of robots to perform minimally invasive operations means that less invasive procedures can be created, thereby reducing postoperative pain and hospitalization. However, there are obstacles to the deployment of these machines. A critical evaluation of their effectiveness and potential risks must be conducted before their widespread use in healthcare settings. There must be cooperation between the healthcare community and the research community to present solid evidence of the effectiveness of healthcare robotics. As stated, "it is imperative that both the industrial and research communities collaborate to provide a strong evidence base for healthcare robotics" (Riek et al., 2017). Nurses are spearheading this transition, making a smooth transition to better surgical practice while safeguarding patient interests. Additionally, system-delivered integrated care facilitates the transformation and utilization of medical technology in medical-surgical nursing. By ensuring the collaboration of healthcare stakeholders, including providers, patients, and payer partners, organizations can guarantee seamless care paths and improved performance measurement. The emergence of accountable care organizations (ACOs) is a significant step towards optimizing patient outcomes while emphasizing the importance of cost-effectiveness. They necessitate the involvement of skilled nursing professionals with the ability to utilize innovative medical technologies under a team-based system. The Brookings-Dartmouth ACO Pilot Program is one such model that integrates this with an emphasis on productive performance measurement and reporting (Citters et al., 2012). As medical-surgical nurses master the use of technology and participate in these innovative models of care, they enhance their value-added contribution to patient outcomes and satisfaction across various healthcare environments (Figure 2.20).

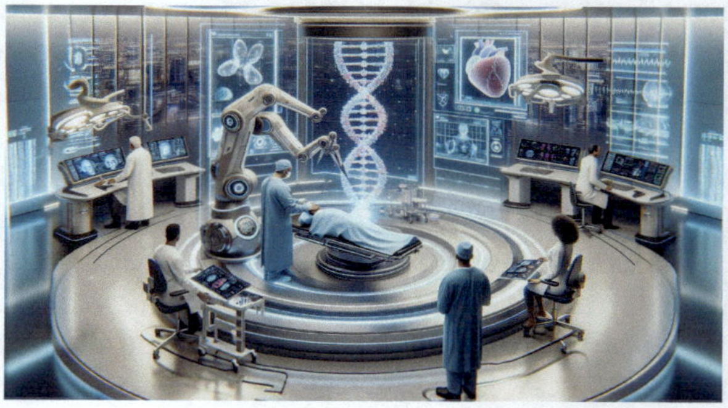

Figure 2.20. The advancements in medical technology.

Source: https://boom-trikes.eu/wp-content/uploads/2024/02/zcndfavqib.jpg.

Test Your Knowledge

1. What are two critical challenges facing medical-surgical nurses in acute care settings?
2. How does dynamic change in patient status impact decision-making in medical-surgical nursing?

SUMMARY

The scope and practice of medical-surgical nursing encompass a broad range of competencies, enabling the provision of holistic patient care. Medical-surgical nurses act as the hub of the healthcare system, both caregivers and educators. Their roles extend beyond direct patient care to include the integration of evidence-based practice, patient safety, and coordination of interprofessional care. With the evolution of the healthcare field, skilled medical-surgical nurses remain essential, especially with the increasing complexity in cases for patients and healthcare systems. Even by following nursing principles, such as adopting patient-centered care and critical thinking, medical-surgical nurses can effectively address the diverse needs of patients, ultimately leading to better outcomes. In addition, the presence of patient safety programs and standardized practices is also necessary to minimize errors and improve the quality of care delivered in operating rooms. A vital aspect of medical-surgical nursing is the use of effective instruments and training models to establish a culture of safety. Continuing development of practical training modules and a focus on accountability keep nurses abreast of best practices and emerging technologies. This patient safety emphasis has played a significant role in shaping today's nursing practice, and healthcare systems have increasingly adopted more patient-centered approaches that enhance nurse readiness and improve patient outcomes. The upsurge in patient safety interventions is therefore an integral component of nursing practice and education, directly impacting care outcomes. The future ultimately depends on the evolving medical-surgical nursing landscape, which demands an adaptable and informed workforce capable of responding to diverse patient needs. A commitment to lifelong learning, mentorship, and teamwork among healthcare practitioners will ensure that medical-surgical nurses are equipped to tackle future challenges. Extensive training and support systems that facilitate the acquisition of skills are essential in sustaining healthcare settings where patient-centered care thrives. As highlighted in the literature, sound healthcare systems have registered significant patient safety improvements through the development of effective training models and tailored interventions—a testament that a solid grounding in nursing fundamentals not only advances individual nurse competence but also systemic healthcare provision improvements (Gianfrede et al., 1963; McCarthy et al., 2011). The future of medical-surgical nursing depends on our collective ability to integrate these principles and deliver quality care to all patients.

Medical-surgical nursing principles encompass a wide range of patient-centered care, safety, and efficient management of various health conditions. One of the key pieces is integrating evidence-based practices that guide nurses in delivering high-quality care. By applying evidence-based practices, nurses can improve patient outcomes and prevent harm resulting from medication errors. As reported by recent studies, the growing use of patient safety interventions in healthcare systems has been a byproduct of developing efficient training procedures and effective tools that help minimize errors. This underscores the need to foster a culture of responsibility and continuous quality improvement in nursing practice, ensuring a systematic approach to patient care that optimizes safety and effectiveness (McCarthy et al., 2011). Moreover, standardized care practices are also at the core of medical-surgical nursing. Protocol-based care has emerged as a primary mode of implementing service improvement strategies, particularly in systems like those in England. The realistic evaluation methods employed here enable a nuanced understanding of how varied protocols affect patient care across different clinical contexts. With a focus on context, mechanisms, and outcomes, nurses can learn what works for their patients and why. This approach, in addition to refining protocols, also underscores the importance of context in delivering effective care. Such evaluations can play a significant role in aiding the understanding of how standardized care pathways can be applied to optimize patient outcomes through the guarantee of high-quality delivery of care (Hunter et al., 2010). Generally, the paradigms and area of medical-surgical nursing are fundamentally intertwined with the paradigms of safety, evidence-based practice, and standardized care protocols. Ongoing progression of nursing practice calls for a good grounding that allows effective application of these principles. As current evidence indicates, the priority given to understanding underlying causal mechanisms in protocol-based care positions nurses to address the changing nature of patient needs and the healthcare environment. By utilizing realistic evaluation outcomes, medical-surgical nursing can remain current, and practice is not only standardized but also made sensitive to the varying contexts in which it is practiced, ultimately enhancing the quality and safety of patient care (Hunter et al., 2010).

KEY TERMS FROM THIS CHAPTER

- Chronic Illness Management
- Health Assessment
- Holistic Care
- Multidisciplinary Approach
- Nursing Standards
- Patient Education
- Preventive Care
- Rehabilitation Nursing
- Clinical Competency
- Health-Illness Continuum
- Individualized Care Plans
- Nurse practitioners (NPs)
- Patient Advocacy
- Physiological Integrity
- Professional Accountability
- Restorative Care

CRITICAL THINKING QUESTIONS

1. **Which of the following best describes medical-surgical nursing?**
   a. Care limited to post-surgical patients
   b. Pediatric and maternity patient care given
   c. Broad-based nursing care to patients of different medical conditions
   d. Emergency nursing care provided alone in hospitals
2. **What is the primary focus of medical-surgical nursing practice?**
   a. Diagnosis of disease
   b. Prevention of illness and the management of acute and chronic health problems
   c. Performing laboratory tests
   d. Prescribing medication
3. **Which of the following is a principle of medical-surgical nursing care?**
   a. Treatment to be decided by the physician
   b. Exclusive focus on the disease, and not the person
   c. Physical, emotional, and social patient-centered care
   d. Regular care for all patients without evaluating individualized needs
4. **What is a medical-surgical nurse's scope of practice?**
   a. Only postoperative wound dressing
   b. Supporting doctors in the outpatient department
   c. Holistic care to adult patients in various healthcare settings
   d. Diagnostic surgery
5. **What is the most critical component in providing quality and safe medical-surgical nursing care?**
   a. Using expensive equipment
   b. Nurse's ability to work independently without teamwork
   c. Clinical judgment, critical thinking, and standards compliance
   d. Avoidance of patient contact to reduce errors

Short Answer Questions

1. Define medical-surgical nursing.
2. Mention any two principles of medical-surgical nursing.
3. What is the fundamental goal of patient-centered care in medical-surgical nursing?
4. Mention two roles of a medical-surgical nurse.
5. Differentiate between acute and chronic illness in medical-surgical nursing.
6. Explain the scope of medical-surgical nursing practice across healthcare environments.
7. Explain the main principles that govern professional practice in medical-surgical nursing. Refer to holistic care and evidence-based practice.
8. Evaluate the expanding role of the medical-surgical nurse in the modern dynamic healthcare environment, including technology, education, and patient advocacy.

Answers to Critical Thinking Questions

1. (c); 2. (b); 3. (c); 4. (c); 5. (c)

REFERENCES

1. Abushaikha, L. (2013). Midwifery education in Jordan: History, challenges and proposed solutions. https://core.ac.uk/download/48828780.pdf (accessed on 28th June 2025).
2. Blumenthal, D., & McCarthy, D. (2006). Committed to safety: Ten case studies on reducing harm to patients. https://core.ac.uk/download/71350251.pdf (accessed on 28th June 2025).
3. Bonica, M., & Students of Health Management 721.01. (2017). *Healthcare Management Primer*. University of New Hampshire. https://core.ac.uk/download/215509297.pdf (accessed on 28th June 2025).
4. Buyanova, I., Chen, S., & Chen, W. (1967). Innovations and experiments in uses of health manpower—The effect of licensure laws. https://core.ac.uk/download/62555863.pdf (accessed on 28th June 2025).
5. Cantara, S. L. (2008). The effect of preoperative stoma site marking on quality of life in patients undergoing ostomy surgery. https://core.ac.uk/download/215515625.pdf (accessed on 28th June 2025).
6. Clark, E., Ross, F., Health Foundation, Ream, M., Lawton, S., & Reeves, S. (2017). Examining the nature of interprofessional interventions designed to promote patient safety: A narrative review. https://core.ac.uk/download/79607957.pdf (accessed on 28th June 2025).
7. Dobrowolska, B., Kane, R., Linsley, P., Pilewska-Kozak, A., et al. (2013). Academic careers: The value of individual mentorship on research career progression. https://core.ac.uk/download/20320977.pdf (accessed on 28th June 2025).
8. Dobson, R. (1995). The persistent vegetative state: Legal and ethical issues. https://core.ac.uk/download/9640426.pdf (accessed on 28th June 2025).
9. Dunnington, G., Hockaday, M., Smith, C., Torbeck, L., et al. (2018). Optimizing the integration of advanced practitioners in a department of surgery: An operational improvement model. https://core.ac.uk/download/161229732.pdf (accessed on 28th June 2025).
10. Fehring, R. (2005). Attitudes, intentions, and ethical stance of advanced practice nursing students toward abortion provision: Part one B quantitative findings. https://core.ac.uk/download/213083346.pdf (accessed on 28th June 2025).
11. Figueroa, M., Katz, L., & Lazes, P. M. (2012). How labor-management partnerships improve patient care, cost control, and labor relations: Case studies of Fletcher Allen Health Care, Kaiser Permanente, and Montefiore Medical Center's Care Management Corporation. https://core.ac.uk/download/33611597.pdf (accessed on 28th June 2025).
12. Fonseca, A., Lopes, M. J., Santos, S. S. C., Silva, R., et al. (2014). Nursing training in Brazil and in Portugal: Similarities and specificities. https://core.ac.uk/download/62470321.pdf (accessed on 28th June 2025).
13. Genereux, T. B., & Ketchen, F. E. (1963). A study to determine the effects of a planned experience on nursing students' attitudes toward patient teaching. https://open.bu.edu/bitstream/2144/29652/1/Genereux_Therese_et_al_1963_web.pdf (accessed on 28th June 2025).
14. Gianfrede, G. H., & Hornick, C. M. (1963). Teaching patients with pulmonary emphysema. https://open.bu.edu/bitstream/2144/30839/1/Gianfrede_Gloria_1963_web.pdf (accessed on 28th June 2025).

15. Hall, M. M. (1959). A study to determine the role of one mental health integrator as she functioned on the instructional staff responsible for the teaching of fundamentals of nursing, Block III, in "X" University School of Nursing. https://open.bu.edu/bitstream/2144/17954/1/Hall_Margaret_Mary_1959_web.pdf (accessed on 28th June 2025).

16. Hunter, B., McCormack, B., Stetler, C., Tolson, D., Bick, D., Department of Health, et al. (2010). A realistic evaluation: The case of protocol-based care. https://core.ac.uk/download/46425.pdf (accessed on 28th June 2025).

17. Lashbrook, A., & Silow-Carroll, S. (2011). Mercy Medical Center: Reducing readmissions through clinical excellence, palliative care, and collaboration. https://core.ac.uk/download/71358658.pdf (accessed on 28th June 2025).

18. Lee-Riggins, A. M. (2014). Nurses' perceptions of structural empowerment: A practice review process pilot. https://core.ac.uk/download/70419786.pdf (accessed on 28th June 2025).

19. McCarthy, D., & Klein, S. (2011). Keeping the commitment: A progress report on four early leaders in patient safety improvement. https://core.ac.uk/download/71358579.pdf (accessed on 28th June 2025).

20. McCarthy, D., & Mueller, K. (2008). The New York City Health and Hospitals Corporation: Transforming a public safety net delivery system to achieve higher performance. https://core.ac.uk/download/71353446.pdf (accessed on 28th June 2025).

21. Nassar, L. M. (1950). A ward teaching unit on the care of the cardiac patient. https://open.bu.edu/bitstream/2144/4842/1/Nassar_Leenda_1950_web.pdf (accessed on 28th June 2025).

22. O'Brien, K. F. (1989). Descriptive analysis of associate degree nursing in Massachusetts: Changing perceptions. https://core.ac.uk/download/220131004.pdf (accessed on 28th June 2025).

23. Riek, L. D. (2017). Healthcare robotics. http://arxiv.org/abs/1704.03931 (accessed on 28th June 2025).

24. Schenk, K. (1959). A study to determine if facts about drugs and drug therapy can be learned as effectively by a patient-centered approach as by classroom presentation. https://open.bu.edu/bitstream/2144/21940/1/Schenk_Katharine_1959_web.pdf (accessed on 28th June 2025).

25. Sheldon, S. (2015). The decriminalization of abortion: An argument for modernization. https://core.ac.uk/download/30710877.pdf (accessed on 28th June 2025).

26. Thibault, A. L. (2016). Home front to war front: The Navy Nurse Corps during World War II. https://core.ac.uk/download/148923599.pdf (accessed on 28th June 2025).

27. Van Citters, A. D., Larson, B. K., Fisher, E. S., Nelson, E. C., Gbemudu, J. N., Kreindler, S. A., & Shortell, S. M. (2012). Norton Healthcare: A strong payer-provider partnership for the journey to accountable care. https://core.ac.uk/download/71358697.pdf (accessed on 28th June 2025).

HEALTH EDUCATION AND HEALTH PROMOTION STRATEGIES

3

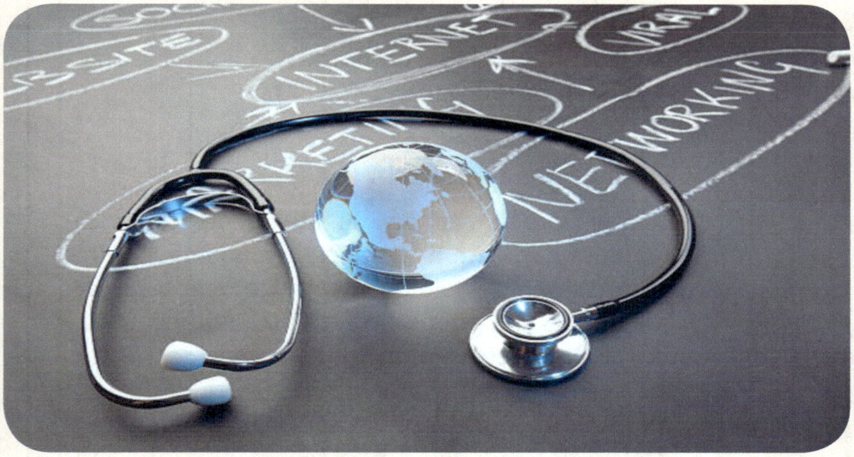

LEARNING OBJECTIVES

After studying this chapter, you will be able to:

1. Understand the role of health education
2. Explain the health promotion strategies
3. Discuss the theories of behavioral change
4. Focus on health literacy
5. Define the health education program evaluation
6. State the challenges in health education and promotion

Introduction

In public health, interventions in health promotion and health education are increasingly crucial to promoting healthier populations. Effective health education empowers individuals with the knowledge and skills necessary for self-empowerment regarding health issues. It encompasses a wide variety of topics from physical activity and diet to prevention of chronic diseases. With the wider dissemination of health information through electronic media, it is imperative that educational programs are evidence-based, relevant, and tailored to address the diverse needs of various populations. Further, health promotion practices complement education by initiating community-based programs for addressing environmental and social determinants of health, thus formulating a holistic approach of health improvement. These approaches aim to empower individuals and populations, and education for health becomes a central process for facilitating successful behavior change. As more is known about the social determinants of health, more attention is focused on integrating these determinants into health promotion and education. The identification of numerous social determinants—e.g., education, socioeconomic status, and cultural beliefs—has provided potential for a revolutionary transformation of the healthcare system. Policy-makers can create environments that promise health equity for all communities through a policy of social determinants. Some examples include programs that enhance access to healthy food and create safe play spaces that directly address social determinants that hinder health. By taking this step, policymakers not only tackle individual behavior that optimizes the health of an individual but also tackle collective resilience and public well-being that ventures into the intricacies of health. Lastly, the determination of these determinants will allow one to understand the potentials of health education and promotion activities as it extends to the nature of the real world (Philip O'Hara, 2005). The "Healthy Universities" initiative is a testament to the institutionalization of health education and promotion within schools, particularly among schools of higher learning, which strive to maximize the well-being of their students. Institutionalizing the Healthy Universities concept enables schools to create learning environments that prioritize both health and learning. The initiative involves critical reflection on how schools as settings can foster health by initiating critical initiatives and policy reform. Thus, universities can make resources like mental health services, food programs, and exercise opportunities available. In addition, institutional collaboration between schools of higher education sets an agenda for Healthy Universities and provides for sustained change, with an emphasis on promoting health education in schools (Cawood et al., 2010). Such promotion of a health culture within universities is thus not just an institutionally mandated practice; it becomes a model for still larger health promotion agendas, ultimately for society as a whole (Figure 3.1).

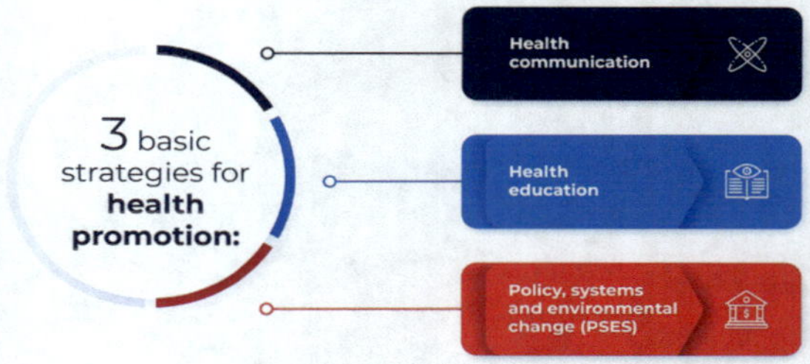

Figure 3.1. Health promotion strategies: A holistic approach in healthcare practice.

Source: https://globalbanking.ac.uk/media/ampaclzh/infographic-1-1.webp.

Definition of Health Education

Health education is one of the cornerstones to healthier population health and wellbeing. It is an interdisciplinary field that deals with empowering individuals and populations with the information and skills necessary to make informed health choices. With the use of various methodologies, health education not only aims at disseminating information, but also empowering individuals to make informed decisions about their behavior. From the provided explanation in the Nairobi Call to Action, the construction of a shared platform of health promotion is necessary in the attainment of competency among practitioners. A shared definition, besides enhancing the cohesion of health education programs, also facilitates the education of future and current health workers, thereby improving the overall effectiveness of health promotion activities (Buja et al., 2015). At the heart of the definition of health education is the understanding that it is more than communication of facts; it tries to influence lifestyle and health behavior through educated decision-making. This necessitates a process of involvement, where students are not mere recipients but active participants in the learning process. Risk assessment is also to blame here, in the sense that individuals can acquire knowledge of potential health risks and make decisions aimed at reducing risks. Good risk communication plays a crucial role here; how information is communicated, individuals' comprehension, and their response towards health risks are largely influenced by it. Health education skill convergence can increase the validity and relevance of information being transmitted, hence a healthier literate population (Ouchi et al., 2025). Health education also provides an opportunity to address broader public health objectives, such as reducing health disparities and enhancing health equity. For this to occur, health education programs must be culturally responsive as well as address the unique needs of different populations. Focusing on social determinants of health enables teachers to examine the interdependency among variables that influence health outcomes. With this integrated strategy, teachers can further develop their understanding of health education's role in health promotion planning, enabling comprehensive and inclusive activities. Finally, teachers must employ a culturally appropriate style of health education to maximize participation and establish sustainable behavioral change among populations (Figure 3.2).

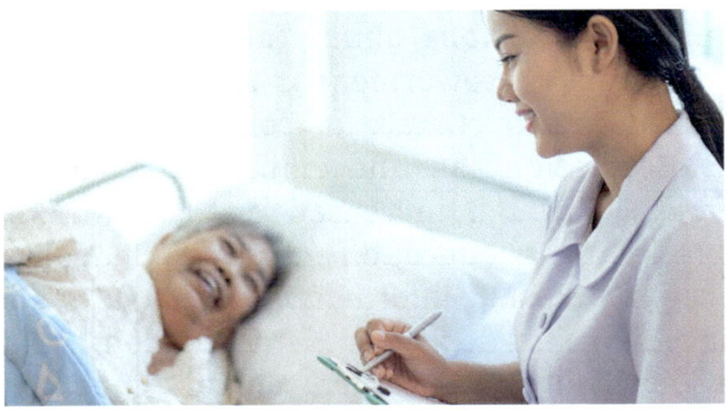

Figure 3.2. Health education.

Source: https://t4.ftcdn.net/jpg/01/89/68/11/360_F_189681193_SZWoBMfEe9pq2453xMKlKn2Mi937uBnD.jpg.

Health Promotion Role

Health promotion is a significant contribution to enhancing the well-being and health of populations and communities. By focusing on preventive health behavior, health promotion intervention works not only to improve physical functioning but also to solve mental health issues, particularly among high-risk populations. For example, depression among adolescents is growing, and disadvantaged adolescents are disproportionately represented. School health promotion schemes can provide appropriate resources and training to facilitate early intervention for both mental and physical diseases (Hari et al., 2017). By teaching depression literacy and help-seeking behavior as part of the school curriculum, interventions aim to provide students with information and competencies critical to their mental health, bridge the gap in health education, and cultivate a culture of support within the learning environment. Lastly, part of what it means to promote health is to focus on building environments that foster health at the community level. Effective health promotion interventions must engage all stakeholders, including policymakers, educators, and healthcare professionals, to co-plan responsive strategies that meet the specific needs of target groups. The World Health Organization's recommendation supports this appeal by advocating for the inclusion of psychosocial risk management in organizational work settings to promote improved mental health (Anand et al., 2015). With an eye on the interconnection of physical and well-being, companies can design interprofessional measures to develop good working environments that promote employee health and adapt to the requirements of modern working life. Not only does it enable a healthier workforce, but it also boosts productivity, citing the wide-ranging benefits of successful health-promoting measures. Finally, the impact of health promotion is not only a matter of individual or social health, but also a reflection of higher social dividends and economic benefits. As rising health expenditure is directly caused by preventable diseases, effective health promotion interventions prove to be a wise investment economically. Through education, lifestyle changes, and the application of preventive interventions, populations can prevent the development of chronic diseases and other health issues, thereby ensuring reduced healthcare expenditures in the long run. These strategies also build a resilient culture and good,reasonable health control, ultimately leading to a healthy population and sustainable healthcare system. Hence, the importance of health promotion cannot be overemphasized as it is one of the essential pillars in shaping improved general well-being and averting future health emergencies, elevating public health to the top of policy agendas and community action.

3.1. The Role of Health Education

Learning Outcome

1. Define the aims of health education
2. Highlight target groups for health education
3. Find ways of delivering health education

Health education is a significant input into individual and community health through the provision of knowledge and skills that enable individuals to make informed health-related decisions. As one of the key components of health promotion interventions, education plays a central role in developing health literacy among groups. By promoting awareness of health risks, preventive behaviors, and healthy lifestyles, health education trains individuals to take ownership of their own health. In addition, by incorporating sensitivity to culture into the educational curriculum, health educators can meaningfully access all demographic groups so that the knowledge is actionable and meaningful. This tailored approach not only enhances the impact of health messages but also fosters community resilience against public health threats, illustrating the interactive dynamics between education and health outcomes, as highlighted in policy recommendations for health equity interventions (Birnbaum et al., 2011). Moreover, the impact of health education is highly enhanced when implemented as part of broader health promotion strategies that address social determinants of health. Health educators are increasingly needed to bridge gaps in access to information and resources, particularly within the most underserved populations, where health disparities are most pronounced. By expanding access to health services and placing greater emphasis on community involvement, health education programs can create an environment that enables the maximization of health promotion activities' results. This comprehensive approach addresses short-term health issues but lays the groundwork for long-term health behavior modification. The compendium of health equity promotion recommendations emphasizes the importance of integrating educational activities with community assets to create seamless and effective, inclusive strategies (Birnbaum et al., 2011). In addition to providing key knowledge in health, health education also fosters critical thinking skills that enable individuals to make informed decisions about their health. This intellectual empowerment is necessary in the current health climate of complexity, where disinformation can undermine public health efforts. Through increased critical thinking capacity, health education enables individuals to recognize credible information, assess risks, and make informed decisions that meet their health needs. Even more critical, health educators bridge the divide for policy transformation in favor of health equity, fostering a synergistic relationship between education and health enhancement at the system level. This campaign is crucial in creating educational systems that promote health among all populations, supporting the need to address health disparities through informed policymaking. As a whole, the convergence of health education and promotion practices is crucial to building a healthier world, as education has been identified as the doorway to realizing the potential for sustainable health improvements (Birnbaum et al., 2011) (Figure 3.3).

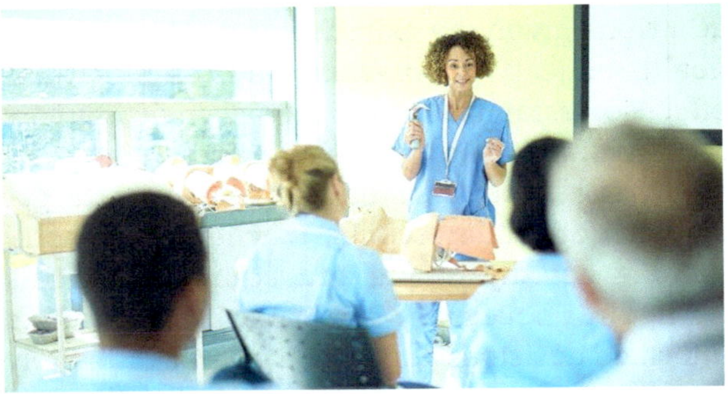

Figure 3.3. Clinical nurse educator career.

Source: https://i.pinimg.com/originals/3a/35/a6/3a35a6acb2dcc69260807f96e8c99f49.jpg.

3.1.1. Objectives of Health Education

Health education is critical in equipping people with information and skills needed to make informed decisions for their health. Awareness of various health issues is among the essential objectives of health education, thus fostering a culture of health and prevention. By focusing on key topics such as nutrition, physical fitness, and disease prevention, health education not only educates individuals but also fosters a culture that prioritizes health. Such learning is essential because the majority of health problems stem from the lack of information or the wrong information regarding health habits. Increased awareness can lead to improved health outcomes, as well-educated individuals who understand the consequences of their decisions are also more likely to adopt healthier habits and behaviors in their communities, ultimately augmenting efforts in public health. Another key objective of health education is to promote positive behavior change in individuals and communities. Effective health education programs implement an array of strategies that target behavior changes, such as the cessation of cigarette smoking, exercise, and healthy consumption. By incorporating messages tailored to the individual and interactive methods, health educators can encourage individuals to adopt healthier behaviors that will lead to a decrease in the prevalence of chronic diseases. For instance, efforts to promote exercise, particularly among elderly persons, have been replicated through varied initiatives aimed at particular groups and their specific issues (N/A, 2001). Hence, promoting behavior change not only adds value to personal lives but also to community health through well-informed decisions that can be contagious and reinforce social norms towards health. Lastly, health education aims to provide a platform for better health policies and practices through the involvement of stakeholders, such as health organizations and community leaders. A significant portion of this objective focuses on the social determinants of health, which play a crucial role in determining the health outcomes of populations (Philip O'Hara, 2005). By addressing the broad determinants of health, such as education, socioeconomic status, and the environment, health education encourages an intersectoral strategy for promoting health. Combined efforts can lead to revolutionary transformations that address root-systemic health issues comprehensively by integrating various competencies and perspectives. Lastly, health education aims are beyond individuals' knowledge and behavior, forming part of a comprehensive strategy that encourages fair access to health opportunities and resources for all.

3.1.2. Target Populations for Health Education

Effective health promotion and education efforts must tailor their approaches to various target populations to fully leverage their potential. Socio-economic status, culture, and level of health literacy present different challenges and opportunities for health educators to address differently. Ethnic minority groups, such as

African-Americans and Hispanics, for instance, present high levels of health disparities, particularly in terms of chronic illnesses such as stroke. There is limited health knowledge among these groups, and they often experience delayed responses to medical emergencies due to cultural barriers and inadequate specialized communication skills. As such, health education interventions conducted in community settings and drawing on culturally sensitive methodologies have proven effective in closing these gaps in perception and knowledge (Booth et al., 2014). Therefore, targeting specific ethnic communities not only enhances individuals' expertise but also benefits overall public health. The other significant population to health education are sexual and gender minorities, including lesbian, gay, bisexual, and transgender (LGBT) populations. This group has had a long history of experiencing health disparities due to systemic discrimination, stigma, and limited access to culturally competent health care. Effective health communication strategies for LGBT populations must be tailored to their specific needs and incorporate their perspectives into the design and implementation of health promotion interventions. Evidence further suggests that multidimensional approaches to health communication—encompassing both community-based interventions and direct engagement with healthcare workers—can have a significant impact on health outcomes in LGBT populations (Drabble et al., 2003). Engaging LGBT communities in the development of suitable health messages not only enhances credibility but also maximizes the potential for effective education programs, underscoring the value of targeted tactics in these pivotal public health efforts. No less essential are adolescents and children, the promise of community health and wellness. Least resilient to any of a variety of health threats, ranging from substance use and obesity to mental disease, this generation deserves targeted health education. When presented through engaging formats, including peer-to-peer dialogue and participatory learning activities responding to their stage of development, initiatives directed at younger generations can be particularly influential. In addition, involving parents and guardians in health education programs can amplify their effects by establishing supportive environments that reinforce healthy behaviors at home. By modifying health promotion strategies to target children and adolescents, teachers can instill lifelong healthy habits and equip individuals with the necessary information to make informed decisions about their health, ultimately contributing to a healthier society (Booth et al., 2014) (Figure 3.4).

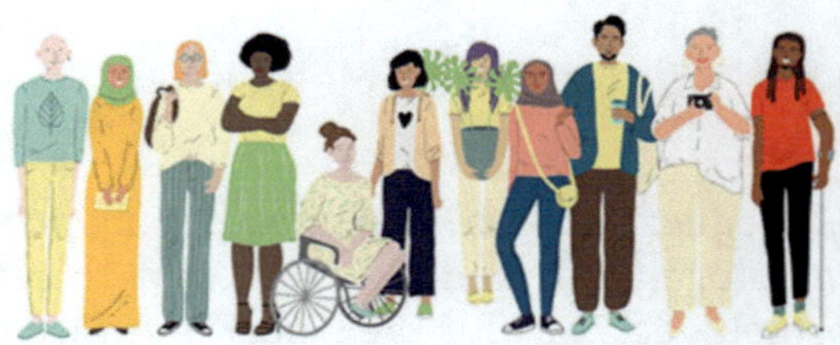

Figure 3.4. Diverse patient populations in clinical research.

Source: https://external-content.duckduckgo.com/iu/?u=https%3A%2F%2Fvertassets.blob.core.windows.net%2Fimage%2F5aff2c7a%2F5aff2c7a-e2c6-4810-b0fd-7355b7cff918%2Fistock_1182497153.jpg&f=1&nofb=1&ipt=90ab6a9dfa44bb489a476e3f68fb2ebdb39cb5f78958e2a74129dc961a897bb8.

3.1.3. Methods of Delivering Health Education

A good health education process must incorporate a variety of delivery methods to most appropriately meet the needs of diverse populations. Lectures and workshops are more structured environments for presenting information, but may not be suitable for all learners. Incorporating interactive approaches, such as group discussions and hands-on activities, can foster greater commitment and enable participants to apply their learning to real-life situations. For instance, in child-centered research, the incorporation of health education into the school curriculum has been a key approach. Programs that are sensitive to the whole needs of students, such as the Health Promoting School Initiative, demonstrate how health education can be contextualized to meet the school setting while enhancing both health and education (Reddy et al., 2015). The synergy of these strategies yields a more comprehensive learning process, fostering long-term behavioral change among students. The new power of technology has also diversified the health education delivery system. Health information can now be accessed in greater numbers through websites, cell phone apps, and social media, which are accessible beyond the traditional settings. For example, social media-driven public health campaigns can effectively reach young people, disseminating vital health messages in a timely and compelling manner. Moreover, e-learning modules offer personalized learning experiences that allow individuals to progress at their own pace, making them particularly useful for those with multiple commitments. However, it is essential that these digital instruments are culturally sensitive and provide access to all population segments. The combination of human intervention and technology-oriented strategies is compelling in enhancing the effectiveness of health education, with the information being relevant as well as practical (Dawson et al., 2017). One of the vital but often overlooked concerns in offering health education is incorporating community and cultural input. Cultural practices and beliefs significantly influence health behavior and attitude. Therefore, health education approaches must consider the cultural setting to make them as relevant and acceptable as possible to the target groups. Engaging community leaders and stakeholders in planning health education efforts can foster trust and enhance communication between health workers and community members. Programs that tailor their content to fit local traditions and customs can encourage participation and adherence to health practices. For example, a study demonstrating how Hong Kong families blend traditional practices with contemporary health advice supports the need for a pluralistic model to promote health (Dawson et al., 2017). By employing culturally appropriate strategies, health educators can maximize the effectiveness of their efforts, thereby creating lasting changes in community health behaviors (Figure 3.5).

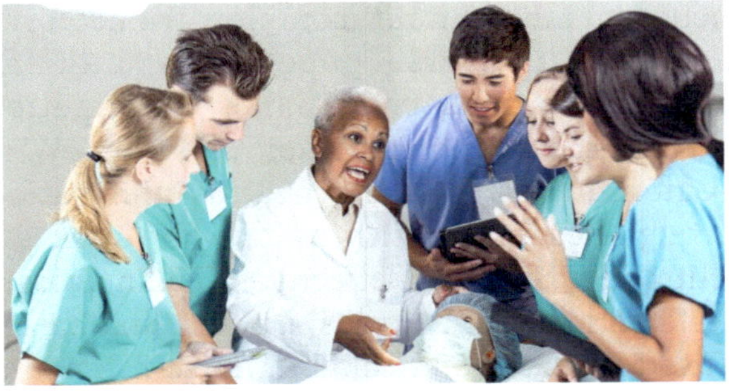

Figure 3.5. Clinical-nursing-educator.

Source: https://www.thechicagoschool.edu/insightadmin/2020/12/tcspp-clinical-nursing-educator-936x512.jpg.

Test Your Knowledge

1. Why is health education an essential responsibility of medical-surgical nurses?
2. Explain how medical-surgical nurses empower patients and families via health education.

3.2. Health Promotion Strategies

Learning Outcome

1. Explain the community-based health promotion
2. Define policy advocacy for health promotion
3. Explain the use of technology in health promotion

Health promotion strategies encompass a wide range of practices that aim to enhance the general well-being and health of individuals and communities. These strategies are vital to health promotion, enabling a proactive approach to health as opposed to responding to disease. Education and empowerment of people to become their own health managers form an integral component of effective health promotion. It involves disseminating health information, providing behavioral interventions, and promoting sustainable lifestyle changes. Facilities must adopt complex frameworks that benefit diverse populations, utilizing methods such as community participation and tailored health education programs. With greater access to basic health information through resources such as the Playbook for Action, agencies can effectively communicate vital health methodologies in a way that makes sense to leaders and community stakeholders, thereby making a significant contribution to overall health outcomes (N/A, 2008). The work setting is an important setting where health promotion interventions should be implemented, particularly in encouraging employee health. Organizations that seriously consider employees' health by investing in health schemes realize positive outcomes, including increased productivity and reduced absenteeism. One effective strategy is health and wellness coaching, which equips employees with the resources to foster self-awareness and manage stress. As evidenced by current studies, employees who undergo wellness coaching report increased levels of participation and empowerment, leading to a healthier organizational climate (Lawson et al., 2019). In creating environments that promote physical and mental well-being, employers not only enhance their employees' quality of life but also foster organizational effectiveness and morale, providing a compelling argument for the inclusion of health promotion strategies in workplace policy. Moreover, the application of custom-made health promotion interventions can mitigate the effects of chronic conditions, which pose a significant challenge to individuals and the healthcare system as a whole. Preventive strategies, such as information campaigns for lifestyles' change and the control of chronic diseases, are key to this process. Engaging communities in interactive information sessions and workshops has the potential to cultivate a culture of support and mutual sharing of knowledge, thereby fostering greater health literacy and healthier lifestyle practices within communities.

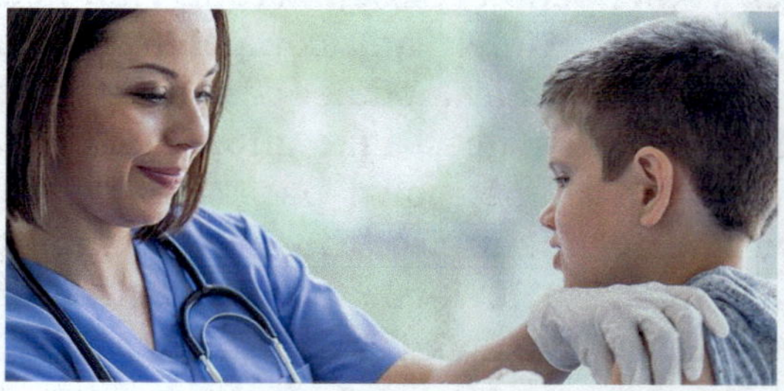

Figure 3.6. Nursing health promotion strategies.

Source: https://external-content.duckduckgo.com/iu/?u=https%3A%2F%2Fwww.nursingwritingservices.com%2Fimages%2FNursing-Health-Promotion-Strategies1.jpg&f=1&nofb=1&ipt=516adee098f99793cfe5833971d9cb6852d422b4414e5bcb87c1159041fef065.

In this context, collaboration between healthcare providers, public health organizations, and community-based organizations is essential.

Through collaborative resources and expertise, a more efficient and sustainable approach to health promotion can be established, addressing the root causes of health issues and promoting sustained health in communities (N/A, 2008) (Figure 3.6).

3.2.1. Community-based Health Promotion

Community-based health promotion is increasingly being recognized as a vital strategy for improving public health outcomes. This approach centers on engaging local communities in formulating and implementing health programs tailored to their specific needs. Progress in health promotion, particularly working through nutrition and habits of lifestyle, has been pivotal in raising awareness and bringing about positive behavior change among communities. For instance, the formulation of interactive media, such as nutrition promotion media, has proven effective in increasing knowledge and influencing healthier food consumption among participants. By prioritizing community participation, such programs not only maximize individual involvement but also foster a culture of shared responsibility for achieving health gains. The success of these programs, as indicated by recent research, highlights the relative importance of local context and community participation in shaping health behavior (Harwanto et al., 2024). Despite the glaring benefits of community health promotion, professionals face serious challenges that can hinder its effective uptake. Among the primary issues is the low level of participation by certain health practitioners, such as occupational therapists, in the community programs. While occupational therapy may contribute significantly to the endeavor of health promotion, Flannery and Barry (2003) found that few occupational therapists were actively involved in community health programs. This disconnect can be attributed to several reasons, including a lack of resources, inadequate training, and uncertainty regarding professional roles. Breaking these obstacles is essential, as the appropriate knowledge and training of professionals are crucial in the design of effective health promotion interventions. Consequently, better education and training on community health promotion among practitioners can lead to more joint efforts towards healthier communities (Sauer et al., 2012), such as a model based on collaboration and integrative education for health workers is of most tremendous significance to the achievement of health promotion activities based in the community. Workshops and training focused on community engagement and resourcefulness can potentially empower healthcare professionals to become active agents of change. Not only do these programs highlight approaches for program implementation and development, but they also equip participants with the resources to fund and sustain their initiatives. By encouraging adult learning principles, these training programs aim to enhance the dissemination of relevant health information to diverse populations. With changing community needs, health professionals who are well-prepared to adapt and respond will become a key success factor in promoting wellness and improving health outcomes. Lastly, ongoing emphasis on community-based health promotion can potentially offer a strategy for sustainable population health enhancement (Sauer et al., 2012) (Figure 3.7).

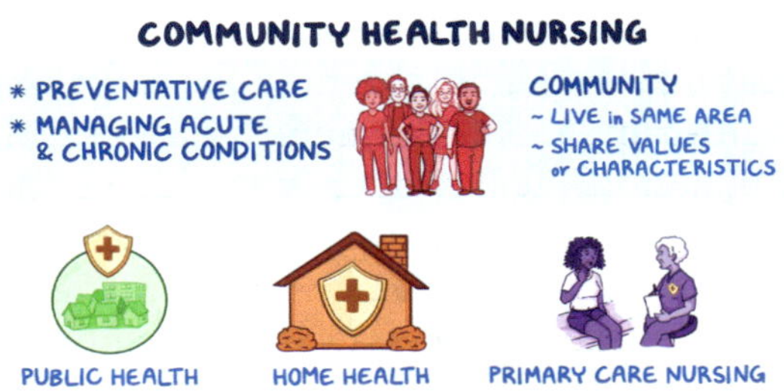
COMMUNITY HEALTH NURSING
* PREVENTATIVE CARE
* MANAGING ACUTE & CHRONIC CONDITIONS
COMMUNITY
~ LIVE in SAME AREA
~ SHARE VALUES or CHARACTERISTICS
PUBLIC HEALTH
HOME HEALTH
PRIMARY CARE NURSING

Figure 3.7. Community-based health promotion.

Source: https://osmose-it.s3.amazonaws.com/WswykXMBTmOY4OhSC78LxV6VRQuzi4hP/_.jpg.

3.2.2. Policy Advocacy for Health Promotion

Policy advocacy is an integral part of health promotion since it affects broader social and political contexts within which public health programs operate. By tactfully coordinating health advocacy, stakeholders will be able to combine their strengths and achieve actual change in health policies. This exercise requires different coalitions of the public, public health professionals, and policymakers united under common ambitions. As demonstrated by the New Mexico for Responsible Sex Education coalition, which formed in response to abstinence-only education policies, the collaboration among various stakeholders plays a critical role in addressing the political dynamics that impact health promotion efforts. The coalition's experiences underscore the necessity of integrating advocacy into health promotion frameworks to tackle systemic barriers and enhance the sustainability of health interventions (Mendes et al., 2016). In an increasingly healthy context, the necessity to improve health promotion strategies for diverse community needs cannot be overstressed. Policy advocacy enables health educators and community leaders to tailor their strategies to target not only the health behaviors of individuals but also the social determinants of health that influence their behaviors. For instance, Integrated Service Post programs bring health services and early childhood education programs together as an example of multi-component community empowerment and enhanced health outcomes. Furthermore, these programs underscore the importance of forming coalitions among stakeholders, as effective social support systems facilitate the implementation of advocacy and can sustain public health interventions in the long term. Therefore, the establishment of partnerships in various sectors aims to increase advocacy and improve health promotion interventions (Farida et al., 2017). Ultimately, integrating policy advocacy into health promotion systems presents both challenges and opportunities in achieving equitable health outcomes. As illustrated in current deliberations, one of the challenges is the issue of political limitations that tend to inhibit public sector employees from actively participating in advocacy work. At the same time, there are hurdles that can be stimuli to innovate, pushing stakeholders into creating new strategies for effective health promotion. An appreciation for the intricate interplay among power, stakeholders, and advocacy channels is key to sustaining health interventions that influence policy reform. By taking an integrated approach that links advocacy and collaborative work, public health workers can cultivate a more practical and sustainable environment for promoting health, one that is responsive to the populations being served (Mendes et al., 2016; Farida et al., 2017) (Figure 3.8).

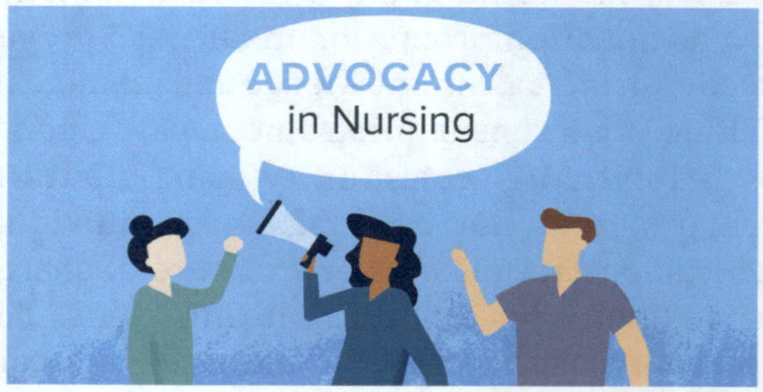

Figure 3.8. Nurse advocacy.

Source: https://nursegrid.com/wp-content/uploads/2018/11/181109_Advocacy_BlogPost.png.

3.2.3. Use of Technology in Health Promotion

The incorporation of technology into health promotion practice marks a significant shift in the delivery and use of health education. Mobile phone apps and internet-based platforms, also known as digital tools, have the potential to increase engagement and access for diverse populations. For instance, the use of mobile technology, such as iPads, has been explored in preventive counseling environments, where it acts as an effective practical tool for training, social marketing, and health promotion. The application of the Indivisible Self-Wellness Model in these settings is a representative example of how technology can be utilized to support tailored health education programs that cater to individual and community needs (Hughes et al., 2015). As health educators and counselors adopt these technologies, they can utilize them to create compelling and interactive experiences that promote overall well-being and motivate active health engagement. In addition, the influence of technology extends beyond education for health to diet and nutrition education as well, particularly in college settings where the health of the students is of paramount importance. Institutions of higher learning must respond to the changing health environment, particularly as teen and young adult obesity continues to rise. The role of college health educators has become increasingly significant in advocating for healthy eating options and developing overall well-being campaigns. A focus group study investigated the potential of using the internet as a channel for disseminating nutritional information and enhancing educational campaigns. The involvement of registered dietitians as members of these campaigns suggests that expert knowledge is essential in designing successful interventions with evidence-based information backing these interventions (Biediger-Friedman et al., 2010). Consequently, technology is not only utilized as a platform for delivery but also as a catalyst for healthier dietary habits in students. Additionally, the success of technology-supported health promotion initiatives often relies on institutional support and organizational policies that prioritize health and wellness. One of the most significant discoveries from interviews with college foodservice directors emphasized the need for healthy eating champions within the college setting. The existence of forward-looking policies contributes significantly to healthy food availability and marketing, as well as an environment that supports better nutrition. The internet remains a key mechanism for disseminating education in nutrition and weight control in reaching a vast body of people. Increased access to information has the power to enable students to make informed decisions about their eating habits and therefore support general health promotion. By carefully leveraging these technological advances, health facilities and educators can reaffirm their commitment to a culture of wellness (Biediger-Friedman et al., 2010).

Test Your Knowledge

1. What is the central goal of health promotion in medical-surgical nursing?
2. Identify two health promotion interventions regularly utilized by surgical recovery or chronic disease care nurses.

3.3. Behavioral Change Theories

Learning Outcome

1. Outline the theories of behavioral change
2. Define theory use in health education
3. Describe the effectiveness of behavioral change strategies

Behavioral change theories are essential elements of health education and promotion interventions, as they explain how people modify their health behaviors. Theories such as the Health Belief Model and the Transtheoretical Model are used to gain an understanding of the psychosocial determinants of health decision-making. For instance, perceived benefit and barrier determinants can be used to inform intervention planning and engage with target populations. Notably, recognizing the influence of social norms on experiences can also further enhance efforts to encourage healthier behaviors. By basing interventions on empirically derived behavioral theories, practitioners can enhance the impact of health promotion activities, which in turn leads to improved public health outcomes. A systematic yet responsive framework enables a rich appreciation of heterogeneous populations, which is critical for mitigating different health risks and behaviors.

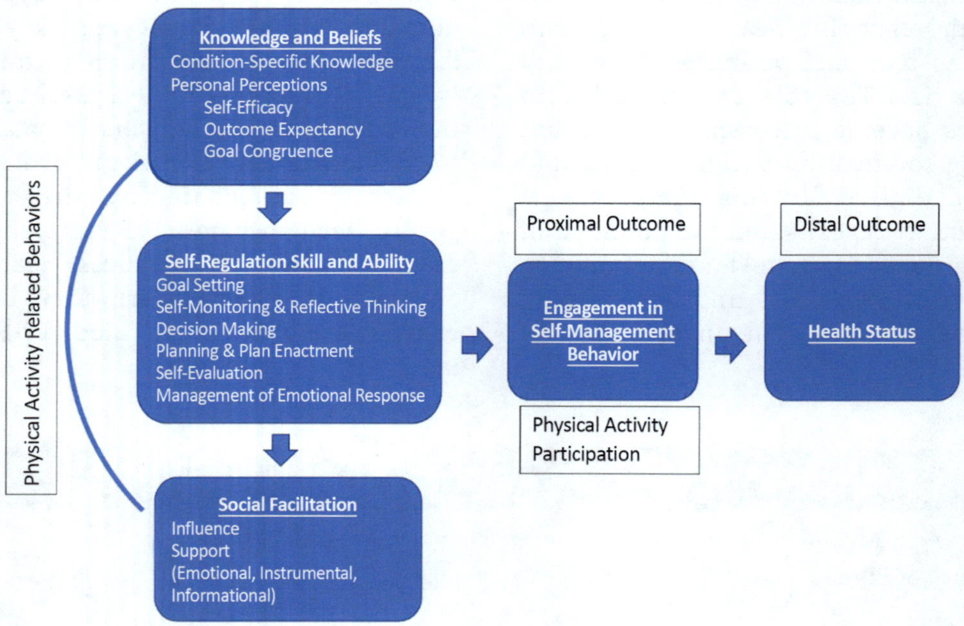

Figure 3.9. The integrated theory of health behavior change.

Source: https://www.researchgate.net/publication/351221215/figure/fig1/AS:1018151957458944@1619757751085/The-Integrated-Theory-of-Health-Behavior-Change.png.

A successful behavior change program is generally characterized by its flexibility by structure, allowing for integration of various models and approaches as used for multiple population groups. This adaptability is highlighted in the development of comprehensive methodologies with a focus on behavioral risk management, particularly in high-risk scenarios like AIDS prevention. With a blend of theories, such as the Social Cognitive Theory, health educators can intervene on various variables influencing behavior change, including self-efficacy and outcome expectations. The interdependence of such variables makes contextual relevance crucial in intervening, ensuring that interventions are tailored to the unique issues of the individuals in question.

Therefore, the use of more than one theoretical orientation not only strengthens health promotion planning but also broadens opportunities for successful behavioral change in diverse settings (Cole et al., 1993). The recent emergence of online health interventions is a testament to the dynamism of theories of behavioral change employed in the field of health education and promotion. With increasing technological developments, such interventions increasingly rely upon theories that adopt behavioral change techniques and principles of persuasive system design. In this age of technology, the integration of various theoretical models may make it possible to develop complex interventions with greater scope and capacity to address complex health issues. Additionally, a combined framework incorporating theories of behavior has the potential to guide developers in creating solid and effective digital health interventions. Such convergence not only enables efficient planning and assessment of intervention, but also facilitates inter-disciplinary collaboration to further augment the overall effectiveness of health promotion initiatives. In light of improvements in the field, health educators must remain acutely responsive to these developments and use them to form sustainable behavioral modifications (Fadhil et al., 2018) (Figure 3.9).

3.3.1. Overview of Behavioral Change Theories

An understanding of behavioral change theories is crucial for developing effective health education and promotion strategies, as these frameworks offer valuable insights into how and why individuals modify their behavior. One of the more well-known models is the Health Belief Model (HBM), which proposes that individuals are more likely to adopt health-promoting behaviors when they perceive a high personal risk associated with a particular health issue and believe that there is some action that can significantly reduce that risk. This model emphasizes the importance of perceived barriers and personal incentives in encouraging behavior change and, therefore, forms a critical element in designing focused health interventions. Furthermore, this model serves as a guide for teachers to create programs that appeal to the aspirations and concerns of the target population, thereby making them more effective in promoting healthy living styles. Another critical method in the domain of behavioral change is the Transtheoretical Model (TTM), which focuses on the steps one goes through when changing one's behavior. These steps—precontemplation, contemplation, preparation, action, and maintenance—help practitioners target their interventions according to an individual's readiness to change. For instance, interventions in the precontemplation stage may focus on establishing awareness of the necessity of change, while those in the maintenance stage may focus on sustaining the behavior change. This structured nature of the models makes it adaptable to many health-related behaviors, and health educators can form strategies that are appropriate for participants' prevailing motivational levels and challenges towards achieving health-related activities. In recent years, the integration of digital health interventions with behavior change strategies has gained increased attention. The interventions are developed based on several behavioral theories and technologies, as they utilize digital platforms to introduce requisite health-supporting behaviors. The integrative framework, which combines behavioral theories, the behavior change technique (BCT) taxonomy, and persuasive system design (PSD) principles, has emerged as a comprehensive tool for intervention developers. This model enables a systematic yet flexible approach to designing, evaluating, and reporting behavioral change interventions, allowing them to meet the individual needs of various population segments. As Cole et al. (1993) detail, the flexibility of such models is critical when strategies are to be appropriately tailored in response to various health threats, e.g., disease prevention, as with AIDS. Moreover, with the application of this systematic strategy, health promotion interventions can be effectively assessed and refined in the future, leading to improved health results (Figure 3.10).

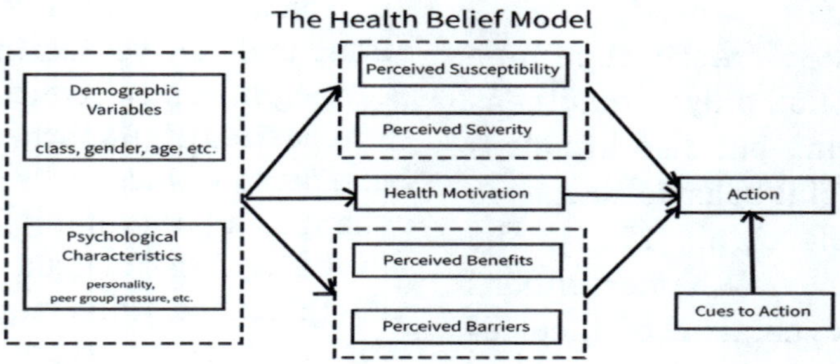

Figure 3.10. Health belief model (HBM).

Source: https://mental-health-matters.org/wp-content/uploads/2023/01/health-belief-model-original-1.jpg.

3.3.2. Application of Theories in Health Education

The integration of behavioral theories in health education is necessary to respond effectively to public health issues. Theories such as the Health Belief Model and the Theory of Planned Behavior provide frameworks that inform the planning and implementation of health promotion interventions. For instance, the Health Belief Model focuses on perceived severity and susceptibility, which are crucial in motivating people to change their health behavior. By this line of thinking, one can personalize education programs to raise awareness of health hazards and the benefits of healthy behavior. Additionally, integrating such theories allows one to learn about the drives and challenges people encounter when adopting healthier living, which eventually results in successful interventions and health education programs. Social marketing strategies guided by behavioral theories have been emphasized in recent studies as a powerful influence in achieving impressive health outcomes. In Greece, research on the feeding habits of young adults has emphasized the importance of understanding motivation and barriers to healthy eating, which can inform effective health education. Health benefits, body image, and mental well-being were ranked as motivation towards healthy intake by the participants, with time constraint and accessibility of fast foods ranked as barriers. The knowledge gained from focus groups enabled the creation of targeted interventions that eliminate such barriers, demonstrating the application of theories in practice. Such is how this illustrates how knowledge of consumer behavior, viewed through a theoretical lens, not only helps disentangle complex health issues but also facilitates the formulation of solutions that resonate with the target market, thereby improving health education and promotion. The need for cooperation and civic engagement is emphasized in health education strategies, that is, through initiatives like University Social Responsibility (USR). USR incorporates ethical values and civic competencies into the study curriculum, promoting a culture of health awareness and responsibility among university students. Evidence suggests that the effective implementation of these strategies relies on effective communication and the involvement of stakeholders. By a methodical procedure of embedding USR in health education, institutions can facilitate an enabling environment for healthy behavior enablers. Such thoughtful incorporation of community-focused theories into health promotion interventions not only enhances the learning process but also creates a long-term model of health consciousness that can be transferred outside organizational limits, ultimately translating to improved health outcomes on a large scale (Bandura et al., 2014; Mart Bínez et al., 2019) (Figure 3.11).

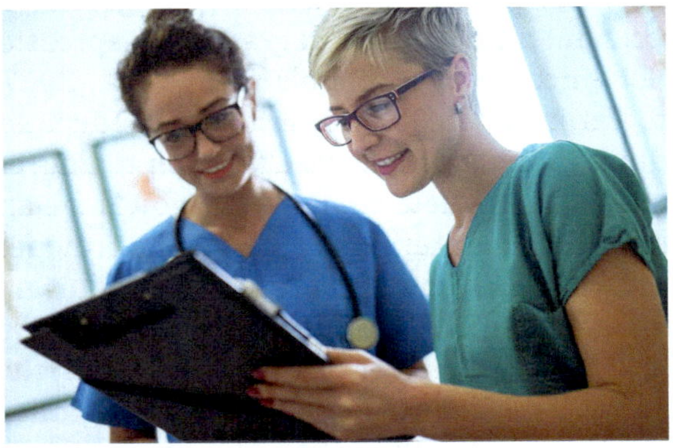

Figure 3.11. Intervention-addressing-communication-in-nursing.

Source: https://anmj.org.au/wp-content/uploads/2022/02/Intervention-addressing-communication-in-nursing-handover.jpg.

3.3.3. Effectiveness of Behavioral Change Strategies

Success in behavior change intervention in health promotion and education is increasingly known as an essential driving force for developing sustainable health habits in communities. Recent advances in health promotion have focused on enhancing awareness of nutritional needs and motivating lifestyle changes. Such interventions utilize technology, communities, and learning infrastructure to transfer health information that is most needed successfully. For instance, initiatives such as nutrition promotion media—spanning pop-up books, educational videos, and interactive puzzles—have proven highly successful in enhancing awareness and changing behavior regarding nutrition. Facilitating the active participation of members of the public through initiatives such as focus group discussions and collaborative meal preparation further substantiates the relevance of these behavioral change strategies in addressing matters of public health (Harwanto et al., 2024). However, demonstrating the effectiveness of such strategies relies on overcoming methodological challenges, including small sample sizes and short intervention periods. Insofar as physical activity promotion is concerned, particularly among university students, behavioral change techniques dominate efforts to enhance long-term health benefits. It is established that university life is correlated with reduced levels of physical activity; however, this can be turned around with specific interventions that promote an active living environment. A review of controlled trials highlights the need to address a multitude of behavioral determinants through personalized methods of encouraging physical activity. Evidence has demonstrated that interventions, in addition to organized PA sessions, can comprehensively increase activity levels among students. Notably, 16 out of 27 studies evaluated showed positive physical activity changes; however, they grappled with study design and participant retention problems that necessitate the adoption of more robust methodologies to ascertain the most effective approaches (Carraro et al., 2018). The inclusion of behavioral change strategies in health education programs not only promotes immediate benefits but also builds positive habits for generations to come. Thus, research on the effectiveness of such interventions should expand through longitudinal studies to investigate long-term outcomes and factors that mediate contextual effects on health behaviors. Under this integrative approach, educators and health promoters will be in a position to develop population-specific interventions, including those targeting vulnerable populations. Furthermore, evaluating community empowerment programs can strengthen local health policies and encourage long-term health promotion interventions. By addressing these challenges and prioritizing innovative solutions, health education can effectively transform community health practices and ultimately enhance overall well-being (Harwanto et al., 2024).

Test Your Knowledge

1. Why is the use of behavioral change theories in nursing practice necessary?
2. Give an example of a commonly used behavior change theory and its concise application in patient education.

3.4. Health Literacy

Learning Outcome

1. Identify the significance of health literacy
2. Define health literacy barriers
3. Describe the methods for improving health literacy

Health literacy is a crucial component of effective health education and promotion interventions, as it empowers individuals to make informed health-related decisions. Health literacy is the ability to seek, process, and understand plain health information, and it is a key determinant of people's capacity to navigate the healthcare system and implement preventive behaviors. The lack of health literacy has also been linked with poorer health outcomes among vulnerable populations. For instance, young individuals who come from vulnerable backgrounds are likely to develop mental health issues since they lack access to essential information and resources that are important in the fight against mental health issues. Therefore, integrating health literacy into curricula for learning, particularly in schools in vulnerable populations, can enhance understanding of health and spur early intervention, especially in mental health facilities, as suggested by successful intervention programs on depression in low-income high schools (Hari et al., 2017). Integrating health literacy into health education requires a comprehensive approach to address multiple health determinants of knowledge and awareness. Teachers and healthcare providers must adopt strategies that resonate with diverse populations, including socioeconomic, cultural, and linguistic differences. The Youth-Physical Activity Towards Health (Y-PATH) program is an example of how specialized programs can promote physical literacy among adolescents, establishing a model leading to lifelong physical activity. This program's holistic, whole-school approach not only fosters knowledge of physical health but also equips students to help create a better sense of overall wellbeing. Embedding physical activity into various subjects and creating enabling settings for movement can indeed improve the extent of health literacy, promoting academic and physical achievement (Belton et al., 2017). Finally, the roles of health professionals extend beyond mere information transmission; they must also be facilitators and champions of health literacy. This involves collaboration with schools, communities, and families to create supportive environments where health information is readily accessible and comprehensible.

Preparing educators to offer health literacy education effectively is pivotal in preparing competent, knowledgeable individuals to speak out on their own behalf for their health. Furthermore, the implementation of holistic programs that align with health literacy goals plays a crucial role in mitigating the disparities faced by underserved groups. With concerted efforts to raise health literacy, health promotion and education interventions can significantly reduce health-related risks, ultimately leading to a healthier society in the long term (Figure 3.12).

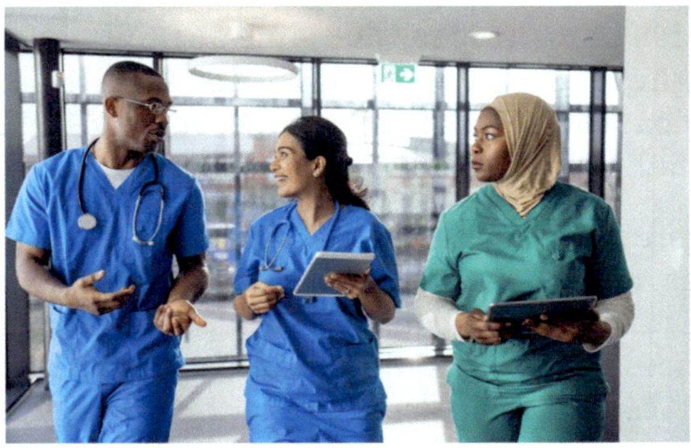

Figure 3.12. The nurse's guide to health literacy.

Source: https://res.cloudinary.com/highereducation/images/f_auto,q_auto/v1665415429/NurseJournal.org/GettyImages-1362936837_6811369943/GettyImages-1362936837_6811369943.jpg?_i=AAupload/c_fill,fl_lossy,q_auto:best,w_448,h_382,g_center/undefined.

3.4.1. Definition and Significance of Health Literacy

Health literacy, or the ability to access, understand, evaluate, and use health information effectively, is crucial for promoting positive health outcomes. It entails a set of competencies that include reading and writing, critical thinking, and the ability to navigate complex health systems. The importance of health literacy cannot be overstated, as it encompasses the ability to make informed decisions about health and well-being. Higher health literacy has been associated with better control of chronic conditions, more consistent use of preventive health behaviors, and improved ability to communicate with doctors. Therefore, health literacy is a crucial determinant of health equity, influencing the quality and availability of care that an individual receives. With an understanding of and addressing health literacy, efforts in health education and promotion can be more effectively tailored to meet the diverse needs of populations. Furthermore, recent studies have revealed a concerning correlation between health literacy and social determinants of health, including physical inactivity and loneliness. The relationship between the variables highlights the challenges faced by individuals with poor health literacy, particularly those who also struggle with social isolation. For instance, studies found that individuals with lower health literacy were more vulnerable to experiencing loneliness, particularly among physically active older adults (Sarmanlu et al., 2024). This means that enhancing health literacy not only equips individuals with appropriate information about health but also addresses broader social issues that contribute to declining health. As such, by incorporating initiatives to enhance health literacy, it is achievable to attain inclusive health promotion interventions that address knowledge gaps and emotional health, which are crucial for effective health education. Additionally, improving health literacy is crucial for advancing equity in health outcomes. The health equity movement emphasizes the importance of reducing social injustices causing health disparities among marginalized populations. By promoting health literacy among these populations, health education interventions can empower individuals to seek healthcare services, identify health hazards, and make informed choices that enhance their quality of life. Evidence suggests that as health literacy initiatives become increasingly prevalent, they can help reverse health inequities, particularly when embedded in community-based programs (Birnbaum et al., 2011). Therefore, embedding health literacy within health education programs not only enriches individual capacity for disease management and self-care, but also further the general goal of advancing health equity across different groups of populations.

3.4.2. Barriers to Health Literacy

Health literacy has emerged as a key factor in determining health outcomes, yet numerous barriers hinder individuals' ability to navigate the complex healthcare system effectively. Among those barriers, educational attainment and socioeconomic status play essential roles. Individuals with lower education levels often struggle to understand medical information, which can lead to misinterpretation of health instructions and ultimately, poorer health outcomes. With over 36% of US adults having low health literacy, healthcare systems pay a greater cost in inefficiencies and expenses in an effort to address the needs of these patients. Additionally, the imbalance between patients' information requirements and providers' communication potential exacerbates the condition, indicating a pressing need for interventions that close these knowledge gaps (Siskind et al., 2016). Cultural factors also play a significant role in health literacy, both as obstacles and facilitators of health communication. Cultural belief systems and practices can condition one's understanding of healthcare, shaping willingness to seek aid or comply with a doctor's orders. As an illustration, members of marginalized groups may distrust health systems, something that could be a byproduct of historical differences and inequities. This critical thinking makes it difficult to promote health literacy, as individuals tend to read health information from a critical angle.

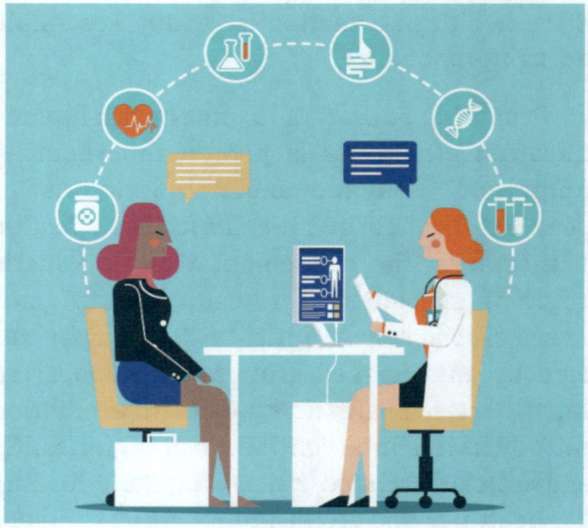

Figure 3.13. Barriers to health literacy.

Source: https://s3.amazonaws.com/higherlogicdownload/HEALTHSTREAM/UploadedImages/TXuKsQEWTeedweWFgv32_HealthLiteracy_CourseImage.png.

Therefore, health education methods must incorporate culturally sensitive approaches that are applicable to diverse populations. Such processes can not only promote understanding but can also inspire trust within healthcare systems, which yields improved health outcomes in a range of cultural groups (N/A, 2004). Secondly, the organization and accessibility of health materials tend to present substantial health literacy barriers. Ambiguous medical terms and poorly laid-out information can disengage patients from becoming engaged and informed. If there are no clear instructions and accessible learning resources, people are less likely to acquire essential health knowledge, thereby preventing them from making informed health decisions. To counter these challenges, it is essential to utilize user-centered resources that focus on simplicity and clarity. Resources such as the Teach-Back method can help assess patient understanding such that individuals grasp the information needed for health management. By prioritizing access to health materials and employing effective communication strategies, healthcare systems have been able to overcome significant barriers to health literacy, facilitating more participatory involvement and improved health promotion outcomes (Siskind et al., 2016) (Figure 3.13).

3.4.3. Strategies to Improve Health Literacy

Improving health literacy is a multifaceted process that involves integrated strategies for good communication and understanding of health information among populations. Education plays a significant role in the process, where specialized health education programs can be developed to meet the needs of specific demographic groups. For instance, health literacy in lower socioeconomic populations requires culturally sensitive, targeted education interventions that are highly accessible. The use of pictorial aids, in-neighborhood workshops, and interactive learning opportunities can significantly enhance understanding and engagement. As the State of Health Equity Movement, 2011 Update states, these strategies have the potential to bridge the gap in health knowledge, enabling people to make informed decisions regarding their health and wellbeing (Birnbaum et al., 2011). Enhancing health literacy also requires another important strategy: the effective dissemination of health messages through technology. Mobile applications and online sites offer new opportunities for reaching young groups, who frequently engage with technology. Health agencies can produce engaging content to encourage individuals to seek information regarding managing health and preventing disease through these media. Furthermore, increasing digital literacy among all age cohorts is essential because it has implications for individuals' capability of searching on-line health resources securely. The cyber safety report emphasizes a shift from safeguarding the user alone to promoting their digital resilience that can help them critically evaluate health information online (Third et al., 2014). The availability and ease of use of technology will also make it more likely to build health literacy. Lastly, sustaining health literacy gains entails the focus on behavior change rather than awareness. Interventions should be designed to facilitate long-term involvement and grasp of health information.

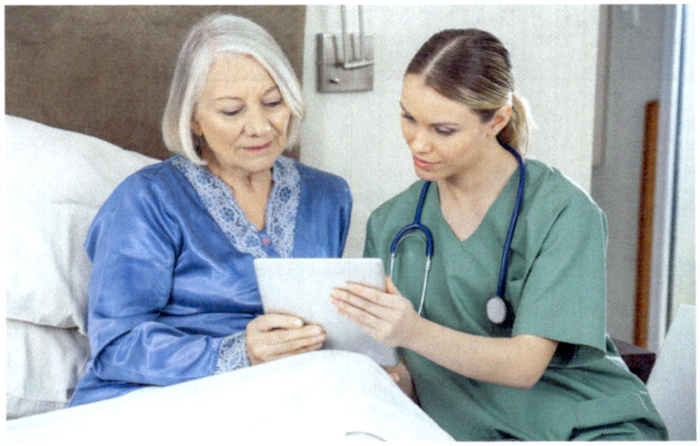

Figure 3.14. Nurses can help patients improve health literacy.

Source: https://s3.amazonaws.com/utep-uploads/wp-content/uploads/2017/04/22150239/Helping-Patients_Image-1.jpg.

This is a recursive process wherein initial educational efforts are supplemented with sustained support and aids, facilitating long-term control of health behaviors. Enabling participatory learning, whereby individuals can share their experiences and coping mechanisms for health management, creates a supportive community and fosters shared knowledge. Furthermore, stakeholder participation from different fields, including education, public health, and technology, will lead to a more harmonized approach towards improving health literacy. With the integration of novel learning methods and community engagement, effective health promotion strategies will thus implement a blend of different approaches to empower people to cope with the complexity of health information in an ever-changing environment (Figure 3.14).

Test Your Knowledge

1. What is health literacy, and why is it so critical in medical-surgical nursing?
2. Give two examples of how nurses can assess and improve a patient's health literacy.

3.5. Evaluation of Health Education Programs

Learning Outcome

1. Describe the importance of program evaluation of health education
2. Define methods in assessing the effectiveness of health education
3. Discuss the case studies of practical health education evaluation

The evaluation of health education programs is a multifaceted process that requires a nuanced understanding of various stakeholder perspectives. Central to this evaluation are the roles of the educator, parent, and community. Their participation is crucial in evaluating the effectiveness and sustainability of the programs, as well as in establishing a shared environment that fosters sustained behavioral changes among participants. By engaging these stakeholders, health education programs will be able to measure their efficacy more comprehensively and develop programs tailored to the specific needs of the population they are addressing. Such incorporation promotes an ecological model of health promotion, as identified in Bishop et al. (2014), whereby interventions address both individual and environmental determinants of educational health behaviors. Hence, evaluating such programs not only emphasizes outcomes but also places more importance on the stakeholder aspect as part of the evaluation process that contributes to the overall utility and efficacy of health education programs. Moreover, the significance of incorporating cutting-edge approaches into health education program evaluations cannot be overstated. Recent technological advances and community activities have significantly changed the manner in which health education is disseminated and assessed. Technologies such as interactive nutrition tools, educational videos, and community involvement contribute to higher understanding and participation by various populations, particularly school children. Results discussed in Harwanto et al. (2024) identify the significant relationship between these innovations and improved nutritional knowledge and behavior. The evaluation of health education programs using these contemporary strategies provides more insight into their outcomes. It facilitates continuous feedback cycles of improvement, allowing both educators and students to foster a culture of awareness that ensures the well-being of the broader community. Finally, effective health education program evaluation must also consider long-term impacts and contextual determinants of success. As noted in existing research, limitations such as a small sample size and methodological flaws may hinder the practical evaluation of program outcomes. It is imperative, therefore, that subsequent evaluations adopt longitudinal approaches involving bigger and more representative populations. It will give a larger perspective on the impact of health education interventions on change over time, particularly among at-risk populations. The suggestions of Harwanto et al. (2024) emphasize the need to draw on cross-sectoral engagement to further enhance community empowerment and mainstream health education into local policy. Ultimately, effective evaluation frameworks will ensure that health education programs are not only theoretically worthwhile but also yield meaningful and lasting benefits in practice, thereby reorienting health promotion activities in communities (Figure 3.15).

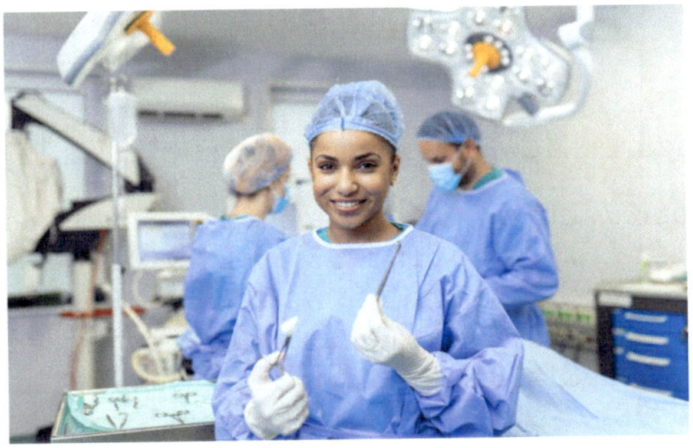

Figure 3.15. Surgical tech bridge program.

Source: https://surgicaltechuniversity.com/wp-content/uploads/2024/11/745-1.jpg.

3.5.1. Importance of Program Evaluation

Program evaluation is also a core component of the health promotion and health education strategy, as it provides a structured method for assessing the effectiveness and worth of interventions. Through the application of program evaluation, stakeholders can identify the strengths and weaknesses of health promotion activities, making informed decisions to improve health outcomes. This evaluation process benefits not just the revision of existing programs to enhance their efficacy but also informs the development of new interventions that are specifically tailored to meet the specific needs of specific populations. With changing public health contexts, the ability to think critically about programs becomes vital in addressing not just general issues of health but even particular concerns in communities, thereby creating a culture of continuous improvement and accountability in health promotion interventions. Program evaluation becomes particularly crucial in multicultural community contexts, such as those encompassing Indigenous youth. A systematic review, with a focus on the characteristics of Indigenous youth-led health promotion initiatives, highlights the need for targeted program evaluation to optimize community engagement and outcomes. While there has been a high level of interest in youth-led interventions, most of the work has shown methodological flaws, necessitating rigorous evaluation to assess the impact of such programs. Increased knowledge of Indigenous peoples' intervention mechanisms can guide future initiatives, specifically the design of culturally tailored health promotion interventions that resonate with Indigenous populations. Understanding such nuances through accurate assessment enables program developers to maximize the potential of peer-based programs, ultimately leading to enhanced health outcomes among vulnerable populations (Aguilera et al., 2018). Additionally, program evaluation helps address the youth's health-related needs, interests, and concerns in schools and colleges. The report on the assessment of health promotion activity in further education highlights evidence-based practice that can be tailored to younger groups. Findings reveal that evaluating current health promotion activity can identify , practical, and novel approaches, as well as identify those showing little or no effectiveness. Such assessments not only contribute to the empirical evidence regarding the dynamics of college students' health but also enable the design of interventions with a special emphasis on various sub-groups, e.g., those with disabilities or those with multiple health issues. Such a differentiated approach, supported by program assessment, ultimately contributes to the efficacy of health promotion strategies, making them more responsive and relevant to the unique needs of different student groups (Aggleton et al., 2008).

3.5.2. Methods for Evaluating Health Education Effectiveness

Evaluation of the efficacy of health education interventions is crucial to ensure that the approaches employed contribute to public health gains. Various methodologies can be utilized, with quantitative approaches typically of the highest priority. These strategies usually involve measuring specific health indicators both before and after the intervention to assess whether there have been any significant changes. Randomized controlled trials (RCTs), for instance, produce high-quality evidence of the effectiveness of health education interventions by comparing the intervention group with a control group. Participants in such studies are randomized in an attempt to minimize biases, allowing the researcher to attribute any improvements in health directly to the educational intervention provided. Besides, systematic reviews can consolidate outcomes from multiple studies, highlighting overall trends in the effectiveness of a given health education strategy, thereby offering a clearer picture of their impact on the populations in question. Qualitative methods also play a pivotal role in measuring the effectiveness of health education by adding depth to the quantitative findings. Through methods such as interviews, focus groups, and observational studies, researchers can measure participants' experiences and perceptions, thereby identifying obstacles to understanding and embracing health behavior change. In culturally targeted health education, for example, qualitative measurement can provide insight into the specific needs and challenges of diverse communities. This is particularly crucial in ethnic minority health programs, as studies have shown that certain groups of people may resist standard health messages. Through the use of qualitative data, health educators can refine their strategies and make interventions more relevant and effective, thereby enhancing the sustainability of long-term behavior change among diverse communities (Booth et al., 2014).

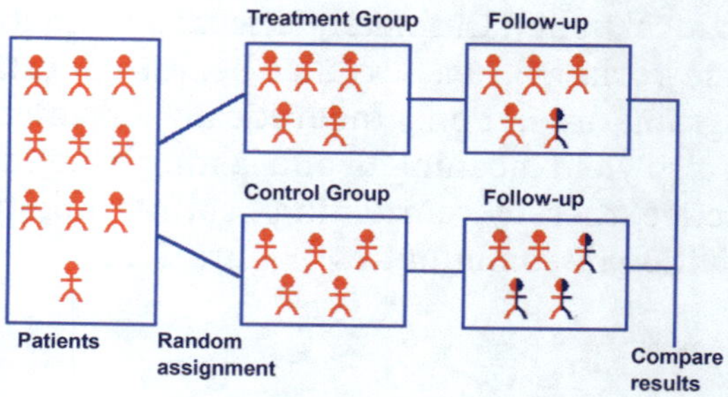

Figure 3.16. Randomized clinical trial (RCTS).

Source: https://external-content.duckduckgo.com/iu/?u=https%3A%2F%2Fwww.statisticshowto.com%2Fwp-content%2Fuploads%2F2015%2F09%2Frandomized-controlled-trial.png&f=1&nofb=1&ipt=342fa83ed85412e250078b7d19fc788cc7e1dca9c66bbaf7bb72dc2a63e979d5.

As a further benefit, mixed methods are also gaining support in assessing health education interventions because they have the capability of triangulating evidence from both quantitative and qualitative data. When numerical information is combined with people's stories, researchers can gain an accurate understanding of the reasons and mechanisms through which an educational intervention works or does not. For instance, evaluating the impact of dietary salt reduction interventions by combining evidence of effectiveness from health indicators with qualitative responses will reveal the underlying motivations and actions that inform adherence to recommended changes. Beyond offering a description of the intervention's immediate impact, this places the findings within the social and cultural contexts where they occur. This simultaneous focus on outcomes, in addition to participant experience, can enhance the quality of design in future health promotion strategies, making them both evidence-based and community-appropriate (Mayaleh et al., 2014) (Figure 3.16).

3.5.3. Case Studies of Successful Evaluations

Health promotion strategy evaluation is crucial for understanding effectiveness and adaptability across diverse populations. Effective evaluation case studies often target interventions that have been demonstrated to improve health outcomes for specific groups. Examples include initiatives to improve the physical and emotional well-being of students in continuing education. Evaluations aim to inform on key issues related to the health-related needs, interests, and concerns of 14–19-year-olds, providing valuable insights into effective health promotion. By uncovering best practices and understanding which approaches resonate most with particular populations, stakeholders can design tailored efforts that meaningfully address students about the importance of caring for their health and well-being. This evidence-informed approach emphasizes the importance of continuous evaluation and updating in health education practices, utilizing successful case studies as guiding tools for future program planning (Aggleton et al., 2008). Additionally, evaluating social and emotional well-being health promotion interventions adds another layer of understanding what works. Among the features of effective evaluations is programs tailored explicitly for Indigenous populations, where the focus on social and emotional well-being is placed solidly in cultural contexts. Interventions that promote mental well-being and mental health, particularly those piloted in urban and rural environments, reveal significant relationships between supportive community systems and beneficial effects on health. Evaluations that record these culturally tailored models demonstrate how context plays a role in health promotion activities and illustrate how community-based interventions can effectively enhance participants' resilience and coping abilities. The findings from these evaluations yield essential lessons that are transferable to contemporary health practice and policy development, reminding us to adapt approaches for varying cultural contexts to maximize overall impact (Papajcsik, 2025). The application of case studies on model evaluations also proves the long-term sustainability of health education programs. When programs are systematically examined, they not only identify short-term results, such as behavior change, but also track the longitudinal effects on health trajectories of participants. For example, techniques that prove successful in smoking cessation among young adults can be analyzed to identify the most prominent elements that lead to long-term behavioral changes. These findings are crucial for planning programs that will endure by creating environments that promote sustained health benefits. Second, having the details of what works for specific groups of people allows for the targeted implementation of best practices, making health education interventions not only efficient but also practical. Ultimately, the exploration of effective evaluations strengthens the debate of health promotion strategies, allowing evidence-based models to thrive across different educational settings (Aggleton et al., 2008).

Test Your Knowledge

1. What is the importance of the evaluation of medical-surgical health education programs?
2. What are the steps for program evaluation of a health education program?

3.6. Challenges in Health Education and Promotion

Learning Outcome

1. Describe the socioeconomic determinants of health education
2. Define the cultural barriers to health promotion
3. Discuss combating misinformation in health education

Health education and promotion are confronted with numerous challenges that short-circuit effective dissemination of vital information to various groups. Among the key challenges is the disconnection between theory and practice. Programs in most institutions focus on theoretical training, which might disengage students and make it difficult for them to apply lessons in real-life situations. This constraint not only affects student involvement but also undermines the effectiveness of follow-up health education interventions. Furthermore, the character of health issues, which routinely require multidisciplinary intervention, calls for robust coordination between schools and community agencies to develop curriculum designs that are meaningfully connected and responsive to community demands. The participation of students through experiential, hands-on instruction, as observed in partnerships between students, faculty, and community partners, can bring legitimacy to health education modules and better equip future healthcare professionals (Kempenaar et al., 2018). Furthermore, addressing health disparities presents an additional layer of complexity for health education and promotion programs. Rural or impoverished communities often have limited access to fundamental healthcare and education, resulting in persistent public health issues. The best example is the under-five mortality rate in developing countries, which is a far too high proportion, and a significant contribution to this has been inadequate health education in communities. Traditional health worker roles, such as "tumpuroo" in Sulawesi, Indonesia, demonstrate the mechanism by which gaps in health education can be bridged through community involvement and the promotion of essential health practices. However, the effectiveness of these initiatives is typically undermined by inadequate governmental support and coordination with local organizations. Thus, incorporating community-based health workers into health promotion strategies has proven crucial in ensuring health education reaches vulnerable populations, ultimately improving health outcomes (Muis et al., 2018). Finally, evaluating the effectiveness of health education programs poses a significant challenge, often leaving educators without adequate feedback on their practices. The nuances of the measurement equation of behavior change and health outcomes may make it difficult for researchers to establish the complete impact of many methods used in education. Conventional measures may not capture the cultural frames of reference that influence and shape health behaviors at both community and individual levels and, therefore, mask the effectiveness of utilized strategies. Thus, health educators need to design new models of evaluation considering the social determinants of health and the needs of specific target populations. With a culture of continuous improvement and adjustment of interventions based on constant evaluation, health education and promotion programs could be enhanced and suitable for various populations (Kempenaar et al., 2018) (Figure 3.17).

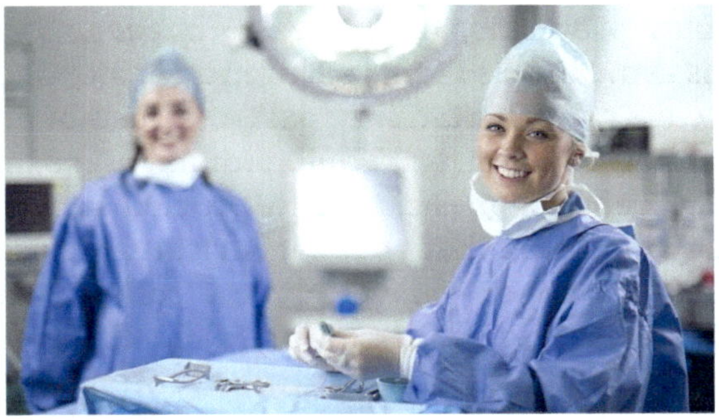

Figure 3.17. Day in the life and duties of a surgical nurse.

Source: https://www.fortis.edu/blog/nursing/a-day-in-the-life-and-duties-of-a-surgical-nurse/_jcr_content/blog/image.coreimg.jpeg/1548460608914/a-day-in-the-life-and-duties-of-a-surgical-nurse.jpeg.

3.6.1. Socioeconomic Factors Affecting Health Education

The overlap of socioeconomic determinants and health education reveals significant disparities that could affect the health outcomes of individuals and communities. There is evidence that health disparities are not entirely the result of biological factors but are, to a large degree, influenced by the social determinants of health, such as income, educational level, and occupation. Increased socioeconomic status is typically associated with higher health literacy, enabling individuals to effectively use and acquire health information. For to a lack of knowledge about health services and preventive interventions among individuals from lower socioeconomic backgrounds. Such disparities require targeted health education interventions that consider the particular challenges faced by disadvantaged groups, and with the resultant demand for policy interventions to address these underlying social determinants and improve equity of access to health education (Bambra et al., 2018). Moreover, community-based health education has also been a crucial method of reversing the negative adverse effects of socioeconomic factors on health. Community initiatives with relevant content that reflects the community's culture are seen to promote participation and have a positive impact. Social enterprises tackling the initiative on community food, for instance, not only provide healthy food but also enhance the social networks for healthy living. In addressing both the determinants of individual behavior and the broader social environment, these initiatives demonstrate how health can be enhanced through community involvement. Similarly, the study maintains that social enterprises impact various levels of social determinants of health, but are particularly effective in building community resilience and capacity when it comes to addressing health inequities, thereby making comprehensive health education even more imperative (Gordon et al., 2017). Lastly, the integration of socioeconomic considerations into health education curricula is crucial for promoting health equity. By recognizing the constraints imposed by socioeconomic disparities, health education can create programs that are both informative and empowering. Implementing health education tailored to the specific health concerns of low-income and marginalized groups can ensure the maximum effectiveness of health promotion programs. Moreover, gathering stakeholders from various sectors, such as education, healthcare, and social services, will foster more holistic health education. This partnership is essential in developing interventions that fill the void created by socioeconomic inequalities, ultimately leading to more equal health outcomes for all. Continuous examination of health education interventions from a socioeconomic viewpoint will ensure that interventions remain up-to-date and effective in addressing the population heterogeneity (Gordon et al., 2017; Bambra et al., 2018) (Figure 3.18).

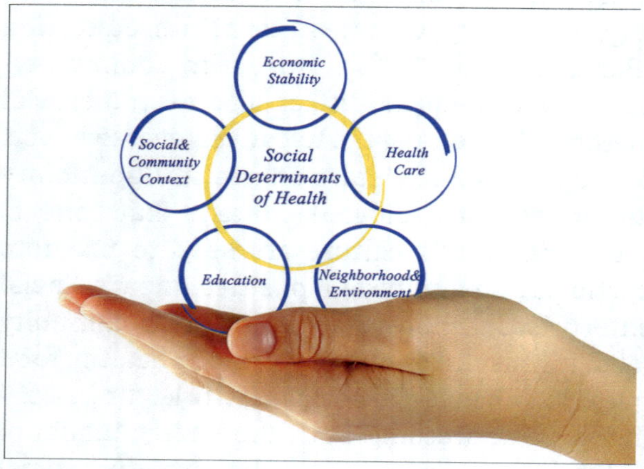

Figure 3.18. Socioeconomic factors play significant role in health.

Source: https://physicians.dukehealth.org/sites/default/files/article/Issue-151_GenMed_Endo_870x300.jpg.

3.6.2. Cultural Barriers to Health Promotion

Cultural barriers significantly impede effective health promotion, often expressed through attitudes and beliefs that influence health behaviors. They result from deeply ingrained societal norms and expectations that shape the way specific groups engage with health education and preventive care. For instance, cultural constructs of masculinity can create resistance to accessing medical services for men, who view vulnerability as unmanly. These views contribute to a denial pattern among men for their health issues, as indicated by the answers during a workshop among behavioral and social researchers aimed at men's health. The agreement exhibited suggests the manner in which societal constructs not only affect individual health choices but also undermine broader public health consequences by sustaining unhealthy lifestyles and enhancing stigma surrounding health management interventions (McHugh et al., 2004). Within specific populations, there may also be cultural barriers, supplemented by socioeconomic determinants, that limit access to healthcare resources. For instance, studies of African American men revealed the Ostrich Behavior phenomenon, in which individuals deliberately eschew resolution of health problems, in this case, hypertension. This avoidance is often rooted in a constellation of cultural orientations, past distrust of the healthcare system, and economic limitations that make frequent physician visits problematic. The study indicated that younger African American men aged 18–45 years have less contact with healthcare practitioners, which shows the need for culturally appropriate interventions that capture the attention of their world. There is a need for health educators to understand these hindrances in order to formulate effective health promotion interventions that address not only clinical aspects but also social and cultural dynamics influencing health behaviors (Slack-Gay et al., 2017). To overcome the cultural barriers to health promotion, it is essential to design health education programs that are responsive and inclusive of diverse cultures. This entails not only identifying prevailing beliefs and practices prevalent among target communities but also engaging them directly in designing health promotion efforts. Culturally appropriate materials attuned to the values and experiences of target groups can help encourage involvement and participation in health programs. Furthermore, building partnerships with stakeholders and community leaders can facilitate the building of trust and promote open dialogue concerning health. Through carefully bridging cultural divides, health promotion interventions can empower populations to adopt healthy lifestyles, hence contributing to improved health among various populations. This integrated approach is crucial in creating a culture of health that transcends divides and fosters integral well-being.

3.6.3. Addressing Misinformation in Health Education

In contemporary health education, misinformation management is of central importance, as digital media facilitate the dissemination of accurate information and the spread of errors. Misinformation, especially regarding vaccines, is a central public health concern, leading to vaccine hesitancy and undermining trust in health systems. McGee et al. (2020) define vaccine hesitancy as being typified by refusal to immunize, often based on complex social and emotional motivations. Health educators must utilize effective communication channels to dispel such myths. This entails the spread of evidence-based information that targets the values and fears of the target group, thus establishing a culture of support for informed decision-making. Through direct and compassionate strategy in conflict resolution, health practitioners can help guide unwilling people to get vaccinations and appreciate their role in public health. The role of healthcare providers in the battle against disinformation extends beyond individual consultation; it involves an active role at the community level. Effective health education must involve reputable sources, i.e., predominantly healthcare providers who are generally regarded as reliable informants regarding vaccines (McGee et al., 2020). Educators may utilize models such as the C.A.S.E. Model, emphasizing clear communication, active listening, caring, and empathy when discussing vaccine hesitancy. Additionally, incorporating community involvement can significantly enhance the success of health promotion campaigns. Encouraging discourse among communities has the potential to demolish barriers of mistrust and misinformation, leading to a common understanding of health practices. Unite as one, health providers can overcome misinformation and reinforce public confidence in vaccinations and other health initiatives. Moreover, financial disinformation expenditures in health promotion should not be overlooked, as evidenced by requests for more funds in effective health education initiatives. Although health promotion programs are currently a significant part of healthcare expenditure, their visibility and impact can spur more investment in countering disinformation. Anti-smoking, pro-exercise, and immunization campaign investment is needed not just to augment health in the population but also to reduce reliance on curative care. As health educators encourage multi-faceted interventions against misinformation, they must also emphasize long-term investment in health promotion activities. Lastly, the development of refined health education models will lead to improved health outcomes and an educated public, capable of understanding the complexities of modern health information (Figure 3.19).

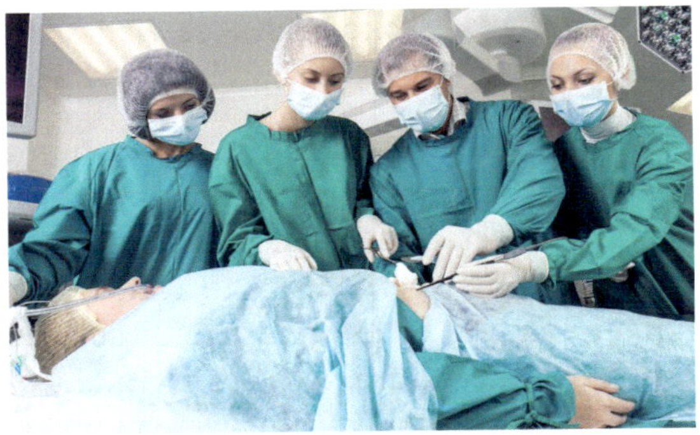

Figure 3.19. Circulating nurse.

Source: https://images.wisegeek.com/team-of-surgeons-in-operating-room.jpg.

Test Your Knowledge

1. What are two common barriers medical-surgical nurses face in providing health education to patients?
2. How can cultural beliefs impact the success of health promotion programs?

SUMMARY

Public health outcomes continue to require effective health education and promotion practices. As the essay demonstrates, the use of social media websites has emerged as a compelling mechanism for disseminating health information in an effective and timely manner. The latest studies reveal that health planners and decision-makers recognize the role of websites in health promotional campaigns. However, the process of balancing getting a large population exposed to health information and overcoming problems like misinformation requires thoughtful planning and strategization. Prioritizing two-way relationships in the communication of public and health promotion workers can potentially create an environment supportive of trust and participation, thereby strengthening the effectiveness of health promotion programs (Alanazi et al., 2025). Additionally, assessment of some health status, for instance, single breastfeeding amongst Arab origins, reflects the types of complexities in promoting health education amongst multicultural groups. Socio-demographic and cultural determinants influencing breastfeeding practices had a critical impact on health education policy. Intervening on the factors of maternal age, religiosity, and geographic heterogeneity will yield better and more targeted public health interventions. This further emphasizes the necessity of health promotion interventions making use of cultural competencies and addressing the unique circumstances of a wide range of populations in order to make health messages audible and recognizable to the very populations that are being addressed (Awawdi et al., 2025). Finally, the necessity of firm policy guidelines to direct health promotion interventions cannot be overstressed. Effective health policy must balance thorough stakeholder perspectives, including those of health professionals, social media outlets, and client populations. As robust networks of allies, they can exchange ideas and best practices and must contend with ethical dilemmas surrounding privacy and misinformation. Through the activation of partnerships, public health programs can create an educated population more inclined to engage in health promotion activities preemptively. Therefore, ongoing evaluation and updating of such strategies remain a high priority for providing long-term improvements in public health, as well as the continuous development of the health environment (Alanazi et al., 2025; Awawdi et al., 2025).

Following the role of health education and health promotion strategies, importance must be assigned to the role of culturally appropriate interventions. It has been evidenced that gaps in knowledge of the particular health needs of various groups, including minority ethnic groups, refugees, and Gypsy Travelers in Wales, exist. A systematic approach to identifying gaps provides an understanding of existing health services and promotes best practices. Of most significance, it is noted in literature, is the enactment of health promotion programs and policy in culturally appropriate and socially inclusive manners (Aspinall et al., 2006). Such well-matched strategies not only enhance participation but also engender trust and efficacy with target groups. Generally, these interventions for specific health promotion issues provide equitable access to health information and services, which further enhances the public health impact among underprivileged communities. Equally urgent is the intersectionality of the environment with health promotion, particularly in the context of water, sanitation, and hygiene (WASH) practices. Increasing evidence suggests that improved WASH conditions have an essential role to play in nutrition, particularly in nations like Bangladesh, where undernutrition is a matter of considerable concern. Through a systematic review of published and grey literature, the impact of improved WASH facilities on nutritional well-being was assessed against an underused determinant of health promotion debates (Mahmud et al., 2016). Through the integration of WASH enhancement and nutrition education, public health can develop a comprehensive model for addressing disease causes through health promotion interventions. Those multicomponent interventions, in turn, aim to break the cycle of poverty and eliminate health inequalities, particularly among vulnerable population groups. Moreover, the effectiveness of health promotion and education interventions relies on continuous monitoring and adjustment of activities in response to new evidence and feedback from the people. This adaptive process makes the interventions effective and appropriate in addressing the ever-evolving health needs of the population. Prioritization of areas to be further explored is necessary, particularly in areas where vulnerable populations are at risk of exclusion from access to health information and services (Aspinall et al., 2006). By fostering an inquiry-based and responsive culture, health education programs can be more effective in developing sustainable health outcomes. As health promotion approaches change, incorporating feedback from various communities ensures that they not only enhance short-term requirements but also enable people to to establish a culture of health extending beyond the program's life. Such an active policy lays the groundwork for long-term improvements in population health.

KEY TERMS FROM THIS CHAPTER

- Barriers to Learning
- Communication Skills
- Cultural Sensitivity
- Empowerment
- Group Education
- Health Literacy
- Lifestyle Modification
- Preventive Strategies
- Behavior Change
- Community Involvement
- Educational Materials
- Goal Setting
- Health Belief Model
- Health Promotion Models
- Motivational Interviewing
- Program Evaluation

CRITICAL THINKING QUESTIONS

1. **What is the fundamental aim of health education?**
   a. To diagnose and treat disease
   b. To cure chronic illness
   c. To offer individuals information that they can apply to make informed choices about their health
   d. To replace physician care
2. **What is one method of health promotion?**
   a. Treating medication
   b. Teaching hand hygiene in schools
   c. Prescribing antibiotics
   d. Surgery
3. **What is one fundamental feature of effective health promotion?**
   a. Treats disease alone
   b. Involves community participation and empowerment
   c. Rely solely on government policy
   d. Targets only healthcare professionals
4. **The Ottawa Charter describes the number of basic action areas for health promotion?**
   a. 3
   b. 5
   c. 7
   d. 10
5. **Which of the following most accurately describes health promotion?**
   a. A hospital-based intervention to treat acute illness
   b. A process of enabling people to gain greater control over and to improve their health
   c. Educating doctors in surgery
   d. Drugs to the elderly

Short Answer Questions

1. Define health education and its overall goal.
2. Mention any two strategies that are practiced generally in health education.
3. What is the difference between health education and health promotion?
4. Mention any two principles of effective health education.
5. What is the nurse's role in health promotion?
6. Identify the key elements of a successful health promotion plan with examples.
7. Identify the five action areas of the Ottawa Charter for Health Promotion.
8. Identify why the participation of people guarantees maximum success of health education programs.
9. Evaluate the application of health education in the prevention and control of non-communicable diseases.
10. Compare and contrast the medical, educational, and socio-environmental models of health promotion.

Answers to Critical Thinking Questions

1. (c); 2. (b); 3. (b); 4. (b); 5. (b)

REFERENCES

1. Mason, H., Shoaibi, A., Ghandour, R., O'Flaherty, M., Capewell, S., Khatib, R., Jabr, S., Unal, B., Sözmen, K., Arfa, C., Aissi, W., Romdhane, H. B., Fouad, F., Al-Ali, R., & Husseini, A. (2014). A cost effectiveness analysis of salt reduction policies to reduce coronary heart disease in four eastern Mediterranean countries. *PLoS ONE*, *9*(1), e84445. https://doi.org/10.1371/journal.pone.0084445Aggleton, P., Statham, J., & Warwick, I. (2008). Healthy and health promoting colleges – An evidence base. https://core.ac.uk/download/pdf/82100.pdf (accessed on 28th June 2025).
2. Aguilera, A., Bauman, A., Bentley, M., Biggs, J., Carpenter, K., Cobb-Clark, D., Cochran, S., et al. (2018). Indigenous youth peer-led health promotion in Canada, New Zealand, Australia, and the United States: A systematic review of the approaches, study designs, and effectiveness. https://core.ac.uk/download/213607663.pdf (accessed on 28th June 2025).
3. Anand, R., Bakhuys Roozeboom, M., Berkhout, S., Boyatzis, R., Braun, V., Bryman, A., Centers for Disease Control & Prevention, et al. (2015). Examples of holistic good practices in promoting and protecting mental health in the workplace: Current and future challenges. https://core.ac.uk/download/33575818.pdf (accessed on 28th June 2025).
4. Aspinall, P. J. (2006). Main findings and recommendations. https://core.ac.uk/download/91082.pdf (accessed on 28th June 2025).
5. Awawdi, K., Yahya, O., Sabbah, M., Bisharat, S., & Tarabeih, M. (2025). Factors influencing exclusive breastfeeding amongst Arab mothers in Israel: Social, cultural, and occupational aspects. *Healthcare, 13*. https://www.semanticscholar.org/paper/ea1b4e216bcafc66e7aece32dd41554a1343dc6c (accessed on 28th June 2025).
6. Bakos, A., et al. (2017). Implementation of the National Partnership for Action to End Health Disparities: A three-year retrospective. https://digitalscholarship.unlv.edu/cgi/viewcontent.cgi?article=1640&context=jhdrp (accessed on 28th June 2025).
7. Bambra, C., Forster, T., & Kentikelenis, A. (2018). Health inequalities in Europe: Setting the stage for progressive policy action. https://core.ac.uk/download/199426311.pdf (accessed on 28th June 2025).
8. Bandura, A., Carroll, A., Drewnowski, A., Kafatos, A., Kirmani, A., Papadaki, A., Richards, A., et al. (2014). Social marketing and healthy eating: Findings from young people in Greece. https://core.ac.uk/download/29843393.pdf (accessed on 28th June 2025).
9. Barrena Martínez, J., Llinàs Audet, F. J., & Ramos-Monge, E. (2019). Drivers and barriers of university social responsibility: Integration into strategic plans. https://core.ac.uk/download/157810895.pdf (accessed on 28th June 2025).
10. Belton, S., Issartel, J., & O'Brien, W. (2017). Promoting physical literacy in Irish adolescent youth: The Youth-Physical Activity Towards Health (Y-PATH) intervention. https://core.ac.uk/download/84073833.pdf (accessed on 28th June 2025).
11. Biediger-Friedman, L., & Reed, D. (2010). An assessment of US college food environments: From food service to college students. https://core.ac.uk/download/43630807.pdf (accessed on 28th June 2025).
12. Birnbaum, N., Masterson, E., & Schoomaker, H. (2011). State of Health Equity Movement, 2011 update Part C: Compendium of recommendations. DRA Project Report No. 11-03. https://core.ac.uk/download/pdf/18491812.pdf (accessed on 28th June 2025).

13. Birnbaum, N., Masterson, E., & Schoomaker, H. (2011). State of Health Equity Movement, 2011 update Part B: Catalog of activities. DRA Project Report No. 11-02. https://core.ac.uk/download/pdf/18491811.pdf (accessed on 28th June 2025).

14. Bishop, D., Evans, A. B., Evans, D., Keegan, R., et al. (2014). The importance of parents and teachers as stakeholders in school-based healthy eating programs. https://core.ac.uk/download/17171089.pdf (accessed on 28th June 2025).

15. Booth, A., Gardois, P., Goyder, E., Ryan, J., et al. (2014). Health promotion interventions for increasing stroke awareness in ethnic minorities: A systematic review of the literature. https://core.ac.uk/download/30269912.pdf (accessed on 28th June 2025).

16. Buja, A., Casuccio, A., Cecconi, R., Contu, P., et al. (2015). Professional competencies in health promotion and public health: What is common and what is specific? Review of the European debate and perspectives for professional development. https://core.ac.uk/download/301569768.pdf (accessed on 28th June 2025).

17. Carraro, A., Gobbi, E., Maselli, M., Ward, P., et al. (2018). Promoting physical activity among university students: A systematic review of controlled trials. https://core.ac.uk/download/154330550.pdf (accessed on 28th June 2025).

18. Cawood, J., Doherty, S., Dooris, M. T., Powell, J., et al. (2010). Healthy universities: Concept, model and framework for applying the healthy settings approach within higher education in England. https://core.ac.uk/download/6113134.pdf (accessed on 28th June 2025).

19. Cole, G. E., Holtgrave, D. R., & Rios, N. M. (1993). Systematic development of trans-theoretically based behavioral risk management programs. https://core.ac.uk/download/72056919.pdf (accessed on 28th June 2025).

20. Connelly, L. (2025). Welfarist and non-welfarist conceptions of "health promotion." https://core.ac.uk/download/pdf/6438637.pdf (accessed on 28th June 2025).

21. Dawson, A., Fowler, C., & Lam, W. (2017). The role of culture in relation to the seasonal influenza prevention practices of Hong Kong Chinese parents with preschool children. https://opus.lib.uts.edu.au/bitstream/10453/123435/4/The%20role%20of%20culutre_HK%20parent%20health%20practices%202017.pdf (accessed on 28th June 2025).

22. Doherty, S. H., & Dooris, M. T. (2009). National research and development project on healthy universities: Final report. https://core.ac.uk/download/6113091.pdf (accessed on 28th June 2025).

23. Drabble, L. A., Keatley, J., & Marcelle, G. (2003). Progress and opportunities in lesbian, gay, bisexual and transgender health communications. https://core.ac.uk/download/70410107.pdf (accessed on 28th June 2025).

24. Fadhil, A., Lange, J. P., Reiterer, H., Wang, Y., et al. (2018). Integrating taxonomies into theory-based digital health interventions for behavior change: A holistic framework. http://arxiv.org/abs/1810.08812 (accessed on 28th June 2025).

25. Farida, S., Priyanto, K. E., & Suhita, B. (2017). Implementation of health promotion strategies in the integrated service post park programs at the Public Health Center Pesantren I Kediry City. https://media.neliti.com/media/publications/236639-implementation-of-health-promotion-strat-9feb0671.pdf (accessed on 28th June 2025).

26. Gordon, K., Shaw, E., Tonner, A., Wilson, F., et al. (2017). How can social enterprises impact

health and wellbeing? https://core.ac.uk/download/77036381.pdf (accessed on 28th June 2025).

27. Hari, G. (2017). Depression in low-income adolescents: Guidelines for school-based depression intervention programs. https://core.ac.uk/download/130354083.pdf (accessed on 28th June 2025).
28. Harwanto, F., Saci, M. A., Arigo, Y., & Indah, Y. (2024). Innovation in nutrition promotion: Literature analysis to increase community awareness and healthy practices. https://core.ac.uk/download/617989014.pdf (accessed on 28th June 2025).
29. Hughes, E., & Rawlins, M. L. (2015). Preventive counseling without borders: Using mobile devices for teaching, training, and wellness promotion. https://core.ac.uk/download/48834700.pdf (accessed on 28th June 2025).
30. Kempenaar, L. E., & Shanmugam, S. (2018). The shared learning journey: Effective partnerships to deliver health promotion. https://core.ac.uk/download/293864909.pdf (accessed on 28th June 2025).
31. Lawson, K., Yocum, S., et al. (2019). Health coaching case report: Optimizing employee health and wellbeing in organizations. https://core.ac.uk/download/223117465.pdf (accessed on 28th June 2025).
32. Mahmud, I., & Mbuya, N. (2016). Water, sanitation, hygiene, and nutrition in Bangladesh: Can building toilets affect children's growth? https://core.ac.uk/download/75783689.pdf (accessed on 28th June 2025).
33. McGee, L. U., & Suh, J. (2020). Communication strategies to address vaccine hesitancy in healthcare settings and on social media. https://core.ac.uk/download/323216373.pdf (accessed on 28th June 2025).
34. McHugh, B., Estrine, J., & Moran, R. (2004). Promoting men's health: Addressing barriers to healthy lifestyle and preventive health care. https://core.ac.uk/download/71356600.pdf (accessed on 28th June 2025).
35. Mende, C. M. (2020). Health promotion for tobacco control. https://core.ac.uk/download/287193231.pdf (accessed on 28th June 2025).
36. Mendes, R., Plaza, V., & Wallerstein, N. (2016). Sustainability and power in health promotion: Community-based participatory research in a reproductive health policy case study in New Mexico. https://core.ac.uk/download/328367411.pdf (accessed on 28th June 2025).
37. Muis, E. W. (2018). Tempura as a local community health worker to support for family with children under five. https://media.neliti.com/media/publications/275350-tumpuroo-as-a-local-community-health-wor-1f6b70fe.pdf (accessed on 28th June 2025).
38. Munoz, C., Rosenoff, E., Sepulveda, E., Coffman, J., Grumbach, K., & Gandara, P. (2003). Strategies for improving the diversity of the health professions. https://core.ac.uk/download/71355240.pdf (accessed on 28th June 2025).
39. O'Hara, P. (2005). Creating social and health equity: Adopting an Alberta social determinants of health framework. https://core.ac.uk/download/71343870.pdf (accessed on 28th June 2025).
40. Ouchi, F. (2025). A literature review on the use of expert opinion in probabilistic risk analysis. https://core.ac.uk/download/pdf/6644569.pdf (accessed on 28th June 2025).

41. Papajcsik, I. (2025). Strategies and practices for promoting the social and emotional wellbeing of Aboriginal and Torres Strait Islander people. https://core.ac.uk/download/pdf/30677387.pdf (accessed on 28th June 2025).
42. Reddy, M. (2015). A framework for integrated school oral health promotion within the Health Promoting Schools Initiative in KwaZulu-Natal. https://core.ac.uk/download/288926112.pdf (accessed on 28th June 2025).
43. Sarmanlu, D., Maindal, H. T., Heuck, I. R., Ryom, K., & Lim, M. H. (2024). Health literacy and loneliness among physically inactive Danes aged 18–65: A cross-sectional study. https://core.ac.uk/download/634250197.pdf (accessed on 28th June 2025).
44. Sauer, L., & Wolsky, L. (2012). Developing an occupational therapy community/client wellness program. https://core.ac.uk/download/235073426.pdf (accessed on 28th June 2025).
45. Siskind, S. M. (2016). Promoting strategies to overcome low health literacy and improve patient understanding in outpatient setting. https://core.ac.uk/download/79664921.pdf (accessed on 28th June 2025).
46. Slack-Gay, D. (2017). African American men and ostrich behavior. https://core.ac.uk/download/70427184.pdf (accessed on 28th June 2025).
47. Third, A., Collier, A., & Forrest-Lawrence, P. (2014). Addressing the cyber safety challenge: From risk to resilience. https://core.ac.uk/download/pdf/30674272.pdf (accessed on 28th June 2025).

ASSESSMENT OF ADULT HEALTH: PHYSICAL, NUTRITIONAL, AND CULTURAL DIMENSIONS

4

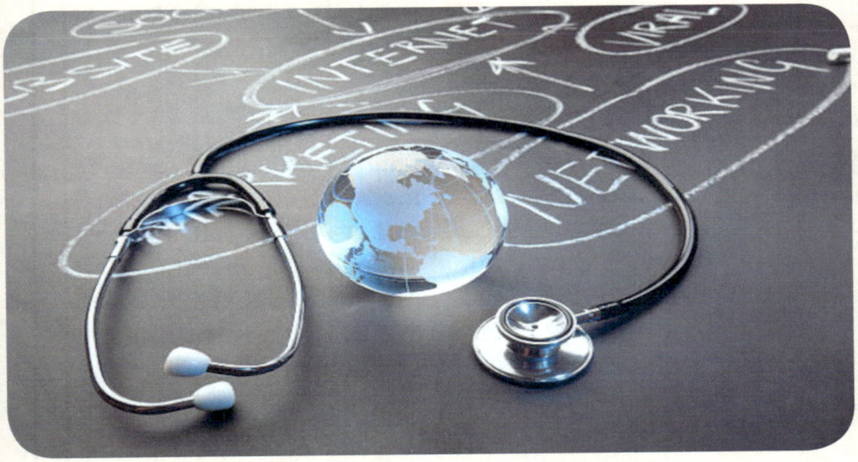

LEARNING OBJECTIVES

After studying this chapter, you will be able to:

1. Understand the physical health assessment
2. Describe the nutritional health assessment
3. Discuss cultural dimensions of health
4. Emphasize the interrelationship between physical and nutritional health
5. Mention socioeconomic factors in health assessment
6. Define technology in health assessment

Introduction

Adult health is an assessment that integrates an account of the physical, nutritional, and cultural. This theoretical background is crucial in understanding how the various determinants interact and impact the health status of the adult population. The assessment is not merely physical; it incorporates lifestyle choice, food intake, and the socio-cultural settings that affect people's health behavior. An understanding of the interaction between these dimensions can guide health professionals in crafting balanced interventions that promote well-being and prevent chronic disorders. Furthermore, this holistic perspective allows for the identification of target populations to intervene upon, highlighting the value of shaping healthcare practice in a way that responds to differing needs. Nutrition is the cornerstone for evaluating adult health and plays a critical role in physical well-being and overall health. Malnutrition leads to numerous health issues like obesity, heart disease, and type 2 diabetes, and hence it is incredibly crucial to be armed with efficient nutritional assessment tools. In consideration of the recent research, climate change and global socio-economic disparity render the nutrition issue elevated and affect the availability of healthy food to the majority of the population. It requires intersectoral coordination to adopt sustainable behaviors towards achieving healthy diets. The relationships between nutrition and health outcomes are pressing and underscore the need to strengthen the evaluation of nutrition in guiding the development of efficient public health policies to address these essential problems.

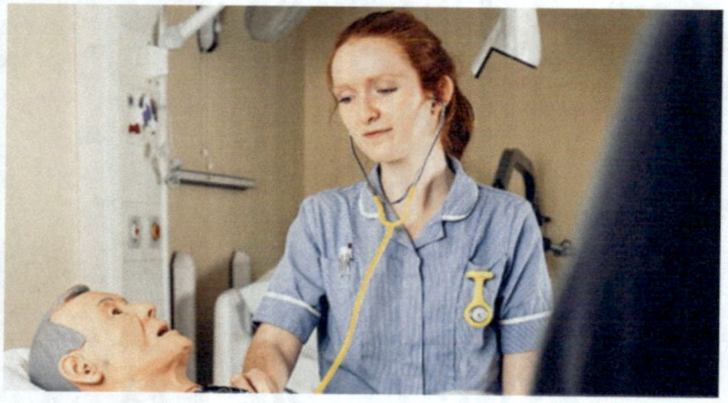

Figure 4.1. Adult health.

Source: https://external-content.duckduckgo.com/iu/?u=https%3A%2F%2Fwww.bournemouth.ac.uk%2Fsites%2Fdefault%2Ffiles%2Fstyles%2Fb_16_9_desktop%2Fpublic%2Fassets%2Fimages%2Fadult-nursing-2-portrait.jpg%3Fitok%3DnrhVYqZy&f=1&nofb=1&ipt=0b8fcb708f944a875d836cec5b1083cfb36f5aaaeac1805b9573a471d20591f0.

Cultural determinants play a vital role in evaluating adult health because they influence individuals' ideas and practices regarding nutrition and health. Cultural beliefs and practices can yield deep insights into diet, food choices, and the utilization of healthcare. Cultural considerations can also affect the effectiveness of health interventions, and therefore, culturally tailored strategies should be integrated into health assessments. The intersection of culture, nutrition, and body well-being recognizes the mechanisms through which social norms influence consumption and overall health. With involved complexities, critical analysis beyond measurement of the physical kind is called for. This is vital in considering how cultural contexts influence lived realities, i.e., in understanding and responding to the implications of issues such as those elaborated in Gillespie et al. (2025) and the United Nations System Standing Committee on Nutrition (2020), which identify determinants of health within a systemic context (Figure 4.1).

Definition of Adult Health

Understanding what adult health entails requires a thorough assessment of its multifaceted nature, encompassing not only physical health but also nutritional and cultural aspects. Adult health can be understood as a state of being physically, mentally, and socially healthy in individuals aged 18 years and above, aside from the mere absence of disease. This definition is system-focused in a holistic sense, knowing that lifestyle choices, psychological resilience, and social support systems are determinants of health outcomes to a great extent. For instance, diets are a determinant of the increasing rates of diabetes and cardiovascular conditions, with adult health implications of intervening in diet behavior being part of it (Vila et al., 2018). Therefore, adult health screening must be multifaceted and take into account physical fitness, nutritional status, and cultural determinants of individuals' perceptions and behaviors on health. Cultural determinants also play a significant role in determining the health of adults. Attitudes and behavior patterns of culture contribute significantly to health behavior formation, access to health care, and overall health. Individuals from diverse backgrounds may hold varying perceptions regarding illness, treatment, and well-being, which can influence their engagement with healthcare systems. Certain cultural practices will promote the use of traditional healing methods over mainstream medicine, with broader implications for health outcomes and patient compliance. Furthermore, cultural determinants such as support networks, household structure, and community resources are significant forces that modify attitudes and behaviors related to health. Changes in health assessment tools, for example, cross-cultural adaptation of Readiness for Hospital Discharge Scale for application in Brazil, show the need for culturally appropriate approaches in health assessment procedures (Vila C et al., 2018). The awareness broadens adult health beyond tight physiological estimates. Nutritional health is a key part of the adult health definition and measurement, as it encompasses food literacy and healthy eating habits that are central to preventing chronic diseases. Food literacy entails an understanding of the complex food environment in terms of food decision, preparation, and knowledge of nutrition that, cumulatively, optimizes health gain. As has been made evident by current evidence, policy, social, and psychological determinants constitute food literacy, which cumulatively build people's food-related skills (Leal et al., 2019). The skills have a direct impact on dietary practice and nutrition status, which indirectly impacts adult health in general. not just quantify physical health, but also assess nutritional behavior and awareness of individuals, so that interventions are made available to enhance food literacy and health awareness in various populations. Incorporating the three components—physical, nutritional, and cultural—into the paradigm of adult health yields a more pragmatic and integrated approach to evaluation (Figure 4.2).

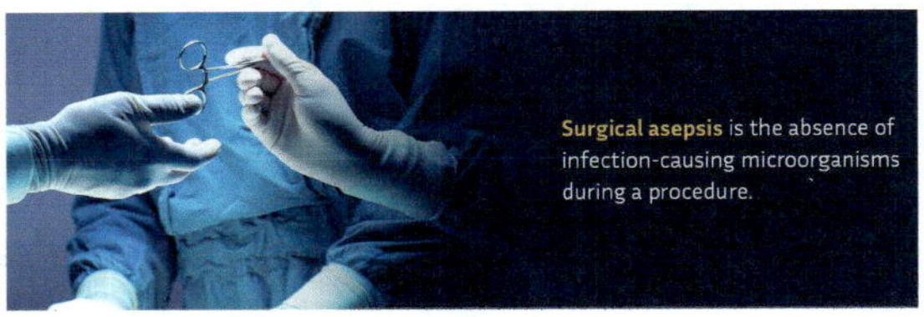

Figure 4.2. Surgical-asepsis.

Source: https://jewelprecision.com/wp-content/uploads/2022/08/02-surgical-asepsis.png.

Importance of a Holistic Assessment

Holistic assessment is essential in the context of adults' health because it provides a complete picture encompassing physical, dietary, and cultural factors. It surpasses traditional evaluation techniques, which can be limited to biological markers, to encompass all the factors in patients' lives that contribute to their well-being. It is this multi-dimensional view that recognizes that health is more than the lack of disease and is shaped by a myriad of influences affecting the quality of individuals' lives. In practice, the nursing role is increasingly recognized to require holistic assessments as highlighted in the majority of conferences and holistic nursing care literature. This is evidence of an understanding that effective care must consider the social, economic, and environmental context of individuals to enable healthcare professionals to design more targeted and effective interventions (Nurmalia (Editor) et al., 2015). Incorporating cultural elements into holistic assessments is particularly relevant in multicultural populations, where health behaviors and practices are highly influenced by beliefs and values. Identifying patients' cultural backgrounds helps clinicians address specific health disparities and optimize the effectiveness of care. To illustrate, food insecurity, as highlighted by recent research, manifests differently across cultures, influencing eating behaviors and health status in subtle yet typical ways. Through ethnographically informed approaches, health professionals gain a deeper understanding of the complex relationship between taken space and food practice, enabling them to provide similarly nuanced dietary counseling that is sensitive to culture (Bleecker et al., 2017). This cultural sensitivity fosters trust and encourages patient engagement, ultimately leading to improved health outcomes and greater equity in the healthcare system. Holistic assessment also promotes interprofessional practice, in which physicians from various specialties collaborate to address the multifaceted nature of patient health. With the exchange of information across such medical fields as nutrition, psychology, and cultural studies, medical teams become more effective at developing more holistic treatment plans that address all facets of a patient's well-being. This collaboration enhances the quality of care and fosters learning, enabling practitioners to nurture and advance their practice through shared experiences and knowledge. As mandated in nursing conferences, such collaborations emphasize nurse education as a whole and building competencies in nursing, so that the provision of care is enhanced in response to new health issues and societal needs (Nurmalia (Editor) et al., 2015). Lastly, holistic assessment acknowledges the interrelatedness of physical, nutritional, and cultural elements, honoring the reaction to health from a multi-dimensional viewpoint.

Overview of Physical, Nutritional, and Cultural Dimensions

Physical health comprises a variety of components, such as physical fitness, body composition, and chronic disease health status. Knowing these parameters is crucial for accurately assessing adult wellness because each has an impact on overall well-being. Regular exercise and a well-balanced lifestyle are essential for maintaining optimal bodily wellness. Inactivity has been shown to increase health threats in the form of obesity, cardiovascular illnesses, and diabetes. To this end, promoting regular exercise and active lifestyles as part of health check-ups becomes a priority for health workers.

By examining physical attributes and health backgrounds on an individual basis, professionals can develop customized health programs that address specific problems and enhance quality of life among adults, ultimately contributing to a comprehensive disease prevention and control strategy (Murphy et al., 2008). Nutritional problems are on the rise in terms of stature, affecting not just physical health but also mental and emotional well-being in adult health assessments. A balanced diet with the appropriate nutrients plays a crucial role in maintaining physiological function and preventing disease. Adults are increasingly faced with access to food and food choice problems whose root causes are socioeconomic determinants. Poor eating habits result in severe health complications like obesity and malnutrition. Healthcare providers should therefore be concerned with both eating habits and physical examination to comprehend an individual's overall health. Aiding nutritional needs through education and support, such as promoting healthy eating, is essential to improving adult health outcomes and reducing the risk of chronic diseases that are often exacerbated by poor nutrition (Sweeney, 2025).

Cultural factors also play a central role in shaping health behaviors and interventions related to physical and nutritional well-being. Nutritional habits, activity levels, and health beliefs are influenced by culture and can vary within and between communities. Sensitivity to these considerations is essential for healthcare professionals interested in implementing successful interventions and community health initiatives. For example, dietary habits influenced by tradition affect individuals' inclinations towards nutrition, and in most instances, this has either positive or negative effects on health. Culturally competent assessment for health helps professionals engage with their patients in ways that are meaningful, ensuring advice is appropriate and respectful of their beliefs. Through the inclusion of cultural awareness in health assessment, providers can develop health promotion strategies that cater to diverse populations, thereby encouraging holistic approaches to adult health (Murphy et al., 2008) (Figure 4.3).

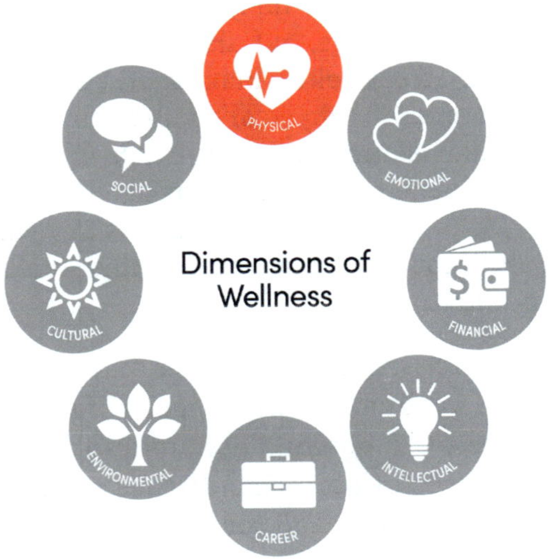

Figure 4.3. Dimensions of wellness.

Source: https://www.uncg.edu/wp-content/uploads/2022/11/Dimensions-of-Wellness-Icons-Physical.png.

4.1. Physical Health Assessment

Learning Outcome

1. Describe the aspects of physical health assessment
2. Highlight mutual evaluation tools and techniques of adult health
3. Obtain facts regarding the contribution of physical exercise to adult health

A comprehensive physical health evaluation is a cornerstone of the overall evaluation of adult health, yielding valuable insights into an individual's well-being. This multifaceted process not only involves examining physiological readings, such as heart rate and blood pressure, but also requires awareness of nutritional and cultural factors that impact health outcomes. By conducting thorough data collection through surveys, physical exams, and patient medical histories, healthcare workers can identify early warning signs of potential health issues, ensuring timely interventions. For example, where the double burden of malnutrition has become a norm for most of the developing world, balanced imagery that considers both undernutrition and obesity is required to represent the various social and economic forces that influence health inequities. When addressing evolving global health landscapes, these aspects need to be incorporated into physical assessments to address the unique health needs of different populations (Aitsi-Selmi et al., 2009). Incorporating nutritional assessments into a holistic physical health evaluation is essential, as these elements are intricately linked. Malnutrition, particularly among vulnerable populations such as the elderly, poses significant health risks, frequently exacerbated by socio-economic challenges. Recent studies indicate that approximately half of all residents in aged care facilities are malnourished, highlighting the urgent need for systematic nutritional strategies in health assessments. Evaluation of food intake and nutrition status can also detect underlying issues affecting not just physical but also cognitive and emotional well-being. Hence, it falls upon health professionals to conduct periodic screenings and provide customized interventions to improve dietary quality and address specific deficiencies. Such a holistic intervention not only boosts the health status but also the overall quality of life across varied care settings (Agarwal et al., 2016). Lastly, cultural determinants of health assessment emphasize the need to make physical evaluations patient-tailored, so that they honor and incorporate patients' cultural heritage. Patients' health beliefs, practices, and diets are usually determined by cultural heritage, which may essentially transform how health data is interpreted and how interventions affect change. Culturally appropriate assessment acknowledges these differences and involves incorporating patients' values and preferences into treatment plans. This not only fosters trust and collaboration between patients and healthcare professionals, as well as compliance and satisfaction with healthcare interventions, but also contributes to improved health outcomes. Ultimately, in the long term, a culturally sensitive approach to measuring physical health is central to ensuring equity, quality of healthcare, and the cross-disciplinary complexity of health shaped by diverse cultural contexts. Understanding the relationship between physical health, nutrition, and culture is crucial for developing effective health interventions among diverse adult populations (Aitsi-Selmi et al., 2009; Agarwal et al., 2016) (Figure 4.4).

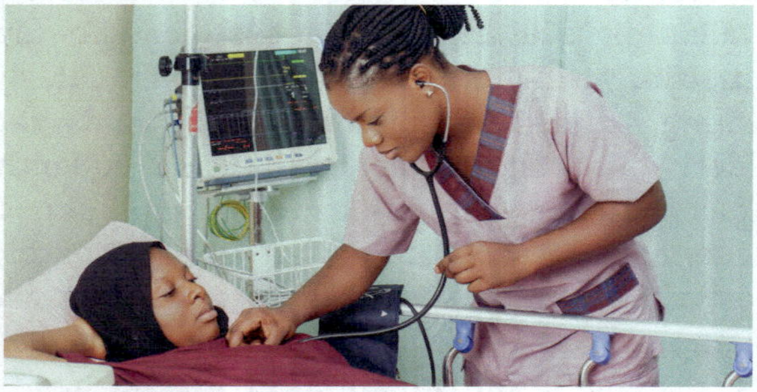

Figure 4.4. Physical health assessment.

Source: https://assets.openstax.org/oscms-prodcms/media/original_images/OSX_Skills_15_00_VitalSigns.jpg.

4.1.1. Key Components of Physical Health

The foundations of physical health comprise several essentials, including regular physical activity, balanced nutrition, and adequate rest. Exercise regularly is also of paramount significance, as it improves cardiovascular function and facilitates healthy weight, with many reports, such as those examined in the CPRC and NICHQ report, indicating physical activity levels are highly associated with all-around health status, particularly in young people and children, demonstrating once more the long-term advantages of cultivating exercise routines from an early age (Murphy et al., 2008). Secondarily, the integration of movement into one's daily life is not simply a weight control issue, but also one of enhanced mood and stress relief, making it a significant factor in overall physical well-being. Proper nutritional balance is at the heart of physical health, influencing everything from energy levels to disease prevention. Having access to a variety of healthy foods is required so individuals can thrive nutritionally.

Research has demonstrated that diets high in fruits, vegetables, whole grain foods, and lean protein can potentially significantly reduce one's chances of acquiring disease states such as obesity, diabetes, and cardiovascular disease. Nutritional education and greater exposure to healthy food sources are thus significant, particularly among socioeconomically disadvantaged groups. Efficient action must be taken against food deserts and promote the idea that all people to make good nutritional choices, which are part of their overall health assessment. The importance of adequate rest and recovery cannot be overstated in the context of physical health.

The nature of sleep has a direct impact on physical performance, mental processing, and emotional stability, underscoring its indispensable role in maintaining health. Growing evidence associates sleep disturbance with many physical health ailments, such as obesity and cardiovascular disease, further underlining the importance of prioritizing sleep. Additionally, economic disadvantage and displacement are two of the stressors identified to noticeably impact the quality of sleep, as referenced in measures evaluating childhood adversity across a variety of cultural contexts (Baker et al., 2008). By examining the intersections of various domains of life and health, an effective plan for physical health can be developed, which is crucial for promoting well-being in different adult groups (Figure 4.5).

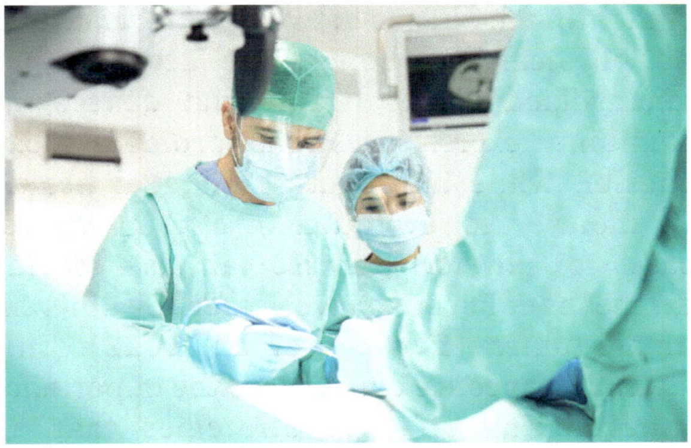

Figure 4.5. Heart surgery.

Source: https://medlineplus.gov/images/HeartSurgery_share.jpg.

4.1.2. Common Assessment Tools and Techniques

Adult health assessment is conducted on a three-pronged basis, encompassing physical, nutritional, and cultural aspects, and incorporates shared tools and techniques as part of the process. They include tools such as health screenings, questionnaires, and diagnostic tests, all designed to provide a comprehensive picture of a patient's health status. Health tests, such as blood pressure and cholesterol readings, provide immediate feedback on physiological health, allowing for the identification of risk factors early. Nutritional screenings, conducted through food frequency questionnaires, also help quantify eating habits, forming the foundation for uncovering the overall relationship between nutrition and health. With the implementation of these test protocols, medical practitioners can develop individualized interventions that address the specific health needs of individuals in various populations. Furthermore, the application of cultural dimensions in health assessments is crucial for effective communication and understanding among diverse populations. Evaluation of cultural beliefs and practices related to health can be achieved through qualitative interviews and culturally validated surveys. These tools not only provide information about an individual's health behavior but also facilitate a deeper understanding of how cultural determinants influence health outcomes. For instance, awareness of local dietary habits allows practitioners to respond and adjust nutrition recommendations accordingly. By incorporating culturally relevant assessment tools, healthcare professionals can maximize their ability to meet the unique needs of diverse populations. Such adherence enables the goal of promoting complete health and well-being while respecting individual histories and beliefs. Furthermore, through the use of new methods, such as principal component analysis, the analysis of poverty and its effects on health status across various populations is enhanced. It determines the relative levels of poverty among populations, which, as noted in the findings, have a significant impact on an individual's nutritional status and overall health. As demonstrated in current literature, the impact of infectious diseases such as HIV/AIDS also complicates dietary needs and health resources within vulnerable populations, particularly in regions such as Sub-Saharan Africa (Gillespie et al., 2025). Its measurement and analysis are crucial for the effective implementation of public health interventions. By applying such sophisticated assessment tools, experts are in a better position to understand the multi-factorial determinants of adult health, thereby promoting more responsive policy and programmatic interventions toward the array of challenges facing diverse communities (Henry et al., 2025).

4.1.3. Role of Physical Activity in Adult Health

Physical activity plays a pivotal role in shaping adult health, serving as the foundation for both physical and mental well-being. Regular engagement in physical activity has been linked to numerous health benefits, including a reduced risk of chronic diseases such as obesity, cardiovascular disease, and diabetes. Some of the mechanisms through which physical activity protects include improved cardiovascular function, metabolic processes, and immune responses. Moreover, the psychological benefits of an exercise routine cannot be overstated: exercise has been shown to reduce depression and anxiety symptoms and enhance mood and cognitive functioning. Given the current epidemic of obesity and related diseases, it is increasingly that we learn about how physical activity affects adult health as we navigate the complexities of modern health problems. Additionally, the financial benefits of promoting physical activity are substantial, as evidenced by studies on the cost-effectiveness of prevention. Investing in physical activity initiatives not only builds healthier populations, but it also reduces the cost of treating obesity and its associated issues. OECD reports substantiate the suggestion that for every dollar spent on prevention, there is a potential return of up to six dollars. This highlights the importance of adopting a whole-of-population physical activity policy, possibly through community plans, worksite health promotion programs, and walkable urban design. All these factors contribute to supporting active living and creating an environment where adults are more likely to engage in regular physical activity. Emphasizing physical health can help societies enhance the quality of life, as well as improve economic returns at the population level (Dwivedi et al., 2022). Culturally, integrating physical activity into everyday life encompasses broader societal norms and values. Different communities embrace different types of physical activities based on cultural beliefs and practices, highlighting the nexus between cultural factors and physical well-being. The activities, as standardized games, traditional dances, or community exercise sessions, promote social cohesion while improving individual health. The metaverses' evolution in offering virtual spaces for physical exercise can also provide new means of boosting involvement by different demographics (Dwivedi et al., 2022). This cultural perspective emphasizes the importance of developing effective strategies that, in addition to addressing health, also resonate with the unique identities of adult populations. By fostering an inclusive environment that makes physical activity accessible and culturally relevant, we can promote long-term engagement in healthier lifestyles and ultimately improve overall adult health status (Figure 4.6).

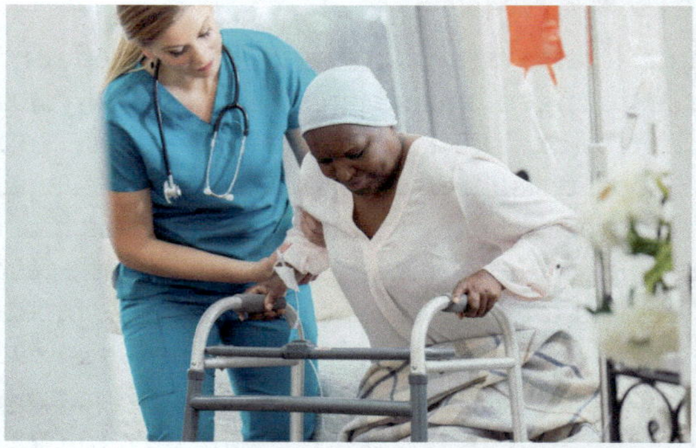

Figure 4.6. Role of physical activity in adult health.

Source: https://www.johnshopkinssolutions.com/wp-content/uploads/2019/03/iStock-932074816-1024x683.jpg.

Test Your Knowledge

1. What are the four basic techniques used in physical health assessment?
2. Why is baseline physical assessment critical in medical-surgical patient care?

4.2. Nutritional Health Assessment

Learning Outcome

1. Describe the importance of nutrition in adult health
2. Specify the processes for assessing nutritional status
3. Describe the influence of food selection on general health

One of the key areas to assess when evaluating adult health is nutritional health assessment, which indicates an individual's dietary way of life, nutritional status, and direction of overall health. Such an assessment helps identify potential nutrient deficiencies and surpluses that may contribute to chronic diseases or affect physical health. Assessment of a person's diet through food frequency questionnaires, 24-hour dietary recalls, and direct observation allows health professionals to tailor dietetic intervention effectively. Additionally, incorporating cultural elements into nutritional assessments makes them more effective, as what one consumes is typically a reflection of their culture and social norms. These cultural influences, being actualized, can lead to more acceptable and personalized dietary advice, ultimately enhancing nutrition recommendations compliance. Also, the role of socioeconomic determinants in nutritional health should not be overlooked. Literature reveals a strong association between individual income levels and food quality, further underscoring the extent to which economic stability influences food choices. Higher income levels are associated with improved cardiovascular health outcomes, as indicated in the Life's Essential 8 Cardiovascular Health Matrix, which encompasses lifestyle components (diet, exercise, body mass index) that can be optimized with greater financial means. Thus, nutritional health assessments that consider economic context are more effective at capturing the details of an individual's health, pointing out where funding or education support can be applied to increase general diet quality. The implementation of such assessments into public health programs can enhance better outcomes and bridge gaps concerning nutrition. Additionally, ongoing research highlights the importance of tailoring nutritional health measures to account for the individual dietary habits and health risk factors of diverse populations. For instance, understanding the impact of mental health on nutrition and vice versa illustrates how psychology may affect diet and nutritional condition. The TUDA study findings highlight the truth that the majority of lower-functioning elderly persons have poorer diets that further deepen them into a cycle of poor well-being. By integrating data from all domains of health, including mental, physical, and nutritional health, professionals can develop comprehensive care plans that consider a person's complete health profile. Thus, integration of all sorts of viewpoints into nutritional health assessments will yield richer insights into health and more efficient interventions that meet the unique needs of various populations (Figure 4.7).

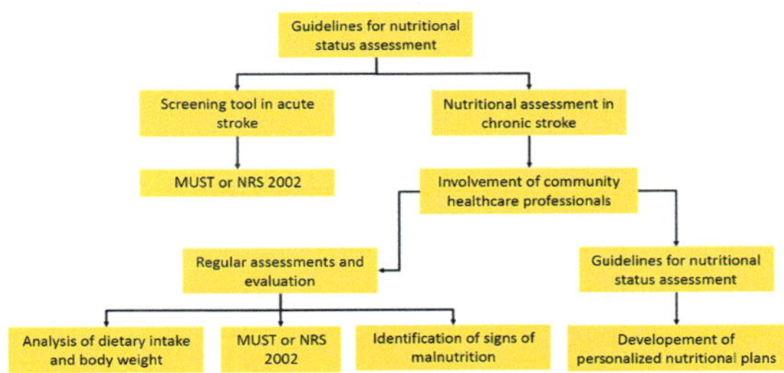

Figure 4.7. Nutritional assessment in stroke patients.

Source: https://www.clinicalnutritionopenscience.com/cms/10.1016/j.nutos.2023.10.010/asset/44f1d154-9825-4ed0-8811-c5509f1e7b37/main.assets/gr3_lrg.jpg.

4.2.1. Importance of Nutrition in Adult Health

Nutrition plays a key role in maintaining adult health, physical health, and quality of life. Good diet is required for the avoidance of chronic illnesses such as obesity, diabetes, and cardiovascular disease that are prevalent among the majority of adults. A diet that is rich in nutrients—such as vitamins, minerals, protein, and fats—is likely to enhance immune function, boost energy, and preserve mental status. Moreover, nutrition plays a significant role in aging, influencing cognitive function and tolerance. With adults leading busy lives, the impact of diet on health becomes increasingly important, prompting well-informed dietary decisions to align with their individual health goals and lifestyle needs. This fundamental aspect of adult health is not merely a question of individual interest, but a universal imperative that shapes healthcare systems and public health programs to improve the health outcomes of populations. The integration of a wide variety of food sources into nutrition guidelines is necessary to address the multifaceted nature of adult health. Cultural elements of nutrition cannot be overlooked, as they significantly impact individuals' eating patterns and behaviors. Public health professionals can plan more effective nutrition interventions by understanding the importance of cultural food practices. The addition of culturally acceptable foods can create a perception of belonging and acceptance, which can positively influence individuals' willingness to adopt healthier food habits. Secondly, creating awareness of the role of nutrition through culturally acceptable education can empower adults to make informed, healthy decisions that improve their health by providing them with the knowledge they need. Thus, a culturally appropriate nutrition policy not only promotes the health of an individual but also strengthens community resilience, supporting the overall objectives of sustainable health promotion (Bangay et al., 2010). The relationship between nutrition and sustainability further emphasizes the importance of nutrition to the health of adults. With the world's challenges, such as climate change, on the increase, the nature of food that adult individuals eat significantly impacts their welfare and the environment. Sustainable nutrition encompasses the concept of healthy eating in balance with environmentally sustainable practices that aim to eliminate waste, conserve resources, and promote biodiversity. Healthy access to food is intrinsically linked to gender equity and resource management, as equal access enables all individuals to make healthy decisions (Herklotz A et al., 2012). It is affect the health of both themselves and the planet. Therefore, nutrition education programs should not only focus on a balanced meal but also promote a holistic concept that relates food decisions to global sustainability, aiming to achieve a healthier population and ecosystem for future generations ultimately (Figure 4.8).

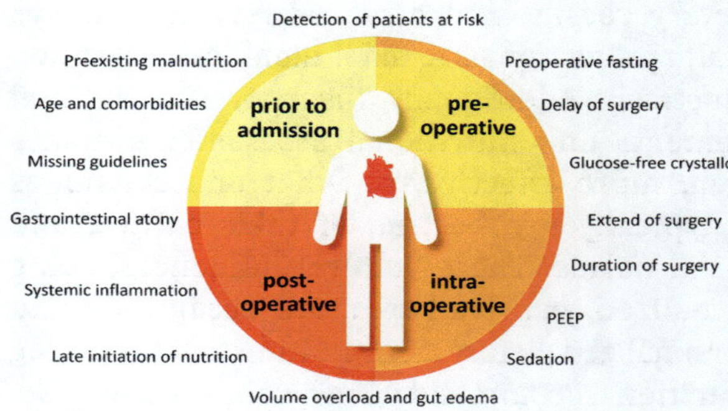

Figure 4.8. Current evidence about nutrition support in cardiac surgery patients.

Source: https://www.mdpi.com/nutrients/nutrients-10-00597/article_deploy/html/images/nutrients-10-00597-g004.png.

4.2.2. Methods for Assessing Nutritional Status

Establishing nutritional status is a complex process that incorporates many methodologies, each designed to provide data on the dietary habits and health of persons. The Dietary

Behaviors Questionnaire is one of the most commonly used measures for assessing how well individuals understand their nutritional needs and adopt healthy dietary habits. This tool is particularly beneficial in clinical settings, for instance, when dealing with patients with type 2 diabetes mellitus (T2DM), whose disease management is central to dietary control. Research has established that enhancing patients' knowledge on diabetic diets is linked with good nutritional intake, which identifies the utility of systematic assessment in determining the need for education (Kritpracha et al., 2011). Lastly, such decisions can inform targeted interventions aimed at enhancing nutritional knowledge and behavior among various groups. Anthropometric measurements are another essential instrument for assessing nutritional status, providing vital information about body composition and physical health. Measurements such as BMI, waist circumference, and skinfold thickness provide data on fat distribution and overall nutritional risk. For instance, a high BMI may indicate obesity, which is a long-term condition associated with conditions such as heart disease and diabetes. Carrying out these tests regularly enables professionals to track how an individual's nutritional status varies over time, enabling preventive health care. Complemented by nutritional assessments, such as the Dietary Behaviors Questionnaire, anthropometric data can help create a comprehensive profile of health that provides greater insight into the interactions between body and nutritional variables in adult well-being. In addition, biochemical analysis provides another level of assessment for nutritional status. Biochemical tests involve analyzing blood, urine, or tissue samples to identify specific nutrients or metabolic end-products. For example, serum levels of vitamins or minerals can be measured to identify deficiencies that may not be detected by dietary analysis alone. Practitioners can then determine the biological impact of nutritional intake and provide more precise recommendations for nutritional modification. The combination of biochemical and clinical parameters can provide a more comprehensive and accurate assessment of a person's health, supporting individualized interventions that consider dietary patterns based on cultural backgrounds and unique health conditions among diverse populations (Murphy et al., 2008). Thus, multiple measures are crucial for accurate assessment of nutritional status (Figure 4.9).

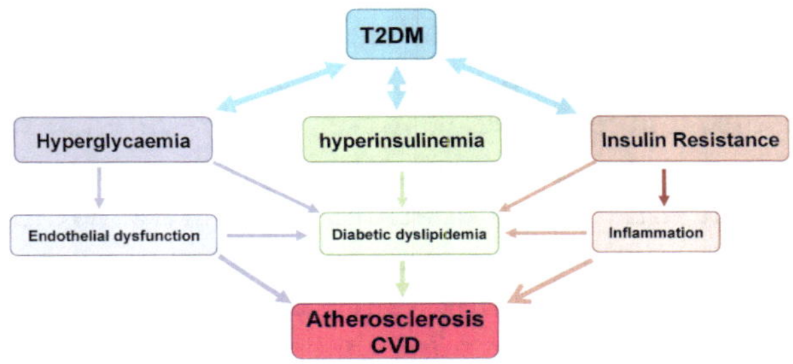

Figure 4.9. Pathophysiology of type 2 diabetes mellitus.

Source: https://www.mdpi.com/ijms/ijms-21-06275/article_deploy/html/images/ijms-21-06275-g006.png.

4.2.3. Impact of Dietary Choices on Overall Health

Food choices have a significant impact on an individual's overall health, both physically and psychologically. There is extensive research that has established a direct link between diet and the avoidance of many chronic diseases, including obesity, diabetes, and cardiovascular disorders. Individuals who eat a diet that includes plenty of fruits, vegetables, whole grains, and lean protein tend to have lower incidences of these diseases than individuals whose diets are made up primarily of processed foods containing high amounts of sugars, fats, and sodium. Furthermore, the mental benefits of eating well cannot be overstated, as nutrition is crucial to mood and cognitive processes. More integrative health can enhance overall quality of life, physical lifespan, as well as emotional balance and mental sharpness, confirming the significance of placing nutrition over other options in schemes to promote adult well-being. The power of food selection is further complicated by the socio-cultural settings within which individuals operate. Access to healthy foods tends to reflect demographic conditions such as socioeconomic status, education level, and availability of foods within their area. In a few populations, primarily those that are characterized as food deserts, individuals have limited access to healthy foods. Research indicates that food shortages may lead to adverse health outcomes, e.g., increased prevalence of obesity and obesity-related diseases among disadvantaged populations, primarily within African American communities. These findings underscore the importance of addressing the socio-economic systems that shape nutritional choices and health outcomes. In the absence of systemic reform of food availability and nutrition education, countless individuals will not be in a position to make more healthy food options, highlighting the importance of widespread public health interventions, including consideration of fair food environments (Smalls et al., 2013). Policy strategies aimed at improving healthier dietary habits and increasing food availability are essential to the overall well-being of diverse communities. Policy action should aim to establish full-service grocery stores within underdeveloped communities, given that exposure to these facilities is likely to have a direct correlation with eating habits. In addition, learning initiatives focused on promoting awareness of nutrition and healthy food preparation can empower people to make informed food choices, positively impacting their health outcomes. Policies also need to take into consideration the complex nature of dietetic impacts, bringing together knowledge from qualitative research that inquires into family structures, cultural habits, and individual tastes for food. In doing this, a more tailored answer can be constructed, leading to improved eating habits and, by association, better health in population groups (Murphy et al., 2008). By prioritizing such methods, we are able to construct environments that promote healthier choices and long-term wellness in adults.

Test Your Knowledge

1. What are two key components of a nutritional health assessment that a nurse conducts?
2. How does compromised nutritional status impact recovery in medical-surgical patients?

4.3. Cultural Dimensions of Health

Learning Outcome

1. Define cultural competence in healthcare
2. Define culture's influence on health beliefs and practice
3. Describe culturally sensitive health assessment strategies

Cultural dimensions are a critical component of adult health assessment as they influence individuals' perceptions, behavior, and health practices. Beliefs about health, rituals, and customs vary considerably across cultures and can significantly influence how individuals care for their health. For instance, in some societies, holistic health incorporates religious practices and social support, which can contribute to overall well-being. Where a culture is more individually oriented, however, the biomedical approach is more likely to be dominant, with medical treatment emphasized over lifestyle changes. Being familiar with these various cultural frames is crucial for health workers who wish to provide effective care and work towards achieving health equity. By incorporating cultural competence into health assessments, clinicians can tailor their interventions to align with the patient's values, thereby establishing trust and supporting improved health outcomes. The concept of allostatic load highlights how cultural contexts influence physical health outcomes, particularly among socioeconomically disadvantaged groups. Studies investigating cumulative stresses in different populations, including the Nepali children examined for allostatic load, suggest that individuals from more adverse environments face an increased risk to their health (Baker et al., 2008). In adults, these same dynamics can play out through chronic stress related to cultural displacement, poverty, or migration and impact physical health indicators such as blood pressure and metabolic function. Thus, understanding these intricate relationships enables health professionals to consider the broader socio-cultural context that influences their patients. Ultimately, addressing such cultural aspects of health can lead to more sensitive and effective methods for adult health check-ups. Nutrition, in conjunction with cultural practices, plays a crucial role in determining adult health and reflects the diverse dietary cultures globally. For instance, the increasing concomitance of undernutrition and obesity in Tangkhul Naga women illustrates how socio-economic change and cultural evolution affect nutritional status (Mungreiphy et al., 2008). Traditional diets may be influenced by local resources, while modernization often leads to a shift towards less healthy food. The duality highlights the importance of culturally sensitive interventions in nutrition, which enable adjustments to local food culture and eating styles for improved well-being. Understanding how cultural determinants influence eating habits is crucial for developing effective public health policies. In this respect, incorporating cultural knowledge into nutrition assessment has the potential to enable people to make informed decisions and enhance their health outcomes (Figure 4.10).

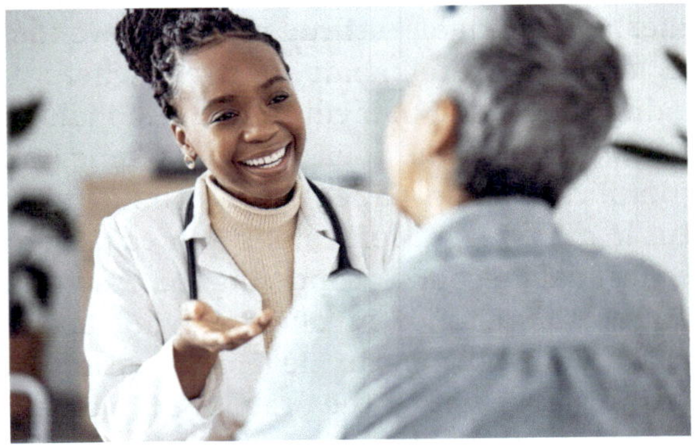

Figure 4.10. Improve cultural competence in health care.

Source: https://publichealth.tulane.edu/wp-content/uploads/sites/3/2021/03/How-to-Improve-Cultural-Competence-in-Health-Care.jpg.

4.3.1. Definition of Cultural Competence in Healthcare

The definition of cultural competence in healthcare has become the essential framework for addressing the diverse needs of patient populations. On a basic level, cultural competence describes healthcare providers' capacity to perceive, understand, and attend to the cultural determinants of health behaviors and outcomes. This involves not only an awareness of one's own cultural biases and values but also a close familiarity with the culture of various groups. As the healthcare system becomes increasingly diverse, practitioners will need to complete continuing education to acquire the knowledge, skills, and attitudes necessary to deliver culturally competent care. This kind of expertise is pivotal in achieving trust and communication between providers and patients, and ultimately, patient and health outcome satisfaction. Given the multidimensionality of cultural competence as a concept, education in healthcare must be tailored to prepare practitioners in the required competencies. Competency in dealing with cultural differences entails knowledge of the various health beliefs, customs, and values that underlie individuals' attitudes toward wellness and health. This demands a system where the coming generation of medical professionals can critically debate the ideas of competency and its implications on patient care. Similar to the focus in more recent competency-based program educational discourse, capturing the essence of cultural competence involves moving beyond technical proficiency to develop relationality and knowledge within the practice environment (Hodges et al., 2013). This integrated model requires providers to treat their patients not only as cases but also as individuals with unique histories that inform their health experiences. Cultural competence is promoted for its role in alleviating health disparities that disproportionately affect specific populations.

Research has shown that culturally competent care can significantly enhance the quality of care by reducing miscommunications and forming an interdisciplinary healthcare environment. This approach not only benefits patients from diverse backgrounds but also promotes the healthcare profession in general through greater inclusiveness and respect. Moreover, conferences such as the 3rd Java International Nursing Conference emphasize the inclusion of cultural competence into nursing and health sciences, reflecting a commitment to improving quality of care through shared knowledge and practices (Nurmalia (Editor) et al., 2015). Essentially, cultural competence must be considered an integral aspect of overall care for adult health assessment, where physical and dietary needs are not only taken into account but also the cultural factors that underpin the health experiences (Figure 4.11).

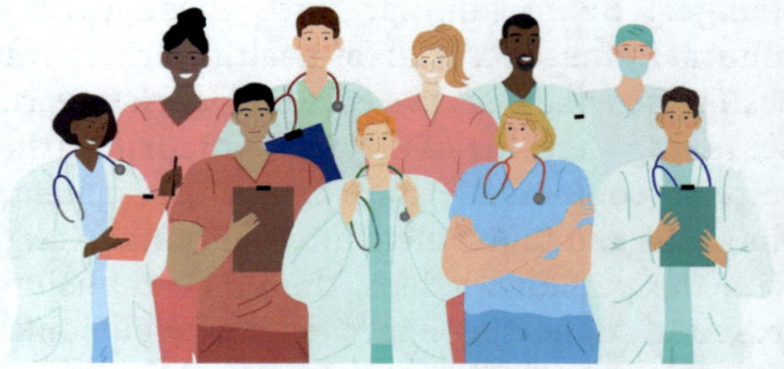

Figure 4.11. Cultural competence in healthcare.

Source: https://www.herzing.edu/sites/default/files/styles/fp_960_480/public/2021-04/Healthcare%20Diversity.jpg.webp?itok=9Ad3N0Ya.

4.3.2. Influence of Culture on Health Beliefs and Practices

Culture has a profound impact on health beliefs and practices, influencing concepts of well-being and approaches to healthcare interventions. In most cultures, illness and health beliefs differ, and these differences influence whether individuals are willing to seek medical attention or adhere to prescribed treatment. For instance, in certain cultures, the practice of traditional medicine, e.g., herbalism or spiritual healing, is prevalent, sometimes even overtaking modern medical interventions. This interplay between health-seeking behavior and cultural practice is central to understanding overall health dynamics among various populations. Proceedings like the 3rd Java International Nursing Conference aim to further inform such cultural influences by providing a platform for discussing whole nursing practice that is culturally attuned and includes the integration of cultural values aimed at optimizing healthcare outcomes among various populations (Nurmalia (Editor) et al., 2015). Furthermore, cultural identity can regulate eating habits, which in turn affect health conditions. Food consumption, cooking methods, and table etiquette are based on dietary habits that are closely tied to cultural traditions. For example, the Mediterranean diet, which includes a lot of fruit, vegetables, and unsaturated fats, is distinct from others, which may largely rely on processed foods. Cultural food consumption patterns should be incorporated into health promotion interventions to create effective strategies for specific groups. Health professionals need to recognize such food consumption patterns and the cultural significance added to them in a bid to form trust and compliance with dietary guidelines.

This approach aligns with the concepts of experts at events like the 3rd Java International Nursing Conference, where the intersection between culture and nutritional health is central to enhancing the quality of care, as well as promoting healthy living (Nurmalia (Editor) et al., 2015). Lastly, cultural beliefs play a role in guiding health practices and preventive health activities and education. Various societies have varying perceptions of disease prevention, which dictate health behaviors like immunization rates and regular health checks. Education plans must be tailored to accommodate these cultural beliefs in order to endorse public health programs effectively. For instance, a society with shared beliefs about health is likely to respond differently to health messages than one that focuses on individual responsibility. Therefore, public health professionals need to adopt culturally sensitive approaches in the dissemination of health messages in a manner that resonates with community values. Such culturally sensitive health interventions are underscored through efforts aimed at reducing health disparities, as documented in joint research studies carried out by agencies such as the CPRC and the NICHQ. By being mindful of cultural settings, healthcare providers are better able to encourage cultural access to care and active health management among diverse groups (Figure 4.12).

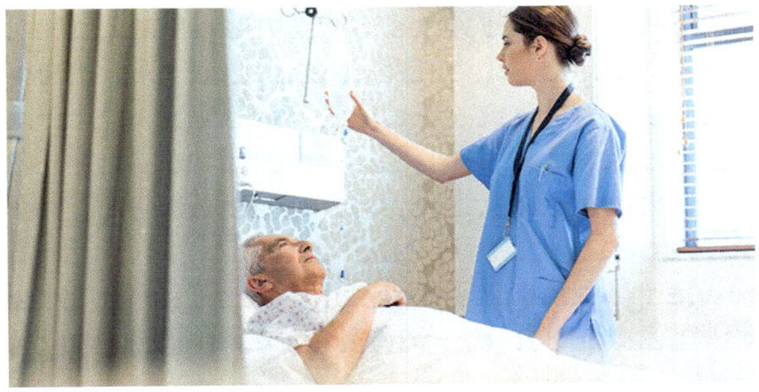

Figure 4.12. Recognizing religious beliefs in healthcare.

Source: https://www.healthstream.com/images/default-source/blog/01761262_cd_904794116.jpg?sfvrsn=4e5a65fe_0.

4.3.3. Strategies for Culturally Sensitive Health Assessments

One of the most critical aspects of culturally sensitive health assessments is the ability to recognize and respond to patients' diverse cultural backgrounds. This involves understanding how cultural values, practices, and beliefs impact conceptions of health and wellness. Some societies, for instance, may focus on holistic practices drawn from ancient healing traditions instead of orthodox medicine. Health practitioners, therefore, need to be capable of active listening in addition to engaging in open-ended discussions that respect and validate patients' cultural stories. These strategies help establish a therapeutic rapport, enabling practitioners to receive accurate health information while fostering trust. Moreover, the implementation of culturally adapted training programs for healthcare providers can enhance their capacity to provide sensitive assessments, hence enhancing the effectiveness of care outcomes among diverse populations. Utilization of culturally adapted educational materials also improves the effectiveness of health assessments. Health literacy among multicultural populations significantly impacts the quality of communication and the uptake of health information. For example,

Aboriginal and Torres Strait Islander health worker projects utilize interactive multimedia resources that are culturally specific, ensuring that information is available and accessible to target communities (Sayed et al., 2011). These intervention efforts are crucial in bridging knowledge gaps and fostering a culture in which individuals feel empowered to discuss their health concerns. Through the implementation of these measures, healthcare providers cannot only improve service delivery but also increase participation among marginalized populations, ultimately leading to improved health outcomes and reduced disparities. Additionally, the assessment methods employed must determine the structural disparities that impact health behavior and access. Knowledge of the general social determinants of health, including economic stability, education, and social context, is essential to the performance of thorough, culturally sensitive evaluations. Healthcare systems can design culturally targeted interventions to meet the specific needs of various cultural groups by using approaches that explicitly take these issues into account (Birnbaum et al., 2011). This, by extension, not only contributes to the reliability of health assessments but also places healthcare professionals in the position of equity advocates. Such advocacy is significant in ensuring that health systems are responsive and reflective of the diverse demographic makeup, thereby fostering a broader agenda for adult health assessments that considers both physical and cultural factors.

Test Your Knowledge

1. Why do medical-surgical nurses have to consider cultural dimensions in caring for their patients?
2. Name two cultural factors that could influence a patient's health beliefs or response to treatment.

4.4. Interrelationship between Physical and Nutritional Health

Learning Outcome

1. Explain the effects of physical health on nutritional needs
2. Define inadequacies of nutrition and their impact on physical health
3. Discuss case studies illustrating the interrelationship between physical and nutritional well-being

The intricate relationship between physical and nutritional well-being is essential in order to meet the complicated nature of adult wellness. Nutrition health significantly influences physical health indicators, such as body mass index (BMI) and overall fitness levels. A proper diet lacking sufficient essential nutrients can lead to various health problems, such as obesity, cardiovascular conditions, and diabetes. On the contrary, a lack of exercise can hurt metabolic processes, exacerbating nutrient deficiencies. The dependencies as mentioned earlier show how a holistic approach in assessing adult health with consideration of the interaction between dietary habits and lifestyle practices is critical. Typical patterns of nutritional intake often correspond to specific health effects; thus, an integrated understanding is helpful in enabling health workers to tailor interventions for overall well-being. Psychological factors also play a significant role in interactions between physical and nutritional health. Studies indicate that certain psychopathological symptoms have the capacity to predict BMI change among participants, illustrating how complexities in psychological health have a direct impact on physical wellbeing (Ballarotto et al., 2017). For instance, emotional eating can lead to weight gain, while restrained eating may be a consequence of depression or anxiety and lead to malnutrition. Such dynamics suggest that psychological health is not a concomitant problem but a component of both nutrition and physical health.

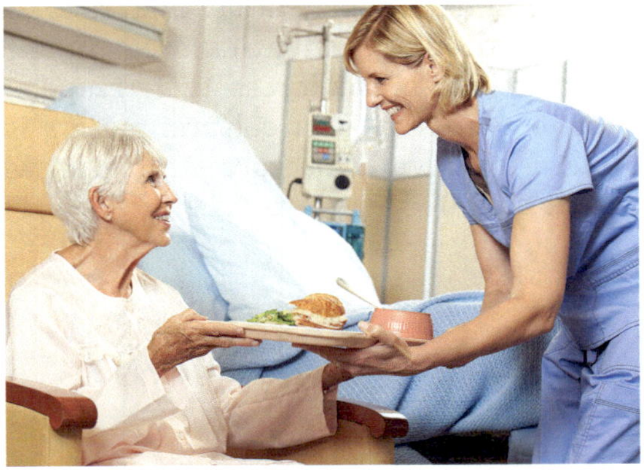

Figure 4.13. Nurse's role in patient nutrition and hydration.

Source: https://cdn.ps.emap.com/wp-content/uploads/sites/3/2015/07/Nutrition-care.jpg.

In assessing adult health, it is crucial to consider how psychological disposition and disorders intersect with dietary and exercise levels. Addressing these determinants holistically in health checks can thus lead to optimal treatment and prevention outcomes. Moreover, cultural determinants also play important roles in the interconnection between physical and nutritional health, particularly for the immigrant population. Variability in food practices, food availability, and beliefs regarding body image can play an important role in nutritional status and health outcomes. For instance, nutritional screening of immigrant communities is useful in identifying high-risk groups for malnutrition or obesity, allowing for personalized dietary counseling (Emanuela, 2015). Sensitivity to these cultural considerations may enable healthcare professionals to develop more effective health promotion programs that reflect diverse dietary practices and preferences. Consequently, combining physical health examinations with culturally adjusted nutritional examinations provides a nuanced understanding of the health dynamics of adults and advances improved health outcomes in diverse populations (Figure 4.13).

4.4.1. How Physical Health Affects Nutritional Needs

The interconnected relationship between physical health and nutritional needs is at the core of comprehending adult health in general. Physical health condition typically dictates an individual's nutritional requirements, as various disease states might alter metabolic and nutrient usage mechanisms. For instance, patients with chronic diseases such as diabetes or cardiovascular disease might require specific nutrient changes in order to manage their disease optimally. These changes can include increased fiber, reduced saturated fat, or controlled carbohydrate intake. Additionally, proper hydration becomes increasingly relevant for patients with poor health, as it enhances the efficacy of drug therapy and supports bodily functions. As such, appreciating the nuances of how certain physical states of well-being influence dietary needs is crucial in maintaining optimal levels of outcomes and preventing further issues among affected individuals. Moreover, physical well-being and dietary needs interact with each other in a complex manner, based on evidence that demonstrates how malnutrition contributes to the worsening of illness. Undernutrition among vulnerable populations is significantly higher in food-insecure countries, such as Mozambique, and leads to a cycle of worsening physical health outcomes (Garrett et al., 2025). This segment illustrates how nutritional deficits can exacerbate susceptibility to illness and impair the capacity for recovery. Satisfaction of the specific dietary requirements emerging from physical health issues therefore acquires an increasingly urgent sense of priority. Nutrition interventions that respect the complex interaction between physical health and nutritional requirements are also capable of significantly enhancing health and well-being, ultimately reducing the cost of avoidable chronic illness. Additionally, cultural dimensions play a crucial role in determining nutritional needs related to physical health. Various cultures have diverse eating habits and belief systems that either support or hinder nutritional adequacy. For instance, cultural preferences may lead to the exclusion of certain food groups that are imperative for individuals with specific health conditions, such as lactose intolerance or gluten intolerance. Concurrently, cultural practices can promote healthy dietary habits that lead to improved physical health and, consequently, overall nutritional status. Understanding these cultural variations enables healthcare practitioners to develop patient-tailored nutrition interventions that are tailored to patients' cultural environments and address their respective nutrition-related health needs. Thus, the appreciation and incorporation of cultural factors into nutritional assessments and interventions can lead to more effective healthcare strategies, with an ultimate result of improved health outcomes (Murphy et al., 2008) (Figure 4.14).

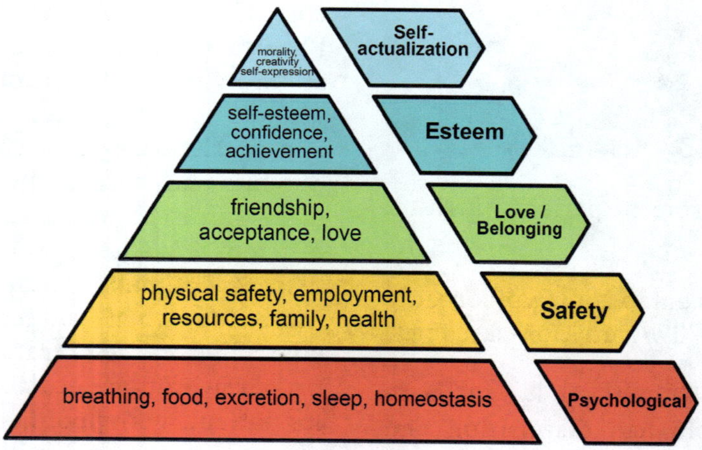

Figure 4.14. Physical health affects nutritional needs.

Source: https://cdn.prod.website-files.com/5babc11099f97ea5dbcf24d5/67339b977e7af2fbc3ff9f8c_AD_4nXeZ6y_CSG_o_9feIIdyLD9LOZ_uG9Mk-NJQ-F7ldEDz81E25vUQ1M9KJdzNJVcoEL8AgN35xaxDlRuqaZmn51mFyM8YCoW_zU6ueS01pNHR2Pc9WJu5fUniCtePRkyB4WVMTweAY2Ysog7qpcH55uA-5em-.jpeg.

4.4.2. Nutritional Deficiencies and Their Physical Health Implications

The relevance of nutrient deficiencies extends beyond individual health to broader public health issues, particularly in adult populations. Deficiencies of essential nutrients, such as vitamins and minerals, can have severe health implications, ranging from impaired immune function to long-term illnesses. For instance, a deficiency of vitamin D results in osteomalacia, a condition that causes softening of the bones and predisposes adults to fractures. Additionally, micronutrient deficiencies may lead to the onset of diet-related chronic diseases, such as diabetes and hypertension, thereby increasing healthcare expenditures and decreasing productivity. These deficits need to be addressed through a multifaceted strategy that combines dietary supplementation and public health interventions to educate populations about the importance of nutrition in maintaining physical health and well-being. This approach enables individuals to make informed food choices tailored to their respective contexts (Flores et al., 2025). The impacts of nutritional deficits extend beyond immediate physical well-being and influence longer-term outcomes such as cognition and mental health. In adulthood, proper intake of essential nutrients is crucial for maintaining cognitive function and emotional well-being. For example, research has shown that deficiencies in omega-3 fatty acids may be linked with symptoms of depression and anxiety. Furthermore, nutritionally imbalanced adults are more likely to develop neurodegenerative conditions, which can compromise their quality of life and autonomy. The psychosocial factors of health are inextricably linked with nutritional status, making it crucial to intervene to promote both mental well-being and physical health. With improved nutrition and management of deficiencies, there is a possibility of enhancing the overall quality of life and resilience among adults (Gillespie et al., 2025). Nutrient deficiencies must be addressed through a multidisciplinary approach, considering the cultural, economic, and social factors that influence food patterns. Socioeconomic limitations in many populations can hinder access to many healthy foods, widening the health cycle of poor circulation. Outreach and education in the community are key components of effective models for enhancing such deficiencies. Culturally appropriate tailoring of programs, along with encouragement towards healthier food intake, can foster community acceptance and sustainability. Furthermore, public policy initiatives that support agricultural practices and food security need to be implemented to address the prevalent nutrition deficiencies among vulnerable populations. Through an understanding of and intervention in the systems of structures that influence nutrition, societies can work to alleviate health disparities and enhance the physical health of adults (Flores et al., 2025) (Figure 4.15).

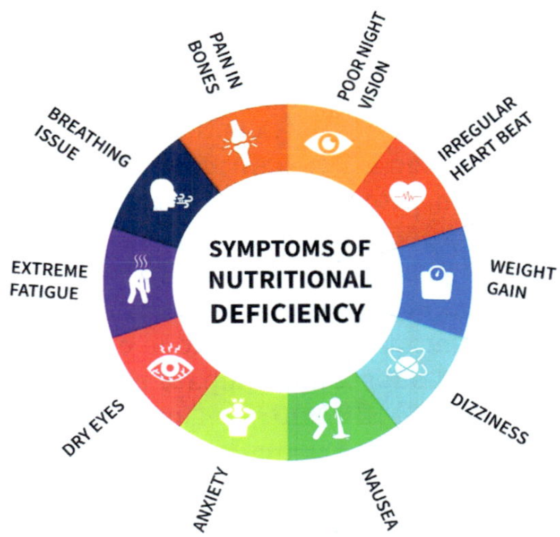

Figure 4.15. Symptoms of nutritional deficiency.

Source: https://www.careinsurance.com/upload_master/media/symptoms-of-nutritional-deficiency.webp.

4.4.3. Case Studies Illustrating the Connection

Case study analysis yields insightful information regarding the intricate relationships between physical health, nutrition, and culture among adult populations. A particularly captivating case is presented in research targeted towards indigenous Argentineans, specifically the Toba and Wichí populations, where socioeconomic shifts have far-reaching consequences for their well-being. Historically, these groups were hunter-gatherers, but political activism and urbanization have caused increased obesity and co-morbidities associated with obesity. Of note, nearly 50% of adult Toba individuals and

34% of overweight Wichí adults were noted, emphasizing the influence of food transition from wild-fared to supermarket food. The study highlights the of biocultural determinantslike political agency and life-course changes in the acceleration of such , such as political agency and life-course changes, on the acceleration of health disparities. It outlines the complex relationship between nutritional health and societal change (Burke et al., 2009). Urbanization also encompasses the interconnectedness of nutrition and health, particularly in nations such as those in Southern and Eastern Africa (SEA). Scientists have documented the interactive dynamics among migration, urban food security, and the HIV/AIDS pandemic. Where city populations increase, rural households increasingly rely on migrant remittances to cover food expenditure, which has a subsequent impact on rural food production. The HIV/AIDS epidemic exacerbates this vulnerability, particularly in the case of mobile populations, as it introduces both short-term and intergenerational health implications that further entangle food security scenarios. The challenge lies in understanding that the urban food security-HIV/migration interface requires integrative policies that consider these interdependencies if communities are to achieve sustainable health benefits (Crush et al., 2007). Synthesizing the case studies offers a valuable template for tackling adult health from a multi-dimensional angle. By examining the intersection of cultural, socioeconomic, and environmental determinants, we are better equipped to identify effective interventions tailored to diverse populations. For instance, interventions that support nutritional education, facilitate access to healthier food and food environments, and reinforce farm-based agriculture can help mitigate adverse health effects observed in both rural and urban settings. Furthermore, the awareness of policy interventions in addressing the underlying causes of health is accompanied by a concerted response that ensures resilience among rural and urban populations. From these case studies, a consideration of adult health is compelled to confront a holistic approach which initially prioritizes physical, nutritional, and cultural factors, ultimately ensuring healthier outcomes in diverse communities (Crush et al., 2007; Burke et al., 2009).

Test Your Knowledge

1. How does nutritional compromise affect physical recovery among med-surg patients?
2. Why is it important to assess physical and nutritional well-being at the same time in patient care?

4.5. Socioeconomic Factors in Health Assessment

Learning Outcome

1. Describe the influence of socioeconomic status on health outcomes
2. Define what keeps individuals from accessing healthcare and nutrition
3. Describe the role of community resources in contributing to enhanced health

Socioeconomic factors play an instrumental role in the health evaluation process, influencing not only access to care but also the individual's overall health status. Economic security in various communities influences eating habits, access to care, and lifestyle patterns, resulting in significant differences in health outcomes. People with lower incomes typically face barriers like limited transportation, fewer healthcare facilities, and higher stress levels, thereby aggravating medical conditions. In addition, incorporating income-related information into health assessments can provide a framework for an individual's health status and identify underlying socioeconomic issues that contribute to chronic illness. Having identified these determinants, health practitioners can then develop targeted interventions and provide resources that maximize the health of population groups disproportionately affected by socioeconomic disadvantage, thereby optimizing health equity among populations. Poverty has significant impacts on diet, and socioeconomic status tends to dictate eating patterns. Individuals with lower socioeconomic statuses have access to less expensive, processed foods that do not include essential nutrients and subsequently experience more diet-related illnesses such as diabetes and obesity. Secondly, options for health-promoting food are often limited in poorer areas, also referred to as food deserts. Recognition of these trends needs to be taken into consideration when designing health measures, ensuring they accurately reflect the dietary component of health. Additionally, understanding the dynamic between food security and economic forces can inform public health interventions aimed at promoting healthy diets among vulnerable populations. Targeted interventions that promote access to fresh, affordable foods can bridge the gap between nutritional well-being and socioeconomic status, ultimately creating healthier communities. Cultural factors are also inextricably linked with socioeconomic forces when shaping behaviors and beliefs surrounding health. Different cultural backgrounds may influence individuals' engagement with healthcare systems, predisposing them to be more or less receptive to accessing appropriate medical interventions promptly or adhering to treatment measures. This intersectionality is crucial under health screenings as cultural beliefs and practices are likely to enhance or undermine the effectiveness of healthcare interventions. For instance, some cultural groups might prefer traditional medicine over modern medical approaches due to belief systems that relate to health. Addressing these cultural nuances requires culturally sensitive approaches to health assessment and intervention planning. In addition, utilizing community strengths and including local leaders may facilitate the bridging of the gap between healthcare providers and ethnically diverse populations, leading to improved health outcomes. By having a comprehensive understanding of these interconnected factors, health professionals can proceed towards more equitable health assessments that truly reflect the nuances of adult health (Figure 4.16).

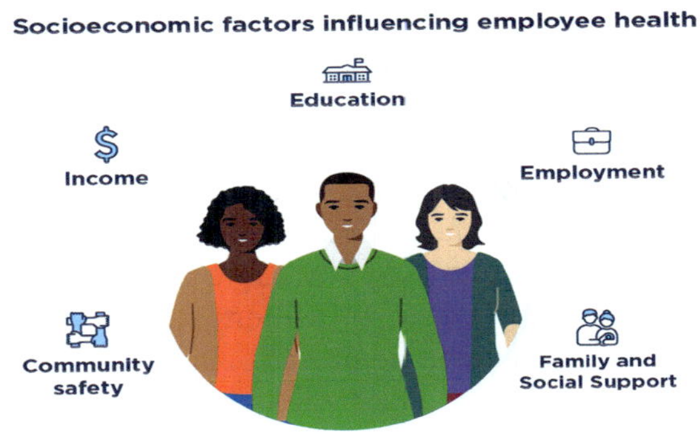

Figure 4.16. Socioeconomic-factors-influencing-employee-health.

Source: https://business.kaiserpermanente.org/wp-content/uploads/2022/12/socioeconomic-factors-influencing-employee-health.png.

4.5.1. Impact Of Socioeconomic Status (SES) On Health Outcomes

SES plays a vital role in determining health outcomes across the life course, influencing physical and mental well-being. Individuals of lower SES often reside in environments with more stress due to economic instability, limited access to healthcare, and inadequate nutrition. This creates long-term disease conditions of obesity, diabetes, and heart disease, which have profound impacts on adult health. In addition, where SES intersects with other social determinants of health, such as education and employment, they compound vulnerability. Understanding how early socioeconomic disparities develop into adulthood underscores the need for integrated health interventions that focus on both short-term interventions and long-term needs, as recognized by the Mitchell Institute. By addressing such natural imbalances, policy measures can be strengthened to ensure equal health outcomes across all socioeconomic strata, ultimately leading to a healthier population (Sweeny, 2025). The influence of socioeconomic status on health is most substantial in the early years of childhood, where early experiences significantly shape an individual's trajectory. Early childhood interventions can dramatically alter the consequences of socioeconomic disadvantage, setting the stage for better adult health and educational attainment. For instance, supportive environments and resource availability can offset the deteriorating effects of poverty for this most vulnerable development period. Children raised in affluent environments are found to develop healthier behavioral habits and coping styles, which lead to better adult health. Conversely, those experiencing child adversity, such as family breakup or poverty, are at increased risk of adverse health in adulthood. Thus, as shown here through evidence from the studies, interventions need to be implemented at an early stage to address and break the cycle of disadvantage and foster resilience (Baker et al., 2008). Additionally, the cultural determinants intertwined with socioeconomic status further widen health inequities. Cultural beliefs and practices can determine eating behaviors, health behaviors, and healthcare use. Marginalized groups tend to experience linguistic and cultural misunderstandings and mistrust of healthcare organizations, leading to underuse of necessary services. The intersection of culture and socioeconomic status, therefore, can lead to increased health risks and decreased health literacy. Addressing these dimensions of culture requires a responsive approach to public health initiatives that recognizes and responds to diverse values within the community. Incorporating cultural competence into healthcare strategies will enable practitioners to enhance communication and care delivery, ultimately leading to improved health outcomes for individuals across diverse socioeconomic levels. Emphasizing this dimension of health equity is critical when addressing the systemic challenges faced by marginalized populations (Sweeny, 2025).

4.5.2. Barriers to Accessing Healthcare and Nutrition

Health care and nutrition access are complex issues influenced by many obstacles that disproportionately affect vulnerable populations. Socioeconomic conditions are of significant significance, since residents in poor communities experience barriers like financial hardship, which restricts their ability to pay for medical services or healthy food. Even where services are available, unaffordable out-of-pocket expenses discourage individuals from accessing necessary care, producing continued cycles of ill health. Further, geographical distances, particularly in rural areas, limit access to healthcare centers, rendering preventive services and nutrition education less readily available. Through these inequalities, then, health inequality is exacerbated, and the most disadvantaged groups are often those that are marginalized. Socioeconomic and geographical barriers must be overcome in efforts to increase access to healthcare and nutrition, ultimately leading to a healthier population that can make a positive contribution to society. Cultural aspects significantly influence the availability of healthcare and nutrition, as beliefs and practices shape how people perceive and utilize healthcare. Populations may experience difficulties accessing the healthcare system due to linguistic and cultural differences, leading to miscommunication. In many cases, traditional concepts regarding nutrition and health are the reasons for skepticism toward modern medical treatment, and hence, patients avoid treatment. Furthermore, cultural stigma may affect the eagerness of an individual to seek care for specific illnesses, particularly mental illness or chronic illnesses. Additionally, cultural dietary preferences may limit access to proper nutrition, particularly in multicultural populations or areas where culturally specific foods are not readily available.

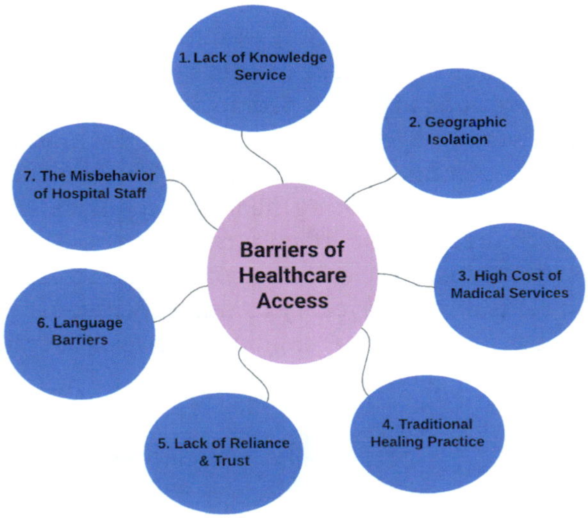
1. Lack of Knowledge Service
2. Geographic Isolation
7. The Misbehavior of Hospital Staff
Barriers of Healthcare Access
3. High Cost of Madical Services
6. Language Barriers
4. Traditional Healing Practice
5. Lack of Reliance & Trust

Figure 4.17. Barriers to healthcare access.

Source: https://www.researchgate.net/publication/373130775/figure/fig1/AS:11431281181614824@1692106994470/Barriers-to-healthcare-access.png.

To establish a more equitable healthcare environment, it is essential to consider these cultural issues and design interventions that respect and incorporate the diverse health practices and beliefs. Access to healthcare infrastructure to medical care and nutritional services cannot be overemphasized. Poor health facilities, lack of skilled health workers, and limited financing create a barrier that prevents people from accessing quality and timely care. For instance, the workload for healthcare workers can overwhelm them, leading to a decrease in the quality of care and patient satisfaction. Nutrition services also cannot receive support or financing to extend services to those in need, particularly among poorer communities. Secondly, integration of healthcare services with other social determinants of health is also essential in overcoming these barriers to healthcare access. According to previous research, strengthening healthcare infrastructure can lead to improved health outcomes and increased access to preventive care and nutrition education. Policymakers must, therefore, take utmost care in developing robust healthcare systems to effectively meet the needs of all these populations (Figure 4.17).

4.5.3. Role of Community Resources in Health Improvement

The role of community resources in health promotion is significant because they play a crucial role in enhancing the physical, nutritional, and cultural dimensions of adult health. Local health programs, fitness programs, and nutrition education services offered by community resources empower individuals by providing them with information and support systems. These resources facilitate the adoption of healthier lifestyles by promoting physical activity and healthy diets that are culturally acceptable and accessible. For instance, neighborhood gardens provide not just fresh fruits and vegetables but also social support and exchange of food preparation and nutrition knowledge. Participation in these activities can lead to greater health benefits through the reduction of the risk of physical inactivity-induced chronic diseases and poor diets, highlighting the importance of community-based initiatives in fostering a culture of health within communities (Murphy et al., 2008). Furthermore, the intersectional nature of community resources and health equity cannot be overstated, particularly in light of the ongoing access inequalities faced by marginalized populations to essential resources such as food, water, and healthcare. Community-based organizations working to mitigate food insecurity, as well as those providing nutrition education, are essential in addressing disparities among diverse populations. Through collaborations with grassroots stakeholders and the utilization of existing infrastructure, such as religious centers and schools, these organizations can tailor their programs to meet the specific needs of the community. These efforts are even more critical in the context of achieving the Sustainable Development Goals, notably SDG 2, Zero Hunger. Failing to make progress towards nutritional adequacy for all, as identified in several studies, necessitates a joint effort by community resources to achieve more equitable health outcomes (United Nations System Standing Committee on Nutrition, 2020). In addition to physical and nutritional health, community resources play a vital role in promoting cultural dimensions of well-being. Culturally responsive health care can enhance the effect of health interventions by recognizing and integrating the artistic practice and preference of different populations. For example, health education programs incorporating culturally appropriate dietary advice not only seem more natural to participants but also promote a sense of community and understanding within the population. Furthermore, the involvement of local leaders and cultural organizations in health promotion enhances its effectiveness by fostering trust and promoting greater community engagement. This holistic approach to promoting health recognizes the interconnectedness of cultural identity, social relationships, and health outcomes, and stresses the central role played by community resources in fostering an environment conducive to overall health gain (Murphy et al., 2008).

Test Your Knowledge

1. What are two socioeconomic considerations nurses need to consider when performing a health assessment?
2. How can socioeconomic status influence a patient's access to and compliance with healthcare and treatment?

4.6. Technology in Health Assessment

Learning Outcome

1. Describe the use of telehealth in adult health assessments
2. Define the digital technologies applied for monitoring physical and nutritional health
3. Identify future trends in health assessment technology

Over the past few decades, the integration of technology in health screening has significantly altered the assessment of adult health on several fronts. Telemedicine, wearable devices, and mobile health apps have revolutionized the collection and analysis of health information. These technological advances enable real-time tracking of vital signs and virtual consultations, overcoming most geographical and socio-economic challenges that previously limited access to healthcare. In addition to this, the ability to track nutritional intake and exercise through mobile applications has empowered individuals to take an active role in their own care, making preventive interventions and lifestyle modifications a reality. This greater focus on an open and accessible model of healthcare shows how technology can drive a proactive health assessment and intervention model, ultimately leading to better patient outcomes and satisfaction. In addition, the cultural aspects of health evaluation are increasingly shaped by technology in several respects. Online platforms have the potential to provide culturally relevant healthcare through the customization of information and resources, making them more effective for culturally diverse populations. This can include everything from multilingual telemedicine to culturally targeted health education materials available online. For example, specific programs can provide nutritional guidance in accordance with the various cultural practices and thereby respecting individual options while addressing nutritional needs. By embracing technology, health professionals can communicate more effectively with patients from diverse cultural backgrounds, thereby fostering greater trust and enhanced communication.

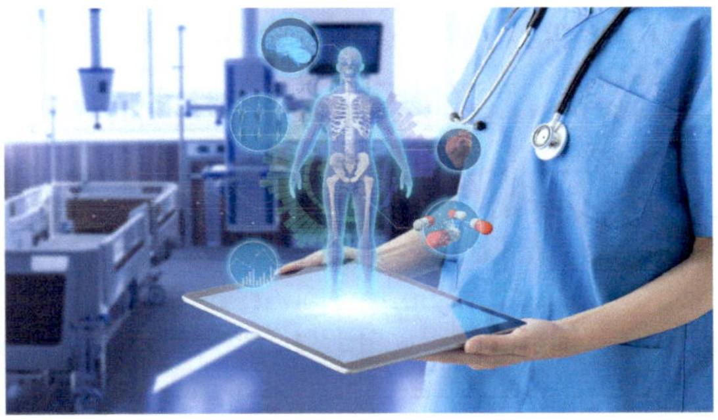

Figure 4.18. Technology changing nursing practice.

Source: https://thedoctorweighsin.com/wp-content/uploads/Nursing-Technology.jpg.

These advances not only improve the effectiveness of health assessments but also increase healthcare system inclusivity, as all individuals are given support in sustaining their health. Technology use is also seen in the advancement of data capture, analysis, and interpretation in health assessments. Electronic health records (EHRs), for instance, facilitate comprehensive documentation, allowing clinicians to document a patient's complete history and social determinants of health. This data-centric approach encourages a deeper understanding of the dynamic interactions among an individual's physical, nutritional, and cultural factors. Furthermore, sophisticated analytics within EHR systems enable predictive modeling, identifying potential health risks and guiding targeted interventions. This becoming increasingly complex and nuanced, making a type of technological bundling necessary. With data and technology, practitioners can enhance their assessment of adult health, ultimately contributing to improved health outcomes through targeted interventions and anticipatory care (Cornell University, 2007; Lohmann et al., 2015) (Figure 4.18).

4.6.1. Use of Telehealth in Adult Health Assessments

The application of telehealth in adult health assessment represents a paradigm shift in how healthcare is delivered, particularly in eradicating barriers to access. The majority of individuals, especially those from rural or disadvantaged areas, face tremendous challenges in accessing healthcare services due to geographic distances and the unavailability of healthcare professionals. This is particularly so in Australia, where the majority of residents must travel long distances in order to access required health services (Bywood et al., 2013). Telehealth addresses these issues through the use of telecommunication technologies for remote consultation, thus providing patients with the convenience of health assessment without the need for travel. Then, the innovation improves access not just to rural populations but also assists healthcare systems by reducing the burden imposed on face-to-face consultations. Moreover, the efficacy of telehealth in adult health assessment is evident in its adherence to modern patient-centered healthcare delivery models. Telehealth technology enables clinicians to gather critical information related to a patient's physical, nutritional, and cultural aspects effectively. Such remote interaction enables the incorporation of multiple evaluation tools that can be implemented in real-time, allowing clinicians to assess an individual's overall health requirements. In addition, as indicated in recent literature, individualized interventions to facilitate equal access to health care are essential in improving the health outcomes among individuals with poor access to health care (Bywood et al., 2011). Telehealth, in addition to its convenience in gathering vital data, helps facilitate patient engagement, ensuring individuals can take an active role in controlling their well-being. Besides, as the telehealth model evolves, it can go a long way toward enhancing the cultural competence of healthcare. By enabling providers to interact with patients in an open and comfortable environment, telehealth encourages trust and openness, which are required for practical health assessments. This is particularly important in diverse populations who may be apprehensive about the conventional healthcare environment. By overcoming these barriers through technology, clinicians can establish improved relationships and rapport with their patients. Through the integrated use of telehealth in healthcare settings, stakeholders must ensure that these platforms are capable of meeting the diverse needs of all patients for equitable outcomes (Figure 4.19).

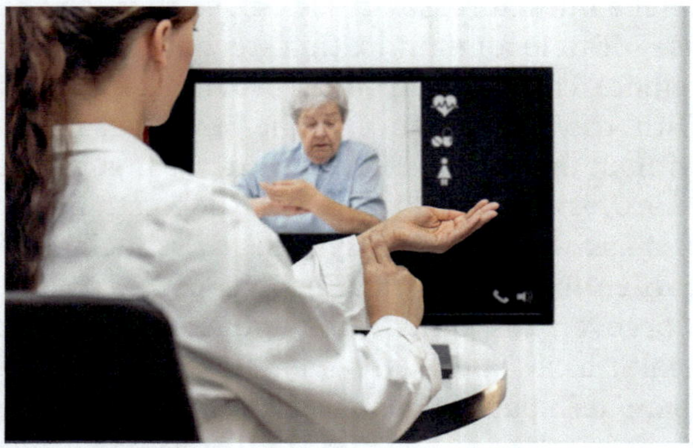

Figure 4.19. Use of telehealth in adult health assessments.

Source: https://surgerylink.com/wp-content/uploads/2020/03/Telehealth-photo-scaled.jpg.

4.6.2. Digital Tools for Tracking Physical and Nutritional Health

The use of digital devices to track physical and nutritional well-being has revolutionized the way individuals monitor their well-being over the last decade. Wearable devices, mobile applications, and websites have enabled individuals to track various health indicators, including physical activity, heart rate, and nutrition. Such technologies offer a unique level of self-awareness, enabling individuals to set personalized health targets and receive immediate feedback on their progress. Importantly, such instruments not only encourage personal responsibility but also provide gateways for insights grounded in data that are potentially beneficial when shared with health professionals. This shift in healthcare is keeping pace with a greater movement toward patient activation, building a culture where patients are actively engaged in their healthcare process, ultimately leading to improved physical and nutritional outcomes. Secondly, the impact of digital health tools extends beyond individual engagement to achieve more macro-level public health objectives. Through the aggregation of large numbers of users, the tools provide very rich data to policymakers and health researchers. Physical activity and food patterns can be viewed on a grand scale to provide information in designing evidence-based interventions. With ongoing health equity remaining an imperative, the use of these tools can inform the identification of populations at risk and support the development of targeted programs aimed at increasing access to physical activity and nutrition services. Apart from this, the adaptability of such web-based systems allows for responsive and sensitive adjustment of intervention for varying lifestyle problems, which encourages greater inclusiveness in health interventions that might otherwise overlook particular needs within a population (Birnbaum et al., 2011). However, the universal application of health-monitoring online technologies over a brief duration interval comes with limitations. There are also issues of data privacy, the accuracy of self-reported data, and heterogeneity in technology access that need to be handled with caution. Most people would gain from these technologies, yet there might be other groups lacking digital literacy or resources to allow them to exploit these opportunities fully, thus thereby perpetuating current health disparities. If these technologies are to benefit health, developers and practitioners must ensure that they are simple to use and have robust support bases behind them. There will also be a need for ongoing monitoring of these technologies as the health monitoring field continues to evolve in response to changing public expectations and constraints within existing frameworks. Being capable of overcoming these methodological and operational issues will be crucial to the long-term success of digital health programs (Raftree et al., 2016) (Figure 4.20).

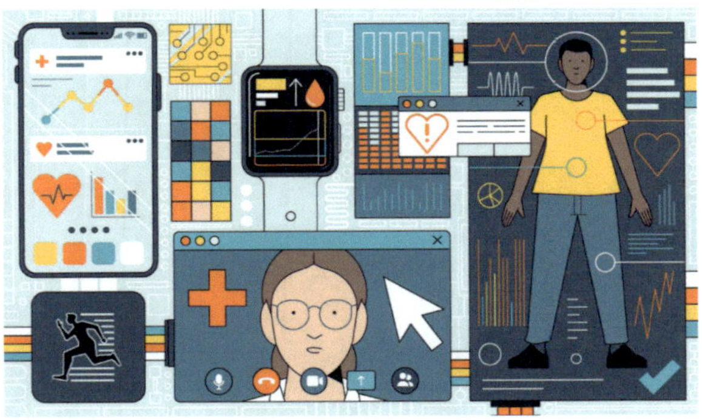

Figure 4.20. Digital tools for tracking physical and nutritional health.

Source: https://media.wired.com/photos/63a1130619e18c9c6297e805/master/w_2560%2Cc_limit/06_Digital-health-tools-need-a-new-benchmark.jpg.

4.6.3. Future Trends in Health Assessment Technology

As technology continues to evolve, the future of health measurement is moving toward an increasingly integrated and personalized approach. Sophisticated devices, such as mobile phones and phone apps, are revolutionizing the way individuals monitor their health markers, providing real-time feedback on physical activity, heart rate, and even calorie intake. They not only make screening more accessible but also make it need-based, thus facilitating proactive intervention rather than reactive. Modern policy discourse has increasingly supported the necessity of addressing multifaceted determinants of health that include physical, nutritional, and cultural determinants in a manner that encourages technology usage to ensure the highest outcomes. By opening the doors to such technological progress, health screening can provide more detailed information about a person's health condition, leading to enhanced-quality care in an era of technological superiority (Murphy et al., 2008). In addition, the combination of artificial intelligence and machine learning with healthcare evaluation processes promises a new future of precision medicine. AI systems are increasingly being applied to sift through complex data streams from electronic health records and wearables, detect patterns, and predict potential health issues before they arise. This capability not only assists clinicians in making informed decisions but also empowers patients to take care of their health by providing them with personalized recommendations and feedback. Of particular importance is the emphasis on the cultural element in the assessment of health, as such instruments can facilitate culturally sensitive care that respects variations in practice and heritage. Policies emphasize intersectoral partnerships among health professionals and technology innovators, ensuring that innovation is not only scientifically sound but also culturally relevant, thereby promoting patient engagement and adherence to health recommendations (United Nations System Standing Committee on Nutrition, 2020). Last but not least, the use of telemedicine in health assessment is expected to expand, particularly with the pandemic-driven transformations globally. Virtual health assessments and telemedicine visits are more flexible and convenient, especially for vulnerable populations in areas with limited access to healthcare. The trend aligns with broader hopes of increasing health equity by eliminating socioeconomic and geography-based barriers. As telehealth continues to expand, it will become increasingly important for platforms to have robust evaluation tools that incorporate physical, nutritional, and cultural measures. This model of integration not only improves immediate health but also leads to long-term success in health management programs. The promise of health assessment technology also has a great deal to offer on the basis of an assured dedication to integrating these various factors of health into an integrative and balanced state (United Nations System Standing Committee on Nutrition, 2020).

Test Your Knowledge

1. Name two technologies that are commonly utilized in health screenings and explain their functions.
2. How have electronic health records (EHRs) improved the accuracy and speed of health screenings?

SUMMARY

The overall assessment of adult health from the physical, dietary, and cultural realms, it is apparent that one needs a comprehensive approach to address health inequities. This review has highlighted the interconnectedness of various parameters that influence adult health consequences. The study work on childhood adversity, as evident in populations like those presented here in Nepal, attests to the additive risk that socio-economic factors such as homelessness and migration pose on people. All these aspects are core to the formulation of intervention strategies that work towards minimizing the stressors of heterogeneous living conditions, as these play a crucial role in determining the health trajectory during the course of adult life (Baker et al., 2008). Secondly, the study highlights the crucial role of nutritional status in adult health, particularly in diverse geographical settings. For instance, while malnutrition is a short-term emergency in rural Mozambique, it has been established that the residents of both rural and urban areas are as susceptible to the determinants of food insecurity. Such a discovery highlights the need to consider localized contexts when addressing nutritional concerns among adults, ensuring that interventions are tailored to the individualized socioeconomic contexts of different populations. By this recognition of such complexity, public health interventions can be improved by harmonizing responses to food security and nutrition as interrelated determinants to overall health (Garrett et al., 2025). Lastly, the total health profile of adults requires the recognition of physical and cultural factors in addition to diet. Practice and belief determine health behavior and access to resources. This requires culturally sensitive and value-based policies to enhance health programs, so that they not only treat but also prevent states of ill health through proper interventions based on cultural context. Subsequent studies must continue to investigate and examine the intricate interplay across these dimensions in order to develop comprehensive and integrative health programs. By bringing together data from physical health assessments, nutrition science, and culture, a more combined model of adult health can be created, providing improved health results across populations.

In assessing adult health, it is necessary to examine how physical, nutritional, and cultural determinants interact with one another. Physical well-being encompasses a range of states, including chronic diseases, mental illnesses, and physical conditions. Health care accessibility, lifestyle, and environmental conditions are all instrumental when estimating the health state of an individual on the physical level. These must be understood during the planning of targeted health interventions. Second, the prevalence of mental diseases, socially, which are usually spread by social stigma, also has to be understood during the construction of integrated health programs that are physical as well as mentally viable. Nutrition is the second significant pillar in adult health assessment, playing a preeminent role in both physical and mental health outcomes. An adequate diet with complete nutrients can ward off the threat of lethal chronic diseases, and malnutrition leads to critical health complications. The divergence in nutritional status among urban and rural communities demonstrates the complexities involved. For instance, undernourishment is more prevalent in rural settings, while food security levels are either equal to or lower than those of urban regions. The trend is a confirmation of the role played by regional variations and socioeconomic influences that govern nutritional access and health conditions, as revealed in fresh studies and verification of the determinants of malnutrition and food insecurity that are not only alike in all environments (Garrett et al., 2025). Cultural factors also play a significant role in shaping attitudes and health practices. Cultural beliefs control attitudes and behavior related to health. For instance, certain beliefs will discourage individuals from reporting to health services until they have established illnesses, thereby precluding screening and health intervention. Additionally, interventions should consider cultural sensitivities to facilitate enhanced health behaviors better. Policies that enhance health outcomes, such as those described in pioneering reports on obesity among children, remind us that culturally appropriate practices must be employed in public health interventions (Murphy et al., 2008). By incorporating physical, nutritional, and cultural components into a unified framework for health assessment, a comprehensive profile of adult health can be obtained, facilitating more informed public health policies and practices.

KEY TERMS FROM THIS CHAPTER

- Anthropometric Measurements
- Cultural Competence
- Dietary Habits
- Health awareness
- Health Risk Factors
- Language Barriers
- Nutritional Assessment
- Religious Food Restrictions
- Body Mass Index (BMI)
- Cultural Dietary Practices
- Dietary patterns
- Health Perception
- Hydration Status
- Malnutrition
- Physical Examination
- Skin Turgor

CRITICAL THINKING QUESTIONS

1. **What is the primary purpose of physical health assessment among adults?**
   a. To identify the patient's education
   b. To diagnose with or without laboratory aid
   c. To establish baseline data on the patient's state of health
   d. To prescribe medication
2. **Which of the following is most frequently employed in nutritional assessment in adults?**
   a. Sphygmomanometer
   b. Body Mass Index (BMI)
   c. Pulse oximeter
   d. Electrocardiogram (ECG)
3. **Which of the following best demonstrates cultural competence in interviewing with adult health?**
   a. Steering clear of talking about cultural practices
   b. Assuming patients have the same beliefs about health
   c. Asking about health practices and being respectful of cultural options
   d. Disregard for linguistic variation in communication
4. **In nutritional assessment, which of the following is an indicator of possible malnutrition?**
   a. Normal hemoglobin
   b. Unintentional weight reduction and muscle wasting
   c. Sufficient food intake
   d. Stable weight for 6 months
5. **On general examination, the nurse observes dry, scaly skin and brittle nails. What could this be a sign of?**
   a. Sufficient hydration and nutrition
   b. Early infection
   c. Possible nutritional deficiency
   d. Normal changes of aging

Short Answer Questions

1. What are the key elements of a physical examination in adults?
2. What is Body Mass Index (BMI) and how is it used in nutritional assessment?
3. What are two physical examination indicators of impaired nutritional status?
4. Why is cultural belief a factor in assessing health?
5. Why is the use of subjective information critical to adult health assessment?
6. Explain the process of conducting a thorough physical assessment of an adult patient.
7. Explain the importance of nutritional assessment in adult health care. Include screening tests and clinical findings.
8. Explain how cultural practices and beliefs influence a person's health behavior and test outcome.

Answers to Critical Thinking Questions

1. (c); 2. (b); 3. (c); 4. (b); 5. (c)

REFERENCES

1. Aberman, N. L., Cohen, M. J., Thompson, B., Tirado, R., et al. (2025). Impact of climate change and bioenergy on nutrition. https://core.ac.uk/download/pdf/6329340.pdf (accessed on 28th June 2025).
2. Agarwal, E., Marshall, S., Miller, M., & Isenring, E. (2016b). Optimising nutrition in residential aged care: A narrative review. *Maturitas*, *92*, 70–78. https://doi.org/10.1016/j.maturitas.2016.06.013Aitsi-Selmi, A., Benova, L., Marmot, M., Sholkamy, H., et al. (2009). Addressing the double burden of malnutrition in Egypt: Do conditional cash transfers have a role? https://core.ac.uk/download/1688696.pdf (accessed on 28th June 2025).
3. Baker, C. M., Worthman, C., Panter-Brick, C., Desjarlais, R., Eveleth, P., et al. (2008). Homeless street children in Nepal: Use of allostatic load to assess the burden of childhood adversity. https://core.ac.uk/download/65673.pdf (accessed on 28th June 2025).
4. Balgir, R. S. (2011). Genetic disease burden, nutrition and determinants of tribal health care in Chhattisgarh State of Central-East India: A status paper. https://core.ac.uk/download/pdf/332892.pdf (accessed on 28th June 2025).
5. Ballarotto, G., Cerniglia, L., Cimino, S., Gnessi, L., et al. (2017). An exploratory study on the influence of psychopathological risk and impulsivity on BMI and perceived quality of life in obese patients. https://core.ac.uk/download/98336136.pdf (accessed on 28th June 2025).
6. Bangay, C., & Blum, N. (2010). Education responses to climate change and quality: Two parts of the same agenda? https://core.ac.uk/download/pdf/83706.pdf (accessed on 28th June 2025).
7. Birnbaum, N., Masterson, E., & Schoomaker, H. (2011). State of Health Equity Movement, 2011 update Part C: Compendium of recommendations. DRA Project Report No. 11-03. https://core.ac.uk/download/pdf/18491812.pdf (accessed on 28th June 2025).
8. Bleecker, M., Krause, C., Linder, K., Moffett, M., et al. (2017). Situating food insecurity in a historic Albuquerque community: The whorled relationship between food insecurity and place. https://digitalscholarship.unlv.edu/cgi/viewcontent.cgi?article=1675&context=jhdrp (accessed on 28th June 2025).
9. Burke, K. M., Fernandez Duque, E., & Valeggia, C. R. (2009). Nutritional status and socioeconomic change among Toba and Wichí populations of the Argentinean Chaco. https://core.ac.uk/download/287881909.pdf (accessed on 28th June 2025).
10. Burton, M. J., Ramke, J., Marques, A. P., Bourne, R., Congdon, N., Jones, I., Ah Tong, B. A. M., et al. (2021). The Lancet Global Health Commission on global eye health: Vision beyond 2020. *The Lancet Global Health, 9*, e489–e551. https://doi.org/10.1016/s2214-109x(20)30488-5 (accessed on 28th June 2025).
11. Bywood, P. T., Katterl, R., & Lunnay, B. K. (2011). Disparities in primary health care utilization: Who are the disadvantaged groups? How are they disadvantaged? What interventions work? https://core.ac.uk/download/14947498.pdf (accessed on 28th June 2025).
12. Carvalho Vila, V. da S., Siqueira, T. H., & Weiss, M. E. (2018). Cross-cultural adaptation of the instrument Readiness for Hospital Discharge Scale–Adult Form. https://core.ac.uk/download/286544020.pdf (accessed on 28th June 2025).

13. Cornell University. (2007). *College of Agriculture and Life Sciences*. https://ecommons.cornell.edu/bitstream/handle/1813/38611/COS_v99_2007_2008_02.pdf?sequence=1&isAllowed=y (accessed on 28th June 2025).

14. Crush, J., Frayne, B., & Grant, M. (2007). No. 3: Linking migration, HIV/AIDS and urban food security in Southern and Eastern Africa. https://core.ac.uk/download/157834934.pdf (accessed on 28th June 2025).

15. Dwivedi, Y. K., Hughes, L., Baabdullah, A. M., Ribeiro-Navarrete, S., Giannakis, M., Al-Debei, M. M., Dennehy, D., et al. (2022). Metaverse beyond the hype: Multidisciplinary perspectives on emerging challenges, opportunities, and agenda for research, practice and policy. *International Journal of Information Management, 66*, 102542–102542. https://doi.org/10.1016/j.ijinfomgt.2022.102542 (accessed on 28th June 2025).

16. El Sayed, F., Soar, J., & Wang, Z. (2011). Cultural matter in the development of an interactive multimedia self-paced educational health program for aboriginal health workers. https://core.ac.uk/download/11047695.pdf (accessed on 28th June 2025).

17. Flores, R., & Gillespie, S. (2025). *Health and Nutrition: Emerging and Reemerging Issues in Developing Countries*. https://core.ac.uk/download/pdf/6288820.pdf (accessed on 28th June 2025).

18. Garrett, J. L., & Ruel, M. T. (2025). Are determinants of rural and urban food security and nutritional status different? https://core.ac.uk/download/pdf/6289471.pdf (accessed on 28th June 2025).

19. Gillespie, S., & Haddad, L. J. (2025). Effective food and nutrition policy responses to HIV/AIDS. https://core.ac.uk/download/pdf/6289466.pdf (accessed on 28th June 2025).

20. Gualdi-Russo, E. (2015). Assessment of nutritional status and body image perceptions on immigrants. https://core.ac.uk/download/54711679.pdf (accessed on 28th June 2025).

21. Henry, C., Lapenu, C., Sharma, M., Zeller, M., et al. (2025). An operational tool for evaluating poverty outreach of development policies and projects. https://core.ac.uk/download/pdf/6289609.pdf (accessed on 28th June 2025).

22. Herklotz, A., Nayar, A., Agarwal, B., Archer, C., Tirado, C., Elson, D., Maceachern, D., et al. (2012). Powerful synergies: Gender equality, economic development and environmental sustainability. https://core.ac.uk/download/75779706.pdf (accessed on 28th June 2025).

23. Hodges, B. D., & Lingard, L. (2013). The question of competence: Reconsidering medical education in the twenty-first century. https://core.ac.uk/download/19958654.pdf (accessed on 28th June 2025).

24. Kritpracha, C., Primanda, Y., & Thaniwattananon, P. (2011). Dietary behaviors among patients with type 2 diabetes mellitus in Yogyakarta, Indonesia. https://media.neliti.com/media/publications/154790-EN-dietary-behaviors-among-patients-with-ty.pdf (accessed on 28th June 2025).

25. Leal, I., Pimenta, F., Rosas, R., Schwarzer, R., et al. (2019). FOODLIT-PRO: Food literacy domains, influential factors and determinants—A qualitative study. https://core.ac.uk/download/322846652.pdf (accessed on 28th June 2025).

26. Lee, J. M., Park, I. K., & Nam, H. S. (2024). Abstract P378: Life's essential 8 and personal income level in Korean adults. *Circulation*. https://www.semanticscholar.org/paper/547e777850747560e6be3d1ea9b218df07118680 (accessed on 28th June 2025).

27. Lohmann, S. (2015). A contribution to the empirics of development and globalization. https://core.ac.uk/download/150155401.pdf (accessed on 28th June 2025).
28. Mungreiphy, N. K., & Kapoor, S. (2008). Overweight, obesity and socio-economic change among Tangkhul Naga tribal women of Manipur, North East India. https://core.ac.uk/download/pdf/287853.pdf (accessed on 28th June 2025).
29. Murphy, C. G., Alendy, C., Cooper, J., & Simpson, L. (2008). Childhood obesity: The role of health policy. https://core.ac.uk/download/71342400.pdf (accessed on 28th June 2025).
30. Nurmalia, D., Padmasari, S., Rokhana, N., Utami, N., et al. (2015). *Proceeding: 3rd Java International Nursing Conference 2015 "Harmony of Caring and Healing Inquiry for Holistic Nursing Practice; Enhancing Quality of Care," Semarang, 20–21 August 2015*. https://core.ac.uk/download/76930906.pdf (accessed on 28th June 2025).
31. Raftree, L., & Bamberger, M. (2016). Emerging opportunities: Monitoring and evaluation in a tech-enabled world. https://core.ac.uk/download/83111958.pdf (accessed on 28th June 2025).
32. Smalls, M. N. B. (2013). A synthesis of the literature on the relationship between food access and overweight and obesity in African American adolescents. https://core.ac.uk/download/12214833.pdf (accessed on 28th June 2025).
33. Sweeny, K. (2025). The influence of childhood circumstances on adult health. https://core.ac.uk/download/pdf/30672978.pdf (accessed on 28th June 2025).
34. Tobin, J., Black, M. M., Ng, J., Rankin, D., Wallace, J., Hughes, C. F., Hoey, L., et al. (2025). Identifying comorbidity patterns of mental health disorders in community-dwelling older adults: A cluster analysis. *BMC Geriatrics, 25*. https://www.semanticscholar.org/paper/228df7f27f1072448a6ae2c245c096721185c1ef (accessed on 28th June 2025).
35. United Nations System Standing Committee on Nutrition. (2020). *Water and Nutrition: Harmonizing Actions for the United Nations Decade of Action on Nutrition and the United Nations Water Action Decade*. https://core.ac.uk/download/288633623.pdf (accessed on 28th June 2025).

STRESS RESPONSES AND INFLAMMATORY MECHANISMS

5

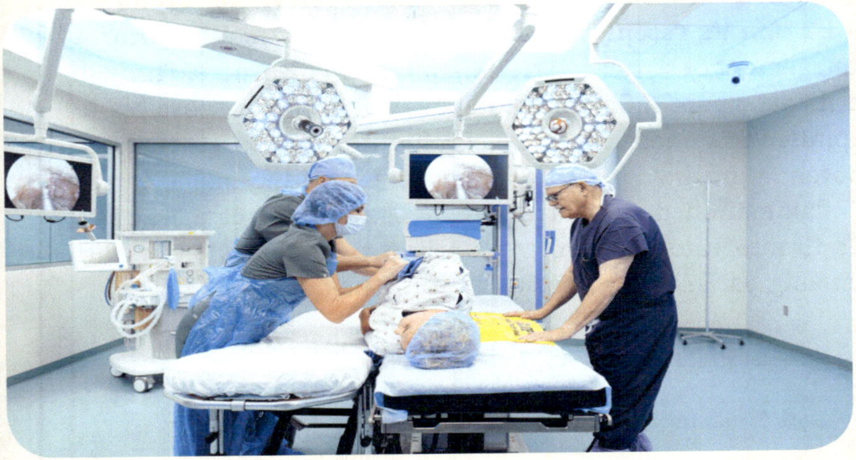

LEARNING OBJECTIVES

After studying this chapter, you will be able to:

1. Know the physiology of stress responses
2. Describe the kinds of stressors
3. Describe the mechanisms of inflammation
4. Highlight stress-induced inflammatory responses
5. Assess the bidirectional interaction between stress and inflammation
6. Recite the approaches to managing stress and inflammation

Introduction

The interaction of stress responses with inflammatory mechanisms is an essential field of study in understanding the body's biological response to stressors. Stress, either psychological or physical, triggers an cascade of HPA-mediated reactions that ultimately lead to the release of glucocorticoids. The function of these hormones is to regulate various body functions, including metabolism and immune responses, indicating that this is a highly developed homeostatic mechanism that maintains the body within a steady state. Nevertheless, chronic stress can lead to the dysregulation of these systems, thereby contributing to the development of various inflammatory conditions. As immediate of inflammation, cytokines and danger-associated molecular patterns, like high-mobility group protein B1 (HMGB1), are particularly pertinent. By inducing inflammation, these molecules have the potential to amplify the body's global stress response, thereby creating a complex feedback loop that can perpetuate a vicious cycle of stress and inflammation. Investigation of the role of HMGB1 in inflammatory responses initiated by stress provides important insights into the mechanisms connecting these two bodily processes. Existing evidence suggests that HMGB1 is a danger signal that is overexpressed in stressed tissues, such as those affected by tendinopathy. Overexpression of HMGB1 results in elevated levels of pro-inflammatory cytokines, such as interleukin-1 beta (IL-1β) and IL-6, which are well-known inducers of inflammation and tissue remodeling. This interaction suggests that HMGB1 not only contributes to the inflammatory milieu that is associated with stress responses but also holds the potential to become a target for therapeutic manipulation. Understanding the manner in which these inflammatory mediators influence stressors can pave the way for new methods of mitigating the pathogenic impact of chronic stress on health (Akbar et al., 2017). The potential implications of modulating the HMGB1-mediated mechanisms are also of immediate clinical relevance. Exploring therapeutic measures that target HMGB1 and its receptor pathways, such as toll-like receptor 4 (TLR4), can significantly impact the management of stress-related inflammatory disorders. Through modulation of HMGB1 expression and its attendant inflammatory sequelae, it may be possible to reduce the severity of conditions precipitated by or accelerated by chronic stress. Researchers have previously reported the therapeutic potential of this approach, citing its use in the management of diseases that are brought on by inflammation due to stress responses (Drew et al., 2014). As technology advances and continues to integrate this information into treatment models, this represents a critical step toward optimizing patient outcomes and overall health (Figure 5.1).

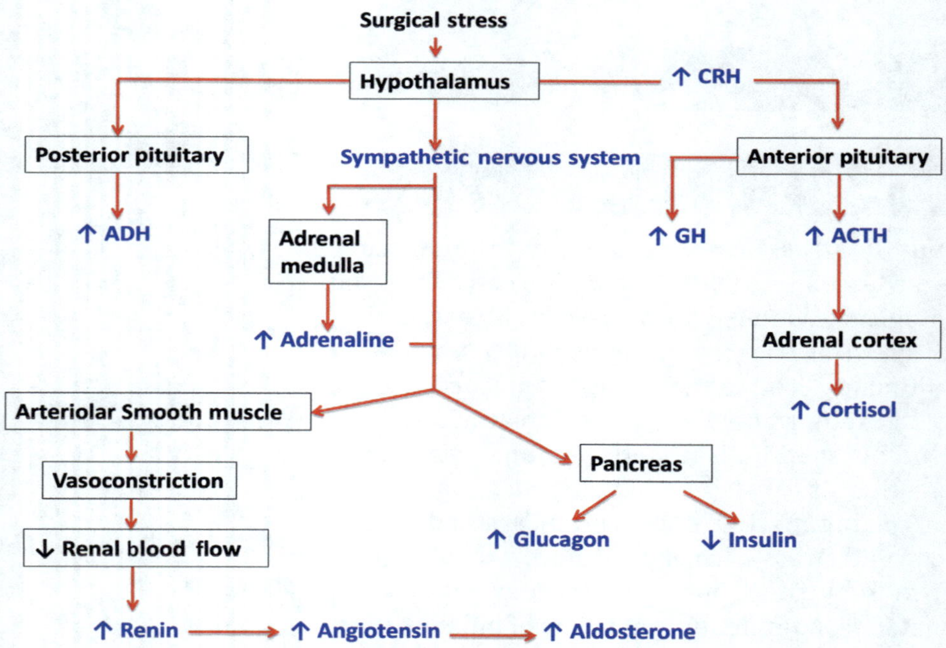

Figure 5.1. Surgical stress response.

Source: https://els-jbs-prod-cdn.jbs.elsevierhealth.com/cms/attachment/5353ee3f-f853-4aaf-91c6-f0a230c7cc68/gr2_lrg.jpg.

Definition of Stress Responses

Understanding responses to stress is essential in deciphering the relationship between stress and inflammatory processes. Responses to stress can be described as physiological, behavioral, and psychological changes that occur in organisms when faced with perceived danger or challenge. The body's stress response is primarily orchestrated by the hypothalamic-pituitary-adrenal (HPA) axis, which results in the release of several hormones, including cortisol. These endocrine changes prepare the body for impending danger by triggering the fight-or-flight response. However, constant activation of stress responses will cause dysregulation, leading to chronic inflammation and contributing to a variety of health disorders. This exchange underscores the importance of in-depth investigations into how stress responses can impact inflammatory pathways, thereby advancing our understanding of diseases such as rheumatoid arthritis and cardiovascular disease, both of which are closely linked to chronic stress. The implications of stress responses extend beyond brief adaptive processes; they fuel long-term health outcomes as they reprogram immune function and strengthen inflammatory processes. For example, chronic stress has been found to increase the release of pro-inflammatory cytokines, which play a crucial role in inflammation and immune response processes. Consistent with recent studies, increased cytokine levels cause tissue damage and increased susceptibility to autoimmune diseases (Ahmed et al., 2017). This association demonstrates that not only does the stress response influence acute reactions to stressors, but it also establishes the foundation for chronic inflammatory diseases. Consequently, understanding these stress-induced changes becomes crucial in developing therapeutic interventions aimed at restoring equilibrium and reducing inflammation, thereby promoting overall health and well-being. Notably, the influence of oxidative stress on stress responses is particularly significant. Oxidative stress occurs when there is an imbalance between free radical generation and the body's antioxidant defenses, and that is usually compounded by repeated exposure to chronic stress. This condition may lead to cellular damage, inducing cascades that promote the synthesis of inflammatory cytokines such as TNF-α and IL-6, which are of central relevance in inflammatory signaling pathways (Cerretani et al., 2015). Consequently, the relationship between oxidative stress, stress signaling, and inflammatory pathways represents a key area of research that sheds light on the pathophysiology of many diseases, including cardiovascular and metabolic diseases. By examining these correlations, researchers can identify potential prevention strategies and treatments that address the root causes of inflammation, rather than merely addressing the symptoms of stress-related diseases (Figure 5.2).

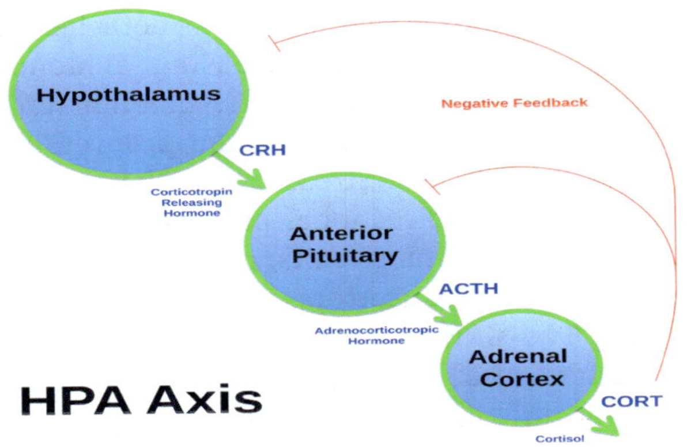

Figure 5.2. A diagram for hypothalamic-pituitary-adrenal (HPA) axis.

Source: https://www.researchgate.net/profile/Pengcheng-Xiao/publication/281995690/figure/fig1/AS:613874227240962@1523370429014/A-diagram-for-Hypothalamic-Pituitary-Adrenal-HPA-axis-In-response-to-stress-the.png.

Overview of Inflammatory Mechanisms

Inflammation is a significant biological defense against injurious stimuli, including pathogens, damaged cells, and irritants. This organized response is a complex interaction of immune cells, mediating signals, and vascular changes that direct the elimination of the offending agents and the initiation of tissue repair. The process may be acute or chronic. Acute inflammation is a rapid process characterized by typical signs of redness, warmth, swelling, and pain, primarily mediated by the activation of vascular endothelial cells and the mobilization of leukocytes. Chronic inflammation, however, persists longer than the standard time frame and can be held accountable for many diseases, like autoimmune disorders and cancer. Stress responses regulate the mechanisms that induce inflammation, particularly through the production of pro-inflammatory cytokines and chemokines, underscoring the importance of understanding these pathways in both health and disease. There is increasing evidence that chronic stress can enhance inflammatory reactions, hence influencing the progression of various diseases. Stress and inflammation converse in a bidirectional pathway involving the neuroendocrine circuits, most importantly those involving corticotropin-releasing hormone (CRH). The CRH family members have been characterized as central controllers of stress, affecting inflammatory mediators to possibly exacerbate diseases like colorectal cancer (CRC) by intricate cascades of signaling. In spite of the obscure molecular pathways through which chronic stress leads to enhanced inflammatory reactions, evidence suggests that such stress-induced effects may impact immune processes and disease pathogenesis. Clarification of this interaction can pave the way for revelations in personalized medicine approaches toward the prevention and control of inflammation-dependent diseases based on stress response (Baritaki et al., 2019). Additionally, the therapeutic role of glucocorticoids (GCs) in modulating inflammatory processes has been thoroughly studied and is known to possess bidirectional mechanisms of action. Upon binding to the glucocorticoid receptor (GR), GCs elicit their anti-inflammatory response primarily through a transrepressive mechanism, which involves repressing the expression of pro-inflammatory genes. Recent findings refute the widespread perception that monomer-mediated functions alone account for their efficacy. Evidence is found in favor of the function of GR dimers in facilitating anti-inflammatory responses, albeit in chronic inflammation. This provides possible implications for new therapeutic drug design specifically targeting GR pathways, calling for a reevaluation of the established paradigms controlling glucocorticoid therapy. These observations underscore the delicate balance between the inflammatory processes and their control through stress-related mechanisms, such as glucocorticoid regulation of immune reactions (Dejager et al., 2013).

Importance of Studying the Relationship Between Stress and Inflammation

It is of utmost importance to investigate the interaction between inflammation and stress in determining the broader implications for human health, particularly in light of the impact of chronic stress on various physiological processes. Chronic stress activates a cascade of biological reactions that can amplify inflammatory pathways, placing the body in an elevated state of systemic inflammation. There is evidence to support this association, as chronic psychological and physical stressors can lead to an overexpression of pro-inflammatory cytokines. These increases in inflammatory markers are associated with a host of health states such as cardiovascular disease, diabetes, and neurodegenerative disorders. As stress is prevalent in today's society, understanding the mechanisms that explain this relationship has the potential to close the gap in intervention development that reduces stress-evoked inflammation and promotes overall welfare. The investigation of stress-evoked effects on inflammation extends beyond physiological monitoring, providing insights into the relationships between physical and mental health. For instance, in research, patients with chronic stress were found to have elevated levels of inflammatory markers, which are suspected to play a pathogenetic role in disease states such as Alzheimer's disease (AD). In particular, stress-induced proinflammatory milieu over time can precondition the brain's microglial cells, which can lead to neuroinflammation and neurodegeneration. This emphasizes the need to respect stress not simply as an emotional process but a significant biological phenomenon with profound ramifications for neural function and cognitive health. Examining these relationships is essential for developing strategies aimed at reducing inflammation through stress reduction, with the goal of improving patient outcomes in various health conditions. In addition, studies assessing the contribution of individual stressors such as sexual minority stress continue to show the intricate dynamic between inflammation and stress. As described in sexual minority stress research, empirical evidence exists for an association between elevated levels of stress and alterations in leukocyte gene expression concerning inflammatory processes (Aouizerat et al., 2018). This indicates the need to consider the psychosocial predictors that increase stress and their physiological effects. By investigating these interactions, researchers can uncover new biological mechanisms that not only explain how stress amplifies inflammation but also inform public health interventions and therapeutic strategies. Lastly, a thorough exploration of these interactions is necessary to understand the complexities of the human stress response and to enable integrated approaches to health management that incorporate both psychological and physical elements of stress (Figure 5.3).

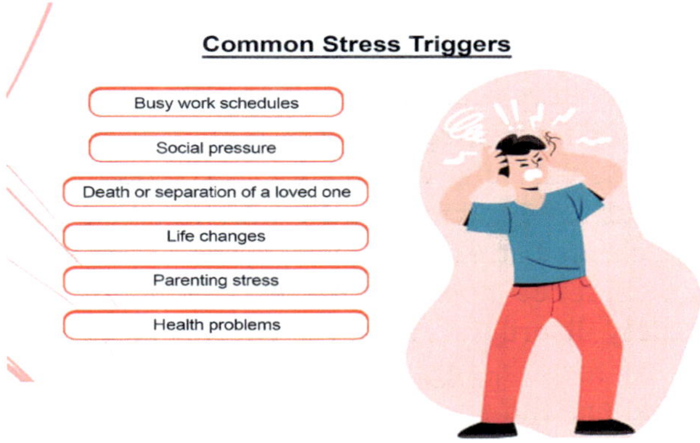

Figure 5.3. Chronic stress triggers.

Source: https://mangoclinic.com/wp-content/uploads/2022/06/What-Causes-Stress-and-How-Does-It-Affect-Your-Life-supporting-image-2.jpg.

5.1. The Physiology of Stress Responses

Learning Outcome

1. Explain the function of the hypothalamic-pituitary-adrenal (HPA) axis
2. Highlight neurotransmitters associated with stress responses
3. Learn about the effects of acute vs. chronic stress on the body

It is essential to learn the physiology of the responses to stress by examining the intricate hormonal and neurochemical mechanisms involved. When an individual is exposed to a stressor, either physiological or psychological, the HPA axis is activated. This leads to the release of corticotropin-releasing hormone (CRH), which stimulates the release of adrenocorticotropic hormone (ACTH) from the pituitary gland. Consequently, the adrenal glands secrete cortisol, a glucocorticoid that plays a central role in regulating metabolism, immune response, and energy mobilization. The cascade not only prepares the body for immediate challenges but also has profound implications for long-term health consequences, since long-term HPA axis activation can lead to dysregulation of inflammatory processes. Dysregulated inflammatory reactions are implicated in many diseases, highlighting the importance of maintaining an optimal stress response system. In addition, the role of inflammatory cytokines in stress reactions must be carefully considered in relation to physiological processes. Pro-inflammatory cytokines, such as interleukin-6 and tumor necrosis factor-alpha, can be elicited in response to both acute and chronic stressors. These cytokines have profound effects on neuronal signaling pathways and can influence mood and behavior, inducing such occurrences as depression resulting from stress or anxiety disorders. Moreover, chronic elevation of these cytokines can cause systemic inflammation, which further aggravates physiological stress. Notably, the interaction between inflammatory cytokines and stress hormones complicates the conventional definition of stress response, as it can influence gene expression and cellular function, thereby initiating a feedback mechanism that can exacerbate chronic inflammatory diseases. This calls for research into prevention strategies for controlling stress and inflammation to prevent harmful health consequences.

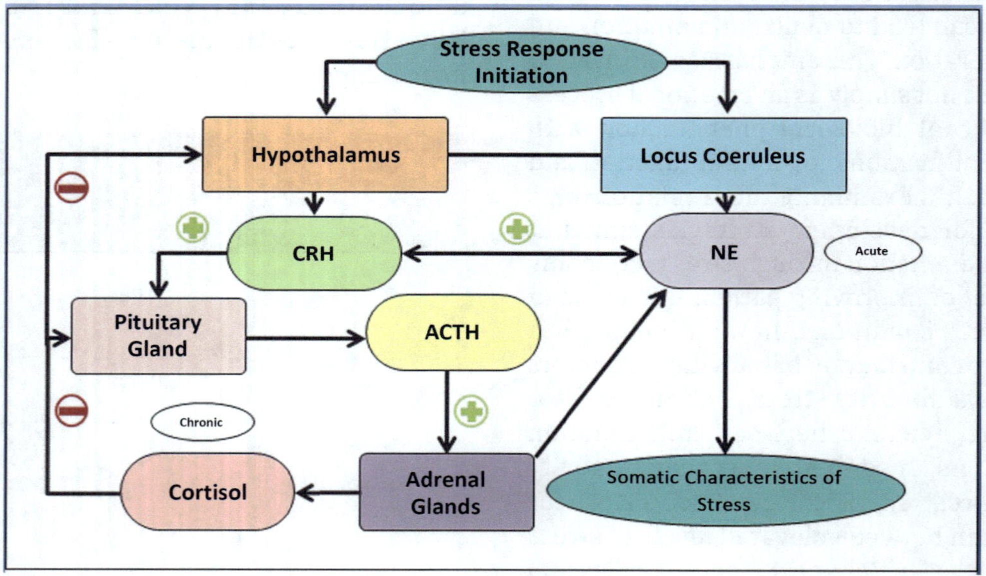

Figure 5.4. The-stress response: CRH (Corticotropin releasing hormone).

Source: https://www.researchgate.net/profile/Mervin-Chavez/publication/326842316/figure/fig1/AS:656692320694273@1533579058286/The-Stress-Response-CRH-Corticotropin-Releasing-Hormone-ACTH-Adrenocorticotropin.png.

The consequences of stress responses are more than the direct physiological importance in that they also impact significantly on muscle integrity and general physical health. Stress can cause sarcopenia, a syndrome characterized by muscle wasting and loss of muscle function. With elevated cortisol levels, the balance between muscle protein synthesis and muscle breakdown is disrupted, thus leading to muscle atrophy. Current evidence suggests that this state might be strongly linked to changes in body composition, including increases in adiposity. Fat infiltration into the muscles can lead to local inflammatory processes that further impair contractility and function of the muscles. These changes mandate interventions aimed at counteracting not just the endocrine consequences of stress but also the inflammatory processes involved in muscle destruction. Strategies that build muscle quality, as opposed to quantity, are critical to the facilitation of resistance to the harmful effects of stress on physical well-being (Chen et al., 2018; Carter et al., 2019) (Figure 5.4).

5.1.1. The Role of the Hypothalamic-Pituitary-Adrenal (HPA) Axis

HPA is one of the primary regulating systems by which the body reacts to stress, integrating the central nervous system with peripheral endocrine processes. Upon presentation of a stressor, CRH is secreted by the hypothalamus, which subsequently activates the pituitary gland to initiate the secretion of ACTH. The hormone then triggers the adrenal glands to release cortisol, a major stress hormone that mobilizes energy reserves and regulates physiological responses. Interestingly, cortisol's impact extends beyond metabolism; it also influences immune reactions, signaling pathways, and other hormonal interactions.

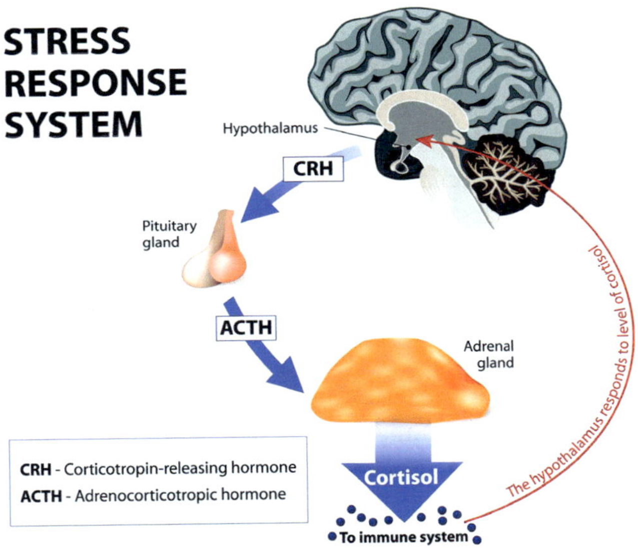

Figure 5.5. Role of the hypothalamic-pituitary-adrenal (HPA) axis.

Source: https://www.verywellhealth.com/thmb/9O0C4Gqktc2yMqY03JRtYRfrQ6I=/1500x0/filters:no_upscale():max_bytes(150000):strip_icc()/cortisol-371314fd2ef34947969e615ee1e75691.jpg.

HPA axis dysregulation, often observed in conditions of chronic stress, may lead to chronically released cortisol that has been implicated in the etiology of various pathologies, including inflammatory diseases and mood disorders, indicating its two-pronged role in both stress response and inflammation pathways. New evidence highlights the intricate relationship between HPA axis activation and inflammation. Chronic stress can lead to a persistent hyperactivity state within the HPA axis, resulting in elevated cortisol levels that paradoxically enhance inflammation rather than inhibit it. For instance, while cortisol is an anti-inflammatory agent at initial stages, it can ultimately lead to tissue damage and other inflammatory reactions when in excess. This is best illustrated by conditions such as major depressive disorder (MDD), where pro-inflammatory states have been linked to HPA axis dysregulation. Both chronic and acute stress responses are mediated by neuropeptides, including those belonging to the CRH family, highlighting their role in linking psychological stress and somatic health outcomes, such as inflammation and disease onset, as in colorectal cancer (Baritaki et al., 2019).

Awareness of this intersection is vital in identifying potential therapeutic options for stress-induced inflammatory disease. Lastly, the impact of the HPA axis on cardiovascular function should not be overlooked, particularly in its connection to MDD and ischemic heart disease. Chronic dysregulation of the HPA axis is associated with overactivity of the sympathetic nervous system and reduced vagal tone, both of which can contribute to risk for adverse cardiac outcomes. The relationship between depression and coronary heart disease (CHD) is a classic instance of such a phenomenon; those systemic factors like diabetes and obesity cross-interact with HPA derangement to enable cardiovascular threats (Budiono et al., 2017). Equally, changes in cardiac response under endocrine stress-induced changes are of concern about the myocardial well-being in depressed individuals. Studying how HPA axis dysregulation exacerbates not just mental disease but also its physiological impact can unveil doors to integrative treatment approaches that address not only psychological well-being but also physical well-being in the context of stress and inflammation (Figure 5.5).

5.1.2. Neurotransmitters Involved in Stress Responses

In the intricate dynamics of stress responses, neurotransmitters play a crucial role in mediating both physiological and psychological consequences. Interestingly, several central neurotransmitters, such as norepinephrine, serotonin, and cortisol, are deeply implicated in the body's adaptive mechanisms against stressors. Norepinephrine, released from the locus coeruleus, increases alertness and prepares the body for the fight-or-flight response, which is crucial during acute stress. Conversely, serotonin not only influences mood but also controls the inflammatory pathways that cause stress-related disorders. The interaction between the two neurotransmitters identifies a delicate balance; while helping to tackle short-term issues, chronic activation due to chronic stress can create adverse effects on health, such as anxiety and depression, thus identifying an obvious link to the inflammatory processes involved during such conditions (Wildeman et al., 2020). The role of neurotransmitters extends beyond immediate responses to stress because they influence longer-term health conditions, particularly in inflammatory contexts. Dysregulation of neurotransmitters by stress has also been implicated in activation, the activation of immune pathways, and the production of pro-inflammatory cytokines. For example, elevated levels of cortisol have been reported to suppress certain immune responses while simultaneously provoking inflammation. This complex relationship is also complicated by the involvement of diet in neurotransmitter balance; diets high in pathological fats and refined sugar can increase inflammation, which can accelerate such diseases as depression, engaged in the modulation of stress response. Therefore, an understanding of the biochemical underpinnings of these interactions allows an advanced consideration of stress-associated disease, where treatments are able to aim at nutritional strategies (Wildeman et al., 2020) and gut microbiome modulation. Furthermore, recent research highlights the interaction between neurotransmitters and the gut microbiota in relation to the stress response. Dysbiosis, or an imbalance of intestinal microbiota, has been found to regulate neurotransmitter synthesis and thereby influence the body's stress response pathways. Specific bacterial genera have the capacity to produce metabolites that can either enhance or suppress the synthesis of neurotransmitters, particularly serotonin, which is primarily synthesized in the gastrointestinal tract. The stimulation of Toll-like receptors by microbial products suggests an instantaneous relationship between gut integrity and neuronal function, highlighting the role of microbiota in regulating stress and modulating inflammatory processes. This interaction provides new avenues for therapy, with potential interventions ranging from dietary adjustment and probiotics to enhancing neurotransmitter balance and inhibiting inflammation induced by stress. Thus, the complex function of neurotransmitters in stress response requires an integrated approach grounded on biochemical, nutritional, and microbiological factors (Figure 5.6).

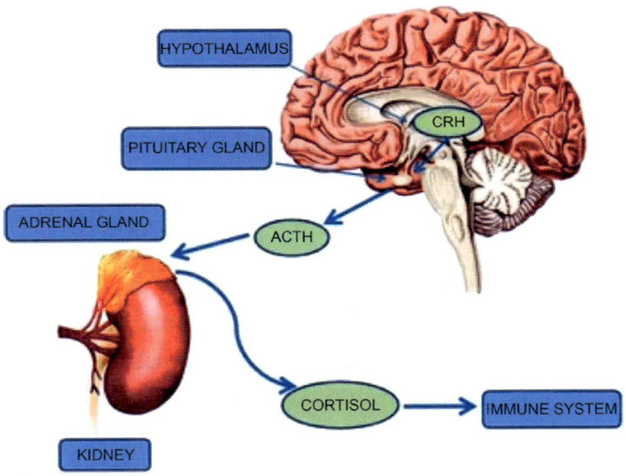

Figure 5.6. Endocrine and metabolic response to surgical stress in the elderly.

Source: https://static.cambridge.org/binary/version/id/urn:cambridge.org:id:binary-alt:20181001232350-50644-mediumThumb-13934fig31_1.jpg?pub-status=live.

5.1.3. The Impact of Acute vs. Chronic Stress on the Body

Stress responses, which can be acute or chronic, have varied effects on the body, particularly through inflammatory mechanisms. Acute stress, typically triggered by immediate dangers, activates the body's fight-or-flight response. The body's physical response is characterized by the release of stress hormones, such as cortisol and adrenaline, which prepare for rapid mobilization of energy and induce alertness. These reactions are beneficial in the short term by boosting survival through increased concentration and bodily performance. However, while acute stress often leads to short-term immunological boosts, chronic stress recurs when repeated stressors persist, resulting in long-term exposure to the hormones that cause detrimental effects on bodily functioning and immune responses. It is crucial to appreciate this duality in order to understand how different types of stress impact health outcomes. Chronic stress, by contrast, is linked to a wide range of pathological conditions, including cardiovascular disease and metabolic syndrome. This persistent exposure to stress results in continuous activation of the HPA axis, ultimately leading to cortisol dysregulation. Surprisingly, chronic stress has been discovered to impair immune signaling and hormonal homeostasis, leading to increased inflammation, a disease risk factor. Such diseases as MDD exemplify interrelationships that the cross-talk between psychological stressors and physiological mechanisms is responsible for cardiovascular morbidity and mortality, as underlined by Budiono et al. (2017). This highlights not only the complexity of stress diseases but also the imperative need for highly sensitive therapeutic interventions that focus on the cardiovascular effects of exposure to chronic stress. Psychosocial stressor studies illustrate the complex relationship between stress, immune dysregulation, and the pathogenesis of chronic disease. Longitudinal monitoring in animals, such as the vervet monkey's response to quarantine, illustrates extensive immune signaling and inflammatory marker alterations following exposure to chronic stress. As indicated by Benjamin et al. (2020), such an immune response involves an organized reduction of critical immune molecules, as well as a marked transcriptional switch, which makes individuals vulnerable to chronic pathologies and enhances their vulnerability to infection. The findings underscore the importance of stress management in preventing the onset of inflammation-associated diseases, thereby highlighting the need for comprehensive information on how acute and chronic stress selectively impact health outcomes at both physiological and molecular levels.

Test Your Knowledge

1. What are the two major systems involved in the physiological stress response?
2. How does the body respond to acute stress at the cardiovascular level?

5.2. Types of Stressors

Learning Outcome

1. Describe the psychological stressors and their impact
2. Describe the physical stressors and their physiologic effect
3. Explain the environmental stressors and their role in inflammation

Stress is typically caused by a series of stressors that can be categorized as either acute or chronic. Acute stressors are normally transient and could be due to an immediate need or danger, for instance, taking an exam or an unexpected death. These stressors tend to switch on the body's fight-or-flight system, causing physiological responses which prepare an individual to confront the challenge. Chronic stressors, however, are due to the process of long-term pressures, such as repeated work problems or deep-seated personal issues. Repeated exposure to stress can lead to significant wear and tear on the body, resulting in fatigue or exhaustion. Significantly, chronic stressors are implicated in several disorders of health, including mental illness and cardiovascular diseases, that require extensive research to understand the role of these long-term stressors in causing inflammation in the body. Among all the categories of stressors, environmental stressors need top priority because they have a far-reaching impact on health outcomes. They consist of various factors such as noise pollution, exposure to toxins, and climatic events. Studies have established that exposure to these environmental stressors is likely to exacerbate chronic stress response systems, triggering an increase in inflammatory markers and leading to adverse health effects in the long term. This is particularly important in urban dwelling, where people are frequently exposed to environmental stressors that result in allostatic load, a term used to describe the total wear and tear on the body's systems due to stress (McCreary et al., 2015). Understanding how environmental stressors function and their probable mechanisms is necessary in order to create interventions that mitigate their detrimental effects on health and well-being. Besides, psychosocial stressors are another vast category that could considerably impact mental and physical health. Such stressors arise as a consequence of interpersonal relationships, social interactions, and role expectations and tend to make one feel inadequate or isolated. MDD's influence, as emphasized in research, demonstrates the complex interaction between psychosocial stressors and cardiovascular disease. MDD patients have a higher risk for CHD, and studies suggest that this can be attributed to psychosocial and biological mechanisms linked with inflammation (Budiono et al., 2017). These psychosocial stressors subject the body to systemic inflammation, which increases the complexity of the stress response and may lead to chronic disease. Therefore, intervention against psychosocial stressors is paramount not only for psychological but also for physical health outcomes, supporting the bi-directional nature of stress and inflammation further (Figure 5.7).

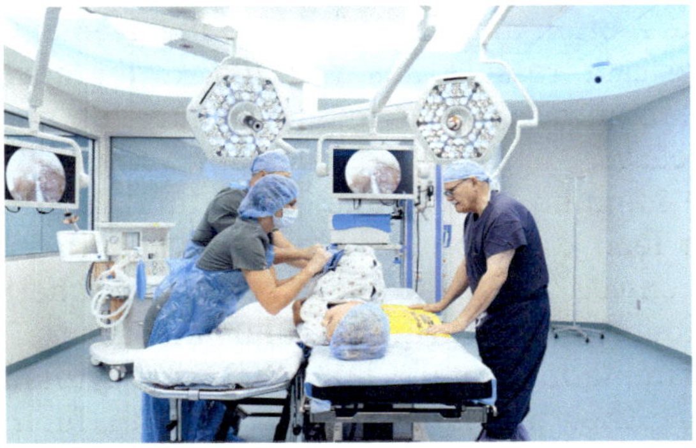

Figure 5.7. Types of stressors.

Source: https://sloanmedical.com/wp-content/uploads/blog-featured-img-250106-SLN-Comparing-Top-Surgical-Safety-Equipment-On-The-Market-v01-MMK.png.

5.2.1. Psychological Stressors and Their Effects

Psychological stressors, encompassing a wide range of experiences from daily hassles to significant life events, elicit complex physiological responses that have the potential to profoundly impact health outcomes. Stressful events trigger the HPA axis to release the stress hormones like cortisol, which can dysregulate immune processes and increase levels of inflammation in the body. This dysregulation can induce a chronic state of inflammation, which plays a role in various diseases, including cardiovascular disease and metabolic disorders. Specifically, individuals with MDD are closely related to heart disease since stress-induced alterations in cardiac function can compromise the heart's own protective mechanisms. The overlap of psychological stress and physiological function highlights the need for coordinated approaches in understanding and treating stress-induced health states and underscores potential intervention targets in managing both psychological and cardiovascular health (Budiono et al., 2017). Most importantly, the impact of psychological stressors extends beyond short-term physiological changes; it also influences health behaviors and contributes to health disparities. Individuals under chronic stress are apt to engage in unhealthy coping behaviors such as drug use, poor diet, or a sedentary lifestyle. These not only contribute to the way stress exacerbates inflammation, but they also create a cycle of worsening health outcomes. Chronic stress is a spectrum of stress forms and longitudinal health effects, an indicator of dynamic interaction between psychological pressure and health behavior across the lifespan. It is thus imperative to understand how various types of stressors affect behavioral response to enhance the development of targeted interventions to break such cycles and promote healthier lifestyles (Crosswell et al., 2018). Moreover, the interaction between stress and inflammation is not only characterized by immediate physiological changes but also by psychosocial processes that can modulate responses to stress over time. The life course perspective on stress recognizes that traumatic and negative experiences have the capacity to make lasting impressions on an individual's health trajectory, stressing the importance of considering an individual's historical context when assessing his/her stress responses. The overall burden of stressors can lead to elevated allostatic load and induce chronic ill health, as well as heighten vulnerability to disease. Through an integrative conceptualization that includes a variety of different kinds of stress—ranging from acute event through chronic exposure—researchers are better able to characterize the processes by which psychological stressors influence health, paving the way for improved therapeutic strategies that consider both psychological and inflammatory dimensions of stress illness (Crosswell et al., 2018) (Figure 5.8).

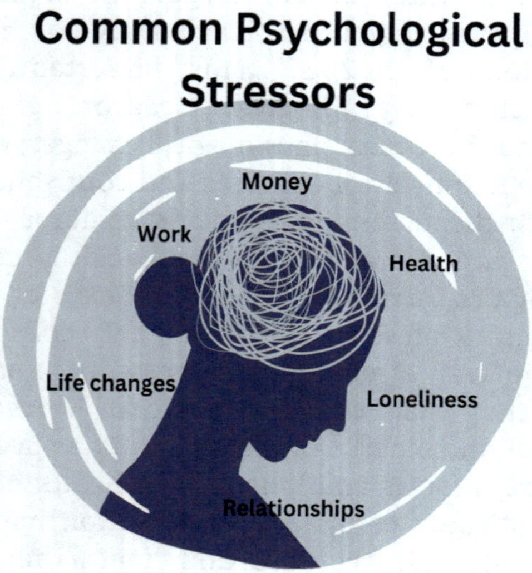

Figure 5.8. Psychological-stressor.

Source: https://www.explorepsychology.com/wp-content/uploads/2023/08/psychological-stressor-1200-x-1200-px.png.

5.2.2. Physical Stressors and Their Physiological Impact

The interaction of physical stressors with their physiological impact is a critical line of enquiry in the study of stress. Various physical stressors, including environmental factors such as high temperatures, noise, and prolonged physical exertion, can have an impact on an individual's health. The stressors elicit a complex cascade of hormonal and biochemical responses, which are primarily mediated by the HPA axis. The body responds to stressors by releasing adrenaline and cortisol, which are stress hormones that stimulate the organism to prepare for a fight-or-flight response. The continuous exposure to frequent acute stressors leads to the chronic activation of the HPA axis, which ultimately leads to maladaptive changes in the physiology, resulting in various conditions like cardiovascular diseases and metabolic diseases. Therefore, a profound understanding of the mechanisms by which physical stressors induce such stress responses is essential to designing successful interventions. In addition, the actions of physical stressors extend beyond acute hormonal effects and into the inflammatory pathways that regulate health outcomes. Chronic exposure to stress, often augmented by the involvement of physical stressors, has been linked to inducing inflammation as a primary cause of many diseases. For instance, constant activation of the immune system due to continuous stress can lead to a condition of pro-inflammatory, which contributes to the conditions of obesity, diabetes, and cardiovascular diseases. The inflammation entails the release of cytokines and other mediators, which lead to further impairment of physiological functioning and an augmentation of responses to stress. Recent research highlights the intimate association of these inflammatory mechanisms with mental health, detailing how diseases like MDD enhance the adverse effect of physical stressors on the organism. Appreciation of this relationship is key to addressing the broader health consequences of chronic physical stressors. Finally, the intricate relationship between physical stressors and their physiological impact necessitates a multidisciplinary approach to studying stress. According to the integrative working model, a better understanding of the interaction between external stressor environments and individuals' responses is needed. By employing a more sophisticated typology of stress that involves various dimensions of exposure—acute, chronic, and event-based—we can better tailor interventions aimed at minimizing the adverse health effects arising from stress. Focus should also be brought to examining underlying mechanisms, such as those of emotional disorders and how they affect the vascular system, as noted in research that associated MDD with extremely high risks of ischemic heart disease (Budiono et al., 2017). As the field evolves, emphasis on an integrative approach to studying physical stressors and their effects on physiology will result in effective prevention and management strategies for enhancing overall health and resiliency despite the presence of stressors (Crosswell et al., 2018) (Figure 5.9).

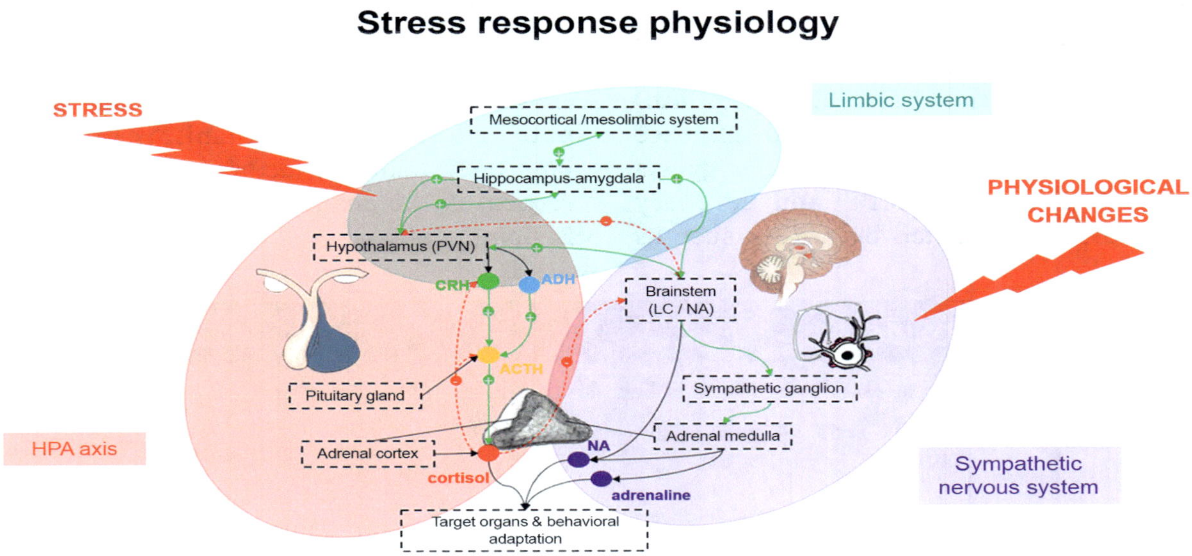

Figure 5.9. Stress response physiology.

Source: https://www.cast-pharma.com/wp-content/uploads/2020/04/nl03_before.jpg.

5.2.3. Environmental Stressors and Their Role in Inflammation

Environmental stressors also play a crucial role in regulating inflammatory responses, typically as the cause of multiple inflammatory diseases. These consist of physical stressors, such as pollution, heat stress, or noise, as well as psychosocial stressors, including chronic stress and depression. Experiments have shown that exposure to such environmental stimuli can trigger the body's stress response mechanisms, resulting in the release of pro-inflammatory cytokines. These cytokines induce a state of chronic, low-grade inflammation, which has been linked to numerous health conditions, including cardiovascular disease and autoimmune diseases. In addition, the connection between environmental stimuli and the physiological response of people illustrates the intricacy of inflammation and suggests that a multidisciplinary comprehension is necessary in order to deal with its public health implications. Other examples of psychosocial stressors include lack of sleep, worry, and anxiety. Environmental stressors also play a role, with the microbiome at the core of inflammatory processes. Environmental conditions, such as diet, antibiotic exposure, and pathogen exposure, may exacerbate dysbiosis in the body's microbial flora. Derangement of the microbiome has been linked to the initiation of systemic inflammation, with specific pathogens contributing to inflammatory processes in other parts of the body. For instance, periodontal microorganisms such as Porphyromonas gingivalis and Treponema denticola have been reported to affect not only oral health but also inflammatory mechanisms related to systemic diseases, including Alzheimer's disease. The interaction among environmental exposures, the health of the microbiome, and inflammation highlights the need to control these factors to mitigate the risk of chronic inflammatory diseases (Crean et al., 2014). The consequences of environmental stressors extend beyond their immediate effects on health; they can have profound long-term impacts on emotional and cognitive well-being. Stressor-induced inflammation has been implicated in mood disorders, with MDD being one such factor that can also influence inflammatory processes. Evidence suggests that the link between MDD and coronary heart disease is mediated by factors such as systemic immune dysregulation and chronic inflammation (Budiono et al., 2017). The link suggests the need to have a comprehensive understanding of how environmental insults can trigger inflammatory cascades that impact both physical and mental well-being. By studying these correlations, scientists can identify potential protective mechanisms that act on both environmental factors and inflammatory responses, thereby improving health outcomes in populations.

Test Your Knowledge

1. What are the two broad stressor categories and how do they differ from one another?
2. What are environmental stressors, and how might they impact hospitalized patients?

5.3. Mechanisms of Inflammation

Learning Outcome

1. Describe the immune response to stress
2. Define the cytokines and their role in inflammation
3. Describe the function of inflammation in chronic disease

Inflammatory processes are a complex interaction between the immune response and various cellular pathways. Proinflammatory mediators, including cytokines and chemokines, are the key elements of this response that orchestrate recruitment and activation of immune cells into damaged or infected tissues. These mediators are activated by exposure to stressors, such as injury or infection, and the subsequent cascade of events signals danger. The early inflammatory phase is characterized by vasodilation and enhanced vascular permeability, allowing for the migration of immune cells to injured tissues. Chronic inflammation resulting from chronic stress or autoimmune disease, however, leads to massive tissue damage and pathology. This is crucial for regulating inflammatory responses to prevent adverse outcomes, particularly in conditions such as rheumatoid arthritis, where chronic stress leads to joint and tissue damage (Ahmed et al., 2017). Chronic stress has been reported to be a critical regulator of inflammatory activities and plays an important role in disease progression. The stress-inflammation interaction is regulated through various mechanisms, some of which involve neuropeptide signaling, such as CRH. These neuropeptides have been shown to influence immune responses by inducing the secretion of pro-inflammatory cytokines. Such interaction can then exacerbate existing inflammatory conditions, necessitating an understanding of the molecular mechanisms that enable this interaction. Chronic stress disrupts homeostasis, leading to an imbalance in immune signaling that favors inflammatory responses. This dysregulation has been implicated in the pathogenesis of numerous diseases, including cancer, wherein inflammation can drive oncogenesis (Baritaki et al., 2019). The interface between stress responses and inflammation thus constitutes an essential area of research in the endeavor to understand disease pathogenesis.

Finally, a complete understanding of inflammation mechanisms necessitates an investigation into the mechanisms by which stress impinges on immune function. Inflammatory mechanisms, although critical in tissue repair and defense, become maladaptive under chronic stress, leading to a vicious cycle of chronic inflammation. Such a cycle can manifest in numerous clinical conditions, making it crucial to have targeted therapeutic approaches that address both the inflammatory response and the underlying causative stresses. New advances in immunotherapy have shown potential not just to manage symptoms of inflammatory diseases but also to restore immune system homeostasis. By exploring how stress responses function to modulate inflammation, new opportunities can be identified to enhance patient recovery in chronic inflammatory disorders and move towards a better model of health that incorporates both psychological and physiological aspects (Ahmed et al., 2017; Baritaki et al., 2019) (Figure 5.10).

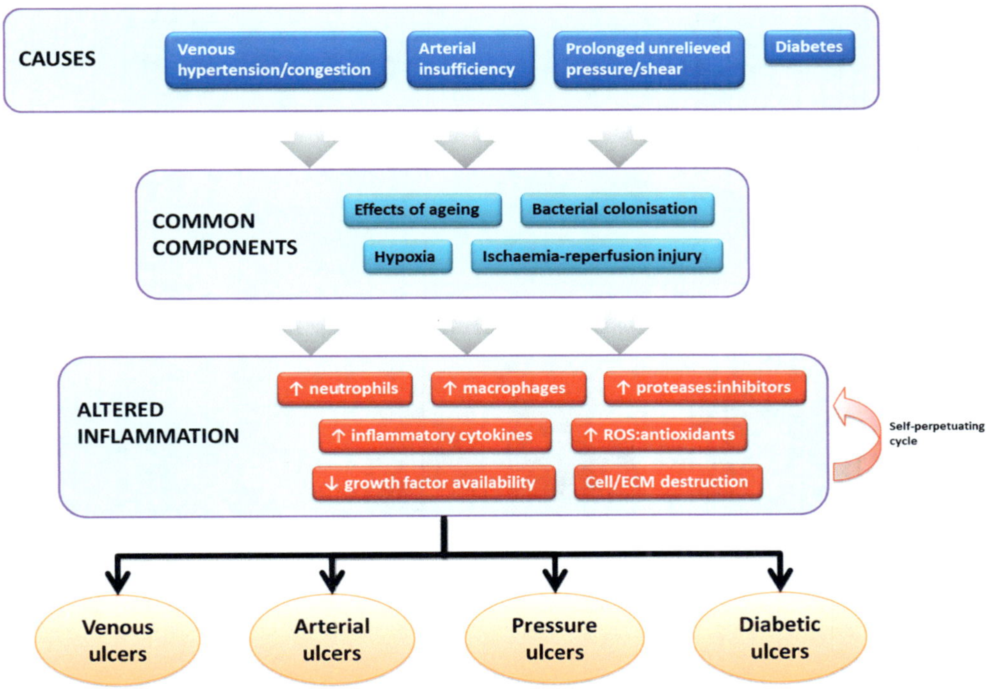

Figure 5.10. Inflammation in chronic wounds.

Source: https://www.mdpi.com/ijms/ijms-17-02085/article_deploy/html/images/ijms-17-02085-g001.png.

5.3.1. The Immune Response to Stress

The immune stress response is a complex interaction that significantly affects overall health and disease susceptibility. Stressors, through the activation of the HPA axis, induce a cascade of hormonal changes, including the release of cortisol, which has immunomodulatory effects. Elevated cortisol is recognized to cause alterations in immune function, including the suppression of pro-inflammatory cytokine expression and the enhancement of anti-inflammatory processes. This is indicative of the body's attempt at homeostasis; nonetheless, chronic stress is more likely to lead to immune dysregulation. To be more specific, long-term exposure to cortisol is linked with the overstimulation of inflammation and the induction of a broad spectrum of conditions that are stress-related, including cardiovascular disease and autoimmune disease. It is essential to understand these dynamics since the immune stress response can either facilitate recovery or augment disease progression, highlighting the need for specific therapeutic interventions directed towards modulating these responses. In addition to hormonal impacts, the role of immune cells during stress also deserves significant attention. Stress promotes the activation of immune cells, such as mast cells, which are widely distributed throughout the body and play a key role in coordinating the initial inflammatory response.

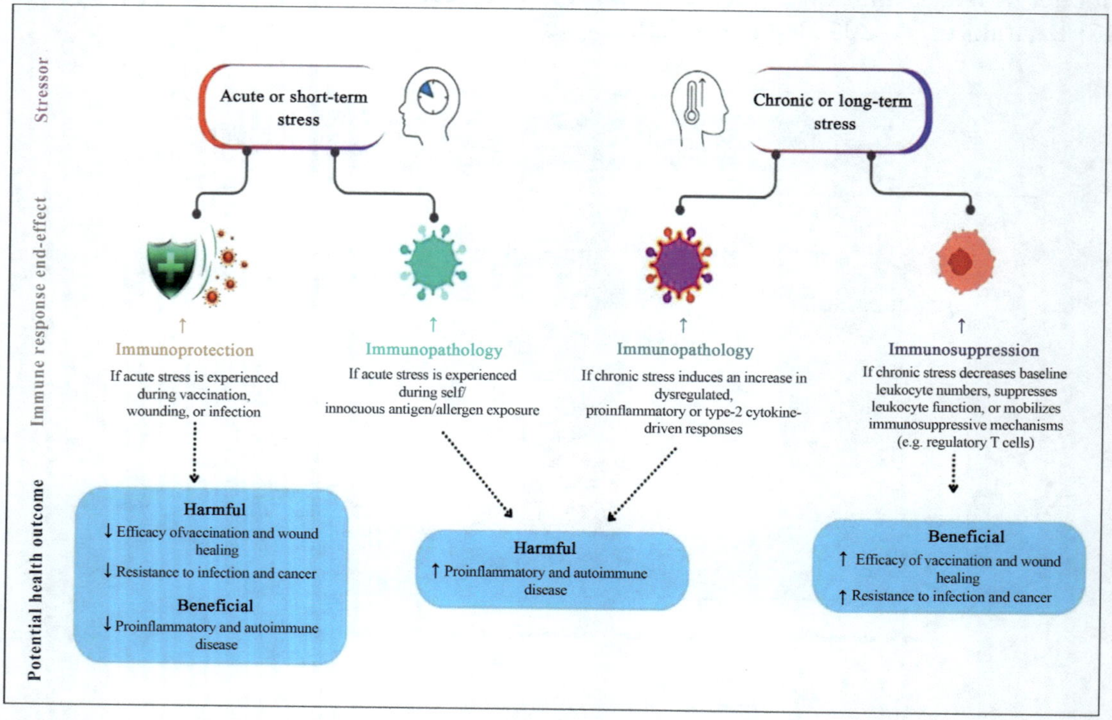

Figure 5.11. Immunology of stress.

Source: https://pub.mdpi-res.com/jcm/jcm-13-06394/article_deploy/html/images/jcm-13-06394-g002.png?1730361384.

The cells remain in continuous contact with the central nervous system and can regulate neuroinflammatory phenomena, particularly through their interactions with glial cells. The crosstalk between mast cells and glia demonstrates how peripheral inflammation can impact the brain, highlighting the importance of neuroinflammation in stress-related pathologies. As these immune cell interactions increase with age or increased vulnerability to stress, they have therapeutic implications. Discovery of the mechanisms to control such immune responses may offer the pathway for new therapies to lower the economic burden of stress-related diseases as illustrated by recent findings on mast cell-glia interaction (Alhouayek et al., 2017). Furthermore, the connection between stress and inflammation is also linked to various disease mechanisms, emphasizing the importance of controlling regulatory pathways. Members of the CRH family have also emerged as central to this end, acting between stress and inflammatory processes. Inflammatory responses can be enhanced through exposure to chronic stress by these neuropeptides, not merely affecting behavioral and metabolic functioning, but by contributing to heightened vulnerability to malignancies such as cancer. The intersection of stress, inflammation, and malignancy necessitates a deeper understanding of molecular signaling pathways regulated by members of the CRH family. This interaction provides an essential insight for advancing personalized medicine strategies in assessing and treating the risk of disease associated with chronic stress and inflammatory processes (Baritaki et al., 2019). Investigation of such pathways presents a firm foundation for further study to reveal the immune stress response and to develop effective interventions (Figure 5.11).

5.3.2. Cytokines and Their Role in Inflammation

Cytokine activity is not one-dimensional, but rather significant milestones in the body's inflammatory reaction to injury and stress. Cytokines are small proteins produced by various immune cells that serve as mediators of interaction between immune cells, influencing the dynamics of inflammatory reactions. Cytokines can either cause or inhibit inflammation, depending on the context and temporal coordination of their production. When tissue infection or injury happens, interleukins and tumor necrosis factor-alpha (TNF-α) are usually upregulated, triggering the recruitment of immune cells to the injured site. There is a need for recruitment to remove the pathogens and initiate tissue repair mechanisms. However, dysfunctional aberrations in cytokine signaling can lead to chronic inflammation, which plays a role in various diseases, including obesity and type 2 diabetes mellitus (T2DM), where inflammation is central to the pathogenesis of metabolic dysfunction (Fu et al., 2020). During chronic conditions, the accumulation of pro-inflammatory cytokines significantly contributes to the impairment of tissue function. For example, overloading macrophage infiltration by local cytokine signaling during conditions of insulin resistance creates a cycle of inflammation.

The high concentrations of cytokines produced in the adipose tissue can create cellular stress, leading to β-cell failure in the pancreas, crucial in glucose homeostasis. Specifically, islet macrophages release cytokines that exacerbate insulin resistance and impair β-cell function. This intricate interaction highlights the paradox of inflammation, where a process intended to heal actually perpetuates a cycle of tissue damage and metabolic derangement (Fu et al., 2020). These results further reinforce the need to target cytokine pathways for therapeutic interventions in managing chronic inflammatory conditions. Furthermore, cytokines are not limited to the peripheral tissue but have significant implications within the central nervous system, causing neuroinflammation. This process often occurs after prolonged inflammation that persists even when the initial insult has resolved, leading to detrimental neurological effects. The communication between immune cells within the nervous system, including microglia and mast cells, demonstrates that cytokines cannot only affect peripheral inflammation but also central inflammatory processes. Release of cytokines upon infections or neuronal injury has the potential to trigger a cascade of neuroinflammatory responses that exacerbate Alzheimer's disease and multiple sclerosis by damaging neuronal structures. Therefore, it is essential to elucidate the mechanisms of cytokine-mediated neuroinflammation in order to develop effective measures to prevent chronic inflammatory reactions that lead to severe neurological disorders (Figure 5.12).

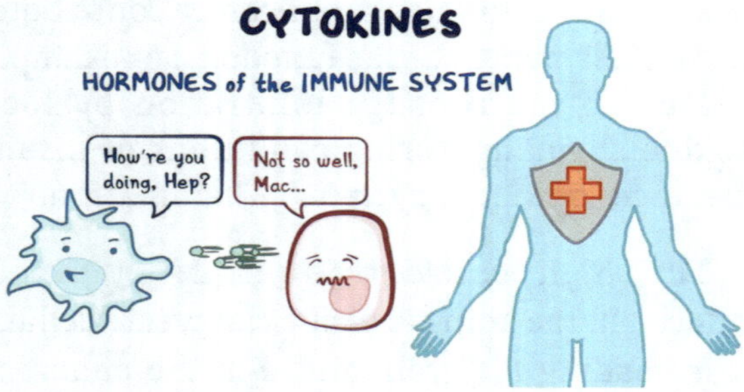

Figure 5.12. Role of cytokines in inflammation.

Source: https://www.osmosis.org/_next/image?url=https%3A%2F%2Fd16qt3wv6xm098.cloudfront.net%2Fd4WEz1pnTLGM5y75KgdTqgV0Q0uM0dvd%2F_.jpg&w=3840&q=75.

5.3.3. The Relationship Between Inflammation and Chronic Diseases

The interlink between inflammation and chronic diseases is a new area of research in the field of medical science and public health. Chronic inflammation is a fundamental pathological process that underlies most chronic diseases, including cardiovascular disease, diabetes, and neurodegenerative disorders. Cellular injury and dysfunction resulting from the persistent state of inflammation ultimately lead to disease progression. For instance, research has provided insight into how chronic low-grade inflammation, which is usually a consequence of lifestyle determinants, environmental stimuli, or infection, contributes to worsening obesity and metabolic syndrome.

The interaction between inflammation and the immune response not only complicates the clinical management of such conditions but also raises concerns regarding whether therapeutic interventions are possible to target and modulate inflammatory processes, thereby restoring immune homeostasis. Of particular interest is the relationship between periodontal disease and systemic inflammatory processes, with significant implications for brain function and cognition. Inflammation induced by periodontal pathogens, such as Porphyromonas gingivalis, demonstrates a very real correlation with diseases like Alzheimer's. The bidirectional quality of this interaction is a classic example of the extent to which chronic inflammatory processes can extend to distant organ systems, leading to neuroinflammatory mechanisms that erode cognitive functions over time. In patients with periodontal disease, ongoing bacteremia from routine activities will perpetuate a cycle of inflammation that not only exacerbates local tissue loss but also primes systemic inflammatory processes that can engage the brain.

This complexity underscores the need for integrative approaches to treating chronic disease, considering both local and systemic inflammation (Crean et al., 2014). Similarly, the term allostatic load illustrates how chronic stress is heavily associated with the inflammatory process and adverse health outcomes, such as preterm birth. Chronic stress over time can potentially result in dysregulation of the stress response with repeated stimulation of the HPA axis. Research has shown that allostatic load causes exaggerated inflammatory response, thereby predisposing to adverse pregnancy outcomes. Chronic stress in mothers can lead to increased inflammation markers, which could impact fetal growth and lead to preterm labor. Knowing the mechanisms can provide revealing hints at prevention and intervention for vulnerable groups with the ultimate aim of reducing the burden of inflammation-related chronic diseases on the health system. The results underscore the importance of integrating stress management and inflammation-oriented therapies into clinical practice (McCreary et al., 2015).

Test Your Knowledge

1. What are the typical signs of inflammation, and what is the underlying cause of each of them?
2. Name two significant chemical mediators of the inflammatory response and provide short descriptions of their functions.

5.4. Stress-Induced Inflammatory Responses

Learning Outcome

1. Describe stress and immune system dysregulation
2. Define the function of cortisol in the inflammatory response
3. Outline the behavioral factors that contribute to enhanced inflammatory responses

The intricate interaction between stress and inflammation can be attributed to a range of biological processes leading to significant physiological changes. Stress in the body activates the HPA axis, leading to the release of glucocorticoids, which play a significant role in controlling inflammation. Chronic stress, on the other hand, may trigger systemic dysregulation of this process and result in a chronic elevation of pro-inflammatory cytokines, such as TNF-α, IL-1β, and IL-6. These cytokines, ubiquitous in all inflammatory responses, induce cellular damage by perpetuating oxidative stress, with wide-ranging consequences to the cardiovascular system and beyond. The pathologic effects of stress-induced inflammation have been well-documented, to the extent that it has been established that individuals who suffer from chronic stress have a higher susceptibility to inflammation-associated disease, such as cardiovascular disease and autoimmune diseases, underscoring the necessity of deconstructing such processes in health and disease conditions. The cross-talk among psychological stressors and inflammatory responses provides essential insights into the pathogenesis of various health diseases. MDD, for instance, is associated with increased systemic inflammation, resulting in a higher risk for ischemic heart disease. Stress not only enhances hyperactivation of innate immune signaling pathways but also impacts behavioral changes that may exacerbate these disorders, such as physical inactivity and dietary habits. The cross-talk between CHD and MDD highlights the multifaceted nature of inflammatory reactions triggered by stress. Researchers have also noted that stress induces changes in myocardial susceptibility to ischemia-induced injury, suggesting neurobiological components involved in immunoinflammatory dysfunction. Understanding the mechanisms in question could provide insight into potential therapeutic targets for suppressing the inflammatory responses caused by chronic stress, potentially enhancing patient outcomes and informing clinical interventions. Moreover, chronic stress may significantly interfere with the body's natural protective processes for the heart, rendering the stress-inflammation connection more intricate. As a case in point, changes in the HPA axis under stress can lead to sympatho-vagal imbalance, where excessive sympathetic activity and diminished vagal tone promote inflammatory responses. This dysregulation not only induces heightened oxidative stress but also disrupts the myocardium's resistance to ischemic damage, leading to deleterious effects such as myocardial infarction. The interaction between oxidative stress and inflammatory mediators further complicates the scenario, as increased free radical production can damage cellular components, perpetuating the cycle of inflammation. The consequences of stress-induced inflammatory responses extend beyond immediate physiological changes, posing long-term health risks. Thus, the study of such central processes is crucial in developing effective prevention and treatment strategies for stress-related diseases, and in highlighting the importance of holistic approaches in managing the dynamics of stress and inflammation in healthcare (Figure 5.13).

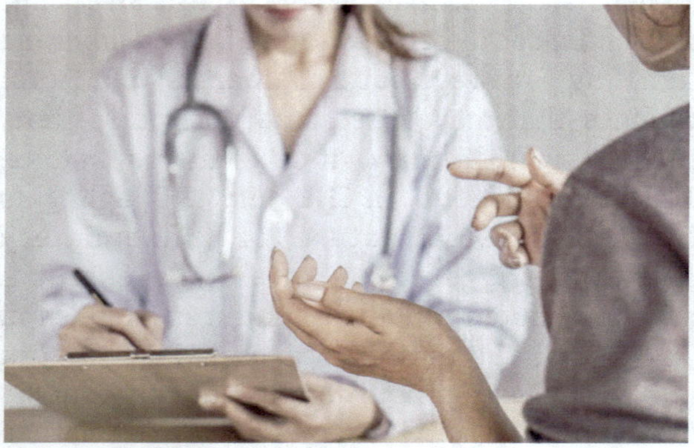

Figure 5.13. Major depressive disorder (MDD).

Source: https://cdn.sanity.io/images/0vv8moc6/ajmc/55711c0510e058d007284678eff5b8741a891c92-1280x853.jpg?fit=crop&auto=format.

5.4.1. The Connection Between Stress and Immune System Dysregulation

The intricate link between stress and immune system dysregulation demonstrates the significant health impact that psychosocial factors have. Both chronic and acute stressful events activate the HPA axis, which releases increased levels of the glucocorticoids, primarily cortisol. The resultant hormonal surge is intended to address current peril, but with the passage of time, can dampen immune function. Elevated cortisol levels impair the functioning of immune cells, yet simultaneously trigger systemic inflammatory conditions. Thus, the body is rendered vulnerable to infections and chronic disease, and a frightening feedback loop of expanding health and stress. Understanding the mechanisms involved provides insight into the ways in which stress affects immunity, a subject that is becoming increasingly important in both clinical psychology and immunology. Research has consistently shown that environmental stressors, such as pollution, tend to exacerbate immune system dysregulation and inflammatory processes. As characterized in current studies, pollutants target the immune pathways and induce pro-inflammatory responses, with an implicit complex relationship between extrinsic stressors and biological health. Pollutants also possess the ability to reorganize gut microbiota, reducing the protective roles of beneficial microorganisms and promoting pro-inflammatory categories of microorganisms. This dysbiosis and oxidative stress synergize to disrupt the intestinal barrier's integrity, ultimately leading to systemic inflammation and increased susceptibility to disease. So where environmental stressors intersect with psychosocial stress, a very new public health arena is highlighted. By addressing these concurrent problems, solutions that assist in reducing environmental ecological toxins can also minimize their adverse effects on the immune system and overall health, facilitating a more holistic approach to healthcare. Empirical evidence further supports the notion that psychosocial stressors inherently disrupt immune signaling and function. A longitudinal study of vervet monkeys in quarantine revealed extensive immune dysregulation, characterized by changes in the blood transcriptome and immune signaling molecules upon exposure to stress. Notably, immune function genes were suppressed, while coagulation and platelet activation pathways were increased in response to acute stress. This is reflective of the body's response to stress at the expense of reduced immune competence. The study highlights the importance of understanding the mechanisms that link stress and immune dysregulation, particularly in the context of chronic disease and susceptibility to infection. The more data that are gathered, however, the more it may be possible to grasp these connections and create properly targeted interventions specific to psychosocial stressor-driven immune-related disorders (Figure 5.14).

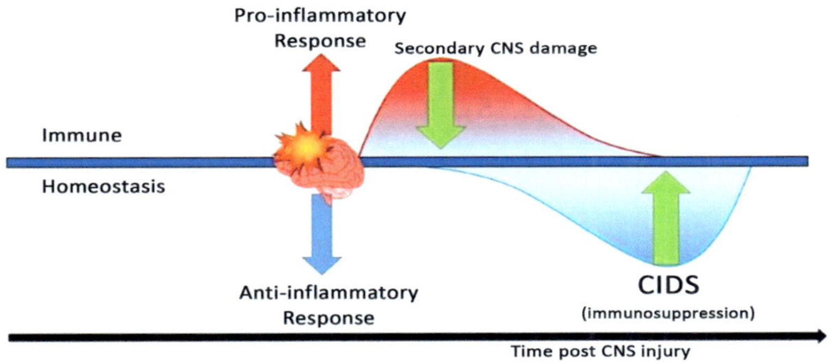

Figure 5.14. A graphical representation of immune dysregulation.

Source: https://external-content.duckduckgo.com/iu/?u=https%3A%2F%2Fwww.researchgate.net%2Fpublication%2F352521783%2Ffigure%2Ffig1%2FAS%3A1036100697083906%401624037064727%2FA-graphical-representation-of-immune-dysregulation-following-central-nervous-system-CNS.png&f=1&nofb=1&ipt=784129ef66e3259a861d71687357bf449beb416b9fd5fa1d08b49c496f935302.

5.4.2. The Role of Cortisol in Inflammation

Cortisol is a steroid hormone produced by the adrenal glands and plays a vital role in managing the bodys reaction to inflammatory and stressful stimuli. With the activation of the HPA axis upon exposure to stressors, cortisol levels increase, triggering certain physiological responses aimed at restoring homeostasis. The hormone is an immunosuppressant, thereby regulating immune activity by suppressing it, hence managing the intensity and duration of inflammatory responses. Elevated cortisol can inhibit the release of pro-inflammatory cytokines, a vital mechanism that helps maintain extreme inflammation at bay, which can cause tissue damage. However, while cortisol's anti-inflammatory effect might work well in acute states, prolonged exposure to elevated cortisol levels can create a paradoxical immune system, as constantly high levels might hamper the immune response and cause inflammation. In conditions such as malaria, cortisol's role is even more complex, as it plays a role in systemic regulation and disease tolerance. Elevated glucocorticoids in infections such as malaria help moderate inflammation and the immune response, again echoing the duality of hormones' roles. By inducing an appropriate inflammatory response, cortisol can enhance resistance to infection while preventing the body from experiencing the damage brought about by excessive inflammation. But the clinical implications of cortisol in disease have long been underappreciated, particularly with respect to its potential use to manage complications of disorders such as sepsis. Appreciation of glucocorticoids suggests that their mechanisms of action could inform better therapeutic strategies, especially when inflammation is a central promoter of morbidity and mortality. Also, the cross-talk between inflammation and stress is essential when attempting to value the longer-term effects of cortisol dysregulation. Chronic elevation of cortisol due to prolonged stress may cause the immune system to become habituated to a state of low-grade inflammation. This condition is most often associated with various chronic diseases, such as cardiovascular diseases and metabolic syndrome, to highlight the significance of studying cortisol's role beyond mere acute responses. In agriculture, the enhanced welfare status of domesticated animals, as indicated by cortisol as a biomarker, may not only signal health but also stress levels, thereby influencing productivity. Further studies into cortisol's function could help explain its role not only in human medicine but also in veterinary medicine, underscoring its importance in understanding stress responses and inflammatory processes in both biological systems (Arkins et al., 2006; Bosscher et al., 2019) (Figure 5.15).

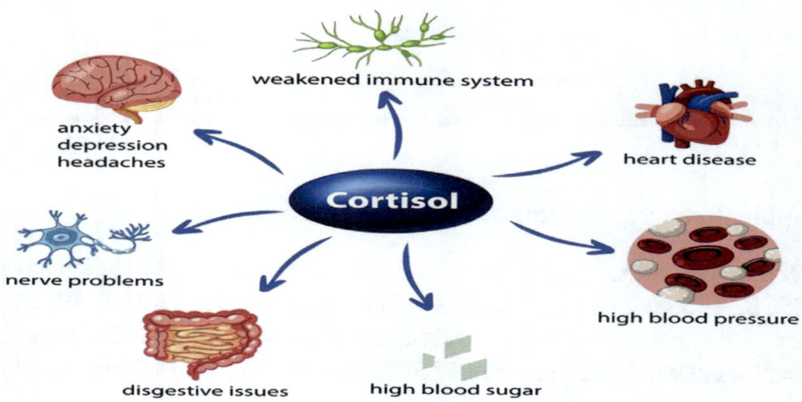

Figure 5.15. Cortisol function.

Source: https://www.drhagmeyer.com/wp-content/uploads/2021/08/5-ways-to-balance-cortisol-levels-in-your-body-4.jpg.

5.4.3. Behavioral Factors that Exacerbate Inflammatory Responses

A comprehensive evaluation of the role of lifestyle in triggering inflammatory responses and their exacerbation, therefore, necessitates the consideration of behavioral factors, including psychological stress and dietary habits. Psychological stress is one of the key instigators of inflammation because it disturbs the body's homeostasis and induces the release of pro-inflammatory cytokines. Repeated exposure to stress hormones, such as cortisol, results in a state of chronic inflammation, which, after a long time, leads to chronic inflammatory diseases. Furthermore, maladaptive coping mechanisms like withdrawal or aggression can also perpetuate stress reactions and produce a cycle of increased inflammation. Inflammatory diseases, such as Crohn's disease and ulcerative colitis, have been linked to behavioral factors, suggesting that stress management is possibly an essential component of inducing therapeutic interventions for managing inflammatory processes (Bitton et al., 2015). Dietary lifestyle is also a key factor in exacerbating inflammatory responses, with effects on immune function and gut microbiota populations. High-fat and sugar dietary consumption is linked to higher pro-inflammatory status, which translates into higher numbers of metabolic diseases and gastrointestinal inflammation. A diet rich in antioxidants and omega-3 fatty acids has been shown to have anti-inflammatory effects. Modulation of food consumption is even more relevant when one considers the mechanisms through which stress could lead to the use of unhealthy diets, raising inflammation levels. Thus, understanding the interaction between diet and psychological health is crucial in developing interventions that target both behavioral and inflammatory processes. As studies indicate, intervention in these aspects of lifestyle may yield significant benefits in managing inflammatory disease (Bitton et al., 2015). Physical inactivity is also a behavioral factor whose influence on inflammatory processes should not be underestimated. Exercise has been demonstrated to reduce the levels of inflammatory markers, boost immune function, and improve mood, whereas inactivity can enhance inflammation, primarily through the detrimental effect that stress has on physiological responses. Individuals with a sedentary lifestyle may exhibit higher levels of anxiety and depression, contributing to their susceptibility to inflammatory diseases. Furthermore, exercise can serve as a stress-reduction method, offering both psychological and physiological benefits that help lower inflammation. The interaction between inactivity, stress, and behavioral factors necessitates a complex health promotion plan focused on physical activity to control inflammatory conditions.

Test Your Knowledge

1. How does chronic psychological stress modify the body's inflammatory response?
2. What is the role of cortisol in regulating inflammation during stress?

5.5. The Bidirectional Relationship between Stress and Inflammation

Learning Outcome

1. Describe how to inflammation may lead to increased stress
2. Define the feedback process between stress and inflammatory markers
3. Describe how implications for mental and physical well-being

The intricate interaction between stress and inflammation has drawn significant interest in the context of psychosomatic well-being. Biological stress reactions, particularly those mediated by the HPA axis, elicit the release of immunomodulatory glucocorticoids. Acute stress may have a regulatory role in inflammation, while chronic stress is more likely to cause dysregulation and a heightened inflammatory response. The pro-inflammatory state can exacerbate many diseases, such as cardiovascular disease and autoimmune disorders. Thus, stress not only impacts inflammation but also introduces a feedback process through which inflammation can trigger additional stress responses, initiating a vicious cycle of deteriorating health outcomes. Further supporting this link, research also indicates that variations in inflammatory profiles can impact psychological health. For instance, cytokines associated with inflammation, such as interleukin-6, have been linked to behavioral changes typical of conditions related to stress. In the examination of postpartum depression, a principal finding was that disruptions in the bidirectional interface between inflammation markers and HPA axis function were identified as predictors of increased risk of developing depressive symptoms. Specifically, biomarkers such as cortisol and the ratio of pro-to-anti-inflammatory cytokines were associated with heightened risks, illustrating how chronic inflammation can provide a physiological substrate for stress-associated mood disorders, as observed in a study of postpartum women (Aagaard-Tillery et al., 2015). In addition, controlled experimental research also confirms the hypothesis that inflammatory states directly influence cognition and regulation. In double-blind experiments, patients injected with a typhoid vaccine showed significant inflammatory reactions, leading to extreme fatigue and confusion.

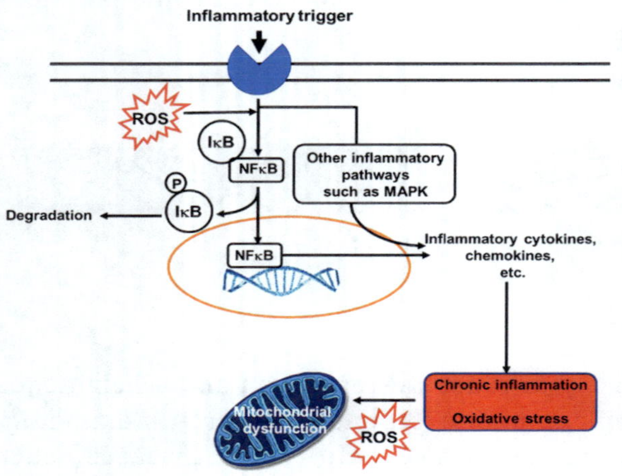

Figure 5.16. Bidirectional relationship between stress and inflammation.

Source: https://www.researchgate.net/publication/352679441/figure/fig2/AS:11431281254447774@1719176178258/The-bidirectional-links-between-inflammation-and-oxidative-stress-Reactive-oxygen.tif.

The interaction not only shows inflammation's impact on cognition but also indicates how the mechanisms behind the role of inflammation in stress experience work. Since the body's inflammatory signals are interpreted by the brain, the signals can reroute motivational states and effectively mold behavior and emotional well-being. The triggering of the respective brain regions in the presence of inflammation highlights the intricate interconnection of physiological activities and psychosocial impact, thereby reiterating the bidirectional interaction between stress and inflammation as a central element in the context of describing mental and physical health (Andrew et al., 2009) (Figure 5.16).

5.5.1. How Inflammation Can Lead to Increased Stress

Inflammation is being viewed more and more as a significant factor in the body's overall stress response, with a complex interaction between immune function and mental health. With exposure to stressors, either psychological or physiological, the immune system is triggered, and pro-inflammatory cytokines are released. The immune response can heighten anxiety and heighten feelings of stress, showing a vicious cycle of stress driving inflammation and inflammation driving stress. In addition, chronic inflammation repurposes the activity of neurotransmitters that modulate mood, basically dictating psychological responses. Thus, as the inflammatory markers increase with chronic stress, psychological responses can further improve, leading to enhanced perception of stress and potential health-related anxieties. The interface between these processes highlights the necessity of understanding how not only physical but also mental well-being is affected by inflammation, thereby necessitating a holistic approach to managing stress. Chronic stress has been shown to have a negative impact on overall well-being, but its interaction with inflammation is a complex and intricate process. Emerging evidence suggests that key modulators of the stress response, such as the CRH family, play a crucial role in mediating inflammation. Higher CRH levels can lead to a response of inflammation that causes most diseases, and it emphasizes the role of stress in initiating sublethal inflammatory cascades. Significantly to note is that the link further blurs the understanding of disease-sustaining inflammation-based diseases, such as colorectal cancer, where inflammation causes progression of disease. By explaining these interactions at the molecular level, scientists believe it will unveil new drug targets that not only contribute to stress management but also to the control of inflammation-based diseases. Unveiling this relationship is crucial for developing effective interventions that address both physical and emotional well-being. New evidence suggests that disorders like periodontitis, an inflammatory chronic condition, are a clear example of how chronic inflammation can maintain stress and anxiety. The presence of periodontal pathogens has also been linked to inflammatory processes that disrupt several bodily systems, including the brain. In their spread, chronic low-grade infections to precondition the brain's microglia, with the result that there is enhanced susceptibility to stressors and a higher risk for neurodegenerative disorders, such as Alzheimer's disease. The implication here is the importance of healthy oral health to reduce systemic inflammation and, therefore, stress response.

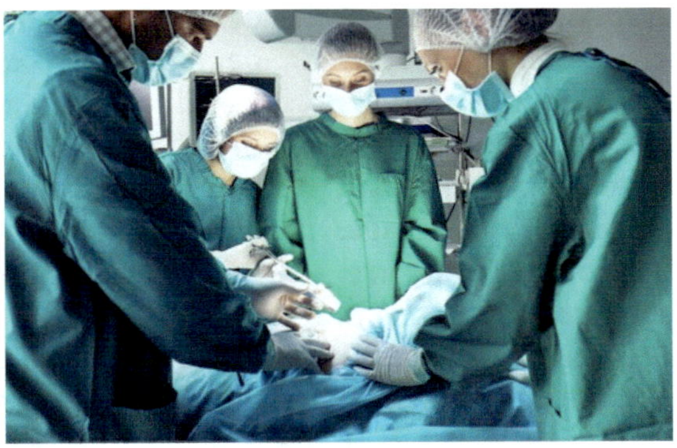

Figure 5.17. Anxiety before surgery.

Source: https://contentpathway.s3.amazonaws.com/surgery-anxiety-full.jpg.

Thus, the treatment of inflammation at its source becomes a vital step not just for relieving physical symptoms but also for preserving mental health. The intricate processes linking periodontal disease, inflammation, and stress can help summarize the overall effects of chronic inflammation on health and wellness (Figure 5.17).

5.5.2. The Feedback Loop Between Stress and Inflammatory Markers

The relationship between stress and inflammatory markers is characterized by a double-sided feedback loop that exerts a substantial influence on physiological health. Psychological stress triggers the HPA axis, resulting in the release of cortisol, a glucocorticoid best known for its role in stress regulation. While cortisol's acute response is to suppress the inflammatory response, prolonged or chronic stress will instead perpetuate a situation where inflammation ensues. High levels of pro-inflammatory cytokines, such as TNF-α and IL-6, result from this stress, thereby aggravating physical and mental health. This interaction is most apparent in autoimmune conditions, where markers of inflammation from stress can contribute to disease initiation or flares, demonstrating how the body's coping mechanisms can have unintended health consequences. Autoimmune thyroid disease studies, namely Graves' disease and Hashimoto's thyroiditis, emphasize this stress-inflammation feedback loop. These conditions chronicle how prolonged stress may activate the immune system and lead to the production of anti-thyroid antibodies. When stress is coupled with inflammation markers like leptin, prevalent in females, the risk of autoimmunity is increased. According to current hypotheses, adipokines play a crucial role in this process by modulating inflammation and immune responses within the thyroid. The function of stress becomes pivotal when one considers how environmental influences can be responsible for initiating the initial breakdown of tolerance to self-antigens, resulting in the onset of autoimmune diseases. Therefore, understanding these dynamics is crucial for creating targeted therapeutic interventions to alleviate stress-related autoimmune diseases among affected groups (Merrill et al., 2015). The influence of stress extends far beyond the context of individual diseases, affecting more general processes, such as inflammaging—an age-dependent syndrome characterized by chronic, low-grade inflammation. Contemporary studies have highlighted the mechanism by which endocannabinoids may influence this condition, with potential for the creation of new therapeutic directions. Synthetic endocannabinoids, such as Isopalmide, demonstrate the ability to enhance stress-induced inflammatory effects on skin models. Through the regulation of inflammation, these substances have been shown to inhibit pathways such as NF-κB, a key player in the inflammatory signaling pathway. This implies that by targeting the interface between stress and inflammatory markers, new therapeutic targets can be identified to reverse the detrimental effects of stress on aging and inflammation. The interaction between inflammatory processes and the body's stress response has far-reaching implications for both clinical care and research, highlighting the importance of further investigation into these interacting systems (Caviola et al., 2019) (Figure 5.18).

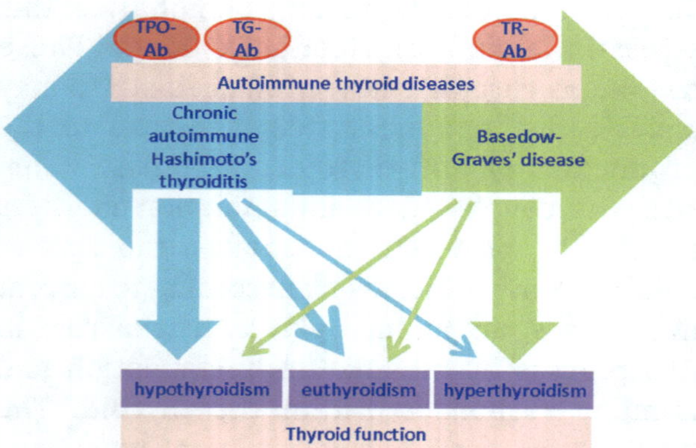

Figure 5.18. Thyroid causes diagnosis.

Source: https://www.creative-biolabs.com/natural-autoantibody/static/img/naa-services-for-anti-tpo-antibodies-1.png.

5.5.3. Implications for Mental Health and Physical Health

The interconnected nature of inflammatory processes and stress responses thus has significant implications for physical and mental well-being. Chronic stress also activates the HPA axis, leading to elevated cortisol levels that fuel inflammation. This biological reaction is not merely a stress aftereffect but has the potential to exacerbate mental illness, such as anxiety and depression. Individuals suffering from chronic stress are caught in a self-perpetuating cycle in which inflammation worsens mood disorders, creating a feedback loop that complicates treatment. It is stressed in current research to respond to mental health care with an understanding of the biological foundation of stress and inflammation to encourage integrated intervention strategies that address psychological and physical health factors. Resilience plays a central role in mediating the effects of stress on mental health. In contrast to previous assumptions that resilience is a stable personality trait, it is increasingly understood as a developing capacity shaped by long-term interactions between psychosocial and biological factors. Self-efficacy and social support are essential factors that foster individual resilience to mental disorder such as LLD. Psychobiological mechanisms involving neuroendocrine and inflammatory processes reciprocally influence risk factors that are associated with the onset and course of LLD. By identifying and bolstering resilience factors through targeted interventions—such as cognitive behavioral therapies and movement-based therapies—healthcare workers can develop more effective interventions to prevent and manage chronic stress-induced mental health disorders (Funes et al., 2019). The more immediate implications of chronic stress extend into physical health, where its functions have been critically assessed. Stress is an factor determining numerous health conditions that usually end in chronic diseases, including cardiovascular disease, diabetes, and metabolic syndrome. The literature underscores that stress does not act solely by influencing health through behavioral mechanisms, including diet and physical inactivity, but also through intricate biological pathways. The interaction between brain function and body health suggests a disconnection between traditional care practices, which often separate mind and body. A model that integrates both can optimize treatment outcomes, promoting a more comprehensive understanding of health that recognizes the two-way relationship between stress responses, inflammation, and wellness (Estrine et al., 2006).

Test Your Knowledge

1. How is stress implicated in initiating or worsening inflammation within the body?
2. How does chronic inflammation impact the body's stress response system?

5.6. Strategies for Managing Stress and Inflammation

Learning Outcome

1. Describe the lifestyle changes to reduce stress
2. Define the nutritional measures to combat inflammation
3. List the relaxation and mindfulness techniques

The convergence of stress and inflammation necessitates a multicomponent management strategy that incorporates psychosocial and biological interventions. An appreciation of resilience as an adaptive capacity influenced by various factors is crucial in the development of effective interventions. There is evidence that available coping mechanisms, social support, and a sense of meaning in life can enhance resilience and thus mitigate the impact of stress on inflammation. Furthermore, mindfulness activities such as meditation and cognitive therapy have been shown to enhance psychological resilience, which can in turn decrease inflammatory markers within the body. With the incorporation of these psychosocial factors in stress management interventions, people can build support that not only alleviates stress but also addresses the inflammation processes of chronic disease. This holistic process aims to enable people to take control of their health by actively managing it through improved mental coping and resilience, creating a two-way positive feedback between physical and psychological health. In addition to psychosocial interventions, physical interventions are essential for reducing stress and inflammation. Regular exercise, including aerobic activities, tai chi, and yoga, has been shown to induce the release of endorphins and produce a positive mood, while simultaneously reducing pro-inflammatory cytokines. Exercise enhances circulation and immunity, allowing the body to combat the physiological impact of stress better. Furthermore, movement practice fosters mindfulness as a strategy of reconnecting with body and stress response, thereby leading to increased emotional regulation. These activities can serve both as preventive measures and therapeutic interventions for stressed individuals, offering empirically based benefits such as reduced inflammation and improved general health. Thus, incorporating exercise into everyday life is a long-term remedy for the complex interplay between inflammation and stress mechanisms. Finally, new biological therapies hold promise as potential interventions against inflammation and stress. Treatments that target intrinsic inflammatory pathways, including anti-inflammatory medications and antioxidant-containing nutraceuticals, are being investigated for their potential to modulate stress-induced inflammation. For example, Myriocin and Fulvic Acid have shown both antifungal and anti-inflammatory activity, implying dual-action therapeutic potential. In this context, suppression of chronic inflammation can not only mitigate signs and symptoms of stress but also prevent the pathogenic sequelae of chronic inflammatory conditions. By combining these biological interventions with psychosocial and physical interventions, a comprehensive management program could be designed. Such an integrated model not only aligns with the prevailing literature on resilience and stress but also addresses avenues that lead to chronic inflammation, ultimately resulting in better health outcomes and quality of life (Borghi et al., 2015; Funes et al., 2019).

5.6.1. Lifestyle Changes to Reduce Stress

To effectively combat stress and its attendant health dangers, lifestyle changes are crucial in their role of building better overall well-being. The inclusion of regular physical exercise in an individual's daily routine is a significant contributor to the alleviation of stress. Exercise triggers the release of endorphins, also known as "happy hormones," to enhance happiness and alleviate tension. Additionally, physical exercise promotes cardiovascular health by reducing hypertension, one of the body's physiological responses to prolonged stress. Hypertension triggers adverse vascular events, including inflammation and endothelial dysfunction, as authored by Cameron et al. (2016). Thus, daily exercise is not only a means of stress relief but also reverses the connected inflammatory processes, which have the tendency to degrade overall health and render a person more susceptible to diseases. Besides exercise, adopting a healthy diet rich in wholesome foods can go a long way in managing stress. Intake of food directly influences biochemical activities in the body, like inflammation and hormonal balance. A diet consisting of fruits, vegetables, whole grains, and omega-3 fatty acids has been shown to support peak brain function and mood. Yet, a diet of high-processed foods and sugars can exacerbate underlying stress reactions through systemic inflammation. Nutrition should be targeted, as the relationship between diet and mood significantly impacts the way the body reacts to stressors and ultimately influences stress-mediated inflammatory processes, as noted in Estrine et al. (2006). Therefore, mindful consumption can be coupled with other lifestyle changes to render it an effective strategy for reducing stress. Mindfulness training and relaxation techniques such as meditation and diaphragmatic breathing are equally crucial for reducing stress.

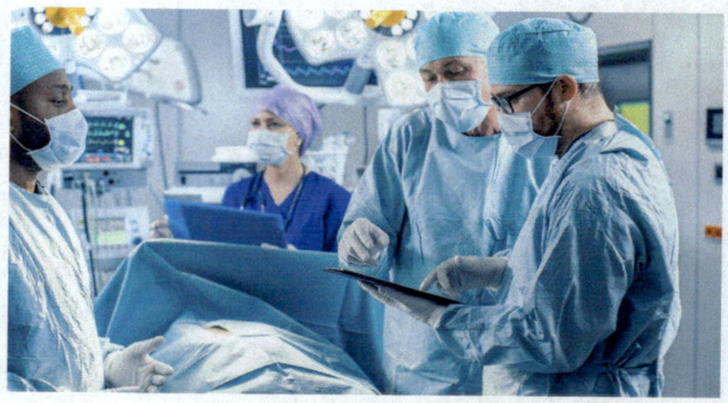

Figure 5.19. Reducing stress and increasing surgical performance.

Source: https://nexgensurgical.com/wp-content/uploads/2022/04/surgical-performance-1024x576.jpg.

Mindfulness practice makes it more possible for individuals to become more aware of their emotions and thoughts, resulting in improved emotional regulation and stress resilience. Research has shown that these practices can help lower cortisol, the primary stress hormone in the body, which has a direct correlation with inflammation and cardiovascular health. As addressed in Cameron et al. (2016), effective stress management can lower vascular dysfunction as well as other negative consequences of chronic stress. By applying mindfulness to everyday activities, individuals can enhance their ability to manage stress and its physiological effects, thereby strengthening the mind-body connection. These lifestyle modifications not only alleviate acute stress but also contribute to long-term health benefits and reduced inflammatory processes (Figure 5.19).

5.6.2. Dietary Interventions to Combat Inflammation

The link between diet and inflammation has emerged as a significant field of research over the past few years, as researchers have discovered how diet can exacerbate or mitigate inflammatory responses. Dietary interventions that incorporate anti-inflammatory foods, such as fruits, vegetables, whole grains, and oily fish, have been shown to reduce markers of inflammation. These foods are rich in antioxidants, vitamins, and omega-3 fatty acids, which can modulate the immune response and overall improve health. A balanced diet can also influence gut microbiota composition, thus playing a role in systemic inflammation. By adopting eating patterns rich in these nutrients for better health, individuals can experience a reduced risk of chronic inflammatory conditions, such as cardiovascular disease and metabolic syndrome. Therefore, food selection proves to be a crucial element within the broader context of stress response management and inflammation. Coupled with the improvement in consumption of anti-inflammatory foods, exclusion or minimization of pro-inflammatory foods also plays a crucial role in food intervention. Processed foods containing high levels of added sugars, trans fats, and sodium have been linked to increased inflammation and oxidative stress. These dietary components are capable of inducing an immune response, which subsequently activates inflammation pathways. Consequently, a diet with excessive consumption of these foods has the potential to cause a vicious cycle of stressful and chronic inflammation. In an effort to counteract inflammation through diet, individuals are cautioned against replacing unhealthy foods with whole foods that are high in nutrients. This approach acknowledges both acute inflammatory markers and health benefits with a long-term impact, documenting the close relationship between nutritional intake and control of inflammation. A second field of interest for dietary interventions is based on the role of specific nutrients and supplements in modulating inflammation. Curcumin, found in turmeric, and polyphenols in green tea, are some examples of substances with a very high anti-inflammatory effect. Supplementation with these and other beneficial foods can lead to significant reductions in inflammatory biomarkers, thereby augmenting overall physiological resistance to stress-induced inflammation. In addition, synergy between different food components can reinforce their health-supporting impact; accordingly, dietary intervention should aim for overall dietary regimens, rather than isolated nutrients. Lastly, evidence now suggests that lifestyle factors, such as physical activity, influence the effectiveness of dietary interventions. By the interplay of conscious food intake and physical lifestyle, an individual can better manage the dynamics of inflammatory processes and stress reactions towards better health results and a greater sense of well-being (Clarke et al., 2015; Cameron et al., 2016).

5.6.3. Mindfulness and Relaxation Techniques

The contemporary view of stress reactions places focus on the strong interaction between psychological processes and physiological effects, particularly about inflammation. Mindfulness and relaxation techniques have emerged as prominent interventions that induce stress reduction and, consequently, modulate inflammatory responses. By creating awareness and promoting relaxation, these techniques enable individuals to disentangle themselves from habitual stress-inducing cognitive patterns.

Research has shown that mindfulness meditation has the capacity to alter an individual's perception of pain, and neuroimaging results have demonstrated that heightened mindful awareness is associated with significant changes in brain areas involved in pain processing. This means that mindfulness not only decreases subjective pain reports but also affects the neuromechanisms underlying them, thereby contributing to a multidisciplinary insight into how such practices might be used to decrease stress-related inflammatory responses (Aguirre et al., 2019). Mind-body treatments (MBIs), such as the practice of mindfulness, yoga, and tai chi, are tools for people who want to better manage stress and inflammation processes. The focus on thoughtful engagement in these practices has been linked to profound changes both at the psychological and molecular levels. Specifically, evidence has been found that MBIs have the potential to lead to downregulation of the nuclear factor kappa B (NF-kB) pathway, an essential component involved in inflammatory responses. This downregulation suggests a protective potential for anti-disease processes, and it highlights the need to examine further how these interventions can reverse stress-induced inflammation. The emerging literature addresses the therapeutic and preventive potential of MBIs, not only as treatments but also as preventive measures against chronic diseases exacerbated by stress (Astin et al., 2017). As relaxation and mindfulness interventions become increasingly popular as stress treatments, their broader public health dimensions come into clearer perspective, particularly with regard to their anti-inflammatory effects. As chronic stress is recognized as a subtle cause of various health issues, incorporating mindfulness training into daily life presents an effective strategy for enhancing well-being and resilience. Schools, employment settings, and healthcare facilities can implement these practices to raise awareness about their worth across various populations. Through emphasizing the need for relaxation and mindfulness in reducing stress responses, participants can practice healthier lifestyles that can help avoid inflammatory diseases. Ultimately, the establishment of a culture that prioritizes mental health can lead to enhanced health outcomes and a significant shift in societal consciousness towards overall healthcare routines, acknowledging the interdependence of mind and body in maintaining health (Figure 5.20).

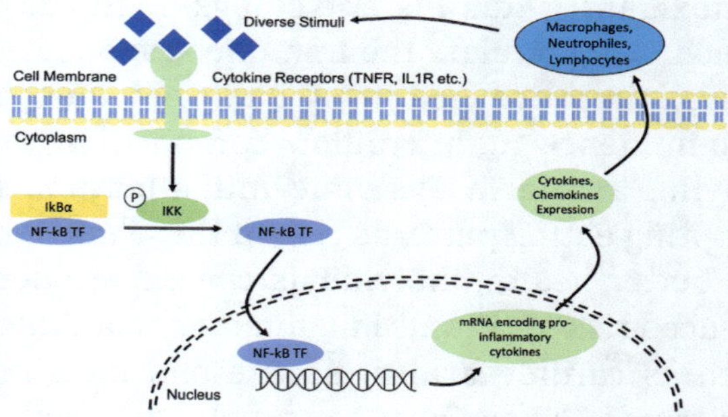

Figure 5.20. Nuclear factor kappa-B pathway.

Source: https://sites.tufts.edu/hkerstjaaalislai/files/2020/11/NFkB2.png.

Test Your Knowledge

1. List two non-pharmacological interventions that nurses may employ to help patients with stress management.
2. How does effective stress management have a role to play in reducing inflammation?

SUMMARY

The association between inflammatory processes and stress responses is a complex but fundamental branch of study, highlighting the effects of physiological stress on overall health. Based on a number of studies, chronic stress activates the HPA axis, leading to the release of glucocorticoids that regulate immune responses. This involves the release of pro-inflammatory cytokines, which are required for an acute stress response but are detrimental when constantly elevated. The emerging concept of stress-induced inflammation necessitates a reevaluation of traditional views on immune function, opening new avenues for research into how stress influences both health and disease at the systemic level. Furthermore, the interconnection between stress and inflammation has significant implications for public health and overall well-being. An awareness of this link can inform the design of interventions to reduce stress and its harmful impact on health. For example, the inclusion of stress management techniques such as mindfulness, cognitive-behavioral therapy, and exercise has been shown to reduce the adverse effects of stress on inflammatory markers. In addition, animal welfare considerations suggest that better conditions for raising animals not only improve their health but can also contribute to enhanced productivity and quality of life, according to some research (Arkins et al., 2006). Finally, any future research must consider the discovery of molecular processes linking stress response and inflammation, as well as the potential therapeutic interventions. The investigation of neuropeptides, such as PACAP in migraine headache, represents an ongoing attempt to understand complex pain processes (Akerman et al., 2018). Clarifying the subtypes of individual receptors and brain circuits responsible for stress-evoked inflammation can inform the design of new therapies to treat stress-related disorders. By advancing our knowledge in this multidisciplinary field, we can better manage the health issues arising from chronic stress and its associated inflammatory outcomes, and thus achieve enhanced integrated health and wellness.

The interconnectedness among inflammatory processes and stress responses manifests the profound impact of psychosocial stress on human health. Relocation, isolation, and extreme changes in social relations are life events that are potent stressors with the capacity to trigger a myriad of physiological responses. In one longitudinal experiment involving vervet monkeys subjected to a 28-day quarantine, the authors demonstrated widespread alterations in immune signaling and gene expression. The findings revealed a coordinated decline of nine immune signaling molecules, indicating that acute stress can cause a rapid, typically dysregulated immune response. This means findings on the biological processes underlying development of chronic health conditions, e.g., those in the cardiovascular system or infectious susceptibility, and as such this is an area worthy of more studies into stress-related interactions within the immune system (Benjamin et al., 2020). Additionally, the impact of stress on the transcriptome reveals a complex interplay between psychological states and physiological responses. The study revealed that stress resulted in a profound dysregulation of gene expression in immune function and inflammatory processes. In other words, some genes associated with chronic diseases and immune defense mechanisms were suppressed. In contrast, genes responsible for blood coagulation and platelet activation were elevated as a reaction to stress. These findings demonstrate that stress not only alters immune signaling at the molecular level but also restructures the entire immune landscape, highlighting an essential avenue for future research. Knowledge of such changes is critical for the design of interventions to reverse the adverse health effects of chronic stress and to investigate its role in stress-associated disorders (Benjamin et al., 2020). Lastly, the impacts of stress cannot be easily categorized, as they encompass both acute and chronic elements of disease risk associated with inflammatory processes. The research strategy in responding to immune response within an artificial environment provides a robust framework for establishing the basis upon which psychosocial stressors can be transformed into unwanted physiological effects. The shifts observed in immunity within the test group reveal the dynamic operation of the immune system against stressors, highlighting potential avenues for preventing various diseases. This information is critical for preventive measures and therapeutic control, particularly since the global dynamics of human social interaction continue to evolve. Explanation of mechanistic relationships between stress responses and inflammatory pathways not only increases the scope of health research but also informs clinical practices to improve patient outcomes (Benjamin et al., 2020).

KEY TERMS FROM THIS CHAPTER

- Acute Phase Response
- Chronic Inflammation
- Cytokines
- General Adaptation Syndrome (GAS)
- Homeostasis
- Immune Modulation
- Inflammatory Response
- Neuroendocrine Regulation
- Allostatic Load
- Cortisol
- Fight or Flight Response
- Histamine
- Hypothalamic-Pituitary-Adrenal (HPA) Axis
- Inflammatory Markers
- Leukocytes
- Oxidative Stress

CRITICAL THINKING QUESTIONS

1. **Which hormone is mainly released during the stress response and is involved in modulating inflammation?**
   a. Insulin
   b. Cortisol
   c. Adrenaline
   d. Glucagon
2. **What is the primary function of the hypothalamic-pituitary-adrenal (HPA) axis during stress?**
   a. Increase glucose uptake in muscles
   b. Increase immune cell proliferation
   c. Control cortisol production
   d. Lower heart rate
3. **Which cytokine is known as a pro-inflammatory mediator?**
   a. IL-10
   b. IL-4
   c. IL-6
   d. TGF-β
4. **Chronic stress is known to have what impact on inflammation?**
   a. Suppresses all immune activity
   b. Prevents cytokine release
   c. Encourages low-grade chronic inflammation
   d. Causes immediate healing of tissue
5. **What immune cells are mainly responsible for initiating the inflammatory response?**
   a. B cells
   b. T helper cells
   c. Neutrophils and macrophages
   d. Natural killer cells

Short Answer Questions

1. What is cortisol's role in the stress response?
2. Name one pro-inflammatory cytokine and one anti-inflammatory cytokine.
3. Which part of the brain initiates the stress response?
4. What is the sympathetic nervous system's role in stress?
5. How is acute stress different from chronic stress when it comes to inflammation?
6. Explain the role of the hypothalamic-pituitary-adrenal (HPA) axis in the response to stress and how it influences inflammation.
7. Explain the link between chronic psychological stress and the pathogenesis of inflammatory disease.
8. Explain the cascade of events for the inflammatory response to tissue injury.
9. How do glucocorticoids influence immune and inflammatory responses?
10. Compare and contrast the impact of acute vs. chronic stress on immune function.

Answers to Critical Thinking Questions

1. (b); 2. (c); 3. (c); 4. (c); 5. (c)

REFERENCES

1. Corwin, E. J., Pajer, K., Paul, S., Lowe, N., Weber, M., & McCarthy, D. O. (2015). Bidirectional psychoneuroimmune interactions in the early postpartum period influence risk of postpartum depression. *Brain Behavior and Immunity*, *49*, 86–93. https://doi.org/10.1016/j.bbi.2015.04.012Aguirre, A., Amanzio, M., Andrews-Hanna, J., Atlas, L. Y., Atlas, L. Y., Basbaum, A. I., Behzadi, Y., et al. (2019). The neural mechanisms of mindfulness-based pain relief: A functional magnetic resonance imaging-based review and primer. https://core.ac.uk/download/323064453.pdf (accessed on 28th June 2025).
2. Ahmed, A., Ai, A., Ai, A., Anzilotti, C., Arend, W. P., Astorri, E., Benham, H., et al. (2017). Immunopathogenesis of rheumatoid arthritis. https://core.ac.uk/download/80696952.pdf (accessed on 28th June 2025).
3. Akbar, M., Crowe, L. A. N., Garcia-Melchor, E., Gilchrist, D. S., et al. (2017). Targeting danger molecules in tendinopathy: The HMGB1/TLR4 axis. https://core.ac.uk/download/84340439.pdf (accessed on 28th June 2025).
4. Akerman, S., Baca, S. M., & Waschek, J. A. (2018). PACAP and migraine headache: Immunomodulation of neural circuits in autonomic ganglia and brain parenchyma. https://core.ac.uk/download/323078275.pdf (accessed on 28th June 2025).
5. Alhouayek, M., Amor, S., Amor, S., Appel, S. H., Bankston, A. N., Biber, K., Biran, V., et al. (2017). Neuroinflammation, mast cells, and glia: Dangerous liaisons. https://core.ac.uk/download/129593018.pdf (accessed on 28th June 2025).
6. Andrew, A., Steptoe, A., Bluthe, R., Bretdibat, C., Brydon, L., Capuron, L., et al. (2009). Neural origins of human sickness in interoceptive responses to inflammation. https://core.ac.uk/download/2710274.pdf (accessed on 28th June 2025).
7. Aouizerat, B. E., Carrico, A. W., Flentje, A., Flowers, E., et al. (2018). Minority stress and leukocyte gene expression in sexual minority men living with treated HIV infection. https://core.ac.uk/download/213085711.pdf (accessed on 28th June 2025).
8. Arkins, S., Boyle, L., Llamas Moya, S., Lynch, P. B., et al. (2006). Effects of husbandry and low-dose lipopolysaccharide challenge on the acute phase response of young pigs. https://core.ac.uk/download/45656698.pdf (accessed on 28th June 2025).
9. Astin, J. A., Baskaran, C., Baxevanis, C. N., Benson, H., Bhasin, M. K., Bierhaus, A., Black, D. S., et al. (2017). What is the molecular signature of mind-body interventions? A systematic review of gene expression changes induced by meditation and related practices. https://core.ac.uk/download/228151455.pdf (accessed on 28th June 2025).
10. Baritaki, S., Chatzaki, E., de Bree, E., Pothoulakis, C., et al. (2019). Chronic stress, inflammation, and colon cancer: A CRH system-driven molecular crosstalk. https://core.ac.uk/download/323076588.pdf (accessed on 28th June 2025).
11. Benjamin, C., Coppola, G., Freimer, N. B., He, Y., et al. (2020). Immunosuppressive effect and global dysregulation of blood transcriptome in response to psychosocial stress in vervet monkeys (*Chlorocebus sabaeus*). https://core.ac.uk/download/323080367.pdf (accessed on 28th June 2025).
12. Bitton, A., Bitton, A., Dignass, A., Kaser, A., Lunderquist, A., Timmer, A., Wakefield, A. J., et al. (2015). Environmental factors in the relapse and recurrence of inflammatory bowel disease:

A review of the literature. https://core.ac.uk/download/29112037.pdf (accessed on 28th June 2025).

13. Borghi, E., Borgo, F., Morace, G., Nile, C. J., et al. (2015). New strategic insights into managing fungal biofilms. https://core.ac.uk/download/42365456.pdf (accessed on 28th June 2025).

14. Cameron, A. C., Lang, N. N., & Touyz, R. M. (2016). Drug treatment of hypertension: Focus on vascular health. https://core.ac.uk/download/46559725.pdf (accessed on 28th June 2025).

15. Carter, C. S., Justice, J. N., & Thompson, L. (2019). Lipotoxicity, aging, and muscle contractility: Does fiber type matter? https://open.bu.edu/bitstream/2144/40625/7/carter_justice_thompson_Lipotoxicity_paper_04302019.pdf (accessed on 28th June 2025).

16. Caviola, E., Galizia, G., Baratto, G., Meloni, M., Semenzato, G., et al. (2019). New synthetic endocannabinoid as anti-inflammaging cosmetic active: An *in vitro* study on a reconstructed skin model. https://core.ac.uk/download/185556582.pdf (accessed on 28th June 2025).

17. Cerretani, D., Di Paolo, M., Fineschi, V., Neri, M., Pomara, C., Riezzo, I., & Turillazzi, E. (2015). Cardiac oxidative stress and inflammatory cytokines response after myocardial infarction. https://core.ac.uk/download/54248089.pdf (accessed on 28th June 2025).

18. Chen, H., Choi, E. T., Cueto, R., Drosatos, K., et al. (2018). DNA checkpoint and repair factors are nuclear sensors for intracellular organelle stresses: Inflammations and cancers can have high genomic risks. https://core.ac.uk/download/213438588.pdf (accessed on 28th June 2025).

19. Cianci, R., Gambassi, G., Gasbarrini, A., & Rio, P. (2024). Pollutants, microbiota and immune system: Frenemies within the gut. https://core.ac.uk/download/613662566.pdf (accessed on 28th June 2025).

20. Cicala, M., Guarino, M. P., Putignani, L., Severi, C., et al. (2016). Gastrointestinal neuromuscular apparatus: An underestimated target of gut microbiota. https://core.ac.uk/download/98336463.pdf (accessed on 28th June 2025).

21. Clarke, S. F., Cotter, P. D., Cronin, O., Molloy, M. G., et al. (2015). Exercise and the microbiota. https://core.ac.uk/download/45656552.pdf (accessed on 28th June 2025).

22. Crean, S., Harding, A., Kesavalu, L., Robinson, C., et al. (2014). Oral inflammation, tooth loss, risk factors, and association with progression of Alzheimer's disease. https://core.ac.uk/download/42137086.pdf (accessed on 28th June 2025).

23. Crosswell, A. D., Epel, E. S., Mayer, S. E., Mendes, W. B., et al. (2018). More than a feeling: A unified view of stress measurement for population science. https://core.ac.uk/download/305124133.pdf (accessed on 28th June 2025).

24. De Bosscher, K., Opdenakker, G., Van den Steen, P. E., Vandermosten, L., et al. (2019). Critical roles of endogenous glucocorticoids for disease tolerance in malaria.

25. De Rosa, V., Marelli-Berg, F., Mauro, C., Solito, E., et al. (2015). Metabolic syndrome and the immunological affair with the blood-brain barrier. https://core.ac.uk/download/30697111.pdf (accessed on 28th June 2025).

26. Dejager, L., Libert, C., Tuckermann, J., & Vandevyver, S. (2013). New insights into the anti-inflammatory mechanisms of glucocorticoids: An emerging role for glucocorticoid-receptor-mediated transactivation. https://core.ac.uk/download/55843668.pdf (accessed on 28th June 2025).

27. Drew, J. E. (2014). Signaling pathways implicated in obesity-associated cancers. https://core.ac.uk/download/29150956.pdf (accessed on 28th June 2025).
28. Estrine, J., & DeLisle, L. (2006). Stress: Putting the brain back into medicine. https://core.ac.uk/download/71356692.pdf (accessed on 28th June 2025).
29. Facci, L., Giusti, P., Skaper, S. D., & Zusso, M., et al. (2018). An inflammation-centric view of neurological disease: Beyond the neuron. https://core.ac.uk/download/154331993.pdf (accessed on 28th June 2025).
30. Fu, W., Lee, Y. S., Olefsky, J. M., Ying, W., et al. (2020). The role of macrophages in obesity-associated islet inflammation and β-cell abnormalities. https://core.ac.uk/download/287622268.pdf (accessed on 28th June 2025).
31. Galley, H. F., Lowes, D. A., McCreath, G., Scullion, M., et al. (2016). Pharmacological activation of endogenous protective pathways against oxidative stress under conditions of sepsis. https://core.ac.uk/download/42130744.pdf (accessed on 28th June 2025).
32. McCreary, J. K., Metz, G. A. S., Ng, J. W. Y., Olson, D. M., et al. (2015). Allostatic load and preterm birth. https://core.ac.uk/download/74559442.pdf (accessed on 28th June 2025).
33. Merrill, S., & Mu, Y. (2015). Thyroid autoimmunity as a window to autoimmunity: An explanation for sex differences in the prevalence of thyroid autoimmunity. https://core.ac.uk/download/213059550.pdf (accessed on 28th June 2025).
34. Pendergraft, B. (2016). The effects of smoking on the calcification of the aortic valve. https://core.ac.uk/download/72841045.pdf (accessed on 28th June 2025).
35. Wildeman, K. (2020). The role of diet in the onset of depression: A biochemical connection between nutrition and mental health. https://core.ac.uk/download/322850898.pdf (accessed on 28th June 2025).

GERIATRIC NURSING: MANAGEMENT OF THE OLDER ADULT PATIENT

6

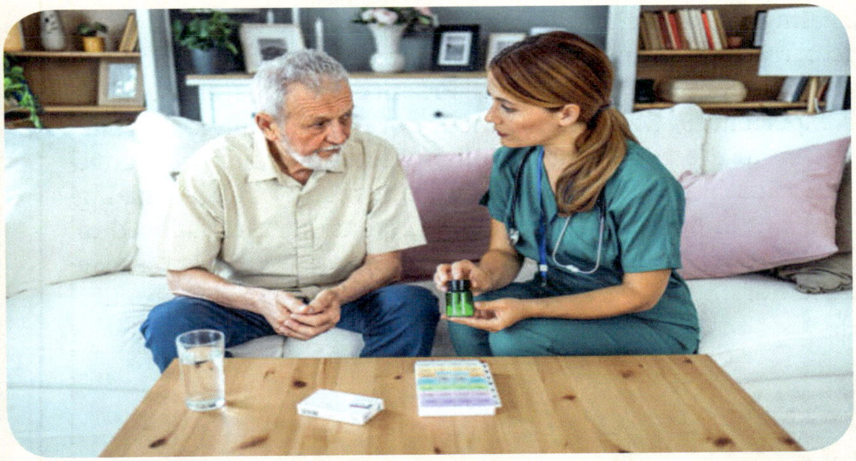

Introduction

Increasing demographic trends towards aging are placing a greater emphasis on the need for specialized nursing care of the elderly. As medical conditions associated with aging become increasingly complex, geriatric nursing has become a vital field of practice in healthcare, specializing in the specific needs and concerns of this population. With the prevalence of more than one co-morbidity and higher vulnerability to functional disability being presented most commonly by older individuals, nurses must possess a refined understanding of both geriatric syndromes and optimal management. The specialty not only brings value to patient outcomes but also meets the importance of holistic care, with physical, mental, and social health dimensions being integrated. Special training for nursing professionals needs to be included in order to be able to transfer to them the skills and knowledge that would enable them to deal with the complexities involved in taking care of older individuals. To meet the complex needs of geriatric

LEARNING OBJECTIVES

After studying this chapter, you will be able to:

1. Understand the role of the geriatric nurses
2. Describe the most prevalent problems of older adults
3. Discuss assessment strategies in geriatric nursing
4. Identify pain relief for older adults
5. Learn about nutrition and fluid requirements
6. Assess end-of-life care and palliative care interventions

patients adequately, nursing education programs are now incorporating specialized training in gerontological care. There is reason to believe that the same would be able to implement substantial care improvements to the aged, primarily acute care facilities. For instance, studies have shown that specialized nursing staff training reduces frailty and improves functionality among older patients in the hospital, with an evident connection between the patient's state and education (Peterson et al., 2025). This training encompasses in-depth elements of geriatric care, including mobility management, medication management, and care for frailty. However, the question remains whether education alone can be sufficient to change workplace practice or nursing practice, particularly in a stressed hospital environment that may constrain the application of learned ideas (Peterson et al., 2025). Additionally, the integration of reflective practices in nursing education, such as simulation-based training, can have the potential to enhance critical thinking and self-reflection among nursing students. Reflective journaling after simulation practice, according to research, helps nursing students comprehend geriatric care more comprehensively, as it exposes them to actual environments where they can apply their theoretical knowledge. Practice like this encourages students to critically think about their experiences, which helps them develop as individuals and enhance their professional capabilities. Due to the complexity of older adult care, such reflective learning practices are indispensable. They instill a workforce trained not merely in recognizing the unique challenges of geriatric patients but in developing creative solutions that are tailored to the unique needs of every patient within diverse health care settings. This strategy for the disease as a whole seeks to redefine the geriatric nursing topography, in the end benefiting the broader population of older adults (Figure 6.1).

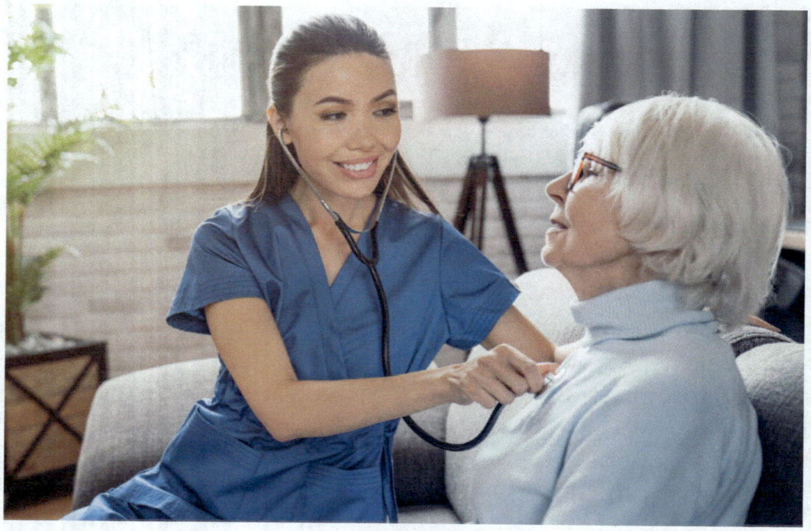

Figure 6.1. Geriatric nursing.

https://www.incrediblehealth.com/wp-content/uploads/2022/06/iStock-1181670520-scaled.jpg.

Definition of Geriatric Nursing

Geriatric nursing is a clinical specialty of nursing that caters to the unique health care needs of the elderly. It accounts for the intricacy of aging, whereby the concomitance of one or more chronic conditions, cognitive impairments, and psychosocial complications is possible. Geriatric nurses are trained to evaluate, plan for, and deliver care that is individually tailored for the elderly, with regard to the physiological changes that accompany aging. Not only is this specialty concerned with the physical care of these patients, but also their emotional and social well-being. Population trends evidence the expanding requirement for gerontological nursing expertise, such as the projection that by 2029, 20% of the United States population will be over 65 (Wynn-Grundy et al., 2016). Thus, geriatric practice nursing plays a vital role in delivering quality healthcare and optimizing the dignity and quality of life for older persons. Geriatric nursing is also characterized by its holistic approach to care, encompassing not only medical care but also support systems for older persons in a general sense. It is through this inter-professional methodology that collaboration with a variety of health care practitioners, such as physicians, social workers, and physical therapists, is needed to address the multifaceted problems of aging patients. Identification and intervention in conditions that are prevalent in older persons but usually go unnoticed, like depression in a potential 40% of chronically ill patients (Wynn-Grundy et al., 2016), is one of the salient features of this profession. Competence to take care of such complications is significant because uninsured mental health complications will hinder the upkeep of vital health education, hence affecting the overall health outcomes of this group. Recognition of such barriers enables geriatric nurses to formulate particular care plans that foster recovery and endurance among older adults. Satisfaction among geriatric nurses is a critical determinant of the care they deliver. What they are content with is the rewarding relationships they establish with patients and the satisfaction of making a meaningful contribution to their lives. Problems do arise, though, with the well-being of patients who have dementia and the stress involved with being able to provide sufficient care. To enhance nursing practice in this demanding specialty, efforts are needed to develop strategies for planning that address the needs of geriatric nursing staff, including special training and ongoing professional development opportunities. Evidence suggests that enhanced nurse satisfaction can have a direct and favorable impact on patient care outcomes, representing a negative correlation between patient disease and nurse health. By making geriatric nurses feel competent and valued, health care systems are able to potentially improve the overall quality of care delivered to the elderly, which responds to the growing number of complexities that they experience.

Significance of Geriatric Care

The growing importance of geriatric care is further influenced by the increasing numbers of the elderly, who have specific health issues requiring specialized handling. As the burden of age-related illnesses, such as dementia, long-term illness, and impairment of function, grows, the healthcare systems must be refashioned to meet the complex needs of this population. Geriatric care seeks to optimize quality and functional ability, engaging a multidisciplinary strategy that is mindful not only of medical issues but also of psychosocial and environmental determinants affecting older individuals. Evidence for the efficacy of person-centered interventions has been shown to enhance health outcomes, with evidence that high-quality geriatric care has the potential to decrease hospitalization and improve patient and family satisfaction. The contribution of family caregivers cannot be overemphasized in the context of geriatric care since they contribute substantially to the care of older adults with activities of daily living and related health tasks. Whilst they have a vital function, caregivers are likely to experience high levels of stress, and this has led to demands for targeted support and provision. There is evidence from literature of limited understanding of hard-to-reach groups of caregivers, such as older or ethnically diverse caregivers, and this is the basis for improved development in policy and practice (Henwood et al., 2017). Since then, medical caregivers have been forced to adopt more coordinated approaches that acknowledge the unique needs of various caregiver groups, so that patients as well as caregivers receive the kind of support they require. This urge for increased caregiver support is consistent with existing research initiatives aimed at better informing policy and practice toward the ultimate objectives of more efficient care coordination and improved patient outcomes. Finally, support for aging adult care depends on policy changes that prioritize evidence-based policies, with a focus on preventive care and care coordination. Policies on patient self-management and palliative care are among those that can enhance the health of older populations, based on available evidence (Morton et al., 2015). Gerontological nursing must tap into such evidence to drive systemic reform that targets both the medical complexities of aging and the overall well-being of older adults. With concerted action on the part of policymakers, health care professionals, and researchers, the form of geriatric care can shift to be better and more effective, and an improved response to the needs of older adults, so that they can receive the holistic and caring care that they deserve (Figure 6.2).

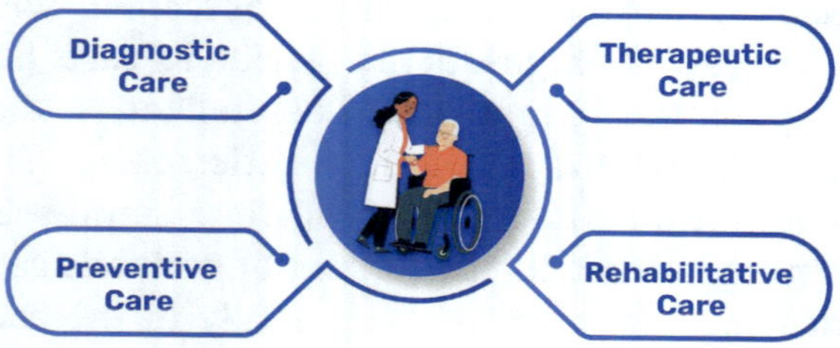

Figure 6.2. Importance of geriatric care.

https://www.theaccesshealthcare.com/images/blog/everything-you-need-to-know-about-geriatric-care/02.webp.

Overview of the Aging Population

The aging population is a demographic shift that is new in character and has worldwide consequences in the field of healthcare, particularly in geriatric nursing. With the forecasts suggesting that by 2029 about 20% of the United States' population will be 65 years and above, there is a requirement for the healthcare providers to understand the dynamics of the demographic change (Colby and Ortman, 2014). With the older person's tendency to experience physical, cognitive, and social health problems, gerontological nursing is much needed to address the complexity of aging. Not only does it address the management of chronic diseases, but it also addresses sensitive healthcare systems that respond to the diversity of needs of this heterogeneous group. To overcome almost all these challenges lies the solution to improving the overall health of the aged and thus their quality of life. Alongside this population trend is the primary challenge of caregiver support, which is a key aspect of the health status of older individuals. Caregivers, according to recent assessments, are diverse in makeup and come with unique challenges that can detract from their efficiency as caregivers. The review confirmed that several caregivers remain underrepresented in policy and research discussion, including older caregivers and the BAME and LGBT groups (Henwood et al., 2017). In gerontological nursing, it is equally essential to be aware of the characteristics and needs of caregivers as it is to identify the older person themselves. Because the care relationship is complex and multifaceted, it is therefore essential to empower the caregivers with appropriate support and resources. This, in turn, leads to improved care among the elderly patients. Geriatric nursing should hence employ a holistic approach that includes the elderly people as well as the caregivers. Undiagnosed diseases such as depression, which are highly prevalent among the elderly, are another imperative factor that determines the success of their health. Research indicates that up to 40% of elderly patients with chronic diseases remain undiagnosed for depression, which can severely complicate learning and memory for vital healthcare information and education (Wynn-Grundy et al., 2016). Depressive symptoms, such as concentration issues, will interfere with the learning process, and putting healthcare in check will be challenging. Geriatric nursing, as such, must include mental health screening as a core part of comprehensive care plans. By treating and diagnosing mental illness at an early stage, nurses not only improve the quality of care but also empower older adults to become active participants in their own healthcare education. This shared process in the war against mental and physical disorder is central to stimulating healthier aging trajectories in this burgeoning cohort.

6.1. The Role of Geriatric Nurses

Learning Outcome

1. Explain the responsibilities and roles of geriatric nursing
2. Highlight skills required in geriatric nursing
3. Learn about interdisciplinary teamwork in geriatric nursing

In the complex healthcare setting for the elderly, geriatric nurses play a crucial role in addressing the unique needs of this population. Their brief includes more than just easy care; they play a significant role in patient-centered assessment, planning, and execution of care interventions, considering the complex determinants of aging. As frontline caregivers, gerontological nurses must possess comprehensive knowledge of the age-related physiological alterations and the complexities of chronic diseases prevalent among the elderly. This enables them to implement evidence-based practices efficiently according to their patients' desires and values. Through comprehensive evaluations that consider both physical health and psychosocial concerns, geriatric nurses significantly contribute to enhancing the quality of life for the elderly, ensuring their care is patient-centered and comprehensive. Geriatric nurses also play a crucial role in education and advocacy within the healthcare delivery system. They provide patients and families with education on the management of chronic diseases, adherence to medication, and lifestyle modifications that promote healthy living. Additionally, gerontological nurses serve as critical intermediaries between various members of the healthcare team involved in a patient's care, ensuring all concerned parties are informed and in concert with their treatment plan. Such interdisciplinary practice is particularly vital in complex cases where elderly patients often have multiple comorbid conditions. In addition, as in the case of recent studies, care for distressed older patients generally tends to make non-pharmacological measures first-line choices, holding off on pharmacological methods like rapid tranquilization as a last alternative (Kumar et al., 2024). This highlights the role of the geriatric nurse in advocating for safer, improved care that is tailored to the unique needs of older adults. Additionally, gerontological nursing extends into the realm of policy and research, where nurses bring their experiences to create evidence-based practices for caring for the elderly. With their immediate contact with the elderly, they are in an ideal position to recognize lacunas in care and areas of improvement, especially in treating cancer and other age-related illnesses (Fang, 2024). With the aging of the world's population, the need for geriatric nursing expertise grows increasingly essential, particularly in meeting the rising incidence of age-related disorders. By participating in interdisciplinary care teams and research projects, geriatric nurses contribute to the development of guidelines that enhance the quality of care while addressing the ethical issues related to the care of elderly patients. This evolving role underscores the importance of specialized training and ongoing education for geriatric nurses, ensuring they remain at the forefront of caring for the elderly (Figure 6.3).

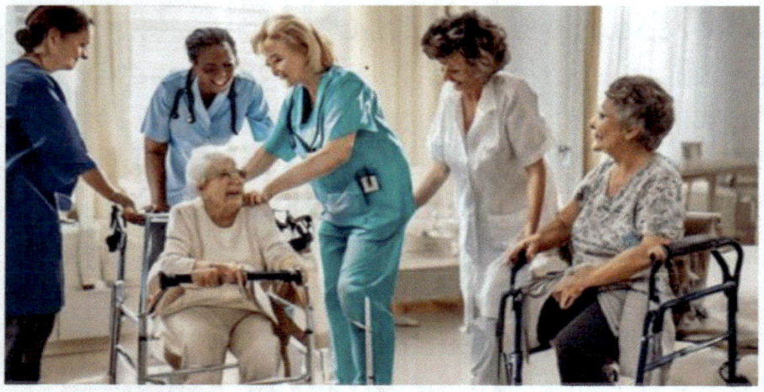

Figure 6.3. Role of geriatric nurses.

https://external-content.duckduckgo.com/iu/?u= https%3A%2F%2Ftse1.mm.bing.net%2Fth%3Fid%3DOIP.nHRfze5oLj3qkfZhJmqrsAHa D5%26pid%3DA pi&f=1&ipt= 07a3 161af 1919 de9884cf36bd94d022c9d8d1 3f8e8843bb3 055afa20f59 d4fe4.

6.1.1. Responsibilities and Duties

In geriatric nursing, outlining duties and responsibilities is essential to facilitating proper management of elderly patients. These nurses must not only offer clinical treatment but also act as advocates for their patients' overall needs. This involves assessing both physical health and psychosocial status, as elderly patients often present with complex problems that require comprehensive evaluation. Geriatric nurses have an obligation to organize care among disparate healthcare professionals so that treatment plans are individually crafted to meet the specific issues of older adults, such as polypharmacy and the complexity of chronic illness. They are also critical in instructing patients and their families on how to handle these situations, thereby promoting autonomy and effective self-management practices. Geriatric nurses' roles extend beyond direct patient care, including fundamental roles in education and supporting families. Due to the heavy emotional work that caregiving entails, knowledge of support dynamics within the family becomes paramount. Over 11 million caregivers care for an Alzheimer's or other dementias individual, demonstrating the heavy utilization of familial support (N/A, 2023). Nurses must educate and prepare families to overcome caregiving challenges, them information about resources and coping strategies that minimize caregiver stress.

This type of education component is especially appropriate in light of the recent evidence indicating an increased risk for emotional distress for family caregivers, particularly under challenging circumstances such as the COVID-19 pandemic, which imposed added stresses in long-term care environments (Rocard et al., 2021). Additionally, the evolving nature of medical care necessitates gerontological nurses to constantly update themselves with new developments in Alzheimer's care and management practices. With new drugs entering the market addressing the underlying biology of Alzheimer's disease, it is essential that nurses constantly update themselves with pharmacologic and non-pharmacologic interventions (N/A, 2023). These professionals are also required to participate in ongoing professional development, including training programs that enhance their skills in chronic disease care and palliative care. Here, gaining knowledge about the broader implications of healthcare policy and the discrepancies in workforce availability is crucial for enhancing the delivery of care. As the geriatric population continues to grow, the role of geriatric nurses in providing enlightened and active care will become increasingly crucial in addressing the immediate needs and long-term requirements of elderly care (Figure 6.4).

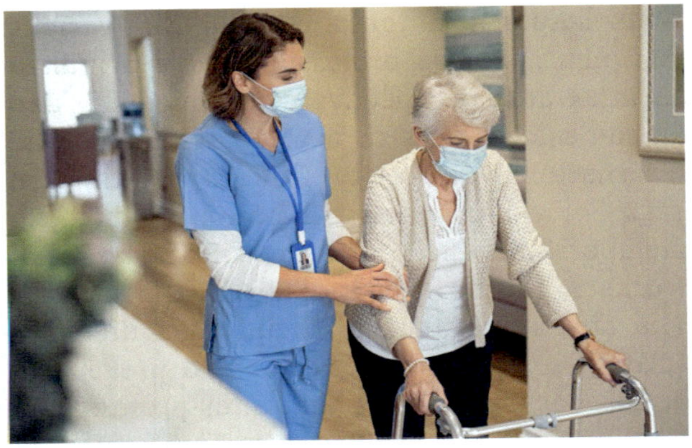

Figure 6.4. Responsibilities and duties of geriatric nurse.

https://nightingale.edu/_resources/images/blog/geriatric-nurse-2.jpg.

6.1.2. Skills Required for Geriatric Nursing

Geriatric nursing care of the older adult patient requires a unique set of skills that distinguish it from general nursing skills. Geriatric nurses must understand the physiological and psychological alterations that are specific to aging. This knowledge is needed to assess and manage complications of complicated health conditions prevalent in the elderly, such as chronic disease and cognitive impairment. Moreover, communication skills are also essential because elderly people are mostly suffering from cognitive mental decline or sensory impairments that blur their ability to communicate their health concerns. Through the development of empathetic and clear communication, geriatric nurses can build trust, enhance patient understanding, and promote adherence to treatment agreements, all of which are vital components of effective geriatric practice. In addition to basic nursing skills, geriatric nursing requires interdisciplinary working competence. The intricacies of caring for elderly patients necessitate an interdisciplinary approach with contributions from a variety of stakeholders in the healthcare community. Nurses are experts in this field as care coordinators, interacting among physicians, social workers, occupational therapists, and families to coordinate holistic treatment. This interdependence is also evident in the Health Care Task Force report, organized by the International Longevity Center, which emphasizes creating a lifespan framework for health preservation and disease avoidance among aging individuals.

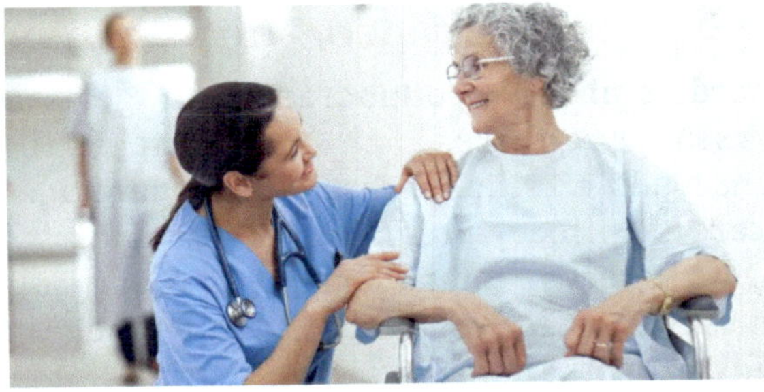

Figure 6.5. Skills to master in geriatric nursing.

https://external-content.duckduckgo.com/iu/?u=https%3A%2F%2Fwww.vivian.com%2Fcommunity%2Fwp-content%2Fuploads%2Fsites%2F3%2F2022%2F10%2FGeriatric-nursing-skills3-scaled-e1664900969302-1024x538.jpg&f=1&nofb=1&ipt=a7ddaa221e6c904e0e74c55e63c05aebdeedd2431102b0479ca56c2b0786dce3.

Through the assimilation of diverse professional opinions, geriatric nurses are well-positioned to advance policies that enhance care coordination and improve patient outcomes for aging patients (N/A, 2006). Finally, geriatric nurses must be skilled patient advocates, fighting for the rights and interests of older individuals within the health care system. Understanding the intricate policies surrounding elder care, as illustrated through the Stern Center's analysis of elderly health policies, enables nurses to navigate the often complex realm of healthcare resources. This advocacy involves lobbying on behalf of family caregivers, who provide care for older adults. Through education and resources provided to families, the geriatric nurse can alleviate some of the caregiving stresses and enhance the quality of life for both patients and their families. Later on, the skills entailed in geriatric nursing—ranging from clinical competence to collaboration to advocacy—are essential for delivering effective and empathetic care to the older adult patient population (Morton et al., 2015) (Figure 6.5).

6.1.3. Interdisciplinary Collaboration

Interdisciplinary collaboration in geriatric nursing requires an approach that transcends traditional disciplinary paradigms. Interdisciplinary teamwork becomes the key to effective management of older adult patients, as it fosters an overall approach that brings together insights from various fields, including medicine, social work, and spiritual care. This teamwork is especially essential when integrating comprehensive geriatric assessments (CGA), in which one not only has to assess the physical well-being but also investigate the patient's psychosocial needs and life stories. Ellingson goes on to emphasize the importance of incorporating spirituality and religious practices into the CGA model, highlighting the importance of addressing these elements to deliver more effective care to the special geriatric patients' needs (Ellingson et al., 2009). Incorporating spirituality and religion leads to more personalized care plans, resulting in improved patient outcomes and overall quality of life. Aware that the management of the elderly is complex, interdisciplinary teams have become an essential component in comprehending and managing the wide array of health conditions in older individuals. With the participation of experts from various disciplines, medical professionals can formulate an integrated perspective of the meaning and outcome of choices in health care today. The International Longevity Centers Health Care Task Force illustrates this notion through its membership, which includes economists, social workers, political scientists, and physicians. The task force aims to focus on a life-span strategy for promoting health and preventing disease, acknowledging that inter-professional relationships can lead to structural shifts in medical care and improve health outcomes and cost-effectiveness (N/A, 2006). With the synergy of the combined expertise of several specialists, geriatric nursing can significantly enhance the quality of care delivery. Furthermore, interprofessional collaboration fosters an environment where continuous learning and communication are encouraged, essential for bridging the gap in caring for an aging population. Such synergy enables caregivers to share information, experiences, and best practices, thereby refining patient care methods. Successful team communication ensures that all dimensions of a patient's well-being —physical, emotional, and spiritual — are considered in the planning of care. Routine interprofessional meetings and case discussions facilitate the convergence of knowledge from disparate specialties, leading to a more comprehensive approach to treatment. Finally, interdisciplinarity among geriatric nursing care can not only promote coordination of care but also community among clinicians, which can invigorate practice and enhance accountability for care.

Test Your Knowledge

1. What is the unifying function of geriatric nurses for the care of elderly adults in the medical-surgical setting?
2. Describe the multifaceted role of geriatric nurses in creating safe and effective care for elderly adults undergoing medical or surgical treatment.

6.2. Common Health Issues in Older Adults

Learning Outcome

1. Define the geriatric chronic conditions
2. Describe the mental health problem
3. Explain the mobility and functional impairments of elderly nursing

Understanding prevalent geriatric health issues among the elderly is crucial for effective geriatric nursing. Some of the most typical concerns include the prevalence of chronic diseases such as diabetes, hypertension, and cardiovascular disease. These conditions not only hamper the physical health of older individuals but also help to lower their mental health. Depression, for instance, typically goes undiagnosed and is estimated to affect about 40% of elderly patients with long-term conditions. This inability to be diagnosed can severely prevent them from being capable of understanding healthcare education, as well as recalling vital information regarding their treatment. Hence, it is essential for geriatric nurses to identify such health issues, as they must devise means that address not only physical ailments but also their psychological impact, to effectively care for patients (Wynn-Grundy et al., 2016). In addition to chronic diseases, cognitive impairment is also a widespread issue usually experienced by the elderly.

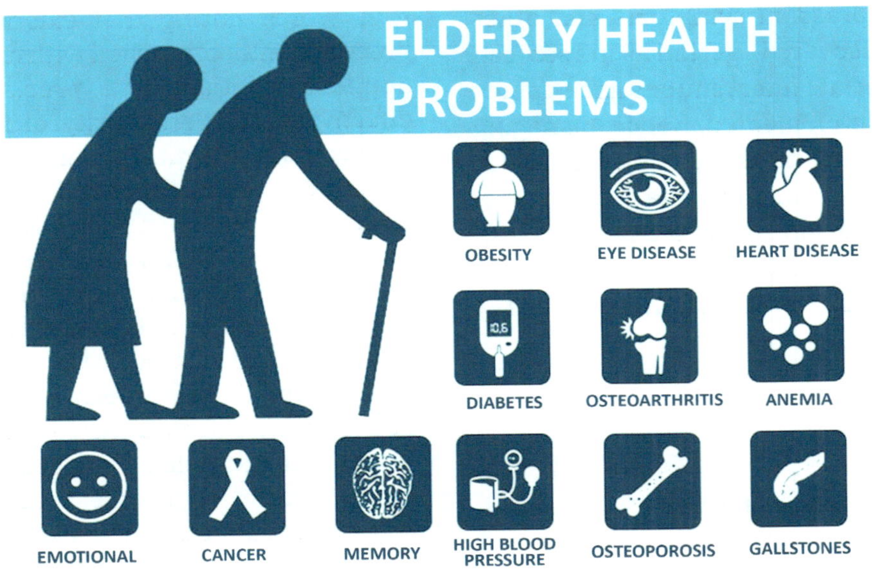
ELDERLY HEALTH PROBLEMS
OBESITY
EYE DISEASE
HEART DISEASE
DIABETES
OSTEOARTHRITIS
ANEMIA
EMOTIONAL
CANCER
MEMORY
HIGH BLOOD PRESSURE
OSTEOPOROSIS
GALLSTONES

Figure 6.6. Common health issues in older adults.

https://drjatintalele.com/assets/img/services/s11.jpg.

Alzheimer's disease and dementia are some of the disorders that pose unique challenges to patients as well as caregivers. The complexities of these cognitive disorders can render their management difficult, and treatment interventions may have to be multifaceted. Geriatric nurses must be empowered with strategies and equipment so that they can interact effectively with cognitively impaired individuals. Secondly, sensitization regarding the psychological and emotional impact of such conditions on both the patient and their relatives will assist nurses in providing holistic care. By encouraging supportive environments and developing individualized care plans, nurses are not only able to assist in lessening the occurrence of cognitive decline but also improve the quality of life in aging individuals with such complications (Vlachos et al., 2012). Finally, the overlap of physical and mental health complications in the elderly supports the importance of systematic geriatric evaluation. Nurses need to adopt an integrative practice that examines the physical well-being of a patient, cognitive ability, and mental health. A general assessment is vital, especially considering the reality that undiagnosed mental illness, like depression, has a significant influence on a patient's adherence to their care and education. If depression symptoms and other diseases are discovered, geriatric nurses can influence appropriate interventions and support measures to be implemented. Hence, managing the multifaceted health issues faced by older individuals not only enhances the health status of this group but also promotes autonomy and empowerment among this vulnerable population (Vlachos et al., 2012; Wynn-Grundy et al., 2016) (Figure 6.6).

6.2.1. Chronic Diseases and Conditions

Chronic disease and conditions are among the biggest challenges of gerontology nursing because old patients tend to have two or more overlapping conditions. Hypertension, diabetes, arthritis, and heart disease are prevalent in them, and these are what create complex care needs. Treating these chronic diseases necessitates an understanding of how the diseases interact and of the unique physiologic changes associated with aging. For gerontological nurses, this entails not only administering drugs and therapies but also carefully observing the patient's reaction to them. Effective management can make a significant difference in the quality of life by decreasing hospitalizations and promoting functional independence. An integrated approach that balances both medical intervention and psychosocial intervention is thus essential to address the needs of older adults with chronic illness (Moghadam et al., 2024). Among the innovations in the care of chronic diseases in older adults is the use of artificial intelligence (AI) in monitoring and delivering care. AI systems enable real-time monitoring of health status, which helps in the early detection of potential complications as well as the customization of treatment regimens. This is particularly important for diseases like heart disease and diabetes, where intervention at an early enough point can avert unfavorable outcomes. Despite the potential that AI poses, it is worth noting that existing research is predominantly concerned with machine learning applications that have precise and limited effectiveness. The majority of research, based on previous literature, targets a narrow set of chronic illnesses, thereby overlooking the wider uses and potential effects of advanced deep learning techniques. Therefore, there is a pressing need for a deeper investigation into a broader range of chronic diseases, so that the technology can be more effectively utilized in the care of the elderly (Moghadam et al., 2024). In the elderly, another determining cause of complicating chronic disease treatment is frailty. Frailty syndrome usually comes with many comorbidities, particularly cardiovascular diseases, diabetes, and other degenerative diseases. This predisposes towards an increased risk of postoperative and underlying condition deterioration during interventions like surgery. The implementation of tailored perioperative care protocols is crucial to managing such complexities and maintaining patient autonomy after treatment. Nurses play a critical role in instituting prevention of complications during the perioperative period, to maintain functional independence despite chronic diseases. With an increasing number of cases of frailty among the younger elderly, geriatric training for nurses is most needed to ensure efficient management measures are implemented (Figure 6.7).

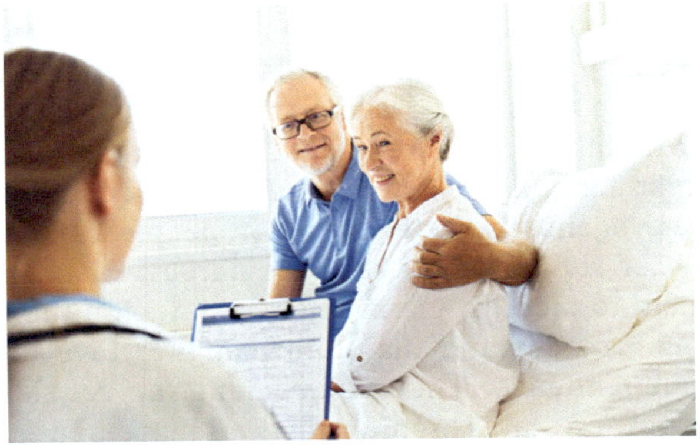

Figure 6.7. Successfully manage chronic diseases in the elderly.

https://hospitalnews.com/wp-content/uploads/2017/02/cover-final-696x464.jpg.

6.2.2. Mental Health Concerns

Mental health conditions in older adults are a key subject of geriatric nursing that significantly influences patient outcomes. With the aging population, mental health complications like depression, anxiety, and cognitive impairment are on the rise. About 40% of older adults with chronic illnesses are estimated to be undiagnosed for depression, which makes it more difficult for them to hold onto vital healthcare education and to participate actively in their treatment regimens (Wynn-Grundy et al., 2016). Depression can also manifest as a symptom, such as poor concentration, a classic symptom that can have a negative influence on an older adult's understanding of their disease and necessary changes in living. Successful care in the geriatric population, thus, depends on routine mental health checks because early detection of such issues leads to better care coordination and better outcomes among the frail elderly. Furthermore, the caregiving context also plays a significant role in the psychological well-being of older adults. The majority of the elderly are cared for by family members, who are likewise under a lot of stress and emotional pressure. The dynamics of power that exist in caregiving relationships have the potential to cause isolation and anxiety in the caregiver and the care receiver. The knowledge of older caregivers' lived experiences remains limited, with many remaining invisible in the field of health policy and research (Henwood et al., 2017). Invisibility has the potential to hinder the development of supportive interventions among the group. Gerontological nursing must consider these conditions by promoting caregivers' resources as well as the mental well-being of the older adults receiving care. By acknowledging and supporting the caregiver role, nurses can encourage more whole-person geriatric mental health practice. Lastly, mental health treatment in the elderly in nursing settings must focus most intensively on person-specific interventions.

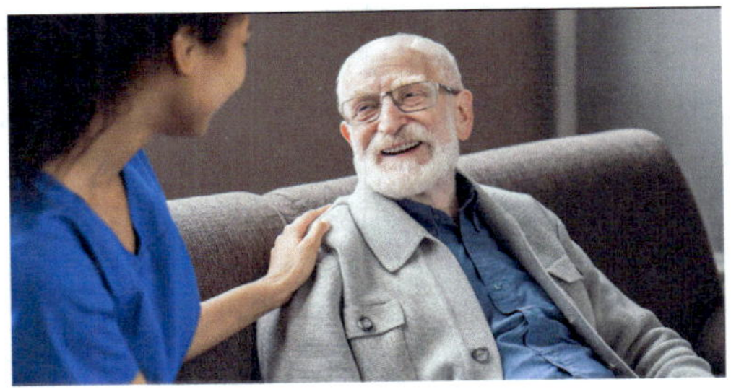

Figure 6.8. Geriatric mental health conditions.

https://keystone.health/images/resources/female-caregiver-chatting-with-elderly-man.jpg.

Not only must these assessments establish mental health status, but they must also analyze each patient's support systems, culture, and co-morbid medical illnesses. Emphasizing individualized plans of care that incorporate psychological support and follow-up can significantly enhance recovery and overall wellness. Further, geriatric nurses who have been educated about the topic of age-related mental health issues can support better communication and foster trust in the patients, leading to better interventions. With the aging population, the management of mental illness has to be part of geriatric nursing practice to deliver quality care to older persons with such needs (Figure 6.8).

6.2.3. Mobility and Functional Limitations

Mobility and functional limitations are priority concerns in geriatric nursing because they have a significant impact on the quality of life and independence of older persons. These are due to numerous physical, cognitive, and environmental factors, so the assessment is important and must be done by healthcare providers. Due to aging, declines in muscle strength, balance, and flexibility naturally occur, and the risk of falls also increases, leading to serious injuries such as fractures or head injuries. Other diseases, such as arthritis or neurological conditions, also contribute to mobility issues, and older people are not able to perform their daily tasks independently. Thus, nurses need to apply targeted interventions that not only address these constraints but also promote methods for maintaining mobility, i.e., physical treatment and customized exercise regimens. Effective management of functional and mobility constraints requires a multifaceted approach that is pharmacological and non-pharmacological in nature. Whereas drugs have the capacity to be utilized in pain and discomfort relief, Reid et al. (2006) emphasize that non-pharmacological treatment is equally essential and suggest that clinical practitioners consider the use of alternative interventions for a holistic approach to pain management. These alternatives may include cognitive behavior therapy, adaptive technique training, and complementary therapies that can complement overall patient health. In addition, the resolution of any psychological issues or misbeliefs related to mobility aids strengthens compliance with treatment plans. Through the inclusion of these heterogeneous methods, older people can be better supported by geriatric nurses, enabling them to mobilize more effectively within their environment and maintain a higher level of independence. The requirement for regular hydration status monitoring is also an essential aspect of dealing with mobility and functional impairment in older people. As highlighted by recent studies, dehydration is a key risk factor in this population, as it is highly associated with compromised physical function and higher morbidity and mortality rates. Ash et al. (2010) identify tongue dryness as one of the practical tools for screening dehydration, exemplifying the effectiveness of careful clinical observation in preventing related complications resulting from mobility issues. Comprehensive examinations, including hydration screenings and mobility assessments, can provide healthcare professionals with the capability to design appropriate interventions that promote the overall well-being of elderly individuals. With the facilitation of ongoing dialogue about mobility challenges and hydration needs, nurses can encourage older patients to take a more active role in managing their own health, improving their quality of life, and functionality.

Test Your Knowledge

1. What are two common chronic diseases commonly seen in older adult patients?
2. Why is the older adult at increased risk of developing complications with surgery or hospitalization?

6.3. Assessment Techniques in Geriatric Nursing

Learning Outcome

1. Explain the extensive geriatric assessment
2. Define the instruments and tools used for geriatric nursing
3. Explain the importance of involving the families of older adult patients

Geriatric nursing assessment techniques are essential in allowing holistic and effective care of older adult patients. They embrace a variety of methods, from extensive health assessments to cognitive evaluation. A thorough health assessment not only considers physical health but also looks at mental, emotional, and social well-being, recognizing that these elements interact with each other. With assessment instruments such as the Katz Index of Independence in Activities of Daily Living (ADLs), nurses can assess the functional status of the elderly. Also, the incorporation of social determinants of health screening can give a picture of determinants that play a role in affecting patient outcomes, and hence geriatric nurses need to conduct thorough evaluation strategies to have more specialized and effective care plans and interventions ultimately. Along with physical and functional assessments, mental health exams are another essential part of geriatric nursing. The presence of a high rate of cognitive impairments, such as dementia and depression, calls typically for special evaluation procedures. Mini-Mental State Examination (MMSE) and the Geriatric Depression Scale (GDS) are some of the standardized instruments that provide tools for quantifying cognitive decline and depressive symptoms. Early diagnosis and treatment of psychiatric illnesses are essential because they can significantly influence the overall well-being and quality of life in elderly populations. Gerontological nurses need to be competent in recognizing finely nuanced patterns of change in mood or behavior and require ongoing assessment as part of the holistic care of older patients and their specific healthcare needs. Lastly, recognition of the caregiver role is an essential aspect of geriatric nursing assessment. Caregivers can endure significant physical and emotional suffering in taking care of the elderly, so it is essential that their needs be assessed in addition to the patients' needs. As the results of various studies confirm, examining the caregiving situation and the specific issues that arise for both the caregiver and the elderly can help create more effective support interventions. Caregiver stress focus and caregiver evaluations integration can be utilized to inform policy and practice, where both parties receive the support and resources they deserve. The two-pronged strategy lends credence to the appeal for interventions targeted at individualized needs that acknowledge the interconnection between patient care and caregiver support, aligning with evidence-based policy guidance on enhancing geriatric nursing (Morton et al., 2015; Henwood et al., 2017).

6.3.1. Comprehensive Geriatric Assessment (CGA)

In gerontological care, the CGA is a primary tool for evaluating the overall needs of older adult patients. This multidimensional intervention not only examines physical health but also psychological status, social circumstances, and functional ability. By employing CGA, healthcare professionals can identify the individual challenges faced by elderly patients, such as comorbid diseases and frailty, which are of essential significance in developing personalized interventions. Existing evidence supports the importance of prevention and care coordination, suggesting that comprehensive assessment can significantly enhance the quality of care for older individuals by identifying gaps and considering the diversity of their health issues (Morton et al., 2015). To this end, CGA promotes a holism approach in which the entirety of the life of an older individual is considered when planning care. CGA implementation plays a crucial role in controlling the high rate of hospitalization and associated complications among the elderly. Older inpatients are predisposed to complications like delirium, which are significant contributors to morbidity and mortality (Chen et al., 2016). The condition needs to be identified and assessed immediately because it is usually overlooked in the event of emphasis on primary conditions. By incorporating tools such as the Confusion Assessment Method (CAM) into CGA protocols, clinical teams will be better equipped to detect and treat delirium and its associated cognitive impairment. Early treatment can minimize adverse consequences, enhance patient recovery, and facilitate a smoother return to their home environment. Ultimately, CGA helps in formulating a more integrated plan of care, prioritizing preventive interventions and support services that can minimize the risks of hospitalization among older patients. More importantly, the CGA process is also multilateral in nature, with an interdisciplinary team sent to offer coordinated care relevant to the needs of older patients. Physicians from various disciplines—such as nursing, social work, and rehabilitation—enjoy diverse expertise that complement the assessment process. This patient-centered approach is significant, as it helps alleviate social determinants of health and the pivotal role of family caregivers (Morton et al., 2015). By facilitating increased communication and joint decision-making, teams can develop a comprehensive care plan that respects the dignity and autonomy of elderly patients. Moreover, research presents an evident connection between the implementation of in-depth assessments and improved health outcomes, also reflecting the importance of incorporating CGA as a standard practice in managing older adults through geriatric nursing interventions (Chen et al., 2016). In doing so, the chances of improved health and well-being among the target population are significantly enhanced.

6.3.2. Tools and Instruments Used

In gerontology nursing, selecting and utilizing the instruments and tools are crucial in assessing the needs of the older adult patients. The Clinical Frailty Scale (CFS) is a significant instrument used to enable nurses to assess frailty levels among elderly patients. The scale is essential because it is an excellent predictor of mortality risk, assisting healthcare providers in making informed decisions regarding interventions and care strategies. For instance, as highlighted in studies, the CFS demonstrated excellent predictive validity in predicting short-term mortality, particularly when complemented with other clinical tools such as the modified CriSTAL framework. Through the effective application of tools such as the CFS, geriatric nurses can screen high-risk patients and tailor care plans to their individual needs, achieving optimal outcomes and improving their quality of life. Another useful resource in the geriatric setting is the use of screening tools for mental status and cognitive status, such as the MMSE and the GDS. These tools are used to detect symptoms of cognitive impairment and depression, which are very prevalent among aging patients. Early detection of these conditions is crucial in ensuring optimal physical and mental well-being in geriatric patients. Utilization of these screening devices allows healthcare providers to develop integral care plans, such as cognitive therapy, medication management, or referrals to specialist service providers. In combination with other actions, such as functional status evaluations and mental health screening data, the information presents a comprehensive view of the patient's overall health and well-being, addressing all considerations of aging in a proper manner. Self-neglect and its cause assessment also play a significant role in older adult care. Self-neglect is usually a challenging topic in family geriatric nursing, as it cuts across with complex problems of health-related issues like mental health and socioeconomic status. Such an assessment requires delicate steps to differentiate between inability and unwillingness to take care of oneself, which has significant implications for intervention. Professionals use standards and models to respond to such challenges effectively, typically by incorporating provisions for enhancing dignity and respect for the patient's autonomy. The subtleties of self-neglect necessitate a human intervention involving the patient and the support system. Understanding the underlying causes of self-neglect, as theorized by studies, can further guide professional interventions, leading to better protection and care systems for elderly at-risk populations (Braye et al., 2011; Silverman et al., 2011).

6.3.3. Importance of Family Involvement

Involvement of family in the care of elderly patients is crucial, particularly from the perspective of geriatric nursing. Families will act as advocates and caregivers, providing emotional support and assisting with the interpretation of communications between the patient and healthcare providers. Family involvement guarantees that medical professionals are aware of patients' special histories, values, and needs, and therefore enhances individualized care. A study suggests that when family members are involved in discussions about care and decision-making, patients are more satisfied with their care, resulting in improved health outcomes. By enhancing family involvement in treatment regimens, nurses can access the experience and knowledge of family members, thereby developing a more holistic geriatric care system. Secondly, provision of families with the geriatric care basics has the potential to influence the elderly significantly. By introducing family education programs into practice settings, families have the opportunity to understand the complexities of aging and the specific care needs of the elderly. Recent research supports that nurses can be trained with special courses to enhance their skills and knowledge in managing elderly patients, but this must also be extended to families. Family involvement through educational programs and resources enables them to become active participants in mobility and fall prevention interventions, as reported in studies on nursing students' reflections on nursing practice with older adults (Kim et al., 2025). Empowered knowledge enables families to develop and implement strategies that promote patient well-being and safety, thereby improving overall health dynamics. Families' emotional and psychological care is also critical in easing older patients' issues. The majority of the elderly patients are frustrated with loneliness and depression when they are transferred to new healthcare units or become independent. Family involvement can temper these issues by establishing relationships that render support to the patient's sense of security. Literature on the experience of nursing care shows that maintaining patients in contact with the family not only sustains patient morale but also enhances patient compliance with treatment regimens (Peterson et al., 2025). Therefore, actively working with family members within care is one aspect that contributes to building trust and resilience for older patients, enabling them to navigate healthcare more confidently and courageously. This multi-criteria intervention highlights the crucial role of family in geriatric nursing and warrants ongoing consideration and integration into care strategies.

Test Your Knowledge

1. What is one of the most common tools used to assess cognitive function in older adults?
2. Why is a functional assessment critical in geriatric nursing?

6.4. Pain Management in Older Adults

Learning Outcome

1. Identify the challenges in assessing pain
2. Describe the pharmacological approaches
3. Describe the non-pharmacological therapeutic approaches

Effective pain management among older adults requires a mature understanding of both pharmacological and non-pharmacological approaches, as the health condition of such individuals is highly complex. Pharmacologic care usually dominates clinical practice, primarily due to the universal expectation of many caregivers that pain relief is initially achieved by medication. Practicing individually with medications, however, leads to suboptimal treatment due to the risk of side effects and polypharmacy, particularly among the elderly. More recently, a review of the literature referred to that, while numerous studies focused on the pharmacological treatment, it is increasingly recognized that non-pharmacological interventions, such as cognitive behavioral therapy and complementary therapies, are effective in managing pain in this group (Reid et al., 2006). The shift is necessary in view of the need for an integrated pain management plan that amalgamates both sets of interventions to provide optimal care to older people. Assessment of pain in older people is difficult in specific ways, particularly where there are difficulties with communication or cognitive impairment. The subjective nature of pain makes self-reporting a cornerstone of good assessment. Still, it is possible for older adults not to be able to describe their pain clearly due to dementia, delirium, or other cognitive impairment. Research indicates that the application of specific measuring devices tailored for the evaluation of older adults will significantly improve the identification and assessment of pain extent (Clarke et al., 2006). The tools not only recognize the physical presentation of pain but also take into consideration psychological and emotional factors that could influence the comfort and general well-being of an older adult. Consequently, nursing assessments must be integrated and incorporate standardized pain scores, combined with observation techniques, to enhance the perception of pain among this population. Education and training of clinicians also play a vital role in improving pain management in older adults. A greater insight into the categories and pathways of pain can inform practitioners, enabling them to design more effective intervention strategies. Unfortunately, conventional education tends to focus on the pharmacological approach, with nursing personnel being insufficiently educated to find alternative means of pain relief. Regular professional education, comprising training in non-pharmacological alternatives, can help close this gap and enhance the overall outcomes of care. Secondly, encouraging the culture of empathy and patient-centered care among the geriatric nursing practice would enable the medical professionals to look for other pain management alternatives, thereby guaranteeing the older individuals receive an all-round and effective care which not only deals with physical pain but also the emotional and psychological well-being (Clarke et al., 2006; Reid et al., 2006).

6.4.1. Challenges in Assessing Pain

Assessment of pain in elderly patients is challenging on a multimodal level due to the complex process of aging and its effect on perception and communication. The majority of elderly patients experience deteriorating cognition that can hinder effective communication of pain. Additionally, physiological alterations in older patients can alter the expression of pain, making it less noticeable to medical staff. The older person will also display stoicism or deny pain to be regarded as not burdensome, again rendering it challenging to measure accurately. Caregivers thus need to apply various strategies, including observational measures and thoroughly tested pain scales specific to the older person, to document pain levels properly. The complexity is also complicated by the presence of comorbidities and polypharmacy in the majority of older adults, which masks pain or generates unusual pain responses, leading to under-treatment or inappropriate treatment of pain (Peterson et al., 2025). Another crucial issue in the measurement of pain among older persons is the variability of pain thresholds and tolerance levels, which such factors as cultural background, previous experience, and psychological factors like depression or anxiety may influence. Older persons may have different pain-related thresholds compared to younger age groups, which makes measurement more complicated. Secondly, the subjective experience of pain necessitates that medical professionals make their decisions based on patients' reports, which can be unreliable in this group. To overcome the barriers, it is essential for geriatric nurses to receive specialist training that equips them with the ability and expertise to assess pain more subtly and in a patient-centered manner. This includes understanding the general context of the health status of older adults and their responsiveness to non-verbal signs of discomfort or pain across different modalities, thus ensuring optimized, individualized pain management strategies (Fang, 2024). Ultimately, the healthcare environment itself poses barriers to practical pain assessment in geriatric patients. Acute care settings have a propensity to foster rapid patient throughput, which can inadvertently reduce the time allocated for detailed pain assessments. This stress can breed inadequate communication between older adults and caregivers regarding pain treatment choices, limiting older adults' potential for proper communication of pain. Institutional policy may also fail to support comprehensive pain evaluation, further exacerbating the issue. Institutionalizing a culture where pain evaluation is prioritized and followed by implementing standardized processes for treating older adults is the way to improve care outcomes. Enrollment in continuous education programs for nursing professionals targeting the geriatric population can promote a deeper understanding of pain complexity and overall quality of care for the elderly, ensuring they receive appropriate pain relief and management (Peterson et al., 2025).

6.4.2. Pharmacological Approaches

One of the most critical aspects of geriatric care is the deliberate selection and management of pharmacological approaches tailored to the unique needs of elderly patients. The older patient is usually characterized by polymorbidity, which demands extensive drug interaction knowledge and understanding of how different drugs influence general health. The most significant problem is heightened sensitivity of the elderly patient to pharmacotherapy, which enhances the risk of adverse drug reactions. Understanding the pharmacodynamics and pharmacokinetics of drugs in this group is essential for nurses to effectively monitor side effects and responses. The role of registered nurses as educators and patient advocates is then central to such a scenario, as they must navigate the complexity of polypharmacy and help patients understand their drug regimens. Active intervention optimizes safety and efficacy, ultimately maximizing patient outcomes. In geriatric health care centers, non-pharmacological interventions usually work as primary interventions to manage behavioral and psychological symptoms of dementia and other mental issues before the implementation of medication. Compliance with interventions such as environmental modifications, cognitive therapies, and the implementation of de-escalation steps will play a significant role in maintaining the well-being of patients without necessarily resorting to pharmacological solutions first. Recent reviews highlight the effectiveness of non-pharmacological strategies, particularly in dementia wards, where staff prioritize the early detection of agitation and the implementation of calming techniques (Kumar et al., 2024). Such an emphasis on non-pharmacological strategies promotes integrative patient care compliance, given that older adults are more likely to respond to individualized, non-invasive interventions. Thus, establishing a strong foundation in non-pharmacological methods can neutralize the use of drugs, therefore eliminating any danger of drug-induced complications. Despite a focus on non-pharmacological methods, there are instances where pharmacological interventions are needed for the management of extreme distress or behavioral disturbance among older individuals. Rapid tranquilization (RT) protocols are therefore utilized under such circumstances, primarily in therapeutic healthcare environments. However, doctors should ensure that they adhere to established procedures to ensure that drugs are used safely, with the patients' interests at heart. Proper training and education of junior doctors, as well as nurses, in RT procedures are said to play a central role in ensuring safety and effectiveness during interventions (Kumar et al., 2024). By balancing the use of RT with an equally strong background in non-pharmacological interventions, the geriatric nurse is a key player in the management of older adult patient care. A subtle balance of knowing when and under what circumstances to implement pharmacological measures can maximize patient outcomes, further stressing the value placed on custom-fit treatment methods in geriatric nursing.

6.4.3. Non-Pharmacological Interventions

In gerontological nursing, non-pharmacologic care is at the core of managing the unique medical challenges of older individuals. These interventions, varying from several different means including behavioral therapy, environmental adjustments, and psychological therapy, concentrate on enhancing general health while attempting to reduce medication usage. For instance, elderly patients with cognitive impairment such as delirium may be assisted to a great degree by structured environmental adjustments and individualized care plans. Nurses' ability to identify delirium with the help of tools like the CAM allows for individualized interventions towards cognitive stimulation and orientation.

Through establishing an environment that promotes mental sharpness and emotional stability, healthcare professionals not only relieve pain but also optimize the quality of life for the elderly, illustrating the critical role played by non-pharmacological interventions in geriatric nursing (Roca et al., 2015). Similarly, psychosocial interventions have been effective in controlling pain for older adults, particularly in those who have dementia. A meta-analysis of randomized controlled trials indicates that such interventions are effective in lowering pain levels to a high degree while concurrently lowering analgesic drug intake. Among non-pharmacologic interventions, sensory stimulation and individual-based counseling have been seen to be highly effective as the perception of pain in these patients is complex. In addition, such interventions provide the option to engage patients meaningfully, hence fostering autonomy and dignity. Although evidence exists for these interventions, careful consideration of the heterogeneity in study quality and results is necessary to encourage geriatric practitioners to integrate psychosocial interventions with caution and a focus on individualized treatment (Jones et al., 2019).

In summary, the use of non-pharmacological therapies within the practice of geriatric nursing helps not only to address acute health problems but also to enhance a holistic approach to patient care. These therapies cover a broad set of ways to improve the quality of care for elderly people and emphasize the need for nurses to be well-versed in these procedures. The integration of these strategies will lead to improved patient outcomes, including reduced hospital stays and better control of mental health conditions. As medical practices continue to evolve, the emphasis on non-pharmacological approaches will surely grow, solidifying their roles as primary components of caring for elderly patients. Ultimately, a solid comprehension and application of these interventions is capable of significantly improving the practice of nursing among the elderly by keeping care patient-centered and effective.

Test Your Knowledge

1. What is one limitation in pain assessment in elderly patients, especially those with cognitive impairment?
2. Describe the basic principles of effective pain management in elderly patients.

6.5. Nutrition and Hydration Needs

Learning Outcome

1. Explain the older adult's diet needs
2. Define the common nutritional deficiencies
3. Discuss the hydration promotion strategies

The nutritional and hydration requirements of elderly individuals are critical components of geriatric nursing care, necessitating tailored methods to meet the unique physiological, psychological, and social determinants influencing this patient population. With increasing age, metabolic alterations, decreased appetite, and the inability to absorb nutrients can predispose to dehydration and malnutrition. It is critically important that such patients be assessed from time to time by medical personnel, particularly because older patients often present with more than one comorbid condition, making their food intake complicated. With the multifaceted nature of nutrition, nurses ought to apply holistic care planning and interventions so they can evaluate and enhance the nutritional well-being of geriatric patients, targeting individualized care based on patient preference and diet restriction, because it treats their own respective ailments. Dehydration, a common yet often overlooked illness among the elderly, brings with it extreme health implications when it goes undetected and is not addressed effectively. The risk of dehydration also increases with age due to various reasons, including impaired perception of thirst, chronic illnesses, and medication side effects, all of which can compromise fluid balance. Appropriate screening for dehydration is essential; research has established that dryness of the tongue is an effective marker of hydration status in older individuals, with high clinical practice sensitivity and specificity (Ash et al., 2010). Geriatric nurses will need to implement systemic measures to keep patients hydrated by reminding them regularly to drink fluids, keeping fluids available at all times, and informing patients about the overall benefits of hydration to ensure optimal health and wellness. Malnutrition among the elderly has to be prevented as well, as poor nutrition will exacerbate existing conditions and slow down recovery from surgery or illness. Research has identified that nearly a third of the elderly are at risk of malnutrition, setting the stage for full-screening and intervention strategies (Beck et al., 2019). Gerontological nursing would entail increasing awareness of nutritional requirements and the necessity of a balanced diet with sufficient quantities of required vitamins and minerals. Practical measures can include nutritional advice, oral dietary supplements, and personalized meal plans to prevent or treat malnutrition and dehydration. By advocating a multidisciplinary policy, for example, nutritional adjustments and exercise, clinicians are best placed to improve the quality of life and clinical outcomes of older patients by addressing their nutritional and hydration needs in the best possible way.

6.5.1. Dietary Considerations for Older Adults

As one grows older, the nutritional needs of the individual change significantly due to changes in physiology and the prevalence of diseases among the geriatric population. The first thing to note is that an elderly person needs a diet rich in essential nutrients, including vitamins, minerals, and fiber, to combat age-related issues such as osteoporosis, cardiovascular disease, and diabetes. Research has shown that older adults typically require fewer calories but more nutrient-dense foods to meet their energy needs without gaining weight. Other preferences for soft foods may develop as a result of dental complications, which necessitate planning the diet to ensure a proper nutrient supply. Therefore, geriatric nursing would need to emphasize tailored dietary advice that incorporates foods rich in antioxidants, omega-3 fatty acids, and complex carbohydrates, while still satisfying the special tastes and preferences of older patients. Hydration is also a crucial aspect of diet management in the elderly, as aging tends to diminish the feeling of thirst and increase susceptibility to dehydration. Dehydration among this population can lead to severe complications, including confusion, urinary tract infection, and kidney dysfunction. Nurses thus need to educate patients on the importance of consuming fluids daily, telling them to drink water, herbal teas, and other high-nutrient beverages throughout the day. Additionally, incorporating foods with high water content, for instance, vegetables and fruits, can help achieve hydration goals. It is also essential for gerontological nursing to assess patients for any condition that can impact fluid balance, such as renal impairment or heart failure, adapting dietary guidance accordingly to enable optimal health results in the older adult (Lumbis et al., 2018). Diet plays a more active role in nutrition than just a passive one; it has a significant impact on the overall quality of life for older adults. Studies have shown that consuming well-balanced meals can improve mood, cognitive function, and energy levels, offering both psychological and physical health benefits. Social interaction during meals may also help mitigate feelings of loneliness prevalent among this group, suggesting the importance of social eating patterns. Geriatric nursing professionals should encourage those social aspects in addition to dietary needs, encouraging meal schemes that provide not only nutritional health but also interaction and support among older persons. By holistically regulating dietary concerns, nurses can influence not only the physical state but also the mental well-being of older patients, successfully overcoming the multifaceted nature of aging and creating a quality of life (Morton et al., 2015).

6.5.2. Common Nutritional Deficiencies

Older people have distinct nutritional needs with age due to physiological changes that affect metabolism and digestion. Older people typically have difficulty with widespread dietary deficiencies due to reduced appetite, altered taste, and chronic illness. Macros and micronutrients, such as protein, vitamin D, vitamin B12, calcium, and iron, are typically excluded in the dietary intake of older adults, which can exacerbate age-related complications. For instance, protein insufficiency can lead to muscle wasting, increased frailty, and decreased functional independence. Therefore, addressing these insufficiencies is crucial for achieving improvements in the health status of older persons and preventing comorbidities related to them, which necessitates a comprehensive approach to dietary care among the elderly. The gut and its associated changes due to age also affect the digestion of nutrients, thereby contributing to malnutrition among the elderly. With increasing age, alterations such as decreased motility of the gastrointestinal tract, modification in the secretion of gastric acid, and enzyme production may slow down normal digestion and the availability of nutrients. The elderly may thus become incapable of absorbing sufficient nutrients despite seemingly adequate intake. Mechanical food breakdown, which is compromised with increasing age, leads to inefficient digestion and absorption, thereby contributing to the risk of malnutrition. It is also essential to explore the connection between GIT function and malnutrition further to implement practical dietary advice specific to meet the special needs of older patients. This knowledge can open the door to interventions to deliver nutrient-dense foods, ultimately preventing the impact of rampant nutritional deficiencies and enhancing the health of older individuals (Bordoni et al., 2015). Furthermore, the relationship between dietary deficiencies and chronic illnesses, such as dementia and osteoporosis, is also a significant area of concern for gerontological nursing. Evidence has established that common deficiencies in nutrients such as vitamins D and K have been shown to coincide with cognitive decline and bone diseases, recording a potential concurrence between the two sets of aging. In fact, patients with dementia are frequently noted to be of poor nutritional status, contributing further to the risk of fracture from osteoporosis. The co-occurrence of these two conditions among elderly individuals necessitates a multidisciplinary approach that considers both the optimization of nutritional status and the prevention of functional decline. Understanding these associations and the biochemical pathways on which they are based can inform strategies for overall care and the prevention of the disease burden associated with aging (Burton et al., 2017).

6.5.3. Strategies for Encouraging Hydration

Effective hydration strategies within geriatric nursing are critical to continued health in the elderly population. One of the difficulties in ensuring adequate fluid intake is the multifactorial basis of factors that influence hydration in this group. Physical limitations, such as reduced mobility and the inability to swallow, can discourage older people from being able to consume enough fluids on their own. Cognitive impairment can also interfere with the sensation of thirst. To overcome these challenges, caregivers must actively assist hydration by implementing structured fluid intake schedules. The use of frequent reminders, offering fluids at meals, and utilizing visual cues, such as water bottles or hydration charts, are key in enhancing fluid consumption. By recognizing and addressing personal impediments to hydration, nurses are able to substantially reduce the prevalence of dehydration and enhance the quality of life for older patients, ultimately resulting in better general health and well-being management (Miller et al., 2017). One of the primary methods of enhancing hydration in older adults involves incorporating flavorful substitutes and personalized options into their diets. Geriatric patients avoid plain water due to unattractiveness or decreased cognitive status, dampening their sense of thirst. By offering a range of diversion in hydrating fluids—herbal teas to thin broths and juices—the nurses are able to cater to every patient's taste and prevent hydration from being uninteresting or unattractive to them, thereby making hydration easier for geriatric patients. In addition, incorporating high-water-content fruits and vegetables in food can provide a secondary method of ingesting liquids. Caregivers also educate patients about the medical benefits of adequate hydration, linking it to improved mood, mental status, and physical well-being, thereby promoting a more assertive approach to fluid intake (Agarwal et al., 2016). Also essential to addressing the systemic issues of dehydration are the use of hydration protocols within residential aged care settings. Research has shown that the overwhelming majority of older individuals who reside in these facilities are at risk for dehydration and malnutrition (Agarwal et al., 2016). A successful hydration protocol would then need to incorporate routine hydration status assessments, individualized interventions, and close monitoring by healthcare professionals. Multidisciplinary care teams can collaborate to ensure that hydration needs are recognized early and addressed effectively. Regular training of caregivers on the importance of hydration and how to promote fluid intake can build a culture of awareness of this essential aspect of patient care. By developing effective hydration strategies and demonstrating dedication from the care team, the risk of dehydration among vulnerable elderly populations can be minimized, leading to enhanced health outcomes and overall quality of life (Miller et al., 2017).

Test Your Knowledge

1. Why are older people more susceptible to dehydration?
2. List two ageing-associated factors that may impact nutritional consumption in older people.

6.6. End-of-Life Care and Palliative Approaches

Learning Outcome

1. Describe the palliative care
2. Describe patient and family communication
3. Outline ethical elements of end-of-life decisions

The provision of end-of-life care and palliative measures is a sobering aspect of geriatric care, with consideration of older adults with the end-of-life's multi-dimensional demands. As the older population continues to grow, healthcare systems must transform to address the increasingly complex care demands of patients. Among the most crucial aspects of such care is ensuring that it aligns with patients' values and preferences, thereby enhancing dignity and quality of life during their terminal stages. Research demonstrates that excellent end-of-life care reduces inappropriate hospitalizations and enhances overall patient satisfaction, thereby highlighting the imperative of incorporating palliative care into standard geriatric practice. In addition, cultural competency and communication training for healthcare workers further enhances the effectiveness of palliative interventions, such that they are individualized to address various patient populations' unique needs and circumstances (Morton et al., 2015). In end-of-life care, family involvement and caregiver support play a significant role in patient outcomes. Facilitating open communication between patients, families, and healthcare workers can significantly enhance decision-making and satisfaction with care. It is essential to recognize the personal dynamics of each caregiving situation, since family members emotionally and physically suffer in this stage. Importantly, research highlights the necessity for specialist support interventions among caregivers, particularly marginalized groups like BAME and LGBT communities, who may feel excluded from existing care systems (Henwood et al., 2017). Effective caregiver participation not only assists in providing enhanced care for the patient but also enhances the well-being of the caregiver, producing a more integrated palliative care strategy. Moreover, systematic review of research results has provided essential policy implications for end-of-life and palliative care service development. Evidence-informed policy aimed at prevention and care coordination has been successful but is prone to overlooking discrepancies in palliative care integration and self-management by patients (Morton et al., 2015). The adoption of traditional models of care overlooks the need for targeted interventions that are tailored to the individual experiences of the older person and their family. Policy makers and healthcare workers must be sensitive to the specific concerns caused by aging populations if they are to develop creative solutions for palliative care. Thus, constructing further research from the experiences of caregivers and effects of supportive interventions will ensure that policy and practice remain informed by the realities of the needs of older people at the end of life.

6.6.1. Understanding Palliative Care

Palliative care is a field of management that is pertinent to the care of elderly patients, particularly those with life-limiting disease. Palliative care is a specialized discipline that aims to alleviate symptoms and enhance the quality of life of patients through addressing physical, emotional, and spiritual concerns. For a geriatric nurse, studying palliative care principles is worthwhile, as they enhance overall practices in patient care. Geriatric nursing palliative care integration has the potential to enable older individuals to benefit from supportive care in challenging phases of illness. Not only does the practice emphasize symptom management, but it also encourages advanced care planning and empathetic communication with patients and families regarding care and treatment preferences. Lastly, palliative care is a model for improving the experience and satisfaction of older individuals with complicated health issues. Despite the perceived benefits of palliative care, adopting palliative care into practice does not always have to be a challenge-free process, especially in geriatric practice. The majority of healthcare providers might not be offered training or expertise to incorporate palliative care principles for effective service delivery and documentation. Within-organization barriers, such as a shortage of interdisciplinary teams or insufficient staff resources, might also hinder integration into practice. Geriatric nurses are best positioned to advocate for greater access to palliative careto provide patients and colleagues with information on the value of palliative care. A body of evidence indicates that the application of integrated health service platforms can facilitate improved outcomes in long-term care environments through potentially inappropriate medication management and improved disease control in older people, as outlined in institutional patient research (Choi et al., 2024). The facilities enable geriatric nurses to address critical palliative care areas, aiming to facilitate successful, multi-domain patient management. An essential component of palliative care education is the learning of its application in the context of end-of-life (EOL) care, particularly among older patients with terminal illnesses like aggressive non-Hodgkin lymphoma. There has been evidence suggesting an alarming trend where nearly all patients have become high utilizers of health care with scarce access to hospice and palliative care services at the end of their life (Markovitz et al., 2021). This emphasizes the role of health professionals, such as geriatric nurses, in facilitating smooth transitions between the curative and palliative phases of care. Prioritizing care conversation initiatives in the initial period of the disease course can significantly boost EOL outcomes among elderly individuals. Enhanced palliative care consultation can lead to enhanced symptom control and increased hospice use, which eventually changes patients' preferences in wanting to receive care in their preferred setting.

The patient-centered and empathic allegiance of geriatric nurses is of utmost importance, maintaining the comfort and dignity of elderly patients during their final days.

6.6.2. Communication with Patients and Families

Communication with patient and family is that area of gerontological nursing that determines the quality of care and patient satisfaction. While health professionals manage the complexities of aging, there is also a need to communicate effectively and compassionately. There are unique needs of elderly people that, in some instances, mean going beyond cognitive or sensory blocks that would be destructive to communication. By using active listening and clarifying questions, nurses can ensure patients feel heard and understood. Additionally, when family members are in consensus, they become part of an environment that supports decision-making, resulting in more individualized and effective care plans. Besides gaining confidence, it also makes the patient and family committed actors in their healthcare process. Family caregivers play a critical role in contributing to the well-being of the older adult, and their integration into processes of communication is vital. The research implies the impact on physical and mental well-being, noting the need for healthcare professionals to provide adequate support to such patients (Henwood et al., 2017). Carers tend to bear the most significant burden, ranging from personal daily care to complex health management activities, which can lead to stress and exhaustion. Open communication with families can thus facilitate easy exchange of crucial information to enable caregivers better to understand medical instructions, treatment plans, and resources. Education classes, support groups, and training resources specifically designed to cater to the needs of non-caregiving family members not only improve care quality but also those of the caregivers themselves and their caregiving effectiveness, ultimately benefiting the older adults in their care. Strategic communication in gerontology nursing also aligns with broader health policies that aim to engage families and caregivers in patient care (Morton et al., 2015). While the connection between healthcare professionals, patients, and their families is of the utmost importance, there are typically systemic impediments to effective communication. The barriers include time constraints, inadequate training in communication, and unfamiliarity with the unique needs of the geriatric population. Bypassing such barriers requires a commitment from healthcare organizations to develop a culture that respects empathetic communication. This involves training employees in the gold standard of communicating with older people and their family members, ensuring a comprehensive understanding of patient care. In closing this gap between clinical practice and policy guideline recommendations in gerontological nursing, the well-being and quality of older persons can be enhanced, with dignity and well-being as the ultimate concerns of care.

6.6.3. Ethical Considerations in End-of-Life Decisions

The ethical basis of end-of-life care in gerontological nursing requires a fine understanding of patient autonomy and informed consent. Older persons often have complex conditions that can compromise their quality of decision-making. Since nurses are health care providers, they must therefore act as advocates for the rights of patients of this type while ensuring that subsequent decisions adhere to their values and wishes. This is even more difficult when the family members do not have similar views about available options for treatment. Good communication skills are thus necessary to provide a platform on which patients' views can be effectively expressed. Also, the patients and their families need to be informed of probable outcomes and what the consequences of different decisions would be, and thereby empower them as active agents in dying. Self-neglect in the elderly is most often the delineating ethical dilemma in the making of end-of-life decisions. The meeting place between autonomy and vulnerability can make the debate tricky, particularly when the subject is opposed to the necessity for assistance or submission to regimes of necessary care. Practitioners are required to negotiate the delicate balance between defending the right of the individual to exercise their own choice and the ethical obligation to step in where health and well-being are at risk. Beneath all this lies the dilemma of how to distinguish incapacity and the overall desire for autonomy, where professionals are torn between their role for safeguarding their clients and upholding their choices in life. Self-neglect can be viewed as a complex interplay of factors, including pride in independence and earlier influences on identity, which further complicates the nursing response to the issues at stake (Braye et al., 2011). The broader caregiving environment is also reflective of the ethical considerations in care at the end of life. Dynamics within care relationships pose one of the most critical challenges in caring for older persons, especially those who are necessarily reliant on their families. The particular dynamics of each case of caregiving must be considered, as they usually shape the form of action by health workers. Older carers are particularly vulnerable to being left out of policy and research talks, when they play a central role in the chain of caring. This invisibility stresses the need for equitable evaluation of carer needs, as well as for recognition by policies of their roles. Through consideration of the extent of carer influences, such as their resilience, well-being, and coping, geriatric nursing can ensure that ethical concerns are always at the forefront of deliberations on end-of-life (Henwood et al., 2017).

Test Your Knowledge

1. What is the primary focus of palliative care in a medical-surgical setting?
2. Name two of the most common symptoms nurses address in end-of-life patients.

SUMMARY

Geriatric nursing care to the older patient must be a multi-trophic approach to meet the many challenges of aging. Effective practice should involve professional education for nurses, reaffirming the values of a broad understanding of geriatric fundamentals such as mobility, drug management, and comorbidities affecting each other. The evidence further shows that the specific training will enhance nursing care, but without working conditions in place to facilitate it, the payback on such educational investment is undermined. This is in line with evidence that shows, despite having the best attitude among workers towards the care of older adults, some constraints make it impossible to use the best evidence, and this calls for change at the system level to improve the quality of care (Peterson et al., 2025). Additionally, the use of enhanced recovery after surgery (ERAS) protocols is promising for maximizing postoperative care in older patients, especially those undergoing procedures such as total hip arthroplasty. The particular advantages of ERAS include lower levels of pain, shorter hospital stays, and enhanced patient satisfaction, which are crucial for the elderly who may have impaired recovery (Liu et al., 2025). The difference between ERAS and typical nursing interventions exemplifies the intervention of necessity which must be individualized and include both physiological and psychological elements. Given the nature of the recovery of this population, such interventions represent an evolution that must occur in geriatric nursing and have the potential to lead to improved health outcomes and cost savings in healthcare. In total, older adult patient management is an evolving and shifting specialty, characterized by continuous improvement and amendments in clinical practice. While specialized schooling and innovative care methods like ERAS drastically improve best-in-class patient outcomes, nursing practitioners must be the proponents of system changes to facilitate the successful implementation of such interventions. Finally, the enhanced quality of care for the aging can only be attained through the concerted efforts of healthcare practitioners, consistent evaluation of care practices, and relentless emphasis on patient-centered care. Through these relentless endeavors, geriatric nursing can advance toward enhanced management practices, ultimately sustaining the quality of life among the aging population.

Effective management of suffering among the aging is critical in geriatric nursing as an attempt to enhance the quality of their lives. One of the critical processes in this context is adherence to pre-set protocols of intervention. A case in point is a recent audit conducted at one psychiatric hospital, which demonstrated that nursing and medical staff on various wards made de-escalation non-medication an initial priority before conducting RT intervention. Staff members recognized the early warning signs of agitation and employed distraction and soothing strategies. Additionally, rigid protocols in geriatric care were found to have patient-centered outcomes. The outcomes stressed the importance of regular training, particularly among junior doctors, who exhibited reduced comfort with RT procedures, reflecting education deficits that could compromise high-quality care for this vulnerable population (Kumar et al., 2024). Involving patients' values and personal history in their decision-making is the other key aspect of geriatric nursing. A photovoice study brought the everyday lives of frail elderly people into focus, highlighting the significant impact their day-to-day problems can have on clinical practice. Qualitative methods enabled participants to take photographs of their surroundings and of what was troubling them, including home hazards and medication. The thematic results of this study, coping adaptations and functional space, emphasize that nursing professionals should take these findings into consideration when planning interventions in care. These interventions, based on individualized needs, not only maximize treatment outcomes but also enable older adults through participation in their own care (Hladek et al., 2024). Finally, geriatric care of older patients needs to be an inclusive process wherein clinical procedure is balanced against the patient's own reality. In light of current research, effective geriatric nursing should encompass two key aspects: one focused on meeting mandated standards of care and the other on recognizing and embracing the unique values of the older adult. Continued education of healthcare professionals in the practice of patient safety and distress management, and attention to the nuances of patients' lived experience, could lead to better outcomes in geriatric patient care. Therefore, incorporating these values will significantly improve the quality of life of older adults in such a way that care becomes not only practical but humane and tailored (Hladek et al., 2024; Kumar et al., 2024).

KEY TERMS FROM THIS CHAPTER

- Activities of Daily Living (ADLs)
- Aging Process
- Cognitive Assessment
- Dementia
- Elder Abuse
- Falls Prevention
- Geriatric Syndromes
- Instrumental ADLs (IADLs)
- Advance Directives
- Caregiver Support
- Delirium
- Depression in Older Adults
- End-of-Life Care
- Functional Assessment
- Incontinence Management
- Pain Management in Elderly

CRITICAL THINKING QUESTIONS

1. **What is a common physiological age change of the following?**
   a. Increased kidney function
   b. Increased bone density
   c. Reduced lung elasticity
   d. Increased skin elasticity
2. **What is the optimal nursing intervention to minimize falls in older adults?**
   a. Encourage independent ambulation always
   b. Keep lights dim to induce sleep
   c. Assess medication side effects and provide assistive devices
   d. Limit fluids to deter nocturia
3. **Which of the following conditions is most associated with confusion or delirium in hospitalized older persons?**
   a. Hypertension
   b. Urinary tract infection
   c. Osteoarthritis
   d. Cataracts
4. **What is the overall goal of geriatric nursing care?**
   a. Full physical recuperation
   b. Lengthy hospital stay
   c. Preservation of functional independence and quality of life
   d. Full prevention of all medications
5. **Screening which is essential in older persons for early identification of cognitive impairment?**
   a. Spirometry
   b. Mini-Mental State Examination (MMSE)
   c. Glucose tolerance test
   d. Colonoscopy

Short Answer Questions

1. What is polypharmacy, and why is it not desirable among older adults?
2. Mention two frequent age-related adaptations in the cardiovascular system.
3. Why must functional status be evaluated in older adults?
4. Identify a screening instrument utilized to screen for cognitive impairment in geriatric patients.
5. Why is it necessary to assess fall risk in geriatric patients?
6. Define the nurse's role in preserving independence and quality of life in older adults.
7. Explain how physiological changes with age influence drug management in geriatric patients.
8. Explain the etiology and nursing interventions for delirium in hospitalized older adults.
9. Describe a comprehensive nursing plan for fall prevention in long-term care.
10. Describe and contrast the expression of illness in younger and older adults using examples.

Answers to Critical Thinking Questions

1. (c); 2. (c); 3. (b); 4. (c); 5. (b)

REFERENCES

1. Agarwal, E., Marshall, S., Miller, M., & Isenring, E. (2016). Optimising nutrition in residential aged care: A narrative review. *Maturitas*, *92*, 70–78. https://doi.org/10.1016/j.maturitas.2016.06.013Ash, S., Harvey, K., & Vivanti, A. (2010). Developing a quick and practical screen to improve the identification of poor hydration in geriatric and rehabilitative care. https://core.ac.uk/download/10895888.pdf (accessed on 28th June 2025).
2. Beck, A. M., Bischoff, S. C., Cederholm, T., Cruz-Jentoft, A. J., et al. (2019). ESPEN guideline on clinical nutrition and hydration in geriatrics. https://core.ac.uk/download/159073557.pdf (accessed on 28th June 2025).
3. Bordoni, A., Dupont, D., Gille, D., Kachal, J., et al. (2015). Understanding the gastrointestinal tract of the elderly to develop dietary solutions that prevent malnutrition. https://core.ac.uk/download/286575279.pdf (accessed on 28th June 2025).
4. Braye, S., Orr, D., & Preston-Shoot, M. (2011). Self-neglect and adult safeguarding: Findings from research. https://core.ac.uk/download/2721774.pdf (accessed on 28th June 2025).
5. Burton, E. F., Downey, C. L., Graham, S. M., MacFarlane, T. V., et al. (2017). Dementia and osteoporosis in a geriatric population: Is there a common link? https://core.ac.uk/download/78902424.pdf (accessed on 28th June 2025).
6. Chen, C., & Saifullah, A. D. (2016). Early delirium assessment for hospitalized older people in Indonesia: A systematic review. https://media.neliti.com/media/publications/155995-EN-early-delirium-assessment-for-hospitaliz.pdf (accessed on 28th June 2025).
7. Choi, J. Y., Kim, H., Chun, S., Jung, Y., Yoo, S., Oh, I. H., Kim, G. S., et al. (2024). Information technology-supported integrated health service for older adults in long-term care settings. *BMC Medicine, 22*. https://www.semanticscholar.org/paper/859556cd0ff482499929e29f7bda9b3ac879b926 (accessed on 28th June 2025).
8. Clarke, A., Dunham, M., Faulkner, M., Howarth, M., et al. (2006). Assessment of pain in older people: Where are we now and what needs to be done? https://core.ac.uk/download/177014.pdf (accessed on 28th June 2025).
9. Ellingson, L. L. (2009). Spirituality within the comprehensive geriatric assessment process. https://core.ac.uk/download/215442322.pdf (accessed on 28th June 2025).
10. Estes, C. L., Yeo, G. W., Molina, L. C., Plumb, M., Hernandez, M., Goldberg, S., Wallace, S. P., et al. (2007). Women, health and aging: Building a statewide movement. https://core.ac.uk/download/71355916.pdf (accessed on 28th June 2025).
11. Fang, Y. Y. (2024). The unique challenges of treating and caring for older adult patients with cancer. *Hu Li Za Zhi: The Journal of Nursing, 71*(6), 4–7. https://www.semanticscholar.org/paper/107e1cf874c12c735401708b8e986947dd4a8d7d (accessed on 28th June 2025).
12. Henwood, M., Larkin, M., & Milne, A. (2017). Seeing the wood for the trees: Carer related research and knowledge: A scoping review. https://core.ac.uk/download/145186527.pdf (accessed on 28th June 2025).
13. Hladek, M., Wilson, D. H., Krasnansky, K., McDaniel, K., Shanbhag, M., McAdams-DeMarco, M. A., Crews, D., et al. (2024). Using photovoice to explore the lived environment and experience of older adults with frailty on their kidney transplant journey. *Kidney360, 5*, 589–598. https://

www.semanticscholar.org/paper/f46cc8e445756b8ecb7dbaad88ce6d4f52ffdd94 (accessed on 28th June 2025).

14. Jones, C., Moyle, W., Pu, L., Todorovic, M., et al. (2019). Psychosocial interventions for pain management in older adults with dementia: A systematic review of randomized controlled trials. https://core.ac.uk/download/196606964.pdf (accessed on 28th June 2025).
15. Kim, G. Y., Son, Y. J., Choi, G. E., & Ahn, J. W. (2025). A qualitative content analysis of nursing students guided reflective journal writing following simulation-based practice for the initial management of falls in older adults. *Korean Journal of Adult Nursing*. https://www.semanticscholar.org/paper/955e3ce2e2c2bbe32d7adfca5e73d9c42ea0572d (accessed on 28th June 2025).
16. Kumar, P., Wild, A., Howells, F., Kumar, T., & Williams, P. (2024). Audit of non-pharmacological and rapid tranquilization practices in managing distress among older adults: A comparative study in Inverness hospitals. *BJPsych Open, 10*, S244–S245. https://www.semanticscholar.org/paper/c54b4c8be8fa32806006fa6a310b176a5fdc47dc (accessed on 28th June 2025).
17. Leach, S. J., Larkin, M., Gras, L. Z., Quiben, M. U., Miller, K. L., Lusardi, M., & Hartley, G. W. (2025). A movement framework for older adults: Application of the Geriatric 5Ms. *Journal of Geriatric Physical Therapy*. https://www.semanticscholar.org/paper/44d43b1b9b6214f6ba8b399fe321e110189a4c79 (accessed on 28th June 2025).
18. Liu, G., Li, L., Deng, J., Cai, L., & He, R. (2025). Enhanced recovery after surgery: Nursing strategy for total hip arthroplasty in older adult patients. *BMC Geriatrics, 25*. https://www.semanticscholar.org/paper/7c5c8c065908e53c225fbcc2842c7c9eaf65fb9e (accessed on 28th June 2025).
19. Lumbis, R. H. (2018). Nourishing dogs and cats through their twilight years. https://core.ac.uk/download/154422917.pdf (accessed on 28th June 2025).
20. Markovitz, N. H., Yi, A., Odejide, O. O., Newcomb, R., Amonoo, H., Nelson, A., Reynolds, M. J., et al. (2021). End-of-life care for older adults with aggressive non-Hodgkin lymphoma. *Blood*. https://www.semanticscholar.org/paper/6e1e9b4eb5ea93d42994fa7d8b28b2ee4b608598 (accessed on 28th June 2025).
21. Miller, C. G. (2017). Dehydration in nursing home residents: A meta-analysis of causes of dehydration, implications, and those most at risk. https://core.ac.uk/download/84674618.pdf (accessed on 28th June 2025).
22. Moghadam, M. P. P., Moghadam, Z. A., Qazani, M. C., Pławiak, P., & Alizadehsani, R. (2024). Impact of artificial intelligence in nursing for geriatric clinical care for chronic diseases: A systematic literature review. *IEEE Access, 12*, 122557–122587. https://www.semanticscholar.org/paper/bee52b8493fbca049f2de3fd099664c1316dedf9 (accessed on 28th June 2025).
23. Morton, S., & Dunn, W. (2015). Addressing the health needs of an aging America: New opportunities for evidence-based policy solutions. https://core.ac.uk/download/75783019.pdf (accessed on 28th June 2025).
24. Peterson, J., Faig, K., Yetman, L., Robertson, C., Flanagan, K., Prosser, J., & Feltmate, P. (2025). 2747 The impact of specialized geriatric 5 M education on mobilization of older adult patients in acute care in five Canadian hospitals. *Age and Ageing*. https://www.semanticscholar.org/paper/9eb02c6b4ef3b93de5b1908877c91b9856723fbc (accessed on 28th June 2025).

25. Reid, D. M., & Schofield, P. (2006). The assessment and management of pain in older people: A systematic review of the literature. https://core.ac.uk/download/177013.pdf (accessed on 28th June 2025).

26. Roca, M. C. (2015). A quantitative study of the effectiveness of the nurse-led delirium protocol on hospitalized older adults utilizing the Confusion Assessment Method (CAM). https://core.ac.uk/download/72840112.pdf (accessed on 28th June 2025).

27. Rocard, E., Sillitti, P., & Llena-Nozal, A. (2021). COVID-19 in long-term care. *OECD Health Working Papers*. https://doi.org/10.1787/b966f837-en (accessed on 28th June 2025).

28. Silverman, M. E., Schofield, D. J., Boyd, K., Cardona-Morrell, M., Samaras, N., Yourman, L. C., et al. (2011). Predictive validity of the CriSTAL tool for short-term mortality in older people presenting at emergency departments: A prospective study. https://core.ac.uk/download/196606831.pdf (accessed on 28th June 2025).

29. Tkacheva, O., Sharashkina, N. V., Balaeva, M. M., Eruslanova, K., Runikhina, N., & Kotovskaya, Y. (2024). Nursing protocol: Management of older and oldest-old patients living with frailty syndrome in the perioperative period. *Russian Journal of Geriatric Medicine*. https://www.semanticscholar.org/paper/cb9d315a32211b6d833f25a4968274a8e6065786 (accessed on 28th June 2025).

30. Vlachos, S. L. (2012). Nursing satisfaction in caring for elders. https://core.ac.uk/download/72047932.pdf (accessed on 28th June 2025).

31. Wynn-Grundy, N. J. (2016). Undiagnosed depression in the elderly and healthcare education. https://core.ac.uk/download/70426926.pdf (accessed on 28th June 2025).

DISABILITY, CHRONIC ILLNESS, AND LONG-TERM CARE

7

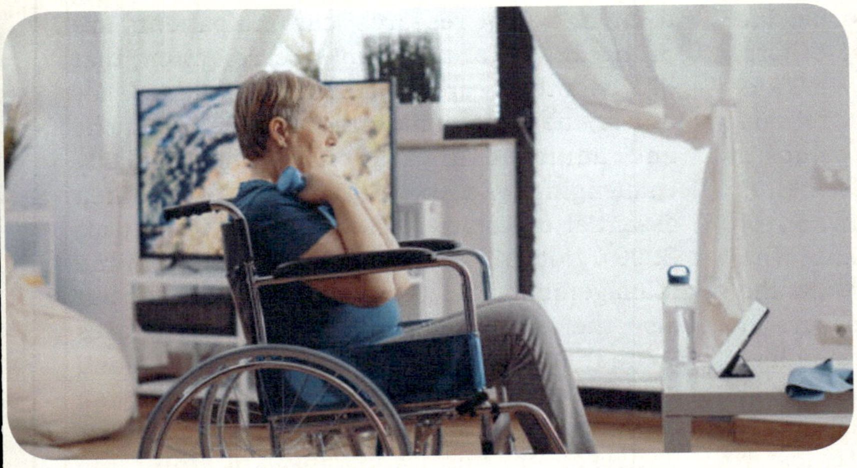

LEARNING OBJECTIVES

After studying this chapter, you will be able to:

1. Understand types of disabilities
2. Describe the chronic illness
3. Discuss the requirement of long-term care
4. Identify challenges in long-term care
5. Learn about policy and law for disability
6. Assess the innovations in long-term care

Introduction

Disability and chronic illness are more relevant than ever before as nations contend with the challenges of population aging and rising healthcare needs. These afflictions often lead to long-term care demands, which can have a significant impact on an individual's quality of life, social functioning, and mental status. Chronic illness tends to limit daily living, reducing independence and increasing reliance on family and care agencies. The social consequences of such reliance can lead to reduced self-esteem and loss in the functioning of valued social roles. It is relevant at this point to understand where disability intersects with chronic disease and long-term care, enabling informed policy and support services. Moreover, current studies suggest that the perception of disability varies significantly across different social structures and cultural contexts. For example, one study conducted in Poland demonstrates the relationship between health condition and social change, elaborating on the fact that functional disability can be a formidable public health policy challenge. As populations are altered and ways of life change, curing the effects of disability and chronic disease becomes paramount in the creation of care policies that are sufficient to cater to varied needs. By integrating empirical data and qualitative results into policy planning, societies are better equipped to deal with the complexities involved with the conditions and enhance the overall well-being of victims. Arts and crafts have been an optimistic area of activity for individuals with chronic illness, as identified in qualitative studies exploring the application of personal accounts. For others, adopting hobbies, such as needlework, is therapeutic and enables them to manage pain and build confidence. It not only provides a means of expressing feelings but also facilitates social interaction and the demonstration of control in illness. The accounts of women who undertook such endeavors later in life reveal the multifaceted benefits of creative endeavors in the context of illness. Overall, an understanding of the importance of psychological and social factors in the management of individuals with disability and chronic illnesses is crucial to foster resilience and optimize long-term outcomes for care.

Definition of Disability and Chronic Illness

The concept of disability defines a broad group of conditions that impair people's physical, mental, or sensory functioning and, in the process, limit their ability to carry out daily activities. The World Health Organization (WHO) categorizes disability in terms of the interaction between the individual and the environment, specifically the manner in which society's attitudes and barriers affect one's experience of disability. Understanding disability is crucial, as it informs policy and practice related to accessibility and inclusion. Chronic illness, typically a condition lasting more than three months, can overlap extremely closely with disabilities, affecting an individual's quality of life and ability to engage with society. The complexity of such definitions reveals not merely the medical but also the social forces behind the marginalization of the afflicted, and it necessitates a holistic approach to care and support. In research into chronic illness, it is observed that such illness can have an immense impact on one's physical, emotional, and psychological health. Chronic illnesses, such as diabetes, arthritis, and heart disease, need to be constantly managed and can lead to significant restrictions if not treated. According to more recent research, chronic patients are in the middle of a disjointed care system that prevents their care from being maintained. For others, the transition process between pediatric and adult healthcare can be particularly challenging, with periods of instability when essential elements of care are lost (Adi et al., 2009). Not only is medical intervention in the management of chronic disease needed, but also the renegotiation of support structures so that individuals can exercise agency and control over their health. The intersection of chronic disease and disability, therefore, underscores the importance of equitable policies and interventions that can enhance job opportunities for vulnerable populations. Empirical data from various nations indicate that socio-economic factors significantly influence opportunities for individuals with disabilities and chronic diseases (Burstrom et al., 2009). Programs that provide specialized assistance can considerably reduce the obstacles faced by these individuals in the labor market, facilitating integration and empowerment. Recognizing the unique challenges posed by these conditions, policymakers can develop solutions that are evidence-informed and tailored to the specific needs of distinct populations. This blended knowledge is essential in the formulation of environments that not only accommodate disabilities and chronic illness but also effectively promote the well-being and livelihoods of those affected (Figure 7.1).

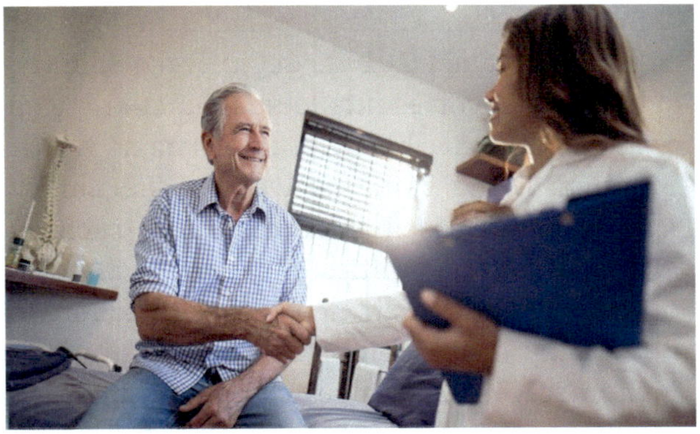

Figure 7.1. Disability and chronic illness.

Source: https://www.cdc.gov/nccdphp/media/images/2024/04/HE-landing-page.png.

Requirement for Understanding Long-Term Care

It is essential to fully appreciate long-term care, especially in light of the increasing prevalence of disability and chronic conditions among elderly populations. Long-term care is a broad category of services designed to meet the needs of individuals who require assistance with activities of daily living for an extended period.

This matters to healthcare professionals and policymakers as they develop optimal care solutions that address the unique issues faced by such individuals. With the ageing population and increasing instances of chronic conditions, long-term care will become increasingly sought after.

It warrants prudent strategies in resource allocation and provision of services. The awareness can translate into higher-quality care, improvement, and ensure equitable access, ultimately enriching the welfare of recipients in their everyday lives.

Moreover, the effects of bad long-term care are not at the individual level but extend to families and broader social institutions. Families often end up taking on caregiving duties, which impose significant emotional and financial costs, particularly as they must navigate complex healthcare systems. An understanding of long-term care enables stakeholders to identify these issues and collaborate towards solutions that ease the burdens on families, providing a supportive environment for both the caregivers and the care recipients.

Furthermore, long-term care facilities need to be designed to meet the various needs resulting from chronic illness and disabilities to ensure not only physical health but also mental and emotional health. Identifying these intricate challenges is half the battle in developing a more coordinated system for long-term care.

Research and evidence-based interventions in long-term care are last but not least important for the purpose of devising efficient interventions that act according to the needs of individuals with chronic illness and disabilities. Research has established the fact that inpatients who are discharged from the hospital to long-term care facilities are likely to develop significant complications without proper follow-up and care coordination.

A thorough understanding of this process is crucial in reducing readmission rates and improving health outcomes. As reflected in recent research, ongoing monitoring and care significantly influence recovery trajectories of patients, as revealed among the individuals with post-acute symptoms following COVID-19 hospitalization (Chopra et al., 2020). By focusing on new models of care and potential interventions, the healthcare sector can develop a caring and responsive long-term care system that actively engages individuals in their own recovery process and is integrated with broader public health goals (Maslach et al., 2016) (Figure 7.2).

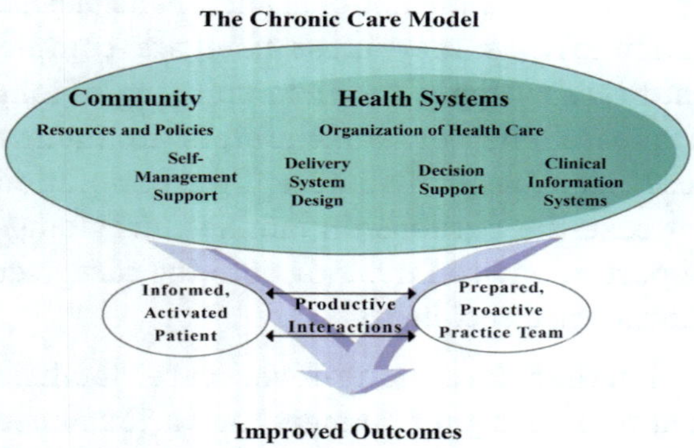

Figure 7.2. Model of chronic care.

Source: https://www.act-center.org/application/files/thumbnails/small/1816/3590/1601/Model_Chronic_Care_Featured.jpg.

7.1. Types of Disabilities

Learning Outcome

1. Describe the physical disabilities
2. Focus on intellectual and developmental disabilities
3. Learn about sensory disabilities

Disabilities can be broadly categorized into various types based on their challenges and the requirements of respective care and support models. Physical disabilities come under those conditions that hinder mobility and physical functioning, such as spinal cord injury, amputations, and diseases like multiple sclerosis.

Individuals with physical disabilities suffer from limitations in accessing public spaces and services, which prolong their physical disability. Supervision of this population includes personalized rehabilitation interventions as well as social programs for improved access in environments. These are critical in building an inclusive society for individuals with physical disability so that they get equal opportunities in occupational and personal development (Chopra et al., 2020). Cognitive disability, however, involves intellectual functioning as well as adaptive behavior impairment, which affects living skills as well as the ability to learn. These include disorders such as intellectual disabilities, Alzheimer's disease, and traumatic brain injury. These disabilities not only pose challenges to the individual themselves but also create significant emotional and financial impacts on families and caregivers. Cognition disability support strategies could involve special education plans and therapy treatment directed at enhancing cognitive function and quality of life.

Furthermore, with an increasing elderly population, the rate of cognitive disabilities is also going to rise, in turn emphasizing the need for combined long-term care interventions to address these complex needs (DePhillipo et al., 2020). Finally, sensory disabilities, i.e., visual and hearing disabilities, represent another vital category. Individuals with sensory disabilities often encounter unique communication and interpersonal challenges within their environment. For instance, blind or visually impaired individuals may require orientation training and assistive devices, whereas deaf or hard-of-hearing individuals may receive sign language services and auditory training. The policy in assisting individuals with sensory disabilities is not merely a matter of providing assistive devices, but also involves raising societal awareness and making communication environments more accessible. As the population grows, it is increasingly necessary to learn about these disabilities to facilitate equal access to education, employment, and social integration for all (Chopra et al., 2020) (Figure 7.3).

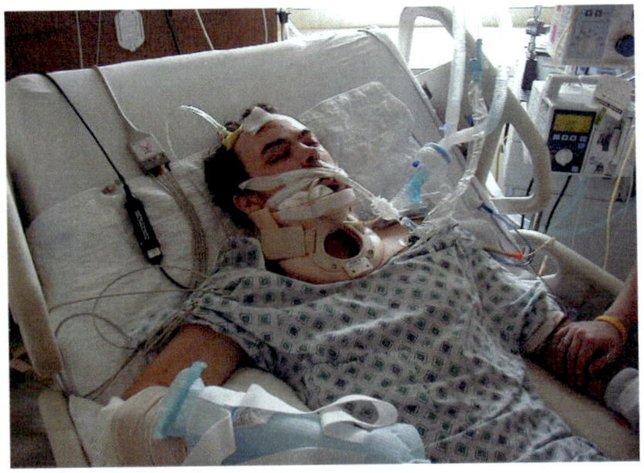

Figure 7.3. Traumatic brain injury (TBI).

Source: https://intensivecarehotline.com/wp-content/uploads/2013/01/bill-ICU-1.jpg.

7.1.1. Physical Disabilities

Physical disability prevalence significantly impacts people's quality of life, typically entailing many chronic conditions that complicate the concerned person's life. Physical disabilities encompass a wide range of impairments, including mobility impairments, sensory impairments, and neurological disorders, each with varying difficulties in conducting daily living activities and accessing general healthcare. The individuals with these disabilities can depend on long-term care services, institutional and community, to facilitate their daily living and integration into society. The support required can stem from the necessity for specialist medical care, rehabilitation services, or simply assistance with activities of daily living, highlighting the complex interplay between chronic diseases and the spectrum of care needed to meet these individuals' needs (Chopra et al., 2020). The intersection of physical disabilities and mental health cannot be ignored, as the latter can be significantly impacted by the former. Physically disabled individuals experience higher rates of depression and anxiety, coupled with their isolation from social, educational, and working life. The long-term implications of this psychological burden demand an active approach to care, with the incorporation of mental health intervention into planning. Furthermore, unequal access to appropriate mental health care for physically disabled individuals can pose the threat of undermining recovery and promoting feelings of alienation. Addressing these issues of mental health is critical, as it will underpin overall welfare in individuals experiencing physical and psychological challenges (Iorfino et al., 2019). Lastly, encouraging better models of care that integrate services for individuals with physical disabilities more comprehensively is of utmost significance. These models should not only respond to short-term health needs but also prioritize independence and quality of life through personalized long-term care planning. Telehealth and community-based innovation can facilitate this integration, providing timely interventions that address both physical and mental health needs. Furthermore, policymakers, healthcare providers, and community organizations must collaborate to establish settings that facilitate accessibility and inclusivity, ensuring that individuals with physical disabilities receive comprehensive care that recognizes and addresses their complex needs (Chopra et al., 2020) (Figure 7.4).

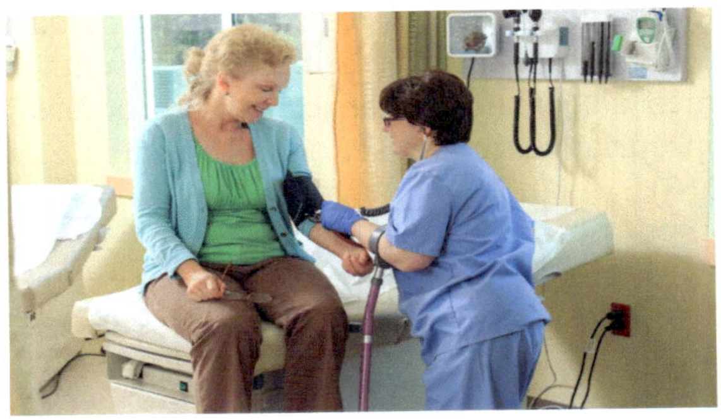

Figure 7.4. Physical disabilities.

Source: https://res.cloudinary.com/highereducation/images/f_auto,q_auto/v1668453213/NurseJournal.org/GettyImages-594831695-1_548367da0e/GettyImages-594831695-1_548367da0e.jpg?_i=AA.

7.1.2. Intellectual and Developmental Disabilities (IDD)

Long-term condition care in individuals with IDD is also a subject of concern equally, particularly from the primary health care point of view. Studies show that the working-age adults with IDD bear more burden for most of the chronic conditions compared to the general population. Still, fewer preventive interventions and screening, thus further enhancing their vulnerability (Allan et al., 2018). Systemic barriers, however, hinder effective delivery of care even in the presence of such established disparities. Notably, the application of routine health screenings has been identified as a probable facilitator of improved health outcomes through early disease detection and control. However, the literature indicates that further efforts are needed to evaluate the long-term impacts of such interventions, suggesting that ongoing research is necessary to establish whether they are effective in supporting healthcare access among the target group. The institutional historical tradition is an expression of a broader cultural disrespect for individuals with IDD. It has solidified their marginalization in health care discourse. Social class prejudice and eugenics have historically contributed to the disabling narrative of mass imprisonment, which also made it harder to gain access to appropriate care and service (Appleman et al., 2018).

This background has created an environment where people with IDD are repeatedly confronted with paternalistic attitudes from medical professionals, which makes self-care challenging for them. Thus, the rehabilitation and integration of people with IDD into community life requires a paradigm shift that encourages autonomy while ensuring overall support. Addressing this policy and practice deficiency in IDD history is essential to equitable health outcomes and furthering an expansive understanding of disability. In addressing the specific needs of individuals with IDD, multi-disciplinary coordination of healthcare provision is critical. This entails tailoring services that not only meet physical and mental health needs but also advocate for the social and emotional well-being of such individuals. An integrated care model involves collaboration among healthcare workers, caregivers, and individuals themselves, with dignity, recognizing their autonomy while enabling self-management. Education for healthcare workers on the unique issues of people with IDD can also break down stereotypes and improve communication and rapport during health interactions (Allan et al., 2018). As awareness keeps rising, the healthcare system must also react by creating accessible paths that allow for effective intervention plans, eliminating barriers, and ultimately improving the health environment for adults with intellectual and developmental disability (Figure 7.5).

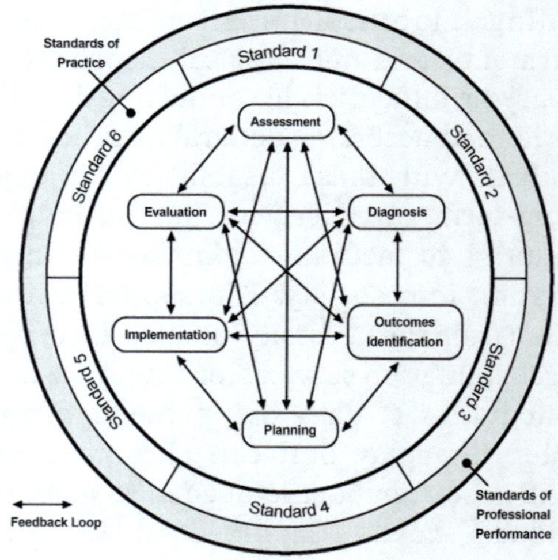

Figure 7.5. Intellectual and developmental disabilities (IDD) of nursing.

Source: https://nursekey.com/wp-content/uploads/2016/07/Scope_of_Intellectual_and_Developmental_Disabilities_IDD_Nursing_Practice-FF1.gif.

7.1.3. Sensory Disabilities

Sensory disabilities encompass a wide range of disorders that interfere with people's ability to process sensory information and significantly impede their lifestyle and relationship with the world. Typically categorized as visual, hearing, and tactile disabilities, sensory disabilities have the potential to impact communication, mobility, and overall participation in social and work environments. With the majority of individuals with sensory disabilities using adaptive technologies and support aids to navigate their surroundings, access to assistive devices and accessible environments in public spaces are vital parameters that favor independence and quality of life among them. Understanding different forms of sensory disability is essential in formulating effective long-term care plans that consider the unique needs of this group, thereby facilitating their integration and active involvement in society. Individuals with sensory disability have specific difficulties that add strength to barriers associated with chronic illness and age in long-term care. Effective long-term care services should not only attend to the health needs of these individuals but also address their sensory impairments in order to enhance safety and comfort. For instance, visually impaired individuals would require that their surroundings use touch markers and auditory signals for safety and navigation. Caregivers also need to be trained on how to communicate effectively with people who are hearing-impaired, thereby eliminating communication gaps that can arise. Based on studies in caregiving, anxieties regarding the safety of sensory disability care recipients are the basis of organizing formal long-term care services, which supports the nature of mainstreaming specialist care in such institutions (Liu, 2024). Through the clear need for adaptive long-term care systems, individuals with sensory disabilities lack access to relevant dental and medical treatment. Research has shown that the prevalence of dental care among long-term care recipients is significantly lower than that of matched groups not affected by these disabilities (Ko et al., 2024). This shortfall exacerbates the existing conditions, as oral health is integral to overall health and well-being. The lack of adequate dental care is symptomatic of a broader pattern of social neglect suffered by residents of long-term care homes, particularly by residents who may already be challenged in some way by their sensory impairment. Closing these gaps requires collaborative efforts to implement patient-centered care approaches that cater to the distinct sensory needs of individuals, thereby improving their access to necessary health services and enhancing the quality of their lives.

Test Your Knowledge

1. Why is it important for nurses to identify some categories of disabilities when planning care?
2. List two wide categories of disabilities and provide an example of each.

7.2. Understanding Chronic Illness

Learning Outcome

1. Describe the examples of chronic illnesses
2. Explain the impact of chronic illness on daily life
3. Discuss the connection between chronic illness and disability

An understanding of chronic illness involves examining the medical and psychosocial aspects that influence people diagnosed with long-term health issues. Chronic illnesses, with duration extended over time and frequently progressive in character, have implications not just for physical but also for emotional and social well-being. Patients suffering from such conditions tend to have greater stress and anxiety levels, as they fight against the necessities of daily life in the backdrop of their condition. This multifaceted aspect of long-term illness requires a complete care approach, encompassing not only the medical treatment but psychological care as well as incorporation in society. The identification of chronic disease as a key public health issue has generated awareness towards interventions that can enhance the quality of life in patients who are suffering from such conditions, and also underlines the significance of healthcare systems that are alert to the nuances of living with chronic disease. The use of specific interventions for individuals suffering from chronic diseases is capable of significantly contributing to their overall well-being. As documented in mindfulness-based stress reduction research, barriers such as unfulfilled expectations and clinicians' lack of knowledge can hinder effective delivery of supportive interventions. For example, qualitative evaluation identified that adapting such programs, such as shortening course length and increasing peer contact, can enhance patient engagement and improve outcomes. By respecting the unique needs of populations with chronic conditions, health professionals can tailor interventions to better meet the specific requirements of this population. Emphasizing flexibility and patient-centeredness can lead to more robust therapeutic relationships and improved management of chronic disease, finally enhancing participation and satisfaction among patients. The socio-economic condition of chronic illness also heavily impinges on the experiences and opportunities for the victims.

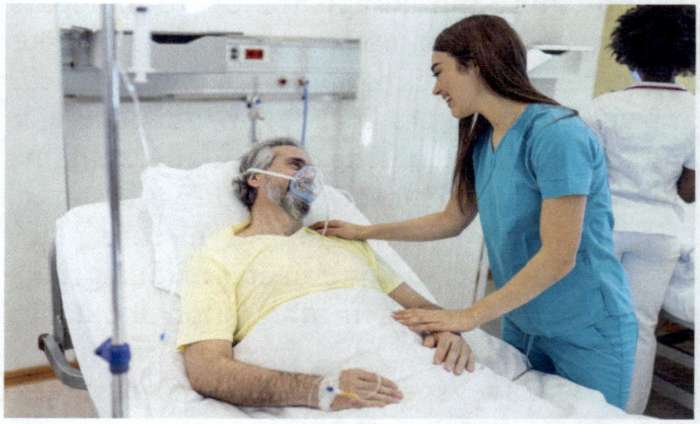

Figure 7.6. Chronic-illnesses in nursing.

Source: https://xpresshealth.ie/wp-content/uploads/2024/02/Addressing-Chronic-Illnesses-in-Mayos-Nursing-Sector-scaled.jpg.

Research has established that macro-level policies can influence the employment levels of individuals with chronic illnesses in various countries, such as Canada, Denmark, and Sweden. By mapping multiple interventions and their impacts, researchers have observed that socio-economic factors play with disability differently and result in varying accessibility to work and support services. This detailed analysis leaves room for strategic thinking in the formulation of national policy to facilitate the socio-economic integration of chronically ill adults. Correctly understanding the intricate dynamic between chronic illness and socio-economic status can play a role in more effective support mechanisms, initiating a culture that embraces inclusion and equitable opportunity for those coping with long-term ill health (Figure 7.6).

7.2.1. Definition and Examples of Chronic Illnesses

Chronic illnesses refer to health conditions that are long-lasting and, in most cases, impede the mobility, normal functioning, and quality of life of an individual. They tend to be differentiated from other conditions by their duration, which typically exceeds three months, and in some cases, they require regular medical attention or control. Some conditions that qualify as chronic illnesses include diabetes, heart disease, asthma, and forms of arthritis. The chronic nature of the disease subjects the patients to repeated flare-ups or exacerbations and necessitates a regular and multidisciplinary approach to treatment and cure. Chronic management also has long-term emotional and financial effects on the patient, their family, and the overall healthcare system. Chronic diseases demand an understanding of their prevalence and multi-dimensionality within modern societies. Six in every ten adults in America suffer from a chronic condition, and four in every ten adults suffer from two or more chronic conditions, according to the Centers for Disease Control and Prevention (CDC). From the above figures, it is clear that the prevalence of chronic conditions is widespread, and as a result, there is an overwhelming need for extensive long-term care planning. For example, chronic obstructive pulmonary disease (COPD) and heart failure necessitate frequent medical visits, lifestyle modifications, and, in most instances, intervention by family members or caregivers. Moreover, long-term care for these conditions typically involves comprehensive approaches that address physical, mental, and social well-being, underscoring the interdependence between long-term care systems and chronic diseases. The consequences of chronic diseases extend beyond individual health complications; they also pose broader social issues that require robust health policies. As individuals attempt to navigate their conditions, health organizations must adapt to provide the necessary support and intervention. Shifts from children to adult healthcare services, for instance, are essential for those with chronic complications, but such shifts are riddled with complications. The lack of standardized transition plans can lead to care discontinuities, bringing still another layer of complexity to the chronic disease management complications (Adi et al., 2009). The definition of disability is also applicable in this context since chronic diseases possess a strong ability to restrict the employee's opportunities and life quality, highlighting the need for policy support favoring inclusion and equal access in the workforce (Gabriel et al., 2000). Thus, knowledge about chronic diseases and their implications is crucial for the development of inclusive disability policies and long-term care policies (Figure 7.7).

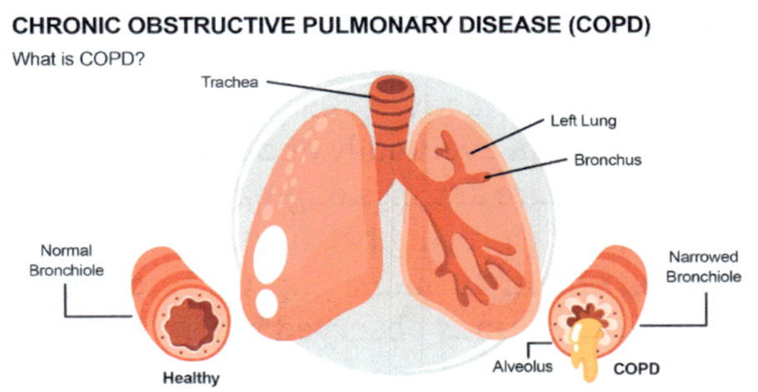

Figure 7.7. Chronic obstructive pulmonary disease (COPD).

Source: https://cdn.sketchbubble.com/pub/media/catalog/product/optimized1/4/6/468a741e356b72201688ca63822e4d0255fbd1a65b331d78f8b7be35a6f92523/chronic-obstructive-pulmonary-disease-copd-mc-slide1.png.

7.2.2. Impact of Chronic Illness on Daily Life

The impact of chronic illness on daily life manifests in multifaceted and profound ways, transforming the patterns and lives of the afflicted in a radical manner. For many, a transition from a state of health to one of chronic illness can evoke a pervasive sense of loss—not just physical capability, but autonomy and social connection as well. Everyday activities that were once taken for granted, such as managing household chores or enjoying recreational activities, become challenging. This shift to a world of restriction significantly affects psychological health, leading to frustration, isolation, and the risk of depression. As explained in research, the experiences of people living with chronic diseases, such as arthritis, highlight the need to better understand how such diseases evolve and affect daily functioning within the broader context of disability and care provision (Smedley et al., 2014). Furthermore, chronic disease can significantly impact social relationships and social functioning. Individuals may become withdrawn from social interaction due to the emotional wear of their illness or due to the physical confinement that the disease has on them. These alterations could create a cycle of isolation, wherein lack of activity exacerbates mental illness and might eventually end in a diminished support structure at times of greatest need. This is particularly worrying because social support will be essential in managing chronic illness. Drawing upon trends observed in Poland, social change over the past two decades has indicated a rising trend in functional and legal disability, which corresponds to the overall implications of chronic illness on community integration and support arrangements (Golinowska et al., 2012). Effective management of the challenges, however, requires not only medical intervention but also concerted efforts in establishing environments that enable social inclusion. The impact of chronic disease extends beyond individual health and influences society's overall systems and health policy. The growing burden of chronic conditions, as evidenced by the shift towards measuring their impact on daily life, requires redesigning systems of long-term care. For instance, Australia's move to the National Disability Insurance Scheme reflects the need for customized support services that address the complex needs of people with chronic illnesses. Having a proper realization of the extent to which such conditions lead to disability can inform policy towards providing sufficient resources to improve accessibility and aid to the affected group. This approach not only aims to enhance the quality of life for individuals but also addresses social issues resulting from an aging population and the rising prevalence of chronic diseases (Smedley et al., 2014). Thus, the combination of disability and care services with chronic illness highlights the individual and collective responsibility for making the environment more supportive (Figure 7.8).

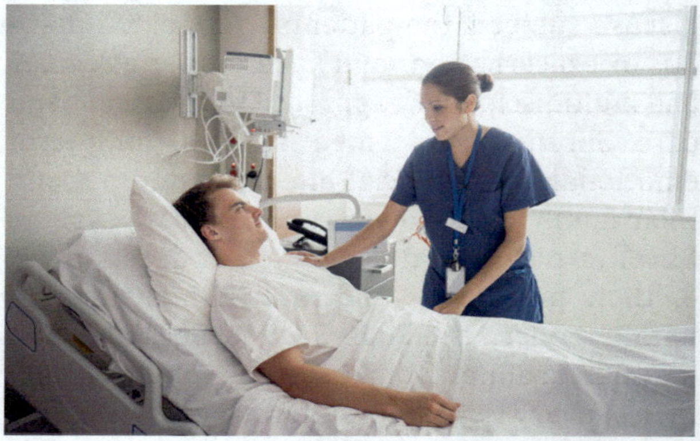

Figure 7.8. Chronic illness on daily life.

Source: https://www.rd.com/wp-content/uploads/sites/2/2016/04/08-50-secrets-surgeon-care-after-surgery.jpg.

7.2.3. The Relationship Between Chronic Illness and Disability

Disability and chronic illness are interrelated conditions that can have a significant influence on individuals' lives and interactions with the health care system. A lot of chronic diseases, such as diabetes, heart disease, and autoimmune conditions, tend to produce extensive amounts of functional impairment, which may lead to disability. This dynamic is indicative of the underlying importance of understanding that chronic illness not only affects physical well-being, but it also affects one's capability to make it through the day as well as social interaction. Acceptance of illness is a significant aspect of this dynamic, as studies have shown that individuals with higher levels of acceptance report higher life satisfaction and functional capacity. Specifically, acceptance was, according to one study, associated with greater life satisfaction among older individuals receiving long-term home care, noting the contribution of psychological adaptation towards coping with chronic illness (Bożena Majchrowicz et al., 2025). Disability experience within the context of chronic illness is also further compounded by the social and environmental factors that constitute individuals' capabilities and options. As identified in research investigating the realities of people with multiple enduring health conditions, the majority of individuals face a dilemma: while they wish to gain significant work, the illness associated with their chronic conditions often makes them unable to sustain work in traditional settings. This self-reinforcing cycle of (un)employment and (ill-)health provides an environment where enduring diseases can drive disability, hence an enabling environment for a disempowered identity among people afflicted by them. The subsequent existential struggle acknowledges the psychological burden of an existence that anticipates production, even for those whose illness severely limits their capabilities (Esca van Blarikom et al., 2025). In addition, the intersection of chronic disease and disability requires an integrated plan for long-term care that incorporates both medical and psychosocial intervention. Effective long-term care models must value the variability in the severity and quality of functional impairment intrinsic to chronic conditions and offer environments that foster autonomy and quality of life, accommodating the inherent variability in the severity and quality of functional impairment associated with chronic conditions. Focusing on care plans that incorporate physical rehabilitation, mental health treatment, and community care can allow health professionals to restrict the disabling effects of chronic disease. Attending to these complex interactions not only promotes patient satisfaction but also enhances the quality of life for individuals living with the challenges of chronic illness and disability, ultimately enabling a more just and compassionate healthcare system (Bożena Majchrowicz et al., 2025).

Test Your Knowledge

1. What is a chronic illness, and how does it differ from an acute illness?
2. Identify two common chronic illnesses commonly managed within medical-surgical settings.

7.3. The Need for Long-Term Care

Learning Outcome

1. Describe the factors that determine the need for long-term care
2. Define long-term care service types
3. Describe the family and caregiver's role in long-term care

The mounting demand for long-term care is intimately linked to the growth of disability and chronic ailments among populations across the world. As populations age or face severe health complications, they often require varying intensities of care to maintain their functional ability on a day-to-day basis. This is compounded by the fact that a majority of disabled people are stuck in a state of long-term poverty, as revealed by evidence from Uganda, which strengthens the close correlation between disability and long-term financial vulnerability (Lwanga-Ntale et al., 2003). The continuous care need is often the product of ongoing disease that necessitates constant care, e.g., mobility assistance or health management, that is not merely a personal matter of wellness but essential to participation in society. Thus, with nations undergoing demographic transformation and soaring healthcare costs, the establishment and building of long-term care infrastructures become part of fulfilling individual and societal healthcare requirements. The complex diseases usually require patients to develop advanced self-management strategies that they can use to control and manage their illness efficiently. These can be medication management, care coordination, and lifestyle modifications, which, in the absence of proper kinds of support, can be intimidating. The disability employment service workforce today is still under-skilled to meet these demanding needs efficiently (Blyth et al., 2013). This deficit in training impacts not only the quality of care provided but also underserves vulnerable groups, i.e., the disabled or chronically ill. Inadequately trained staff, for instance, may struggle to implement integrated care models, which are crucial for addressing the complex problems of such individuals. Therefore, enhancing the quality of long-term care and increasing its availability to the level where individuals receive the kind of care they need is contingent upon developing care providers' skills by equipping them with specialized training in chronic condition self-management. Secondly, intergenerational transmission of poverty and disability is a compelling reason for inclusive and comprehensive long-term care systems.

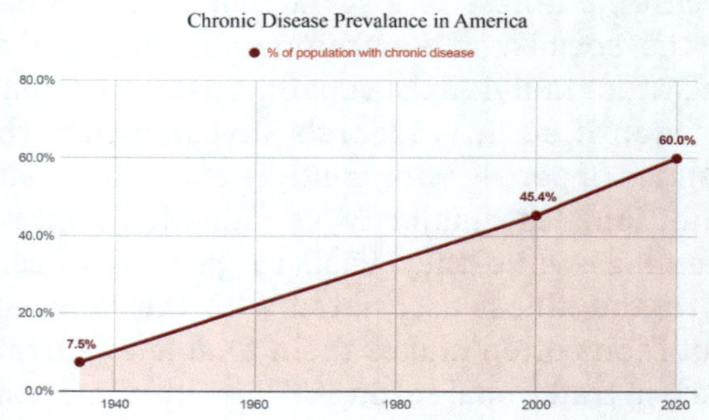

Figure 7.9. Driving chronic disease.

Source: https://uploads-ssl.webflow.com/5e20f576d0e9d12be5abc763/5e8267fbe910250e5b199afc_Chronic%20Disease%20Prevalence%20in%20America.png.

According to evidence, individuals with disabilities are prone to chronic poverty, and this presents barriers that block their access to essential resources and care (Lwanga-Ntale et al., 2003). This cycle not only perpetuates individual hardship but also presents significant challenges to societal progress. Systems of long-term care must respond to such crosscutting needs by having policies that enable them to avoid the pitfalls of chronic poverty while accessing the care and support they require. By shifting their focus to inclusive practice and specific interventions, policy systems can both support the management of individuals with disabilities according to their condition and provide mechanisms for enhanced economic and social integration, best reflecting the fundamental requirement of a reformed approach to long-term care (Figure 7.9).

7.3.1. Factors Influencing the Need for Long-Term Care

The need for long-term care is proportionally influenced by the number of chronic health conditions and disabilities that increasingly affect people's everyday functioning and independence. With the increase in the elderly population, conditions such as arthritis, heart disease, and diabetes are gaining more prevalence, necessitating ongoing assistance for activities of daily living (ADLs). This complication is compounded by the fact that most older patients carry multiple comorbidities that interact synergistically to exacerbate physical and cognitive impairment. Moreover, chronic pain has become endemic in developed countries; some have debilitating conditions that ultimately lead to poor quality of life and higher care requirements. The emphasis on early intervention and self-care in the treatment of such conditions implies that immediate medical attention can avert disabling outcomes. Still, the system boundaries invariably limit complete healthcare access, highlighting the immediate need for long-term care options that meet physical and psychosocial wellness needs (Souza et al., 2001). Another significant determinant of long-term care need is the social and environmental circumstances of the chronically diseased and disabled individual. Caregivers typically carry most of these burdens, and how far they can provide care depends on their own physical and psychological health. The availability of supportive resources, such as healthcare services and community programs, controls how dependent one can become. For instance, studies have evidenced that mixed expectations between clinicians and patients will serve as a barrier in the application of care interventions such as mindfulness-based stress reduction, which have been found to improve mental health for chronically ill persons (Mair et al., 2018). Hence, facilitating a supportive community infrastructure is key to reducing the caregiving burdens and ensuring individuals have enough access to available resources that help to support their long-term care needs.

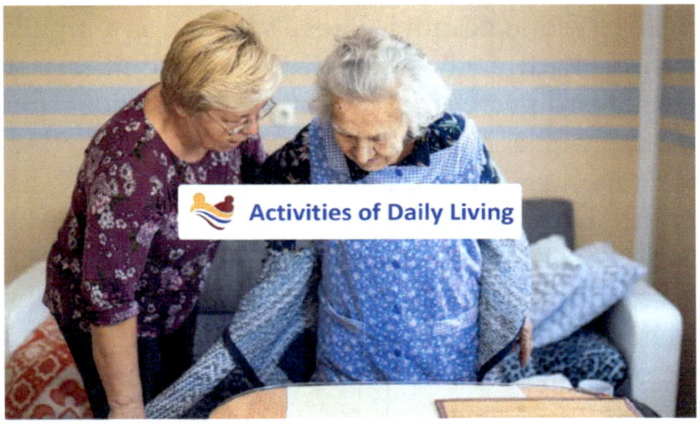

Figure 7.10. Activities of daily living (ADLs) in caregiving.

Source: https://familycaregiversonline.net/wp-content/uploads/Activities_of-Daily_Living_FISM.png.

Finally, economic factors are also pivotal in the demand for long-term care, further shaping the scope of disability and chronic disease management. The cost of healthcare can be prohibitive, particularly for long-term care that is often not fully covered by insurance or government support. As out-of-pocket expenses increase, families are likely to accept inferior care or forgo service altogether, enlarging the person's health problems. In addition, the socioeconomic disparities also compound access to quality long-term care, and the marginalized groups in society bear a disproportionate disability burden and concomitant chronic disease. It is essential to be aware of these economic barriers in developing effective policies to improve access to long-term care while promoting health equity for all individuals facing the consequences of chronic illness and disability (Figure 7.10).

7.3.2. Types Of Long-Term Care Services Available

Long-term care services are required for individuals with disabilities and long-term illnesses, providing care that aids in living their lives to the maximum. These services are highly varied, with each being designed for different needs and preferences. Home care services, for instance, provide assistance while at home. This kind of care can include personal care, such as bathing and dressing, and skilled nursing care for those who need medical attention. Informal care can also include care from family members, although they may need to be supported and resourced to perform their roles effectively. According to research, the transition to models like the National Disability Insurance Scheme highlights the need for home care services tailored to the specific needs of individuals with conditions such as arthritis, which significantly impacts daily function and health (Smedley et al., 2014). Another typical type of long-term care service is assisted living facilities, which offer clients who require more extensive support but do not need the comprehensive medical attention provided in nursing homes. Assisted living provides a continuum of care that bridges the gap between independence and support, offering services such as meal preparation, medication management, and social interaction. These environments are designed to bring together individuals and promote social interaction, which is essential for emotional and mental well-being, particularly among those with chronic conditions. These facilities also require adjustments to services to address the diverse needs of individuals with varying disabilities, enabling them to receive appropriate support (Goodman et al., 2007). It is essential to understand these differences among long-term care settings to effectively advocate for service enhancements that can meet the complicated needs of such populations. Finally, skilled nursing facilities are the more intense type of long-term care and are frequently used by individuals with serious chronic conditions or severe disabilities.

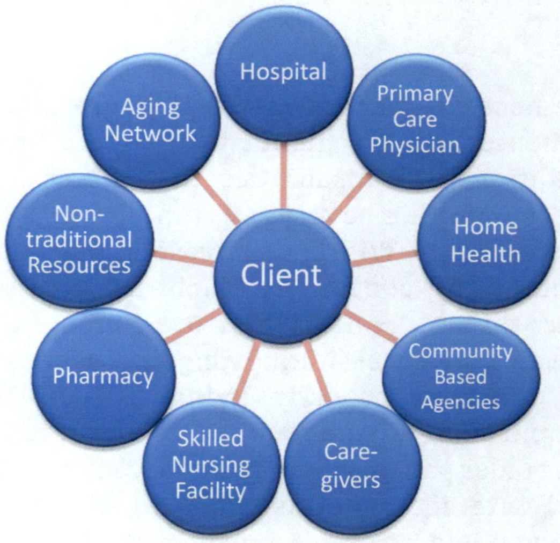

Figure 7.11. Long-term and post-acute care providers engaged in health information exchange.

Source: https://aspe.hhs.gov/sites/default/files/private/images-reports/long-term-and-post-acute-care-providers-engaged-health-information-exchange-final-report/4_1.PNG.

Skilled nursing facilities offer around-the-clock medical treatment and monitoring, catering to individuals who require continuous observation or rehabilitation care. In such a setting, physicians are best equipped to handle complex medical issues, and thus it is particularly well-suited for patients recuperating from surgery, a stroke, or a serious disease. Such facilities are necessitated by the shortcomings within existing arrangements for healthcare financing, which may fall short of crucial service aspects that are key to maintaining patients' quality of life (Goodman et al., 2007). With increasing demands for long-term care, there is a need to break down systemic barriers that prevent accessibility, ultimately providing better integration and coordination of services critical to the well-being of individuals with disabilities and chronic diseases (Figure 7.11).

7.3.3. The Role of Family and Caregivers in Long-Term Care

Caregiver and family engagement is key in long-term care, especially for the chronically ill and the disabled. Families are typically first of all in support, providing the physical assistance and emotional care that professional carers cannot individually replicate. Data indicate that more than 11 million family carers provided an estimated 18 billion unpaid care hours to individuals with Alzheimer's and other types of dementia in 2022, highlighting the important role families play in the care continuum (N/A, 2023). This family engagement not only constructs the caregiving situation but also has a considerable bearing on the quality of life of the patients with chronic diseases, providing a sense of belonging and emotional well-being necessary for the well-being of the mind. Additionally, caregivers often face numerous emotional and psychological issues. The responsibility for care of a valued individual can lead family caregivers to report greater levels of stress, anxiety, and depression, particularly when dealing with more complex health conditions or behavioral issues associated with long-term illnesses. Caregivers are more likely to suffer adverse mental health outcomes, which could be exacerbated by the stress imposed upon them through caregiving (N/A, 2023). The psychological burden of caregiving, combined with insufficient support systems, underscores the need for systematic models of care that incorporate caregiver well-being. Since family members are more likely to be involved in long-term care, interventions designed to support them with resources and assistance become crucial in mitigating such stresses. Training and education programs for family members and informal caregivers would be necessary to promote effective long-term care strategies. Data on the specific medical conditions of their loved ones, such as Alzheimer's or depression, can enhance caregivers' competence to provide high-quality care, thus preparing them to address the particular challenges in long-term care scenarios. Informed caregivers are more likely to be able to communicate with healthcare workers, which leads to better coordination of care and improved patient outcomes. In addition, engagement of family members in the planning process acknowledges their central role and allows them to become the spokespersons for their relatives, making the process of long-term care more integrated, which emphasizes family involvement more.

Test Your Knowledge

1. What are two common conditions that most often lead to a need for long-term care among older people?
2. Why is long-term care planning important in the management of chronic or disabling conditions?

7.4. Challenges in Long-Term Care

Learning Outcome

1. Describe the economic barriers to accessing care
2. Define patient safety problems and the quality of care
3. Describe emotional and psychological issues for patients and families

The issues that emerge in long-term care are glaringly evident by structural variations in access to services, which have a determining impact upon the quality of care received by individuals who are disabled and chronically ill. Research indicates that geographic inequities in non-acute care service provision exist, such as in Ireland's healthcare system, where some counties are significantly under-serviced. The uneven distribution of primary and long-term care exacerbates healthcare inequities, making it challenging for clients with ongoing care needs to access necessary services. As the Irish Health Research Board's healthcare study shows, it is required to fill these gaps if strategies are to be developed for shifting care out of acute hospitals and into more sustainable, community-based systems. In doing this, the shift not only supports health reform goals of the new century but also makes the imperative case for coordinated planning for enhancing the overall quality of long-term care. A second critical component of long-term care concerns is the psychological and emotional well-being of caregivers and recipients of care. For individuals with chronic disease, such as those with multiple sclerosis, the addition of supportive interventions—such as mindfulness-based stress reduction—can be transformational. However, barriers to the uptake of such interventions often arise, citing incompatible expectations among stakeholders, a lack of awareness about access to utilized resources, and rigid mechanisms of care that do not support the specific needs of patients with disabilities. Qualitative studies enumerate that successful integration of mindfulness interventions into routine care demands flexibility and responsiveness that includes adapting programs to match varied levels of disability and comorbidity. Thus, there is a need to value and address the psychological obstacles to accessing and using health services, in order to ensure high efficiency in the delivery of long-term care services.

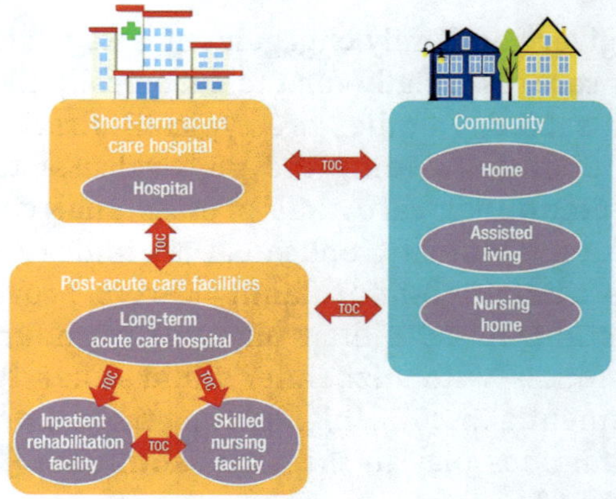

Figure 7.12. Postacute care, rehabilitation, and long-term care systems.

Source: https://i0.wp.com/nursekey.com/wp-content/uploads/2021/06/f46-01-9780323654166.jpg?w=960.

Long-term care also continues to face inherent workforce capability challenges regarding training in specialized areas. In facing the challenge of disabilities and chronic illnesses, the demand for specialization in training is apparent. Clinicians may lack the necessary information on new care approaches and supportive therapies, and consequently may be skeptical of their use. The implementation of new models of care, such as mindfulness-based interventions, requires not only revising existing curricula but also providing continuous support to clinicians through professional development programs. Providing quality outcomes will require a culture of continuous learning for the healthcare workforce, where practice and knowledge sharing will foster a culture conducive to adopting best care approaches. Until these workforce challenges are addressed, having opportunities to improve the quality of care and patient outcomes in long-term settings remains primarily limited (Figure 7.12).

7.4.1. Financial Barriers to Accessing Care

Accessing healthcare services is a challenge for the disabled or chronically ill individuals, founded on several financial constraints. It is typical for the majority of members in the above groups to incur added medical expenses that originate from both the cost of treatment and indirect fees of managing their illnesses. For instance, individuals with long-term illnesses tend to incur recurrent charges for medication, therapy, and frequent visits to physicians, which may be costly. The financial cost can be compounded by changes in earnings due to the inability to work or work part-time, leading to a cycle of debt and dismal health outcomes. In countries such as Australia, where arthritis is a prevalent cause of disability, understanding the economic cost that such conditions impose on an individual's life takes precedence over other factors, especially against the backdrop of a transition towards newer models of healthcare, like the National Disability Insurance Scheme (Smedley et al., 2014). Furthermore, the lack of general insurance coverage forms a major factor that restricts access to necessary medical treatment. The majority of public and private insurance plans place restrictions that do not fully accommodate the different needs of patients with disabilities or chronic illnesses. These restrictions are in the form of high co-pays, limited access to certain specialists, or exclusion of specific treatments and act as deterrents to care. For older individuals navigating various life events, such as retirement or declining health, the lack of insurance can add another layer of complexity to their ability to access necessary services. Research has indicated that such fiscal obstacles disproportionately affect marginalized populations, including low-income older people and persons with disabilities, with enormous gaps in current support (Kusch et al., 2025). Thus, surmounting such fiscal obstacles is crucial in policymaking to facilitate access to care. Fundamentally, where finance meets access to healthcare, issues of social justice and equity arise. When individuals cannot afford necessary medical treatment, their lives and health are compromised, frequently leading to higher utilization of costly emergency services in the long term. Systemic reform is required to remedy these inequalities; some of the systemic reforms that can be encompassed include policies that increase coverage, reduce costs, or subsidize disadvantaged groups. Community support services also have to be made more robust so that individuals can cope with their healthcare needs without sinking into financial adversity. The incorporation of strong support systems that recognize the barriers individuals with disabilities, chronic conditions, and long-term care needs encounter is crucial for achieving a balanced healthcare setting (Kusch et al., 2025) (Figure 7.13).

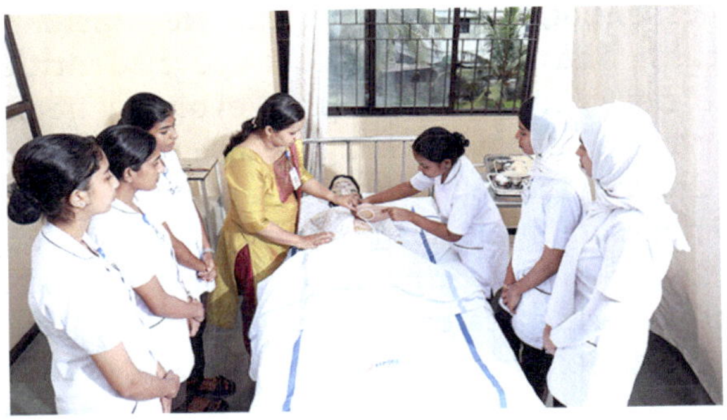

Figure 7.13. Community support services in surgical nursing.

Source: https://babymemorialcollegeofnursing.org/wp-content/uploads/2024/08/medical-surgical-2-1.jpg.

7.4.2. Quality of Care and Patient Safety Concerns

The quality of care provided to individuals with chronic conditions and disabilities is of the highest priority because it has a profound bearing on patient outcomes and overall well-being. Substandard care can cause a myriad of complications, exacerbating linked health issues and reducing patients' quality of life. Furthermore, organizational problems such as health disparities and limited access to services are likely to be contributing factors to differences in care. Overall, an overview of the varied healthcare systems reveals that effective quality improvement interventions are required to enhance patient safety and care coordination (N/A, 2011). Managing such issues requires a holistic approach, such as the implementation of evidence-based practices and stringent patient-focused care, which can reduce the risks of suboptimal quality care. Patient safety concerns are highly related to the long-term effectiveness of care for patients with chronic diseases. In this group, the consequences of patient safety mishaps can be most serious, such as hospitalization unnecessarily, suffering unnecessarily, and mortality at an elevated level. Comprehensive health system assessments are necessary in ascertaining where change is essential; for instance, the New Zealand Health and Independence Report identifies the necessity of developing evolving health services in line with changing health needs and addressing the implications of the burden caused by non-communicable diseases (N/A, 2025). By focusing on enhancing patient safety protocols and fostering a safety culture within healthcare organizations, providers can effectively reduce untoward events and improve overall patient experiences in long-term care settings. Having health information technology incorporated as well plays a significant role in enhancing the overall quality of care and ensuring patients with disabilities and chronic illness are kept safe. Advanced technologies, such as electronic health records, facilitate the coordination of care between various healthcare providers, ensuring that vital patient information is readily available when needed. Such availability can prevent medication management and care transition errors, resulting in better health outcomes. Additionally, facilitating evidence-based practice in health systems not only enhances the quality of care but also cultivates a culture of continuous improvement (N/A, 2011). By investing in technology and upholding superior standards, health care providers can create a safer care environment for their patients, thus contributing to better health outcomes among individuals living with disability and chronic diseases (Figure 7.14).

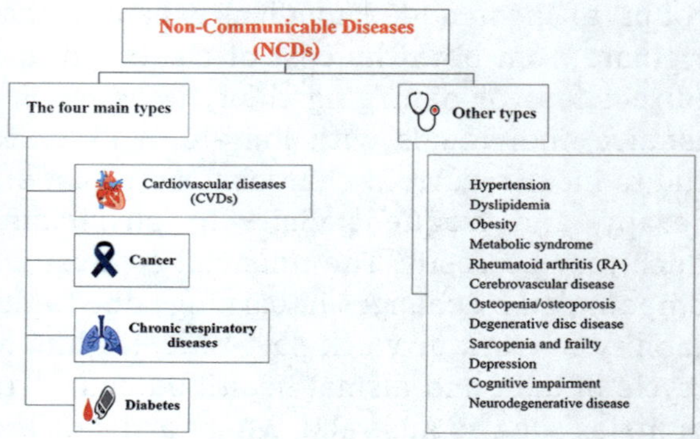

Figure 7.14. Management and prevention strategies for non-communicable diseases (NCDs).

Source: https://images-provider.frontiersin.org/api/ipx/w=1200&f=png/https://www.frontiersin.org/files/Articles/574111/fpubh-08-574111-HTML/image_m/fpubh-08-574111-g001.jpg.

7.4.3. Emotional and Psychological Challenges for Patients and Families

The psychological and emotional load carried by patients and their kin who experience disability and chronic illness is profound and multifaceted. Patients often have to contend with a feeling of loss—loss of normalcy, identity, and independence—which can lead to severe emotional distress. This is compounded by the nature of their illness, which often includes chronic pain, exhaustion, and ongoing medical care. As parents tread the thin line of caregiving, they experience anxiety, depression, and burnout. The emotional environment is volatile, resulting in a world where both patients and caregivers continually redefine their position within the family as they navigate the intensity of long-term care while dealing with their own feelings of loss and anger (Henwood et al., 2017). Moreover, caregiving also extends beyond the immediate emotional issues to cover the mental well-being of informal carers. Evidence shows that 2.7 million Australians provide informal care, and 770,000 of them are the principal carers for people with extensive disabilities (Piccenna et al., 2025). All this heavy investment not only wears out the physical and emotional resources but also the mental well-being of the carers. Caregiving experience is a solitary experience and involves a feeling of loneliness and subjective isolation. The informal caregiver then suffers extreme emotional exhaustion and impaired quality of life because they prioritize the needs of their loved ones above their own well-being. It is essential to understand these experiences so that effective support systems can be developed to cater to the psychological needs of patients and caregivers (Henwood et al., 2017). Chronic illness requires holistic support mechanisms that understand the complex interrelationships between patients and caregivers. Interventions need to target caregiver resilience because research highlights that maximization of support maximizes not only the benefit for the caregiver but also the overall efficacy of the care provided (Piccenna et al., 2025). Both points underscore the importance of psychosocial interventions, educational programs, and family support systems that can promote emotional well-being. In addition, facilitating open communication between health care staff, patients, and families can create more compassionate environments, enhancing coping styles and reducing feelings of isolation. Prioritizing these emotional factors can help alleviate some of the psychological burdens associated with disability and long-term illness, ultimately contributing to an enhanced quality of life for all concerned (Henwood et al., 2017).

Test Your Knowledge

1. How can communication barriers impact care in long-term facilities?
2. Discuss the key challenges of providing long-term care to the elderly.

7.5. Policy and Legislation

Learning Outcome

1. Describe the relevant legislation and regulations for disability
2. Define the role of government programs in funding care
3. Discuss the movement for improved policy and resources for people with disabilities and chronic diseases

The disability, chronic disease, and long-term care policy and legislative framework is evolving because of increased demands by the aging population. As the number of individuals aged 65 and older grows, mainly due to medical innovations and public health policies, the level of cognitive impairment and subsequent diseases has also escalated. It is the responsibility of policymakers to address such rising challenges through creative legislative solutions that prioritize the needs of persons with disabilities. Notably, the development and introduction of adult day services (ADS) represent a key intervention that serves to postpone the need for long-term care home admissions for older adults with cognitive impairment. However, the lack of previously established research on the efficiency of ADS supports the importance of ongoing research and legislative support to solidify their standing in enhancing the quality of life for this group, ultimately deciding on improved policy (Udeh et al., 2025). In addition to promoting services like ADS, policy must also recognize the diversified needs of individuals who receive long-term home nursing care. These patients, often weighed down by chronic illness or acute disability, require comprehensive support systems that encompass medical as well as psychological aspects. Studies have established that patients' acceptance of their illness strongly predicts how satisfied they are with life when placed in long-term home care. Policy intervention should therefore target to foster settings that provide not only medical treatment but also encourage psychological and emotional wellness. By implementing policies that promote functional independence alongside mental health care, lawmakers can facilitate greater subjective satisfaction with life and achieve better outcomes for individuals with long-term conditions (Bożena Majchrowicz et al., 2025). Second, developing effective long-term care policy also needs the conceptual integration of multidimensional disability and chronic illness realities. Legislators must engage with stakeholders, including healthcare providers, patients, and their families, so that policies are reflective of the experiences of those affected. Empowering citizens through participatory policymaking is critical in the struggle for rights and access in the healthcare sector. With an aging population whose cognitive function is at risk, as well as other disorders, the legislative framework must be adaptive to these evolving populations. Finally, a firm, well-educated policy structure can lead to improved models and support systems of care that not only cater to immediate healthcare but also strive to bring about long-term societal change (Bożena Majchrowicz et al., 2025; Udeh et al., 2025) (Figure 7.15).

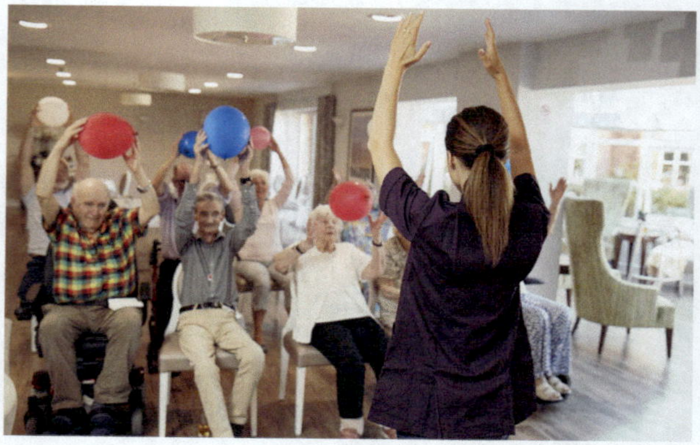

Figure 7.15. Adult day care options.

Source: https://dlyhjlf6lts50.cloudfront.net/app/uploads/2019/02/AdultDayComparison.png.

7.5.1. Overview of Relevant Laws and Regulations

Understanding the discipline of laws and regulations that impact disability, chronic illness, and long-term care is paramount to optimizing the well-being of those affected and their families. Many federal and state codes address the rights and services offered for individuals with disabilities, including the Americans with Disabilities Act (ADA) and the Rehabilitation Act. These laws operate towards preventing discrimination from being practiced and guaranteeing equal access to public services, with a direct bearing on the quality of life for chronic illness sufferers. Furthermore, the provisions of Medicare and Medicaid have important impacts on the financial aid given to long-term care services, which in turn affects the accessibility and quality of services delivered to elderly patients and those suffering from chronic illnesses. With a growing population, an increasing number of individuals experience these problems and thus require more investigation into the adequacy and efficacy of such legal systems in meeting contemporary healthcare demands. State regulations may be somewhat varied, and variations can lead to discrepancies in the availability of resources and the quality of treatment across different regions. These discrepancies may arise as a result of states embracing long-term care policy and financing disability services differently. For instance, other states have introduced new programs to integrate care services for elderly patients in a manner that allows them to experience a richer, more efficient care continuum. Gaps still exist, however, particularly in service coordination for patients with multisystemic illnesses, according to recent reviews of critical care outcomes (Santangelo et al., 2024). These policies and service needs emphasize the need for constant assessment and policy revision to better meet the subtleties of chronic disease and disability management, particularly in an increasingly aging population. Integrating extensive long-term care delivery systems is essential in addressing the multi-faceted needs of elderly patients with chronic disease. Recent innovations envision a shift towards community-based systems that involve the family and informal caregiver, as evident in ongoing efforts in various states (Khongboon, 2025). These models aim to facilitate better coordination of care, enhance the quality of care, and offer a facilitative environment for both patients and caregivers. Involvement of formal training for the informal caregiver is also required to bridge the skills gap uncovered in the majority of the studies. Effective regulatory frameworks should consider not only accessibility but also the assurance of quality in service provision. This vision can eventually translate to improved overall effectiveness of long-term care systems, resulting in improved health outcomes for individuals who have difficulty with disabilities and chronic illnesses.

7.5.2. The Role of Government Programs in Supporting Care

The mature disability and chronic illness care system largely relies on the active engagement of government programs in providing essential support services. The programs are vital, particularly for addressing the needs of those individuals who otherwise have prohibitively high barriers to care and social integration. Through the provision of financial assistance, health services, and rehabilitation services, government programs play a key role in promoting independence among individuals with disabilities and chronic illnesses. For instance, deinstitutionalization programs, as discussed in Koyanagi (2007), not only help move away from institutionalization to community-based care but also emphasize the importance of customized care through which individuals can live without dependencies within their communities. Moreover, government initiatives also play a role in implementing inclusive policies that provide equal opportunities for individuals with disabilities. These initiatives act to eliminate systemic barriers that restrict access to available resources such as vocational training and employment placement. These objectives are given top priority by the International Labour Organization (ILO) in its Disability Charter, with the aim of developing strategies that enable individuals with disabilities to pursue their professional interests while raising awareness among policymakers and employers of these concerns (Gabriel et al., 2000).

By creating a framework that emphasizes diversity in the workforce, government programs effectively address the structural disadvantage that exists for individuals with disabilities and highlight the critical need for supportive care within broader societal contexts. The effectiveness of government programs in caring is underscored by their emphasis on continuous participation and responsiveness to meet the evolving needs of persons with disabilities and chronic conditions. With a changing society and advances in medicine, programs must be adaptable so that they can accommodate new problems.

Not only do these programs provide necessary resources, but they also demonstrate an obligation that is the basis of respect and dignity for those facing long-term care challenges. Investing in community-based initiatives and prioritizing person-centered measures, government schemes can ensure that individuals enjoy a quality life, thereby upholding and enforcing the policy of equal treatment and work as formulated under the ILO Convention 159 (Gabriel et al., 2000). Ongoing assessment and refinement of these schemes will be necessary as society grapples with the complexities of care across an increasingly heterogeneous population (Figure 7.16).

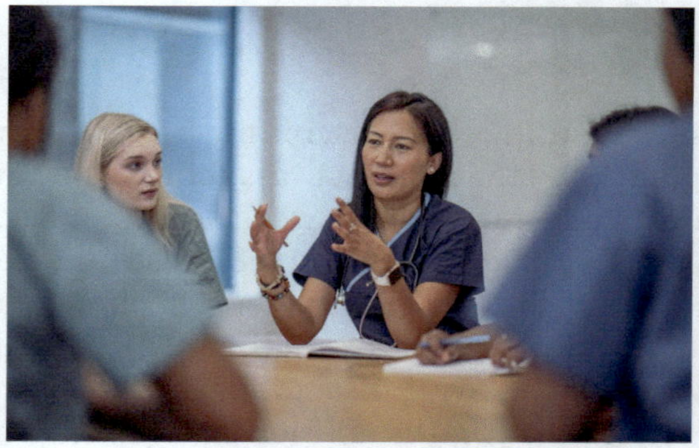

Figure 7.16. Nurses meeting.

Source: https://campaignforaction.org/wp-content/uploads/2023/01/GettyImages-1411002384-1-scaled.jpg.

7.5.3. Advocacy for Improved Policies and Resources

Advocacy for better policies and resources is essential in addressing challenges that face people with disabilities and chronic diseases. As the population of this group continues to grow, the need for systemic change becomes increasingly urgent. Of particular note, the employment gap remains wide, with people suffering from chronic illnesses facing higher unemployment levels compared to their non-ill counterparts. Effective interventions, such as Individualized Personal Support (IPS), are effective at facilitating employment among people with severe mental illness, as noted in a systematic review of employment interventions in the UK. Closing this disability employment gap not only advances economic independence but also moves toward societal goals of inclusion and equity. Therefore, collective advocacy is necessary to bring to the forefront the various concerns that this population faces and to drive policy changes that support more positive employment opportunities and care systems for individuals with disabilities and chronic illnesses (Pennington et al., 2024). Apart from employment, the need for more effective long-term care policies is particularly pertinent for older individuals with chronic illness, especially in low- and middle-income nations. With the population getting older, healthcare systems are faced with greater pressures to provide respectful care that taps into the complex needs of older individuals. In Nepal, for instance, the existing healthcare system reflects significant loopholes in providing long-term care services due to the economic strain and dearth of professionals. The country lacks a competent geriatric workforce, which aggravates the challenge of addressing the growing disease burden of conditions such as cardiovascular and musculoskeletal diseases in older people. Hence, encouraging sustainable financing and the mobilization of resources is crucial for the development and implementation of an extensive long-term care policy that ensures access to sufficient healthcare services for the vulnerable age group (Dhakal et al., 2024). Second, advocacy must go beyond work and health services to encompass an integrated treatment of meeting the complex needs of individuals with disabilities and chronic illness. This includes increased awareness and education about the social determinants of health that disproportionately affect these groups, such as housing stability, access to public spaces, and integration into communities. Effective advocacy involves collaboration across different sectors, including healthcare practitioners, policymakers, and community organizations, to develop an integrated system that benefits people with disabilities. Through advocacy for resource allocation that encompasses not just medical treatment but also social care and integration, advocates can create an environment where individuals with chronic illness and disability can have successful lives. Hence, with the well-established advocacy networks, the impacted will be able to join the policymaking process, and their voices will be among those in shaping the policies that directly affect their lives and neighborhoods.

Test Your Knowledge

1. Why is it essential that nurses should be familiar with healthcare policy and legislation?
2. Name one law that protects people with disabilities or chronic illnesses.

7.6. Innovations in Long-Term Care

Learning Outcome

1. Elaborate on the care delivery technology advancements
2. Clarify the community-based care models
3. Evaluate the impact of telehealth on long-term care

The future of long-term care is rapidly evolving, with significant influence from innovations that improve the quality and accessibility of care for individuals with disabilities and chronic illnesses. With the rise in the prevalence of diseases like Alzheimer's disease, which had an estimated 6.7 million Americans aged above 65 years in 2023, pioneering solutions to address the care needs of these patients are necessary (N/A, 2023). Technological advancements through the delivery of telehealth services have also become a vital tool by allowing medical professionals to deliver remote consultations and monitoring. This not only enhances patient access to specialized treatment but also alleviates the load for family caregivers, most of whom suffer from stress and potential health deterioration due to caregiving pressures (N/A, 2023). With the growing number of the elderly population, such innovations assume a critical role in developing long-term care solutions that are sustainable and accommodate both the needs of patients and the characteristics of healthcare systems. In addition, value-based models of care represent a core shift in how long-term care is treated, with a focus on improved health outcomes rather than the volume of services. The inclusion of SDoH screenings within Medicaid programs has further brought this transformation to the forefront, acknowledging the indivisible link between a patient's social circumstances and their health. By focusing on the whole person, encompassing both medical and social needs, long-term care can be better individualized, ultimately leading to a better quality of life for patients and increased efficiency in the healthcare system. Incentivized programs that encourage health care providers to screen for and treat SDoH contribute to a model of comprehensive care, particularly useful for vulnerable populations that endure extreme health disparities.

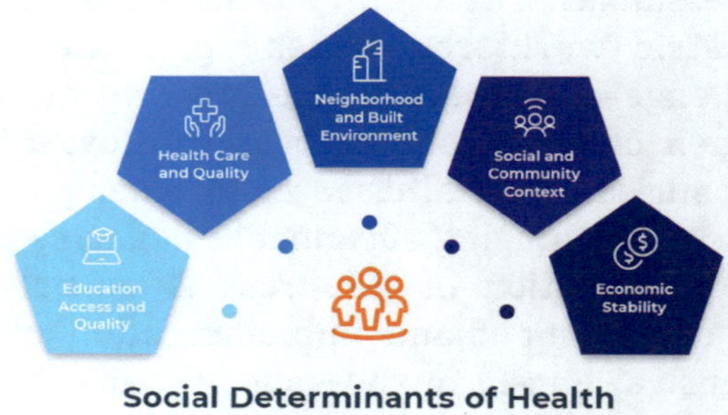

Figure 7.17. Integration of social determinants of health (SDoH).

Source: https://www.johnsnowlabs.com/wp-content/uploads/2023/03/img_blog.jpg.

This paradigm shift not only aligns with equitable healthcare practices but also addresses the challenge posed by controlling chronic diseases in a multicultural society. Furthermore, the role of technology integration in chronic care centers cannot be overstated. Technologies such as electronic health records (EHRs) and mobile health applications are being increasingly employed to facilitate ease of communication among healthcare providers and aid in more personalized care plans. These technologies enhance coordination and ensure that health workers are well-informed about a patient's medical history and current needs, particularly essential for patients with chronic diseases who may require multiple interdisciplinary approaches (N/A, 2023). The changing dynamics of long-term care, driven by technological innovation and policy changes, highlight the need to reimagine a system that values innovation and empathy. With the ever-evolving healthcare landscape, a continued focus on improving long-term care for individuals with disabilities and chronic illnesses remains crucial, promoting a better and more inclusive caregiving environment (N/A, 2023) (Figure 7.17).

7.6.1. Technological Advancements in Care Delivery

The integration of advances in technology into care delivery has brought about far-reaching change in the disability, chronic illness, and long-term care environments. New technologies such as telehealth systems and EHRs enable close monitoring and active management of the health status of patients. These technologies enable doctors to maintain constant contact with their patients, providing timely support and customized care plans tailored to their individual needs. These are valuable improvements, especially for individuals who have physical, psychiatric, and intellectual disability, since they lead to a more encompassing healthcare regime. The International Labour Organization emphasizes the importance of such advancements through its endeavors in empowering individuals with disabilities by providing them with access to appropriate healthcare services, which is closely aligned with their working wishes as described in foundational handbooks, such as the ILO Convention 159 (Gabriel et al., 2000). Furthermore, advancements in assistive technologies are recasting the way individuals with disabilities and chronic diseases engage with their environment. From independent living equipment to mobility-enhancing accessibility aids, these technologies not only facilitate day-to-day functioning but also feed a sense of autonomy. For instance, wearable healthcare monitoring systems can track vital signs and alert caregivers to potential health issues, thus acting as an essential safeguard for individuals with long-term illness. As recognition grows of just how effective these devices are, they are increasingly being integrated into long-term care planning to enable improved patient outcomes. It is worth noting that research has shown that these technological developments can counteract the previous dominance of disability by treating chronic diseases more effectively, leading to healthier, longer lives for those affected (Howell et al., 2025). Finally, technology's impact on care delivery extends beyond mere medical control, into domains of social support and community engagement. Mobile apps and online platforms provide disability support networks, offering opportunities for mutual aid and resource sharing. They can empower users by establishing relationships with peers, overcoming social isolation often experienced by chronic patients. Furthermore, employability-embedded assistive technologies also enhance the professional capabilities of people with disabilities, aligning with the ILO's commitment to using inclusive labor strategies. Alongside such developments, the ongoing innovation of such care delivery systems will increasingly enhance the quality of life and potential of persons living with ongoing health problems, ultimately changing the general public's perception of disability and chronic illness (Gabriel et al., 2000).

7.6.2. Community-based Care Models

Community models of care are increasingly being recognized as an effective strategy in addressing the needs of disabled individuals, chronic illness, and long-term care challenges. These models place a greater emphasis on localized care, which requires a merging of social and healthcare services in community settings. They thus not only promote greater accessibility but also strive to deliver more person-centered care, which is more applicable to individuals facing more complex health challenges. Its potential for health improvement is excellent, particularly among marginalized communities that have been exposed to the health disparities of accessing healthcare for a long time. The preventive and holistic care focus helps address the overall social determinants of health, thereby enhancing the community's overall wellbeing, while mitigating the tide of chronic disease and disability (N/A, 2025). Moreover, the effectiveness of community-based care models is also bolstered by the incorporation of strategies that facilitate inter-actor collaboration among various actors, such as health professionals, community organizations, and families. Through cooperation, a better-organized response to patients' complex needs can be achieved by tapping into the potential and capabilities of every actor within the community. Research shows that with these systems coordinating care effectively, it leads to optimized resource utilization and improved patient satisfaction. This coordination of efforts not only serves the current healthcare needs but also develops sustainable community infrastructures that can evolve with changing demographic trends, such as an aging population, hence striving towards long-term sustainability of care delivery models (N/A, 2001). In traversing the terrain of disability, long-term illness, and long-term care, policymakers and health administrators must make it their top priority to build supportive infrastructure for community-based care. This involves investing in workforce training, developing funding models that support preventive care, and implementing technological advancements that enhance communication among providers. A forward-looking strategy requires a commitment to enhancing the quality of care through measurable outcomes and developing leadership to drive systemic change. As explained in N/A (2025), making community care models responsive, effective, and flexible will be key to assisting individuals with disabilities and chronic diseases in achieving healthier, more productive lives in their communities (Figure 7.18).

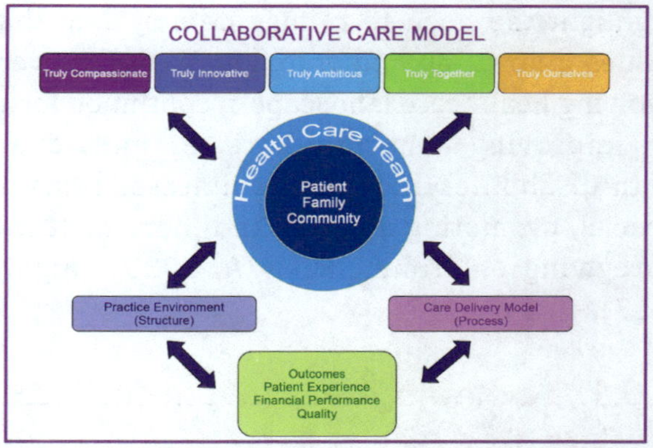

Figure 7.18. Collaborative care.

Source: https://dam.northwell.edu/m/41c20df28b7a4205/Drupal-web_Collaborative-Care-Model_NSUH.jpg.

7.6.3. The Impact of Telehealth on Long-Term Care

Having telehealth services as part of long-term care is a revolutionary opportunity for individuals with chronic illnesses and disabilities. Telehealth minimizes the barriers presented by geographical location and mobility problems by allowing remote consultations, which are often magnified in the lives of individuals with ongoing health conditions. It is pretty helpful for those living in rural areas, where specialist medical care might be limited. There is evidence to suggest that telehealth can improve health outcomes by offering stable monitoring and timely treatment, which is critical for patients with intricate chronic conditions to cope with. Specifically, studies have shown that telehealth can contribute to improved disease control and reduced hospital readmission rates, ultimately enhancing the quality of care delivered in the long run. The application of such technologies essentially reverses the approach to chronic illness management, promoting more patient-centered care in healthcare delivery. Furthermore, the impact of telehealth in long-term care is amplified by its potential to enhance the communication process between patients and healthcare providers. Effective communication is imperative in chronic disease management because it helps ensure that treatment plans are adjusted in a timely manner to address fluctuating health status. Through telehealth sites, health care professionals can easily communicate with patients and provide information, motivation, and counseling on self-management techniques, which are essential skills for individuals with chronic conditions. For instance, telehealth has been shown to significantly reduce emergency department use among poor homebound older adults with depression and chronic disease. With the use of telehealth, healthcare providers are better equipped to address the unique needs of medically frail groups and ultimately achieve improved overall health outcomes. This active reengineering of health communication in long-term care is a powerful key to continued effective management of chronic diseases. The economic impact of telehealth in long-term care should also be carefully watched, particularly within Medicaid systems. As the North Carolina Medicaid Reform project noted, the utilization of telehealth services can lead to a more efficient allocation of limited resources while concurrently addressing affordability gaps prevalent among low-income communities. Telemedicine can simplify care provision, ultimately reducing hospitalization and emergency care expenditures associated with poorly managed chronic conditions. Moreover, initiatives that enhance telehealth reimbursement and regulation can also significantly impact the expansion of access to essential services for individuals with disabilities. Expanding access and keeping costs under control, telehealth not only addresses budgetary challenges but also requires continued efforts towards achieving health equity. Effectively, telehealth integration within long-term care is symptomatic of an overarching policy intended to enhance the delivery of care and support health outcomes for individuals with disabilities and chronic ailments, thus influencing the future of healthcare access.

Test Your Knowledge

1. What is one technology innovation that improves the quality of care in long-term care facilities?
2. What is the role of person-centered care models in today's long-term care?

SUMMARY

The intricate dynamic of disability, long-term conditions, and long-term care underscores the necessity of comprehensive health care strategies that are responsive and sensitive to the distinct needs of populations. Understanding the intricate dynamics of multiple long-term conditions (MLTCs) in populations, particularly individuals with intellectual disabilities, unearths prime insights into trends in health and co-morbidities. For instance, research indicates high rates of mental illness throughout the adult lifespan for individuals with intellectual disabilities, reflecting several physical conditions, including gastrointestinal conditions, coexisting with mental health issues. Such an overlap leaves it glaringly apparent the pressing need for healthcare models that emphasize holistic approaches integrating solutions to physical and psychological health in various patient populations. In addition, the implementation of person-centered care models that empower patients to exercise self-care can significantly improve health outcomes among the population that requires long-term care for chronic conditions. One systematic review identifies the advantage of such models by highlighting correlations between self-care training and enhanced individual health metrics. By focusing on patient experience and involving them in decision-making about their care, healthcare providers can help foster a supportive care environment conducive to better management of chronic conditions. This paradigm shift is particularly important, as it not only promotes patient autonomy but also has long-term implications for reducing healthcare costs and improving the overall quality of care within long-term care settings. In summary, the implications of disability, chronic disease, and long-term care need to be addressed in a multifaceted approach that is empathetic as well as evidence-informed. Given the prevalence of MLTCs within at-risk populations, the embrace of self-care and mental health education strategies is crucial for enhancing outcomes. The findings of the latest research substantiate the idea that person-centered models and individually tailored interventions can lead to substantial health gains and improvements for individuals, their families, and healthcare systems as a whole. By acknowledging the individualized needs of individuals with disabilities and chronic disease, stakeholders can make sure that there is a more inclusive and functional long-term care setting that honors the dignity and self-determination of every individual.

Chronic disease and disability often create heavy burdens on the individual and family, particularly in the context of long-term care. The interplay between chronic health disease and disability emphasizes the necessity for the recognition of the unique needs of these populations. Emerging research demonstrates that elderly patients most frequently develop a multitude of physical, psychological, and cognitive issues following critical illness, which can significantly affect their quality of life and functional status. Of most concern are the multidimensional morbidities that such health crises can be preceded by. The repercussions are not just for the patients but also for their caregivers, who undergo heightened stress and emotional strain, often necessitating intervention involving the care of both the patient and the caretaker. Understanding of these dynamics is necessary for the formation of overall care plans that maximize the maintenance of quality of life and optimization of outcomes for the individuals involved and their families. Central to the response to disability and chronic illness is the recognition of long-term care as a central aspect of health strategy. As recognized in current evidence, interventions for enabling the recovery of geriatric patients from life-threatening illnesses must be multimodal, integrating into the baseline patient health trajectories. The research indicates that avoiding prolonged morbidity requires a multimodal and longitudinal approach, including continuous monitoring that helps inform treatment and care recommendations (Santangelo et al., 2024). These results reveal how the interconnected dimensions can lead to enhanced or worsened health outcomes, which directly impact not only recovery trends but also the quality of long-term care. Moreover, the importance of family involvement is brought into focus, as support mechanisms are a crucial aspect in ensuring the enhancement of recovery and the quality of life in the elderly suffering from chronic health conditions. In the field of chronic diseases, innovations in treatment modalities are also revolutionizing patient experiences and outcomes. For instance, treatments for conditions such as psoriatic arthritis (PsA) are demonstrating potential to significantly improve health-related quality of life (HRQoL) in patients. Current studies show that early clinical improvement is positively correlated with long-term benefit and social reintegration, reflecting a central goal of contemporary therapeutic procedures (Mcinnes et al., 2023). This also brings to the fore the implication that management of both physical and mental components of health is crucial when considering therapy for patients suffering from chronic diseases. By focusing on holistic management, incorporating early intervention and ongoing care, we can significantly enhance the quality of life for individuals with disabilities and long-term illnesses, underscoring the importance of considering these factors when planning long-term care.

KEY TERMS FROM THIS CHAPTER

Activities of Daily Living (ADLs)
Care Coordination
Chronic Disease Management
Disability Assessment
Instrumental Activities of Daily Living (IADLs)
Multidisciplinary Care
Patient Advocacy
Quality of Life (QoL)
Respite Care
Assistive Devices
Caregiver Burden
Chronic Pain
Home Health Care
Long-Term Care Facilities
Palliative Care
Psychosocial Support
Rehabilitation Services
Self-Management Support

CRITICAL THINKING QUESTIONS

1. **What is a chronic disease best described as?**
   a. A condition that will take a few days and will easily be cured
   b. A temporary condition that will require surgery
   c. A condition that will last forever but can be controlled, not cured
   d. A contagious disease that occurs rapidly
2. **What is the broad purpose of long-term care services?**
   a. Cure acute medical conditions
   b. Provide emergency medical treatment
   c. Help individuals with disabilities or chronic diseases with activities of daily living
   d. Give short-term rehabilitation
3. **Which law protects workers' rights with disabilities and public services?**
   a. Health Insurance Portability and Accountability Act (HIPAA)
   b. Patient Protection and Affordable Care Act
   c. Americans with Disabilities Act (ADA)
   d. Social Security Act
4. **Which of the following is a typical psychological consequence of having a chronic disease?**
   a. Increased immunity
   b. Improved physical endurance
   c. Depression and anxiety
   d. Enhanced cognitive function
5. **What is the place of rehabilitation in long-term care for disabled persons?**
   a. It provides short-term hospital stay for acute conditions
   b. It facilitates individuals to return to maximum attainable functioning and independence
   c. It is strictly concerned with medication compliance
   d. It eliminates the necessity for any personal care

Short Answer Questions

1. Define disability and provide an example.
2. What are two common issues faced by those with chronic illness?
3. List two goals of long-term care services.
4. What is the role of assistive devices in disability care?
5. List two government programs that serve individuals with chronic diseases or disabilities.
6. Explain the difference between acute and chronic illness with examples.
7. Describe the impact of long-term disability on mental well-being and interpersonal relationships.
8. Explain the principles and importance of person-centered care in long-term care facilities.

Answers to Critical Thinking Questions

1. (c) 2. (c) 3. (c) 4. (c) 5. (b)

REFERENCES

1. Doug, M., Adi, Y., Williams, J., Paul, M., Kelly, D., Petchey, R., & Carter, Y. H. (2009). Transition to adult services for children and young people with palliative care needs: a systematic review. *Archives of Disease in Childhood, 96*(1), 78–84. https://doi.org/10.1136/adc.2009.163931Allan, L., Cooper, S. A., Hanlon, P., Macdonald, S., et al. (2018). Long-term condition management in adults with intellectual disability in primary care: A systematic review. https://core.ac.uk/download/153444579.pdf (accessed on 28th June 2025).
2. Appleman, L. I. (2018). Deviancy, dependency, and disability: The forgotten history of eugenics and mass incarceration. https://core.ac.uk/download/213020817.pdf (accessed on 28th June 2025).
3. Blyth, C., Byrnes, A., Ganley, M., Hernandez, D., Hudson, J., Loumidis, K., Lawn, S., et al. (2013). Disability employment services in Australia: A brief primer. https://core.ac.uk/download/14947685.pdf (accessed on 28th June 2025).
4. Bruce, M. L., Choi, N. G., Kunik, M. E., et al. (2012). Relationship between depressive symptom severity and emergency department use among low-income, depressed homebound older adults aged 50 years and older. https://core.ac.uk/download/211337832.pdf (accessed on 28th June 2025).
5. Burstrom, B., Clayton, S., Dahl, E., Diderichsen, F., et al. (2009). Helping chronically ill or disabled people into work: What can we learn from international comparative analyses? https://core.ac.uk/download/42136539.pdf (accessed on 28th June 2025).
6. Cano, F., Alves, E., João, A., Oliveira, H., Pinho, L., & Fonseca, C. (2023). A rapid literature review on the health-related outcomes of long-term person-centered care models in adults with chronic illness. *Frontiers in Public Health, 11*. https://www.semanticscholar.org/paper/037e6acf3af2e36a6aef980c7aa0466128c80420 (accessed on 28th June 2025).
7. Chopra, V., Flanders, S. A., O'Malley, M., Malani, A. N., & Prescott, H. C. (2020). Sixty-day outcomes among patients hospitalized with COVID-19. *Annals of Internal Medicine, 174*, 576–578. https://doi.org/10.7326/m20-5661 (accessed on 28th June 2025).
8. Cosma, G., Abakasanga, E., Kousovista, R., Shabnam, S., Kaur, N., Akbari, A., Kiani, R., et al. (2025). Comorbidity patterns and temporal associations of multiple long-term conditions in adults with intellectual disability: An observational study in the United Kingdom. https://www.semanticscholar.org/paper/d48cb9616adebc4b6bf6245d7d1cda8ebc4041aa (accessed on 28th June 2025).
9. De Souza, L. H., & Frank, A. O. (2001). Conservative management of low back pain. https://core.ac.uk/download/333411.pdf (accessed on 28th June 2025).
10. DePhillipo, N. N., Larson, C. M., O'Neill, O. R., & LaPrade, R. F. (2020). Guidelines for ambulatory surgery centers for the care of surgically necessary/time-sensitive orthopedic cases during the COVID-19 pandemic. *Journal of Bone and Joint Surgery, 102*, 933–936. https://doi.org/10.2106/jbjs.20.00489 (accessed on 28th June 2025).
11. Dhakal, U., Briceño, E., Sharma, U., Bogati, U., Sharma, A., Shrestha, L., Ghimire, D., et al. (2024). Health care systems and policies for older adults in Nepal: New challenges for a low-middle income country. *Discover Public Health, 21*. https://www.semanticscholar.org/paper/989e94285f40c4622e6d08a94d7db8a7169c3bbc (accessed on 28th June 2025).

12. Estes, C. L., Yeo, G. W., Molina, L. C., Plumb, M., Hernandez, M., Goldberg, S., Wallace, S. P., et al. (2007). Women, health and aging: Building a statewide movement. https://core.ac.uk/download/71355916.pdf (accessed on 28th June 2025).
13. Gabriel, P., & International Labor Office. (2000). Mental health in the workplace: Situation analyses, United States. https://core.ac.uk/download/5129345.pdf (accessed on 28th June 2025).
14. Garg, A., Homer, C. J., & Dworkin, P. H. (2019). Addressing social determinants of health: Challenges and opportunities in a value-based model. *Pediatrics, 143*. https://doi.org/10.1542/peds.2018-2355 (accessed on 28th June 2025).
15. Golinowska, S., & Sowa, A. (2012). Health status, functional limitations and disability: Changes in Poland. https://core.ac.uk/download/30436254.pdf (accessed on 28th June 2025).
16. Goodman, N., Livermore, G. A., O'Day, B., Stapleton, D., et al. (2007). The health care financing maze for working-age people with disabilities. https://core.ac.uk/download/5121173.pdf (accessed on 28th June 2025).
17. Grover, S., Gautam, S., Jain, A., Gautam, M., & Vahia, V. N. (2017). Clinical practice guidelines for the management of depression. *Indian Journal of Psychiatry, 59*, 34. https://doi.org/10.4103/0019-5545.196973 (accessed on 28th June 2025).
18. Henwood, M., Larkin, M., & Milne, A. (2017). Seeing the wood for the trees: Carer related research and knowledge: A scoping review. https://core.ac.uk/download/145186527.pdf (accessed on 28th June 2025).
19. Howell, B., Burton, J., & Wilson, S. (2025). Work and the disability transition in 20th century America. https://core.ac.uk/download/pdf/6607025.pdf (accessed on 28th June 2025).
20. Iorfino, F., Scott, E., Carpenter, J. S., Cross, S., Hermens, D. F., Killedar, M., Nichles, A., et al. (2019). Clinical stage transitions in persons aged 12 to 25 years presenting to early intervention mental health services with anxiety, mood, and psychotic disorders. *JAMA Psychiatry, 76*, 1167. https://doi.org/10.1001/jamapsychiatry.2019.2360 (accessed on 28th June 2025).
21. Khongboon, P. (2025). Elderly disability in Thailand: Recommendations for long-term care policies in the coming ERAS. https://www.semanticscholar.org/paper/4542be60e150200542d27c317eedfa1a54acaf10 (accessed on 28th June 2025).
22. Ko, K. A., Lee, B. A., Kim, Y. T., & Lee, J. S. (2024). Professional dental care and survival rates in long-term care recipients: A cohort study of 1 459 163 individuals in South Korea. *Gerontology, 42*, 216–224. https://www.semanticscholar.org/paper/9553debf7e49f467aafa82543b4db1e5b55e31fb (accessed on 28th June 2025).
23. Koyanagi, C. (2007). Learning from history: Deinstitutionalization of people with mental illness as precursor to long-term care reform. https://core.ac.uk/download/71348081.pdf (accessed on 28th June 2025).
24. Kusch, K., & Denton, M. (2025). Well-being throughout the senior years: An issues paper on key events and transitions in later life. https://core.ac.uk/download/pdf/6354730.pdf (accessed on 28th June 2025).
25. Liu, Y. C. (2024). Considerations of Taiwanese working carers on choosing long-term care services for relatives with disabilities. *Practice, 36*, 291–308. https://www.semanticscholar.org/paper/60a305e49746a08fb3fdc86feb74a623d6fa6bc9 (accessed on 28th June 2025).

26. Lwanga-Ntale, C. (2003). Chronic poverty and disability in Uganda. https://core.ac.uk/download/5124587.pdf (accessed on 28th June 2025).

27. Mair, F. S., Mercer, S. W., Simpson, R., Simpson, R., et al. (2018). Using normalization process theory to understand barriers and facilitators to implementing mindfulness-based stress reduction for people with multiple sclerosis. https://core.ac.uk/download/151208739.pdf (accessed on 28th June 2025).

28. Majchrowicz, B., Kowalczuk, K., & Tomaszewska, K. (2025). Acceptance of illness and quality of life of patients under long-term home nursing care. *Frontiers in Public Health, 13*. https://www.semanticscholar.org/paper/242ab2a203fd4bcdfde1f6bdd40a3d4a7e0fda84 (accessed on 28th June 2025).

29. Maslach, C., & Leiter, M. P. (2016). Understanding the burnout experience: Recent research and its implications for psychiatry. *World Psychiatry, 15*, 103–111. https://doi.org/10.1002/wps.20311 (accessed on 28th June 2025).

30. Pennington, A., Newbold, D., Yu, Y., White, J., Barr, B., & McHale, P. (2024). A systematic review of evidence on the effectiveness and health impacts of interventions to promote employment rates among people with chronic illness and disability in the UK and Ireland between 2003 and 2023. https://www.semanticscholar.org/paper/be3c42644464a94b89cefb9d7ab807a69fc451bc (accessed on 28th June 2025).

31. Piccenna, L., Pattuwage, L., Bragge, P., & Gruen, R. (2025). Optimizing support for informal carers of the long-term disabled to enhance resilience and sustainability. https://core.ac.uk/download/pdf/30672597.pdf (accessed on 28th June 2025).

32. Reynolds, F. (1997). Coping with chronic illness and disability through creative needlecraft. https://core.ac.uk/download/334645.pdf (accessed on 28th June 2025).

33. Reynolds, J. M. (2017). Merleau-Ponty, world-creating blindness, and the phenomenology of non-normate bodies. https://core.ac.uk/download/159074133.pdf (accessed on 28th June 2025).

34. Rice, A., & Richman, B. D. (2017). N.C. Medicaid reform: A bipartisan path forward. https://core.ac.uk/download/84098969.pdf (accessed on 28th June 2025).

35. Santangelo, E., Wozniak, H., & Herridge, M. (2024). Meeting complex multidimensional needs in older patients and their families during and beyond critical illness. *Current Opinion in Critical Care, 30*, 479–486. https://www.semanticscholar.org/paper/d9cce4ce31e802e0d931c1de4ebbe24b3e041bc7 (accessed on 28th June 2025).

36. Smedley, C., Fisher, K., Wong, M., Kayess, R., & Bates, S. (2014). Arthritis and disability. https://core.ac.uk/download/pdf/30673486.pdf (accessed on 28th June 2025).

37. Udeh, K. C., & Menne, H. L. (2025). Impact of adult day service on long-term care placement: A scoping review. *Dementia*. https://www.semanticscholar.org/paper/ea4610b72d9ed350224f80760e0837b5edcb4592 (accessed on 28th June 2025).

38. van Blarikom, E., Fudge, N., & Swinglehurst, D. (2025). Living "out of the loop": Unemployment in the context of long-term illness. *Anthropology of Work Review*. https://www.semanticscholar.org/paper/f414441c11d288f0dafcee5e7c31445954b1f235 (accessed on 28th June 2025).

8

GENETICS AND GENOMICS IN NURSING PRACTICE

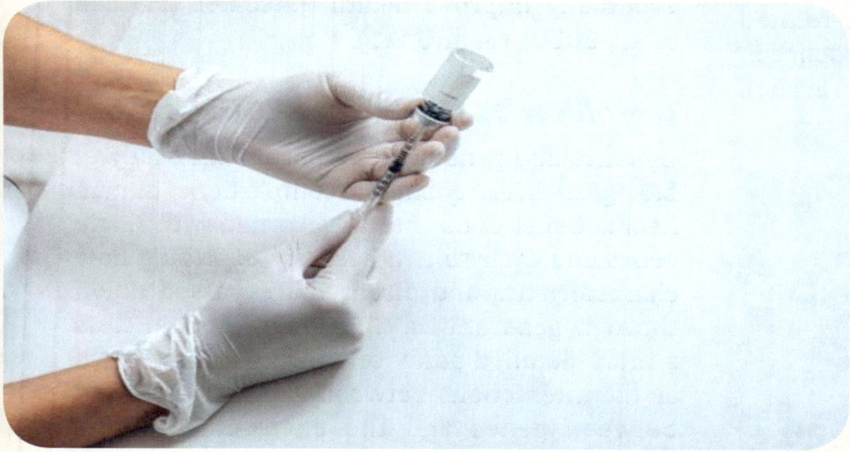

LEARNING OBJECTIVES

After studying this chapter, you will be able to:

1. Attempt the history of genetics in nursing
2. Expound on the genetic testing and implications
3. Explain the genomic medicine and patient care
4. Highlight the nursing roles in genetic research
5. Learn about education and training in genetics for nurses
6. Enunciate the future trends in genetics and genomics in nursing

Introduction

As the healthcare landscape continues to evolve, the role of genetics and genomics in nursing practice has become increasingly vital. Genetic and genomic literacy, with an understanding of the human genome, inheritance patterns, mutations, and their effects on health, is central to current nursing education and practice. Although significant, some evidence demonstrates that few nursing curricula adequately prepare graduates to address genomic health issues. The outcome of a DNP project highlights this imbalance, illustrating that advanced practice nurse students show slight improvement in genomics literacy despite targeted education interventions. Thus, this indicates the pressing need for an integrated and stringent curriculum that promotes genome-based education in nursing education, thereby enabling future nurses to acquire the necessary competencies to integrate genetic knowledge into patient care (Palomera et al., 2023). Genomic competency is one such fundamental role contributed by nurses, but practically, they are primarily unable to apply genomic information. These difficulties are rooted in a variety of sources, some of which include a lack of preparation through their education and training, and insufficient supportive resources after graduation. Research has determined that obstacles, such as adequate knowledge and inadequate access to geneticists, present barriers to nurses providing ideal genomic care. Furthermore, although attempts at education aim to bridge the gaps, they are frequently ineffective, suggesting that genomic-related knowledge and skills should take precedence in nursing education through curriculum revision (Hassen et al., 2020).

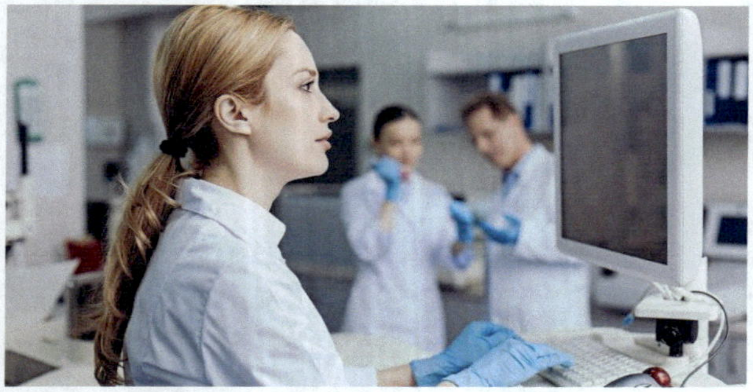

Figure 8.1. Nurses using genomics and genetics in healthcare.

Source: https://s3.amazonaws.com/utep-uploads/wp-content/uploads/DUQ-MIG/2018/07/03102032/Nurse-working-at-computer.jpg.

These issues need to be solved if patient care is to become enhanced and the nursing profession is to be capable of using genetic information judiciously. The need to incorporate genetics and genomics into nursing practice is also aided by the shift in the healthcare sector to individualized medicine. With increased individualized care, genetic inclinations will allow nurses to tailor interventions that respond to specific patient needs. The HCG model is one of the frameworks used to underscore the connection of genetics, education, clinical testing, and the ethical considerations of genomic information. This model requires nurses not only to possess knowledge but also to have critical thinking skills, in order to navigate ethical dilemmas surrounding genetic testing and therapeutic decisions. With this integrative process of nursing and education, the profession can look forward to an improved capacity to respond to the dangers posed by an increasingly genetically diverse patient population and eventually improve health outcomes (Hassen et al., 2020) (Figure 8.1).

Definition of Genetics and Genomics

Genetics and genomics are part of the study of biological diversity and the complexity of human health. Genetics has been concerned with single genes and their role in heredity, exploring how characteristics and diseases are passed down through generations. Conversely, genomics is a more detailed study of entire genomes, such as the interactions between various genes and between genes and the environment. This shift from genetics to genomics represents a fundamental evolution in our capacity to analyze complex biological data, thereby enhancing diagnostic accuracy and therapeutic approaches to disease in clinical practice. With the growing body of science in these fields, the importance to nursing practice increases even further since nurses stand ready to apply this knowledge to patient care and to interdisciplinary teams for improved health outcomes. Of particular interest, the advent of genomics addresses the needs of healthcare in the modern era in such a way that nursing practitioners must have an understanding of genetic principles and the application of genomic technologies. The latest studies have underscored the significance of genetic counseling and multidisciplinary teams in delivering personalized patient care (Norris et al., 2015). The integration of genomic information into nursing practice enables improved risk assessment and targeted interventions. However, the education of nurses regarding the subtleties of genomics remains a priority. For example, one survey revealed that a significant percentage of public health professionals reported varying degrees of comprehension regarding genetic testing and its role in care provision (Baccolini et al., 2020). Thus, providing nurses with the appropriate genomic literacy puts them in a position to champion patient-centered care while also navigating the intricate ethical complexities inherent in genetic information. As genetic and genomic knowledge evolves, it is increasingly critical that nursing education covers these subjects comprehensively. Nurses, by learning about definitions and consequences of genetics and genomics, will be in the best position to engage in collaborative decision-making with patients regarding their genetic health data. This competence is important and vital in patient populations who may be at higher risk for genetic disease, highlighting nurses' educational role within health care teams. Furthermore, as genomic services are increasingly demanded, nurses' ability to interpret and explain genetic findings will significantly enhance their contribution to the clinical setting. Hence, it is clear that incorporating genetics and genomics into nursing education and practice is critical not only for developing nursing competencies but also for enhancing overall patient care outcomes within the context of personalized medicine.

Importance of Genetics in Healthcare

The incorporation of genetics within healthcare represents a revolutionary change in the etiology and control of diseases. It enables health professionals to personalize interventions with a patient's individual genetic makeup, leading to tailored care that optimizes patient outcomes. In practice nursing, empathy and sensitivity towards genetic factors can significantly contribute to the quality of care delivered. For instance, nurses with education on genetic testing are best placed to advise patients on preventive factors and potential health hazards and, therefore, empower patients to make optimal healthcare choices. Moreover, developing a framework that enables patients to receive information about their genetic predispositions also facilitates the proactive management of health, thereby supporting the pivotal role genetics plays in disease management and prevention in healthcare plans (Baccolini et al., 2020). The need for greater genetic education among nursing practitioners cannot be overstressed, as evolving genomic technologies are revolutionizing how patient care is managed. Evidence-based history reveals that many nursing professionals lack knowledge about the contribution of genetics to healthcare (Burton et al., 2013). This gap represents a gigantic public health problem, as poor knowledge can hinder proper integration of genomics and genetic testing into patients' care guidelines.

By incorporating genetic education into the curriculum, future healthcare professionals can develop the skills necessary to address emerging healthcare needs. Greater proficiency in genetics could lead to a more comprehensive assessment of patient histories and presentation, enabling nurses to locate and incorporate vital information to offer suitably personalized interventions. Furthermore, the application of genetics in healthcare extends beyond individual case treatment to encompass public health programs. According to research among public health professionals, there is high demand but significant knowledge gap when it comes to genetic factors influencing population health (Baccolini et al., 2020).

To maximize the potential of genomic data for public health, nursing practice must transform to incorporate genetic information into global health assessments and interventions. Through cooperative ventures with multidisciplinary groups, nurses can advocate for policies that promote genetic screening and counseling, ensuring equal access to genomic data for diverse populations. Ultimately, the successful incorporation of genetics in healthcare relies on the cooperative action of nursing experts to engage in continuous education and promote interdisciplinary collaboration, focusing on both individual and community well-being (Figure 8.2).

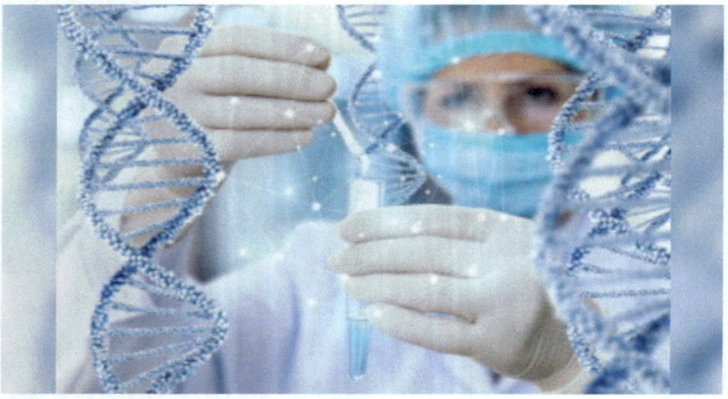

Figure 8.2. Importance of genetics in healthcare.

Source: https://pediatrics.queensu.ca/sites/pediatrics/files/gbb-uploads/Untitled%20design%20(14)-abe1r5.png.

Overview of the Nursing Function in Genetics and Genomics

The nursing function in genetics and genomics is becoming increasingly significant as healthcare moves toward precision medicine, thereby emphasizing nurses' understanding of genetic concepts. Nurses are main facilitators of the interpretation of genetic information, education, and decision support to aid patients in making evidence-based decisions regarding their health. This diverse role has a wide-ranging set of responsibilities, including family history assessments, identifying patients who require genetic counseling, and integrating genomic information into care plans. As complex as genetics is, and as profound as the implications of treatment and prognosis, integration of genetic data into nursing practice is the cornerstone of delivering excellent patient care and initiating an integrative approach to health management. Despite the expanding contribution of genetics to nursing practice, research has shown that nurses often lack the necessary preparation to incorporate genomics into their practice. In a quality improvement project identifying obstacles to incorporating genetics into nursing practice, educational lack and confidence were among the significant obstacles confronting nurses in this field. A survey of the Ozarks Veterans Healthcare System revealed a discrepancy between expected competencies and actual knowledge levels among nurses. This is evidence of the critical need for more educational interventions and supportive systems to offer nurses the necessary genomic literacy. These kinds of projects are essential to facilitate enhanced patient outcomes and ensure nurses can manage comfortably the evolving world of genetics within healthcare, as outlined in the Essential Nursing Competencies and Curricula Guidelines for Genetics and Genomics, which provide expectations for nursing education across any specialty or level of preparation (Guillory et al., 2022). To address the identified gaps in genetic and genomic education, nursing curricula at institutions of higher learning should include specialized training on these essential topics. Evidence suggests that current faculty lack the necessary knowledge to adequately teach genetics and genomics, which contributes to the inadequate preparedness among nursing students (Palomera et al., 2023). Recent attempts to increase genetic literacy have met with limited success, underscoring the need for more effective education methods tailored to varying degrees of nursing education. Broad-based training programs and the development of a robust genomic nursing curriculum will be crucial in enhancing nursing competency in this field. By prioritizing genetics education for nurses, the field can become a dynamic influence on patient care, ultimately enabling nurses to become knowledgeable patient advocates for those with complex genetic health issues.

8.1. Historical Context of Genetics in Nursing

Learning Outcome

1. Describe the evolution of genetic knowledge in medicine
2. Identify milestones in genetic research impacting nursing
3. Discuss the integration of genetics in nursing education

The development of genetics in nursing reflects a transformative progress that parallels progress in the biological sciences and technology. The function of genetics in nursing practice has changed from an ancillary to a central focus. During the early period, nurses were often not formally educated regarding genetic principles, which limited their ability to provide care that addressed the genetic aspects of patient care. With the growth of knowledge of genetic disorders through the 20th century, the demand for nursing practitioners to learn about genetic principles also increased. This led to the development of advanced nursing roles and educational structures that aim to equip nurses with the knowledge needed to manage complex genetic information competently. Therefore, this progress has led to a generation of nurses trained to integrate genetics into patient assessments, thereby providing personalized care based on genetic information. Throughout the latter half of the 20th century, collaboration within healthcare gained increasing importance, particularly in genetic counseling. This discipline emerged as a response to the growing need for patient education regarding hereditary diseases and the implications of genetic testing. The emphasis on collaboration among health workers, including clinical geneticists, nurses, and genetic counselors, has been crucial in delivering effective genetic services. As the evidence in a longitudinal study of service delivery in the UK demonstrates, explicit variations were revealed in the management of genetic referrals by clinical geneticists and genetic counselors. These findings underscore the distinct contributions of each professional in facilitating informed decision-making for patients with genetic conditions (Norris et al., 2015). Such collaboration underscores the pivotal role of nursing within multidisciplinary teams, enabling holistic care that incorporates genetic considerations. The context of genetics within nursing practice is also embodied in community-based interventions that seek to promote genetic literacy. Projects such as the "Talking Glossary of Genomics Terminology," intended for American Indian communities, reflect the importance of culturally appropriate genetic literacy.

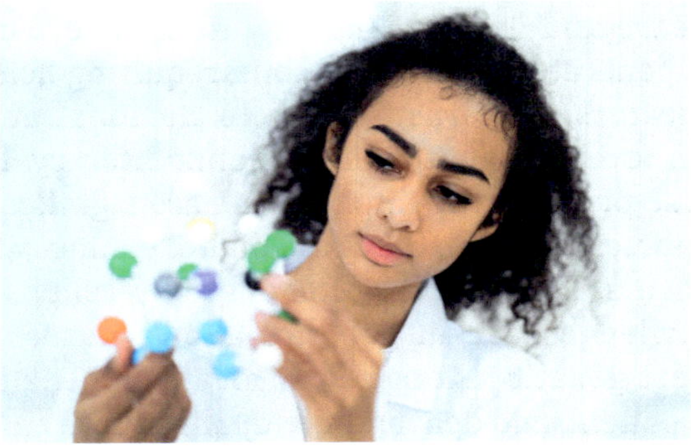

Figure 8.3. Genetics nursing.

Source: https://res.cloudinary.com/orbis-education/image/fetch/f_auto,q_auto/dpr_auto/https://findnursingschools.com/app/uploads/2022/06/Genetics-Nursing.jpg.

Not only does this innovative tool enhance genetics literacy, but it also addresses health disparity gaps that impact disadvantaged groups. With the use of multimedia technology, such projects help close the gap between complex genetic information and community understanding, thereby enabling patients to make informed health decisions. Also, the collaboration of various stakeholders, including educational institutions and health agencies, has made educational resources available and usable across diverse populations (Coe et al., 2012). These earlier initiatives have laid the groundwork for contemporary nursing practice regarding genetic education and advocacy, opening doors to more inclusive healthcare (Figure 8.3).

8.1.1. Evolution of Genetic Understanding in Medicine

Revolutionary advancements have dramatically influenced the history of genetic information in medicine in the field of genomic science. The conclusion of the Human Genome Project in 2003 marked a significant turning point, enabling physicians to better comprehend the intricacies of human DNA and its role in disease and health. This new field of research has generated a paradigm shift, requiring health educators and practitioners to demonstrate a high level of genetic and genomic literacy. For nurse practice, the implications are significant, as nurses are often the first point of contact with patients. Thus, the creation of a comprehensive knowledge base in genetics allows nurses to assess genetic risk better, advocate on behalf of the patient, and deliver individualized care based on genetic risk, ultimately improving patient outcomes and healthcare efficiency. However, a significant disparity remains in education and expertise regarding genetic knowledge among healthcare providers, particularly nurses and allied health professionals. As are documented in recent opinion surveys, physician assistants (PAs) themselves are not feeling suitably prepared to incorporate genetic and genomic thought into patient care. Outcomes of these assessments indicate that while some genetics content is being added to training programs, variability and limited exposure continue to challenge the effectiveness of education in this critical area. Without adequate training, healthcare professionals struggle to handle the complexities of genomics in practice, making it crucial to reform the curriculum to enhance genetic training and ensure that all medical professionals are prepared to address the evolving challenges of genomic care (Patterson et al., 2022). Furthermore, similar trends in other areas of healthcare, such as speech-language pathology, reflect the need to address educational deficits in genetics and genomics. Speech-language pathology program directors recognize the importance of genetic literacy, but there is a substantial disparity between projected competencies and actual readiness of graduates. This inequality suggests that while advances in genetics could influence clinical practice, many healthcare providers lack the necessary knowledge to utilize these advances optimally. To cultivate an educated and engaged healthcare provider, it is essential to implement comprehensive education reforms that incorporate genetics and genomics into healthcare training. Last but not least, through this, nurses and other healthcare providers will be empowered to confidently and competently apply genetic knowledge in practice, thereby enhancing patient care and advancing the integration of genetics into medicine (Leblanc et al., 2012) (Figure 8.4).

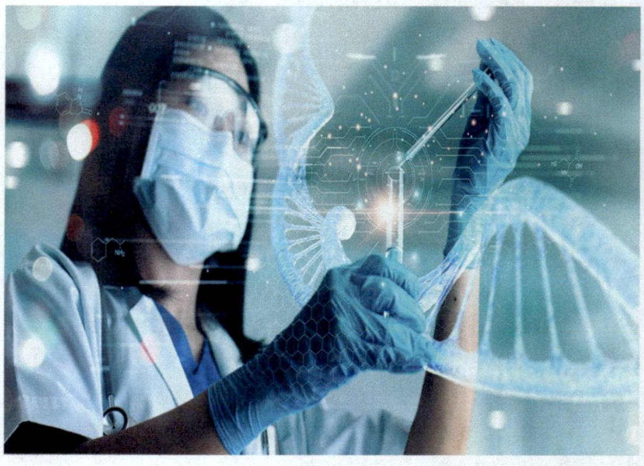

Figure 8.4. Transforming health care with genomics.

Source: https://healthenews.mcgill.ca/wp-content/uploads/2023/07/2023-07-06_Genome-Institute_1080x566.jpg.

8.1.2. Milestones in Genetic Research Impacting Nursing

Advances in genetic studies have had significant implications for nursing practice, particularly in patient assessment and intervention strategies. One critical landmark is the advancement in genetic testing technology, which has led to the development of precision medicine. Nurses are increasingly being called upon to interpret genetic information and formulate personalized care plans tailored to patients' genetic backgrounds. This change is observed in oncology nursing, with an understanding of genetic mutations affecting the treatment plan and the use for prognostic purposes. The advent of genomics-aware nursing policy, as evident in studies comparing US and UK guidelines, illustrates the need for education in nursing to accommodate such advancements. Here, nurses play a vital role in utilizing genetic information to deliver patient-centered care effectively by integrating technology and practice, ensuring that patients receive individualized education and intervention strategies tailored to their genetic background (Calzone et al., 2024). Yet another significant cornerstone in genetic research affecting nursing is the identification of the complex gene-environment interactions that are accountable for the majority of health disorders, such as Autism Spectrum Disorder (ASD). Studies have shown that environmental factors can significantly modify genetic risk to result in diverse clinical presentations among individuals with ASD. Nurses play a crucial role in understanding the nuances, as they must stay up-to-date with new genetic data to provide accurate information and support to families. Not only is this an early intervention and identification method, but also a method to make nurses vocal advocates for resources that facilitate genetic counseling and testing. By incorporating genetic knowledge into their practice, nurses are better equipped to address the multifaceted needs of patients and their families, ensuring they are offered the necessary interventions and support to achieve optimal outcomes (Johnson et al., 2013). The crossover between genomics and nursing practice is also illustrated by competency frameworks that have been created to guide genomics-informed care. These competency frameworks are essential for standardizing the integration of genomics into practice and ensuring nurses have the knowledge to function effectively in this new landscape. By promoting the policy of enhancing the education and training of nurses in genomics, institutions can ensure the incorporation of genetic awareness into the everyday practice of nursing. This includes the development of educational curricula that utilize genetic literacy, enabling nurses to engage patients in discussions regarding their genetic well-being actively. The integration of nursing competencies with genomic data ultimately enhances the quality of practice, enabling nurses not only to provide patient care but also to be prepared to lead the genomics-informed healthcare sector, thereby fostering a culture of safety and equality in nursing practice (Calzone et al., 2024).

8.1.3. The Integration of Genetics into Nursing Education

The integration of genetics within nursing education is an urgent need in current healthcare, primarily due to the rapid advancement of genomic sciences. Nurses, being instructors and caregivers, have an ethical obligation to be aware of the potential of genetic and genomic information for patient care. Not only does this enhance patient outcomes, but it also improves the ability for individualized interventions based on genetic risk. However, research indicates that many nurses feel they are not sufficiently prepared to handle genetic information with confidence (Guillory et al., 2022). A well-staged plan for integrating genetics in nursing education is essential. Guided training can equip nurses with the knowledge and skills required to act as integral bridges between patient care and genetic information. Moreover, educational models have been developed to address the challenges that accompany genomic healthcare. A revised framework based on a consensus model emphasizes the importance of adapting educational models to meet the modern requirements of education in genomics and genetics (Burton et al., 2013). The framework assigns great importance to essential skills such as follow-up care and advocacy, which are paramount for nursing practice today. By applying real case studies and stakeholder feedback, nursing education can be made more responsive to the genetic needs of diverse populations. The direct involvement of nursing leaders in such educational transformation will guarantee that nurses attain competence that will enable them to effectively deal with genetic disorders as well as provide holistic patient care. Moreover, the challenges faced by nursing specialists in genetics highlight the importance of ongoing professional development and support. Nurses have also identified barriers, including a lack of sufficient knowledge, self-efficacy, and resources, in the implementation of genetic information in patient care (Guillory et al., 2022). As genetics continues to play an increasingly prominent role in determining health outcomes, assume a leadership role in genetics and genomics preparation within its core curriculum. The integration of genetics into nursing education not only prepares nurses with the knowledge to meet immediate healthcare needs but also instills in them a culture of lifelong learning and development. Ultimately, this assures nurses can better manage the complexities of genetic information, thereby enhancing the quality of care delivered in the clinical setting (Figure 8.5).

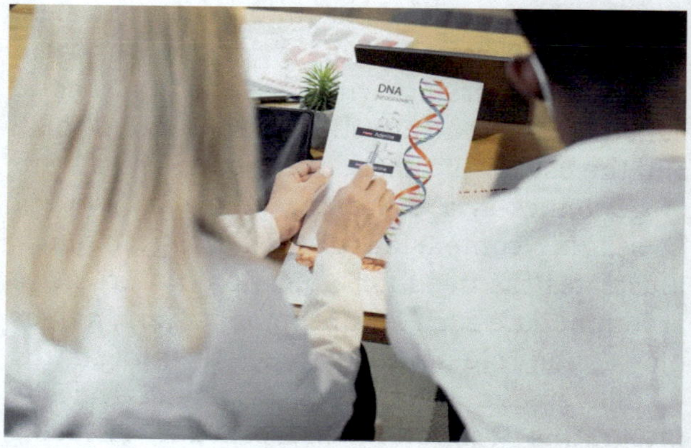

Figure 8.5. Integration of genetics into nursing education.

Source: https://elitenp.com/wp-content/uploads/2023/04/multiracial-genetics-having-meeting-about-gene-engineering-1024x682.jpg.

Test Your Knowledge

1. What is the role of a nurse in genetic education and counseling?
2. How can family history be used to assess genetic risk in nursing practice?

8.2. Genetic Testing and Its Implications

Learning Outcome

1. Describe the types of genetic tests that are available
2. Define the ethical questions in genetic testing
3. Discuss nurses' roles in genetic counseling

The integration of genetic testing into nursing practice is a revolutionary shift in healthcare that has far-reaching implications for patient care and professional practice. Because genomics is an expanding field, nursing professionals must stay current with developments to provide informed, accurate, and compassionate care. The importance of empowering nurses with a firm understanding of genetic principles cannot be overstated, as it is directly linked to their ability to inform patients about genetic test choices, interpretations, and outcomes. Understanding the nuances of genetic testing fosters a reflective process of patient advocacy, enabling nurses to effectively address the ethical dilemmas and psychosocial impacts of genetic information on families and individuals. Moreover, paradigms of nursing education must be altered to incorporate advancements in genomics and genetics. Traditional practices in nursing education overlook the rapid advancements in genetic knowledge and their implications for practice. A reformed curriculum with integrative omics education is called for, as outlined in recent articles that request these ideas be introduced into PhD curricula in nursing (Anderson et al., 2015). Educating future nursing leaders with a strong background in genetics will enable instructors to prepare new generations of nurses to apply this information in diverse clinical environments, ultimately enhancing patient outcomes. This educational change is not only necessary at the individual level but also crucial for the professional advancement of nurses in addressing modern healthcare demands. In addition to educational change, professional advancement in genetics through ongoing education is needed for practicing nurses in order to remain effective practitioners. The rapidly evolving nature of genetic testing technology, including pharmacogenomics and predictive analytics, necessitates an ongoing commitment to learning and adaptation. Nurses must receive continuous education that addresses the competencies required in dealing with the diverse needs of patients seeking genetic testing (Burton et al., 2013). This includes knowledge of the ethical considerations and implications of genetic data, as well as the advocacy role nurses play in ensuring the well-being of patients following genetic testing. Ultimately, the integration of genetic testing into nursing practice is contingent upon a comprehensive strategy that encompasses education, continuous professional development, and ethical preparedness to adapt to this rapidly evolving profession (Figure 8.6).

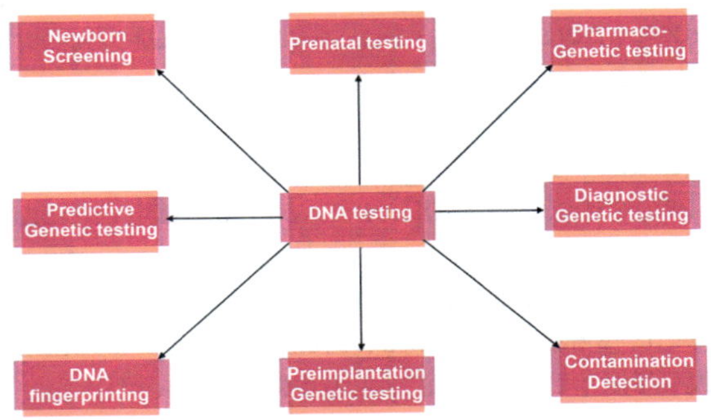

Figure 8.6. Genetic testing.

Source: https://geneticeducation.co.in/wp-content/uploads/2019/10/genetic-testing-.004-e1569989548382-768x490.jpeg.

8.2.1. Types of Genetic Tests Available

Genetic testing has undergone significant development, offering various techniques that cater to multiple clinical needs. Diagnostic tests, which aim to diagnose or confirm a specific genetic disease, are among the most common types of tests. These tests are beneficial when symptoms are indicative of a genetic disorder so that early treatments and management could be initiated. There is also predictive testing, which identifies susceptibility to the development of a genetic disorder in the future. This comes in useful in disorders like Huntington's disease, where early diagnosis could direct lifestyle changes and family planning. In addition, carrier testing indicates whether individuals carry a gene for a recessive condition, which is useful for couples planning to have children. All these types of tests are essential in the field of genetics and genomics in nursing practice, providing tailored patient care and focused health measures. Along with diagnostic, predictive, and carrier testing, pharmacogenomic tests are increasingly used in the field of genetics. These tests examine the impact of genetic makeup on an individual's response to specific medications. With tailored drug prescriptions based on an individual's genetics, health practitioners can optimize therapeutic benefits while minimizing drug side effects. For instance, drug-metabolizing gene variant testing helps in guiding the choice of drugs to treat mental illness, cancer, and other diseases. Consequently, pharmacogenomic testing holds the promise of shifting pharmacotherapy from an empiric, one-size-fits-all approach towards more personalized care. This becomes particularly pertinent in the realm of nursing practice, where genetic data can enhance patient safety and outcomes, illustrating the growing interconnection of genetics with clinical decision-making. Lastly, newborn screening represents a valuable application of genetic testing for the early diagnosis of congenital disorders. This proactive process enables the identification of genetic disorders that are curable if detected early, such as phenylketonuria (PKU) or cystic fibrosis. A few states require newborn screening programs to ensure that infants are screened shortly after birth, allowing for early interventions that can significantly alter their health trajectories. In reality, the implications of finding genetic disease in newborns extend past the resultant health considerations in terms of immediate health, such as long-term care needs and family healthcare management. As nursing professionals grapple with the complexities of such genetic issues, they constitute an essential component of not only coordinating testing but also educating families on the applicability of such tests and the implications of healthcare that ensue, hence making the core connection between genetics and nursing practice authoritative (Figure 8.7).

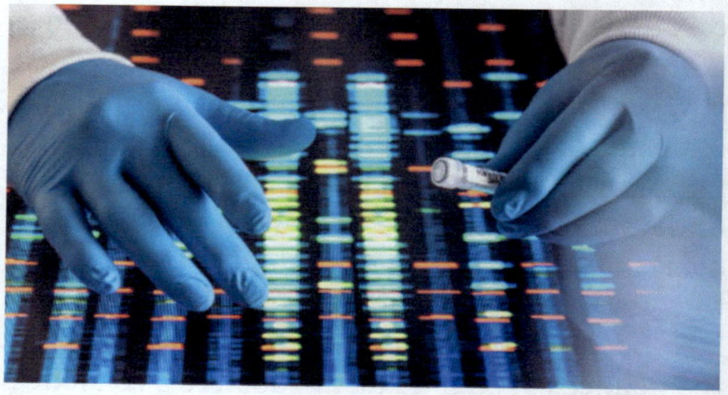

Figure 8.7. The role of pharmacogenomic testing in precision medicine.

Source: https://external-content.duckduckgo.com/iu/?u=https%3A%2F%2Fwww.cvshealth.com%2Fcontent%2Fdam%2Fenterprise%2Fcvs-enterprise%2Fimages%2Fingestion%2F2021-3%2Fcvs-health-the-role-of-pharmacogenomic-testing-in-precision-medicine-1-16x9.jpg&f=1&nofb=1&ipt=55d1ed9b0f90c587b78411bd2ab2aded25742256369c6f82e3710f1633302ab1.

8.2.2. Ethical Considerations in Genetic Testing

Ethical issues are at the heart of genetic testing, particularly as the direct-to-consumer genetic testing market continues to expand. Increasing access to personal genomics services raises significant concerns regarding informed consent, data privacy, and the potential for the abuse of genetic information. Patients requesting genetic testing may not be aware of the test's consequences, especially in the absence of genetic counseling. Pre- and post-test genetic counseling must be an integral part of such services to facilitate informed choices and worry reduction regarding possible health outcomes. Furthermore, genetic counselors' visibility across various sites is evidence of a shift in their professional roles, from teachers to risk interpreters and lifestyle guides, signifying that they ought to be brought into the spotlight regarding their functions within the evolving market of genetic testing (Harris et al., 2012). The implications of widespread carrier screening further complicate the moral aspects of genetic testing. While ECS provides a single process for screening multiple genetic disorders simultaneously, it is flawed as a measure of whether or not an individual should be screened, as opposed to couples. Ethical concerns also surface when considering informed consent, particularly with outside pressures potentially influencing future parents' decisions to test. This serves to highlight the necessity of genetic counseling, as individuals are fully informed of their choices and are not influenced to undergo testing. Furthermore, the ethical principle of adequate counseling emphasizes the ethical obligation to facilitate autonomous decision-making in reproductive contexts. Resolving these problems is crucial to implementing ECS ethically in healthcare settings, with an emphasis on the wellbeing of individuals and their families (Borry et al., 2017). Last but not least, the ethical context of genetic screening is relevant also to the broader contexts of nursing practice. Nurses play a crucial role in educating patients about genetic testing and its implications, drawing on a thorough understanding of ethical principles. Professional nurses must navigate sensitive situations, including confidentiality, patient autonomy, and the psychological impact of test results. Furthermore, ethical principles should guide the provision of genetic testing services to ensure that all patients, particularly marginalized groups who may require support to access testing, have equal access and support. Through a patient-centered model of genetic testing, nurses can help minimize ethical challenges and help patients make informed, voluntary choices about these services. Ultimately, responsible integration of genomics into practice depends on continuing the ethics dialogue on genetic testing (Figure 8.8).

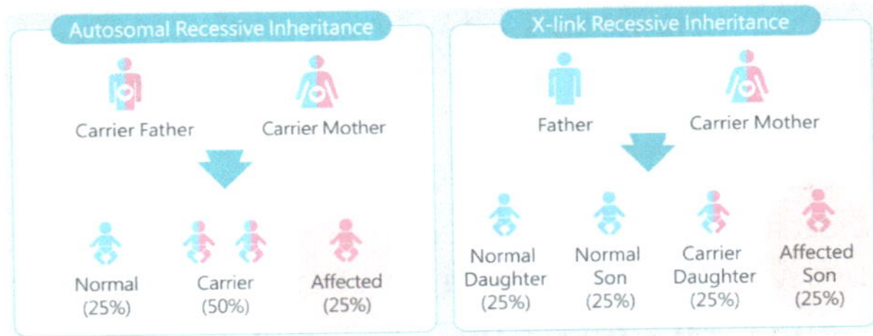

Figure 8.8. Expanded carrier screening.

Source: https://www.ggasia.com.my/wp-content/uploads/2021/01/Expanded-Carrier-Screening-1.png.

8.2.3. The Role of Nurses in Genetic Counseling

The evolving genetics and genomics landscape significantly increases the role of the nurse in genetic counseling. As guardians of primary healthcare, nurses bridge patients with multifaceted genetic information to the complex terrain of genetic testing and subsequent repercussions. Their functions extend far beyond mere information dissemination; nurses have the burden of assessing individual patient requirements, understanding family patterns of inheritance, and counseling through the testing phase. Their specialized role within the healthcare team enables them to explain complex genetic concepts in simple terms, ultimately allowing patients to make informed decisions about their health. As more individuals undergo genetic testing, the need for highly qualified nursing staff with specialized expertise in the field becomes paramount in ensuring patient comprehension and adherence to care schedules. In a recent study on the collaborative function of genetic services, results have shown that non-medical genetic counselors, including nurses, play a role in patient communication and overall service delivery. Genetic counselors represented 95% of all contact with patients according to the statistics, with a complete 50% of new patients seen by nurses or genetic counselors as lead clinical professionals. This highlights their role in managing patient load and ensuring continuity of care. The research highlights the need for interdisciplinary interaction, indicating that nurses have the necessary ability to promote communication, ensure smooth referral processes, and be involved in holistic management of genetic health. With increasing numbers of patients, the integration of nursing professionals into genetic counseling not only enhances care but also facilitates the delivery of services in genetic clinics, making it a key component of contemporary healthcare practice (Norris et al., 2015). Furthermore, genomic information use in the care of patients necessitates that nurses acquire a solid foundation of knowledge of genomics and its applications in the clinic. Advances in DNA sequencing present both opportunities and challenges, necessitating that nursing practitioners be proficient in handling complex datasets to interpret them accurately. By taking proactive roles in counseling patients about their genomic information and its implications for their health, nurses depersonalize genetic concerns. This shift encompasses the entire process, from the initiation of genetic testing through to post-test counseling and intervention planning, aligning with the goal of providing enhanced patient-centered care. As the evidence presented indicates, nurses' ability to translate genomic information into actionable recommendations plays a central role in achieving enhanced genetic counseling outcomes, thereby ensuring their pivotal position in multidisciplinary healthcare teams (Hickey et al., 2017).

Test Your Knowledge

1. What are the risks and benefits of genetic testing in patients and families?
2. How does genetic testing influence disease prevention, diagnosis, or treatment decisions?

8.3. Genomic Medicine and Patient Care

Learning Outcome

1. Explain the personalized medicine and its advantages thereof
2. Define the case studies demonstrating applications of genomic medicine
3. Explain the problems in applying genomic medicine in nursing

The integration of genomic medicine into clinical care represents a paradigm shift in healthcare practice, with a focus on the accuracy and personalization of treatment strategies. This shift is especially pertinent to nursing practice where understanding and incorporation of genetic data has a direct bearing on patients' outcomes. Nurses play a pivotal role in interpreting and translating genomic information to patients. By bridging the gap between complex genetic data and understanding, nurses enhance genomic literacy access so that patients are informed and empowered to make appropriate decisions regarding their health. The incorporation of genomics into nursing education plays a significant role in fulfilling the need for a workforce adept at deciphering the complexities of genetic information, hence empowering nurses to offset the disadvantage of an increasingly complex healthcare environment (Conley et al., 2015). Furthermore, genomic medicine has significant implications for the complex patient population, as it provides for tailored treatment and prevention. Genetic screening could reveal disease predispositions, facilitating targeted intervention capable of preventing or reducing the occurrence of disease. However, the current healthcare system is being tested by the lack of access to genetic services, particularly in underrepresented populations. This background highlights the importance of nurses lobbying for equitable access to genomic resources and promoting initiatives that enhance patient health literacy.

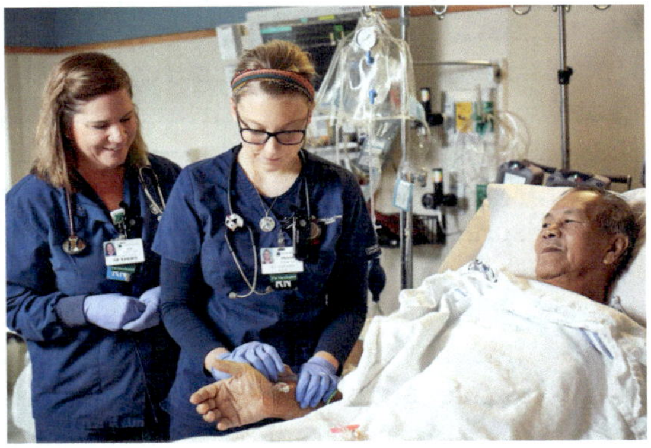

Figure 8.9. Genomic medicine and patient care.

Source: http://news.christianacare.org/wp-content/uploads/2015/01/Cover-story_1.jpg.

As principal providers of healthcare, nurses can advance initiatives to integrate genomic information into daily care, enabling all patients to benefit from advancements in precision medicine (Bastola et al., 2019). Ultimately, the effective integration of genomic medicine into clinical care relies on ongoing education and interprofessional collaboration among clinical staff. To make this possible, nursing education must be developed with genomic competencies that equip nurses with the knowledge to accurately interpret genetic data and provide effective patient counseling. Interprofessional practice between geneticists and nurses can further enhance patient care through expert assistance in the interpretation of genetic testing. With the advancement of genomic medicine, it is essential for nursing practitioners to remain up-to-date and engaged with emerging research and innovations. Embracing this dynamic field will not only enhance patient care outcomes but also place nursing as a part of the precision medicine field (Conley et al., 2015) (Figure 8.9).

8.3.1. Personalized Medicine and Its Benefits

Personalized medicine represents a paradigm shift in medicine, leveraging the promise of genetic and genomic information to tailor treatments to individual needs. By examining the genetic makeup of an individual, healthcare providers can identify potential risks to health and tailor preventive measures or treatment to the individual patient. This individualization can significantly enhance the outcomes of treatment, eliminating the trial-and-error strategies commonly associated with standard treatment protocols. Personalized medicine also enables the identification of the most suitable drug therapies for specific genetic patterns, thereby reducing the occurrence of side effects and increasing overall efficacy. Implementation of these genomic findings in practice is invaluable, allowing nurses to provide effective, patient-centered care that results in better quality of care and patient satisfaction. While there is hope for personalized medicine, there are still challenges to be overcome to provide the best implementation in practice. A recent survey highlighted the knowledge and attitude differences between healthcare practitioners and genetic testing, as well as the uptake of genomic practice (Baccolini et al., 2020). This highlights the importance of additional education and training in genomics, enabling greater confidence among nursing practitioners. As nursing practice evolves, practitioners must be best-positioned to interpret genetic information, communicate effectively, and inform patients on their options.

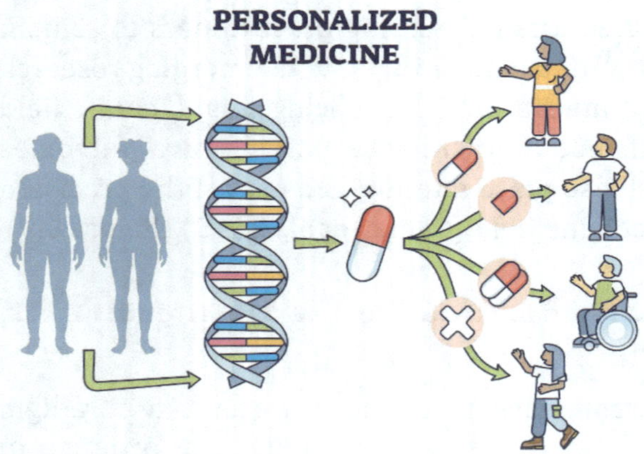

Figure 8.10. Precision and personalized medicine in healthcare.

Source: https://www.medznat.ru/uploads/images/post_content/7182/image_3/1690458980image_3.webp.

Developing the nursing workforce's genomics skills will not only enhance patient outcomes but also stimulate more integrated delivery of healthcare with a focus on genetic considerations, paving the way for more advanced public health efforts that account for diseases with a genetic basis. Furthermore, genetic counselors and specialists' work remains centrally crucial in the days of personalized medicine. While primary care physicians show competence in genetic test result interpretation with the study showing 74.4% versus specialists at 83.4% (Bastola et al., 2019), aspects of genetic counseling still demand specialist expertise. Genetic counselors learn to guide patients' comprehension of complex genetic material, promoting informed decision-making regarding treatment. With the help of genetic specialists, nurses can assist their patients more effectively in coping with customized care pathways. This joint effort not only enhances the nursing profession but also equips patients to become empowered with the knowledge and tools required to participate in their healthcare process in an era increasingly influenced by genetic and genomic determinants (Figure 8.10).

8.3.2. Case Studies Demonstrating Genomic Applications

The application of genomics within nursing practice has been significantly enhanced by case studies that describe its use in patient treatment. One very vivid example is the use of genomic technologies to identify genetic mutations in hereditary breast and ovarian cancer syndromes. Such applications enable nurses to provide personalized risk assessments and prescribe preventive measures based on patients' genetic profiles. Through genomic testing, medical practitioners are capable of identifying individuals who can benefit from enhanced screening or preventive operations, thereby contributing to improved health outcomes. This case study focuses on the need for nursing education to incorporate genomic science, enabling future professionals to accurately interpret genetic information and discuss significant patient care options with patients, thereby contributing to the development of a personalized nursing practice system (Anderson et al., 2015). Another relevant case study illustrates the application of genomic tools in managing chronic diseases, such as diabetes. Genomic information can inform treatment by identifying patients who are more likely to respond better to drugs based on their genetic makeup. Pharmacogenomics, for example, enables nurses to adjust dosing or choose alternative medications based on how a person's genetic variations affect drug metabolism. This tailored approach to treatment not only enhances treatment effectiveness but also minimizes the risk of drug side effects, which shows how genomics can transform the practice of nursing. Furthermore, the application of genomic data in chronic disease management highlights the importance of ongoing education and training for nursing professionals to align with emerging scientific evidence and the skills required in the evolving healthcare setting (Baccolini et al., 2020). Finally, public health programs' case studies emphasize the role of genomics applications within community health settings. These initiatives often incorporate genomics as a means of addressing health disparities by targeting populations with a higher genetic risk for specific diseases. A prime example is initiatives to enhance screening for genetic diseases in underserved populations, which have proven the value of genomics to public health. Nurses play a pivotal role in these initiatives by educating patients on genetic testing and how they can access resources. The data from such case studies substantiate the incorporation of genomic content into nursing education, empowering clinicians to bridge the divide between genomic science and public health practice. Such alignment enhances not only nursing practice but also serves the larger goal of increasing community health through evidence-based genomic interventions (Anderson et al., 2015) (Figure 8.11).

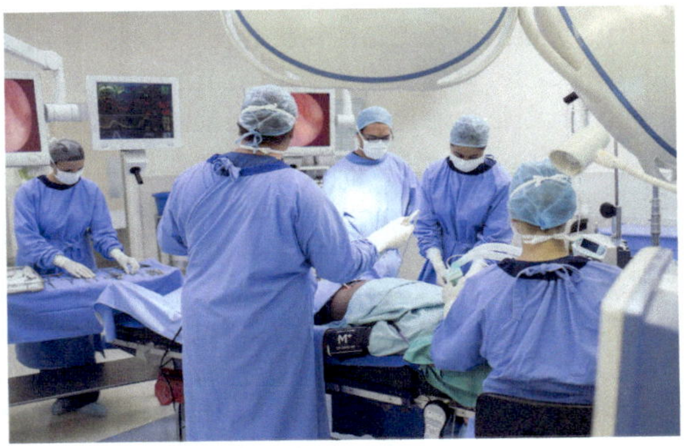

Figure 8.11. Prophylactic surgeries.

Source: https://www.verywellhealth.com/thmb/ku9xo9T8Tu8yo5Yh0baK9DI6bDo=/1500x0/filters:no_upscale():max_bytes(150000):strip_icc()/GettyImages-5306855671-5953be875f9b584bfe98b4a3.jpg.

8.3.3. Challenges in Implementing Genomic Medicine in Nursing

Its implementation as practice among nurses is severely hindered by numerous hurdles, including the need for more education and preparedness among nursing staff. Despite the growing importance of genomic data within clinics, nursing schools are poorly placed to make genomics a part of their root curriculum. This gap complicates nurses' ability to fully engage with genomic tools, which are increasingly becoming a necessary component of customized patient treatment. A work group sponsored by the Council for the Advancement of Nursing Science emphasized the importance of incorporating omics content, including genomics, into PhD nursing programs, ensuring that future nursing scientists are prepared to address these innovations. Without a solid genomic science background, nurses may not be adequately equipped to apply, interpret, and communicate genomic information accurately, potentially with consequences for less-than-ideal patient outcomes and care (Anderson et al., 2015). In addition to education deficits, translation of genomic medicine into nursing is also hindered by the lack of standard guidelines and protocols. As genomic testing becomes increasingly prevalent in the clinical environment, nurses are uncertain about the ethical considerations and optimal practices surrounding genetic information. This is evident from the findings of a survey conducted by the European Public Health Association, which identified that even among individuals working in public health genomics, a high percentage lacked full familiarity with the related medical conditions associated with genetic testing. This knowledge deficit leads to an unwillingness to utilize genomic information, which can lead to the process of personalized medicine initiatives in nursing practice being brought to a stop. There is, therefore, a critical need to develop and disseminate clear-cut guidelines that clearly delineate the roles of nursing professionals in genomic medicine to assist them in making sense out of the complexity of this new field (Baccolini et al., 2020). Furthermore, the implementation of genomic medicine in nursing practice is also hindered by far-reaching systemic obstacles, such as resource allocation and teamwork. Prioritization of genomic projects by most healthcare organizations proves challenging amid competing resource pressures, which can slow the implementation of genomic care into nursing procedures. Additionally, interprofessional collaboration is an integral part of the successful implementation of genomic medicine. Nurses must work closely with geneticists, bioinformaticians, and other healthcare professionals to ensure that proper patient assessment and information sharing occur. Existing limitations, including absence of appropriate communication and lack of team-based training, tend to form silos to counterproductive collaboration. Overcoming these system-wide challenges is crucial to creating an environment where genomic medicine can thrive within nursing, ultimately enhancing patient care and health outcomes (Anderson et al., 2015).

Test Your Knowledge

1. In what ways does genomic information increase the accuracy of diagnosis and treatment?
2. How may nurses integrate genomics into personalized patient care?

8.4. Nursing Roles in Genetic Research

Learning Outcome

1. List the roles of nurses in genetic studies
2. Develop a working relationship with researchers and geneticists
3. Describe the importance of evidence-based practice in genetics

The involvement of nurses in genetic research is increasingly being recognized as a core component of effective healthcare delivery within the domains of genetics and genomics. Nurses, by their access to patients and their families, are uniquely positioned to provide care that extends from physical health to genetic counseling, education, and advice. With multidisciplinary teams becoming the standard in genetic services, nurses assume essential roles in facilitating integration and coordination of care among geneticists, genetic counselors, and other clinicians. The integration of nursing into genetic counseling creates possibilities for bringing innovative models of care that directly address the challenges of genetic diseases and their impact on patients' lives. In addition, collaborative work behaviors detailed in studies demonstrate the manner in which nurses contribute significantly to patient outcomes, reflecting their roles as educators and advocates within the realm of genetic health (Norris et al., 2015). These roles emphasize the need for ongoing professional development and genetics competence within nursing practice. Educational models for nursing practice in genetics have evolved significantly over the years, reflecting the rapid advancements in genomic healthcare. Traditionally, nurses would not have had formal education in genetics, which limited their ability to interact with patients productively regarding genetic information. However, more recent studies suggest that updated frameworks addressing competency in genetic counseling, advocacy, and follow-up are necessary to enhance nursing practice in this field (Burton et al., 2013).

The continuous consensus-building process used to revise educational curricula facilitates a deeper understanding of the individualized patient needs of individuals with genetic conditions. Because nursing education incorporates genetic competencies, practitioners are better able to assist in informed decision-making, thereby empowering patients and their families as they navigate the often complex realm of genetic health. Additionally, implementing updated competencies within nursing, particularly in genetic research, has potential impacts on patient-focused care. Nurses who are trained and equipped with an understanding of genetic information have the potential to make a significant difference in the healthcare encounter for patients. Through genetic research, nurses not only expand their scopes of practice but also guide a more responsive healthcare system that recognizes the unique challenges of genetic disorders. Notably, this paradigm enables the integration of genetic issues into daily nursing practice, ultimately enhancing the quality of care patients receive. As demonstrated by the high participation of genetic counselors in medical practice, nurses play a crucial role in evaluating patient needs and facilitating effective communication within the medical team, thereby ensuring an efficient patient flow through the realm of genetic services (Norris et al., 2015). These roles are evidence of how nursing practice evolves to meet the challenges of modern genetic research and patient care (Figure 8.12).

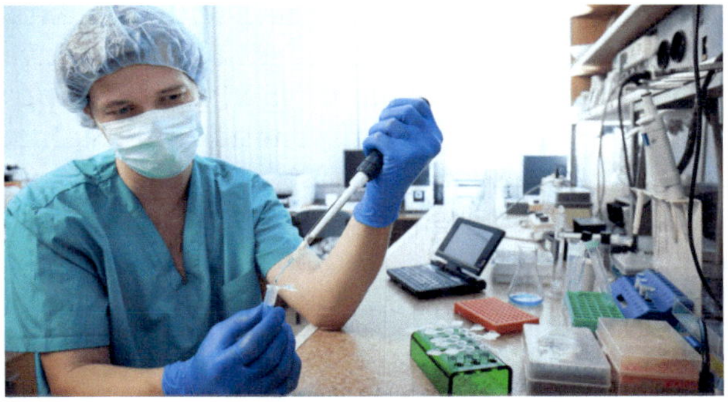

Figure 8.12. Nursing roles in genetic research.

Source: https://external-content.duckduckgo.com/iu/?u=https%3A%2F%2Feverynurse.org%2Fwp-content%2Fuploads%2F2021%2F06%2FGenetics-Nurse-Featured.png&f=1&nofb=1&ipt=1af726059f6b30030e53e05e7e5e646d8ccaa54c500b232aa8c9601f27e6fb57.

8.4.1. Contributions of Nurses to Genetic Studies

Nurses' contributions to genetic studies are increasingly recognized as vital, particularly with the growing trend toward more personalized care. Nurses are, in some instances, at the interface of patients, acting as the middlemen between patients and genetic professionals. Their patient education and advocacy expertise enable them to provide critical support to individuals who undergo genetic testing and counseling. This assistance extends beyond merely informing patients about test procedures; nurses aid in the interpretation of genetic information and guide patients through the emotional complexities of genetic findings. In bridging the gap between patients and genetic care, nurses facilitate successful genetic consultations, ensuring that individuals receive holistic care tailored to their specific genetic needs. This multifaceted interaction highlights the importance of nurses as active members of the genetic study team and fosters a deeper appreciation for patient needs in the genomic era. Nurses play central roles in genetic research through roles in data collection and patient recruitment strategies. Through repeated interaction with patients, they are in a position to identify prospective study participants and facilitate proper follow-up, essential for genetic longitudinal studies. Additionally, nurses typically assist in administering surveys and questionnaires regarding genetic susceptibility, collecting vital health histories and family records to inform research results.

In the process, they help develop robust datasets that maintain the integrity of genetic studies. Furthermore, the acquired knowledge enables nurses to contribute to the design and conduct of research procedures, ensuring studies remain patient-centered and address pragmatic concerns. Their practice not only enhances the standards of genetic research but also sheds light on how genetic factors influence patient care. Education in genetics and genomics has become a flagship of nursing practice, keeping pace with the increasingly complex nature of genetic information. New studies focus on strengthening nursing education models to incorporate today's genetic competencies, thereby positioning nurses more effectively to respond to patients' needs in genetic healthcare.

A consensus approach in 2010 went back to the foundational model of genetics education for nurses and identified deficiencies in skills such as advocacy and ongoing care, particularly in patient and family management with genetic disorders (Burton et al., 2013). Through overcoming such deficits, nurses' education can equip nurses to take more active roles in genetic research, which adds more value to their work. As nurses expand their knowledge in genetics, not only are they developing their professional practice, but they are also significantly improving patient outcomes, illustrating the critical integration of nursing practice and genomic medicine (Figure 8.13).

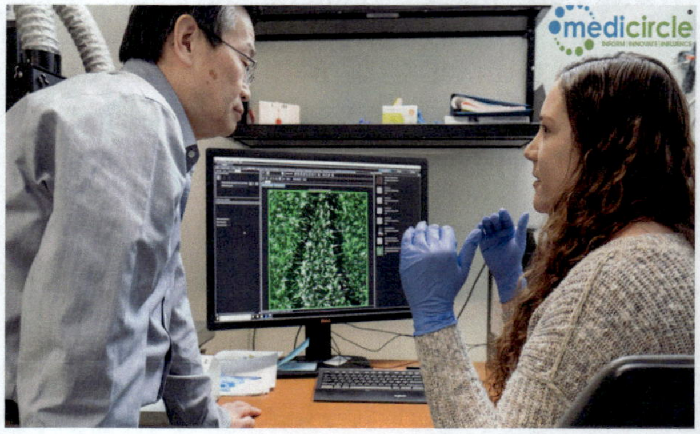

Figure 8.13. The role of genetic profiles in Alzheimer's therapy.

Source: https://medicircle.in/uploads/2024/may2024/artboard_899.jpg.

8.4.2. Collaboration with Geneticists and Researchers

In the increasingly dynamic healthcare landscape, the nurse-geneticist interface plays a central role in integrating genetics and genomics into patient care. With increasing involvement of nurses in genetic information, their ability to provide individualized care is enhanced by working with geneticists who specialize in deciphering complex genetic data.

This collaboration is essential as it enables nurses to identify genetic vulnerability to diseases, thereby providing early interventions and individualized treatment plans. The linkage of nursing practice and genetic science benefits not only the clinical environment but also enhances the quality of care offered to patients, particularly in the management of inherited conditions such as cancers and metabolic disorders. By developing these relationships, the nursing profession can provide a holistic approach that emphasizes both patient education and patient empowerment in genetic health decision-making. Additionally, the participation of nurses as part of collaborative research efforts with geneticists can lead to significant advancements in the field of genomics. Nurses frequently face the real-world implications of genetic information and are well-positioned to acquire the necessary data through their patient interactions. This firsthand experience can be invaluable to inform researchers' agendas aimed at improving genetic counseling services, such as with developing intervention-based research to identify patients better and make genetic counseling more available, as outlined in objectives for relevant research (American Nurses Association (ANA). Consensus Panel on Genetic et al., 2015). By participating in research, nurses can create a connection between genomic science and clinical practice, ensuring that findings are effectively translated into healthcare policy. By doing so, not only is the creation of evidence-based practice eased, but also the practice culture of continuous learning within the nursing profession is promoted. Finally, education efforts to enhance the genetic and genomics skills of nurses illustrate the necessity of multidisciplinary cooperation among geneticists and nurses. With demand for genetic services exceeding supply, developing relationships that teach curricula is increasingly crucial, particularly for non-genetics healthcare providers. Current literature suggests a high demand for genetics education in nursing programs (Patterson et al., 2022).

Collaboration with geneticists to create standardized training modules will enable nurses to know to manage genomic care complexities with confidence. Such a foundation in education will enable nurses to effectively educate patients about genetic risks and benefits, ultimately leading to improved health outcomes and a more competent healthcare system that recognizes the pivotal role of genomics in contemporary medicine.

8.4.3. Importance of Evidence-based Practice (EBP) in Genetics

In the rapidly evolving field of genetics, EBP provides a foundation for ensuring that healthcare practitioners apply interventions that are scientifically grounded and ethically sound.

This methodology requires the integration of the finest existing research evidence, clinical judgment, and patient values, a process that is particularly vital in genetic nursing practice. With medicine increasingly based on genomic information in patient treatment, nurses well-grounded in EBP can make appropriate decisions about genetic testing and counseling such that these treatments are aligned with accepted guidelines and improve patient outcomes. EBP also facilitates identifying probable interventions that can be more effective, thereby eliminating the risks associated with genetic susceptibility to various diseases.

Furthermore, the application of EBP to genetics is emphasized by a growing body of literature that highlights the need for more training and knowledge among nursing practitioners. A study demonstrated that only 28.9% of public health practitioners were capable of recognizing evidence-based conditions where genetic testing can be utilized, which emphasizes a significant knowledge gap among practitioners (Baccolini et al., 2020). This shortfall highlights the necessity of continuous education in genetics, encompassing both technical competence in testing and the appropriate clinical use of genetic information.

Greater awareness fosters good attitudes and practices towards the integration of genomic data into public health and nursing guidelines, encouraging professionals to apply genetic resources efficiently to meet patient requirements. Furthermore, a new model of genetics education for nurses has been proposed to address the above gaps, demonstrating the evolving character of genetic nursing education (Burton et al., 2013). Through its emphasis on competencies such as advocacy, management of information, and ongoing care, the model is not only reflective of the complexity of genetic conditions but also of the evolving character of nurses' work in genomic health care. Nursing leadership is crucial to the effective implementation of this model, as nurses are well-trained to represent their patients and navigate the complexities of genetic data. The integration of EBP and strategic education initiatives develops a nursing infrastructure to deliver comprehensive, evidence-based genetic care, enhancing the quality of patient interactions and public health outcomes (Figure 8.14).

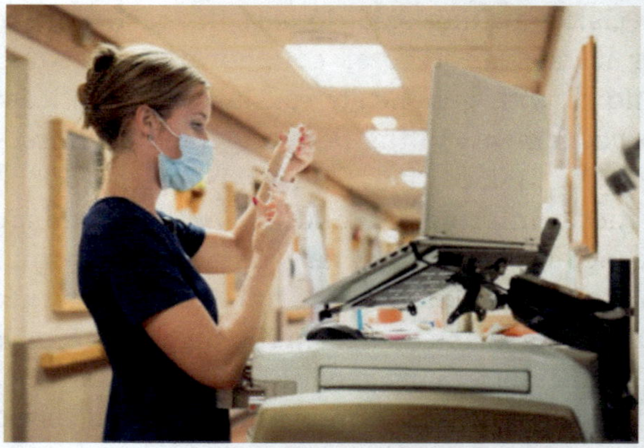

Figure 8.14. The importance of evidence-based practice in nursing.

Source: https://external-content.duckduckgo.com/iu/?u=https%3A%2F%2Fnursingcecentral.com%2Fwp-content%2Fuploads%2F2021%2F04%2F4_2_2021_Evidence-Based-Pract ice-in-Nursing_Body-2-1024x727.jpg&f=1&nofb=1&ipt=baa7452fbe3f5dce4603f9e34ecc3269272666898ad9007847741daecf5c1f10.

Test Your Knowledge

1. What are the possible roles for nurses in recruiting participants and obtaining consent for genetic research studies?
2. How do nurses assist in ensuring ethical practice and patient protection in genetic research?

8.5. Education and Training in Genetics for Nurses

Learning Outcome

1. Describe the current curriculum requirements for genetics in nursing
2. Outline continuing education choices in genomics
3. Describe the impact of training on nursing practice

The nursing practice is evolving at a rapid rate, and it is therefore necessary that genetic education and training become an integral part of nursing education. As genomics continues to expand, it has never been more essential that schools of nursing incorporate better genetic concepts and advanced high-tech devices into their curricula. This incorporation not only acclimatizes prospective nurses to the intricacies of patient care but also equips them with the tools to interpret and use genetic information effectively. Historically, most nurse curricula have not placed significant emphasis on the importance of omics, including genomics, proteomics, and other relevant scientific fields.

The integration of such ideas into training programs has the potential to significantly enhance nurses' contributions to the healthcare industry, as well as empower them to communicate more effectively with interprofessional teams, thereby promoting holistic practice in patient-centered care and closing the gaps in current education programs (Anderson et al., 2015). Additionally, the rapid progress in DNA sequencing technology has shifted the health paradigm, placing a spotlight on the critical role of nurses in applying sophisticated genetic data. As the initial contact person for patient care, nurses are most apt to educate patients regarding genetic testing and its significance in managing health. This position requires a strong understanding of the clinical application of genomic data, as well as the ethical considerations of genetic testing. Genetic training enables nurses to support patients in making informed decisions about their care, informed by genetic data, thereby enhancing patient autonomy and self-empowerment. To achieve this role effectively, nursing curricula must concentrate on practical, yet comprehensive, genetics education, bridging the gap between practice and technological development (Hickey et al., 2017).

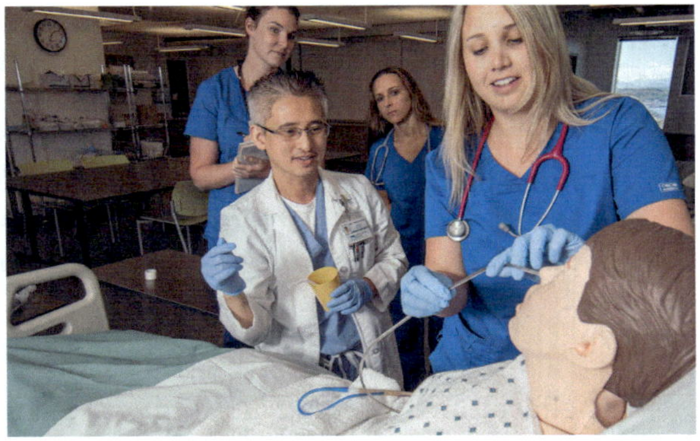

Figure 8.15. Nurse aide training.

Source: https://healthcare.seattlecentral.edu/sites/alliedhealth.seattlecentral.dev/files/inline-images/nursing-students-and-faculty-seattle-central.jpg.

Interdisciplinary approach in genetics education is needed, concentrating on teamwork between genomics experts and nursing educators. With clinical practitioners and nurse scientists increasingly engaged in genomic research and its application, collaboration can strengthen educational programs. Integrating findings of multi-omic research into nursing education enables instructors to provide a more robust and relevant training experience based on contemporary healthcare practice. Such collaborations can provide novel pedagogical strategies that involve experiential training with genetic technology, which is valuable for both instructors and students. Lastly, investing in nursing education in genetics is not a cerebral endeavor; it is a commitment to the quality of care for patients and to equipping nurses to successfully handle the realities of today's healthcare environments (Anderson et al., 2015) (Figure 8.15).

8.5.1. Current Curriculum Standards for Genetics in Nursing

Incorporating genetics into nursing education became increasingly crucial as breakthroughs in genomic medicine redefine healthcare practice. Current curriculum demands for genetics address not only the basics of genetics but also the application of these basics in practice within clinical settings. Nursing schools are being challenged to incorporate integrated genetics education that covers everything from inheritance patterns to ethical issues in genetic testing.

This educational shift is crucial in preparing nursing professionals for meaningful interactions with patients by utilizing genetic information to inform care and decision-making. The disparity between the speed of scientific advancement and an antiquated curriculum has sparked debates on whether there is a need for uniform models of education to facilitate uniform genetics education among nursing schools. In response to the evolving requirements of healthcare, professional organizations are establishing competencies that nursing education programs must achieve to prepare graduates to meet the challenges of genetic and genomic care. These competencies aim to enable nurses to understand the application of genetic risk factors and the impact of genomics on personalized care. By integrating genetics into core nursing education, educators can ensure that nurses of the future not only possess knowledge of genetic concepts but also have the ability to apply genomic data in practice. This emphasis also aligns with broader public health goals of improving healthcare delivery by creating a workforce capable of addressing genetic issues in diverse populations, thereby contributing positively to overall patient outcomes in managing genetic diseases (Ahankari et al., 2016). A successful genetics curriculum does more than teach nurses how to provide direct care to patients. It also emphasizes the importance of interdisciplinary collaboration within healthcare teams. With the incorporation of genomic information into healthcare becoming increasingly mainstream, nurses play a critical role as bridges between patients and the complexities of genetic knowledge. Through enhanced communication competencies and interprofessional attitudes, nursing education can leverage improved collaborative work that enhances genetics and genomics-related quality of care. Furthermore, with the advancement of the nursing profession, the integration of genetics standards has great potential for increasing healthcare efficiency and patient involvement, thereby enabling well-informed health decisions. Thus, the development of genetics education in nursing is essential not only for the individual nurse's capability but also to address larger issues in public health that rely on sound genetic literacy (N/A, 2005) (Figure 8.16).

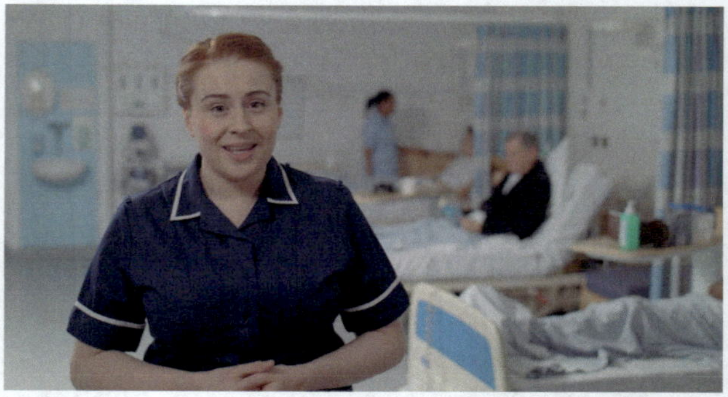

Figure 8.16. Curriculum standards for genetics in nursing.

Source: https://www.genomicseducation.hee.nhs.uk/wp-content/uploads/2018/09/Nursing-film-1138x640.jpg.

8.5.2. Continuing Education Opportunities in Genomics

The transition to genomics as a non-negotiable component of healthcare necessitates that nurses undergo ongoing education to enhance their competencies. Genomics continuing education programs are designed to equip nursing professionals with the fundamentals and advanced competencies necessary to incorporate genomic data into patient care effectively. For instance, accredited internet workshops and courses provide nurses with an accessible learning platform where they can become educated on the fundamentals of genetics, the meaning of genomic testing, and the ethical concerns surrounding genetic information. Through such initiatives, nurses not only improve their knowledge of genomic science but also acquire the skill of distilling complex genetic data to explain it to patients and their families. Such comprehension is significant as the integration of genomics into practice can assist in the generation of more personalized patient care interventions, hence improved overall health outcomes. To address the growing need for genomics education, various organizations offer specialized resources focusing on the relevant skills in nursing practice. Webinar-based courses, certification courses, and interactive conferences permit collaboration among healthcare providers and engage an interdisciplinary model of learning. The International Summit on Medical Nutrition Education and Research highlighted good practices of cross-national sharing of education resources and best practices, where emphasis was laid on utilizing the combined effort to improve medical nutrition education, along with the development of genomics. These avenues not only provide a vehicle for professional growth but also, in conjunction with the commitment of the nursing profession to evidence-based practice. By embracing these scholarly innovations, nurses can effectively stay up to date with the rapidly changing field of genomic medicine, thereby becoming aware of the technologies and techniques that define today's healthcare. Moreover, incorporating genomics into nursing education programs highlights the importance of maintaining nursing relevance within healthcare facilities through ongoing education. The American Academy of Nursing and numerous influential nursing organizations have advocated for the inclusion of new fields of science, such as genomics, into PhD nursing education, underscoring the necessity for formal training in this field. This integration of genomics into educational frameworks not only readies future nursing leaders but also offers a system that encourages lifelong learning for working professionals. With nurses seeking higher degrees and specialist qualifications, they are optimally positioned to lead the charge in championing genomic literacy among healthcare professionals. Lastly, commitment to continuing education in genomics is a fulcrum for advancing nursing practice to the next level, whereby nurses are well-equipped to negotiate and implement genomic innovations into practice for patients and public health programs (Alt-White et al., 2015; Ahankari et al., 2016) (Figure 8.17).

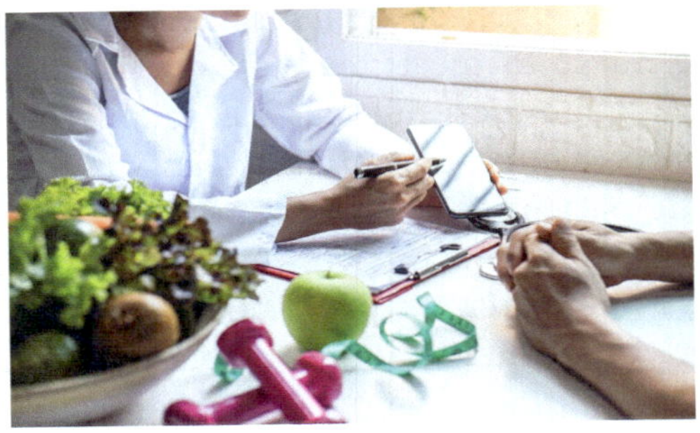

Figure 8.17. Nutritionist giving consultation to patient with healthy fruit.

Source: https://external-content.duckduckgo.com/iu/?u=https%3A%2F%2Fwww.oncozine.com%2Fwp-content%2Fuploads%2F2019%2F08%2FFotolia_274813027_Subscription_Monthly_M.jpg&f=1&nofb=1&ipt=031e861d238879d239bbc3421ffa72913d36fd56364de004b86cf1c209ec17f7.

8.5.3. The Impact of Training on Nursing Practice

Training is core to enhancing nursing practice, particularly in the domain of genetics and genomics. In the evolving health environment, the integration of omics into nursing practice necessitates a workforce competent in these emerging scientific fields. Classical nurse education, being short on large amounts of genomic content, must reform to incorporate training that is sensitive to contemporary healthcare requirements. The incorporation of genomics training not only equips nurses with the exposure to the data that they will need to translate genetic information but also enables them to implement this information into practice. Creating a workforce that can accurately interpret genetic data will ultimately lead to improved patient outcomes and more specific care approaches. As illustrated in current research, healthcare curriculum needs to expand to incorporate generous content on genomics as a key component for educating nursing professionals in order to fulfill the needs of contemporary healthcare delivery (Anderson et al., 2015). Furthermore, the impact of training on nursing practice extends well beyond the single nurse to the extended healthcare team. Skilled genomics nurses are ideally placed members of multi-disciplinary teams, facilitating holistic patient assessment and care planning. Training centered on working in partnership across healthcare professions fosters a culture of mutual skill and whole-person care, essential for the successful management of multifaceted health issues. This collaborative framework not only enhances patient care but also boosts continuous professional development among nursing colleagues. Engagement with genomic data through training courses can foster a shared understanding among all healthcare professionals, creating synergies for optimal patient care plans. The Council for the Advancement of Nursing Science has underscored the merit of such an interprofessional approach, cultivating competent nurses who interlink genomic science and practice (Conley et al., 2015). Finally, the call for greater education in genetics and genomics is a testament to a respect for nurses' influence on paradigms of patient care. As genomic information becomes increasingly accessible, nurses are well-positioned to spearhead the integration of genetic screening, risk analysis, and personalized treatment plans into everyday practice. High-quality education programs need to be in place to ensure that nurses are not only users of genomic information but also engaged participants in bringing this information into everyday professional practice. This revolution is the path to a more personalized practice in nursing, wherein genetic data informs decisions and results. Thus, when nursing education is integrated with genomics, the profession as a whole will benefit, with enhanced quality of care being administered and empowered nurses serving as leaders in the genomic era of healthcare (Anderson et al., 2015).

Test Your Knowledge

1. What is the value of having genetics education for nurses in today's healthcare settings?
2. What are the optimal ways to enhance genetic literacy and skill of nursing personnel?

8.6. Future Trends in Genetics and Genomics in Nursing

Learning Outcome

1. Understand hotel maintenance management and its impact
2. Perform preventive maintenance
3. Discuss about breakdown maintenance

As nursing continues to evolve, the application of genetics and genomics is poised to transform clinical practice. The most prominent trend is the increasing use of whole-genome and exome sequencing (WGS/WES) in healthcare settings.

This technology provides vast amounts of data on a person's genetic makeup, enabling nurses to assess genetic susceptibility to a wide range of diseases and tailor care accordingly.

As Blazkova et al. (2020) believes, the WGS/WES report on a large scale is warranted through the potential for better patient outcomes by way of personalized medicine. Further, the ethical concerns surrounding the handling of genomic data have necessitated policies that ensure patients' rights to their raw genomic data.

Hence, nurses must be aware of both the technical capabilities of such devices and the paradigms governing their use, so that they can effectively collaborate with the intricacies involved in the genomic use of data.

Additionally, future nursing practice will demand an adequate supply of a genetically literate workforce. As medicine shifts towards precision medicine, the ability to understand genetic information is crucial for nurses. Educational institutions must adjust their curricula to include in-depth training in genomics, equipping nursing professionals with the expertise to interpret genetic information and communicate its meanings to patients. Increasingly, people are recognizing that an educated nursing workforce is crucial to achieving optimal care outcomes in genomic medicine. Initiatives aimed at upgrading genomic education for healthcare workers will also impact the demand and supply of the workforce in the pharmaceutical sector, where there is a shift towards more genetically focused therapies (N/A, 2005).

Hence, bridging the education gap will be key to equipping an educationally competent nursing workforce to meet the challenge contributed by genetic and genomic developments. Ultimately, nurses' contributions toward promoting ethics and policy for genomic data become increasingly relevant as technology advances.

Nurses often become the initial and optimal point of contact for patients undergoing the oft-confusing outcomes of genomic testing. Thus, they are well-positioned to advocate for more straightforward guidelines on access and use of genomic data at the practice level. The very evidence from specific sequencing centers raises to the forefront the immediate issues of managing genome access requests and highlights the need for consistent policies (Blazkova et al., 2020).

By facilitating a conversation about the implications of genomic data, nurses can play a crucial role in ensuring patient autonomy while safeguarding against potential misuse of sensitive genetic information. This campaign promotes the overall goal of integrating genetics and genomics into nursing practice, underscoring the central role of nurses in shaping the future of healthcare systems (Figure 8.18).

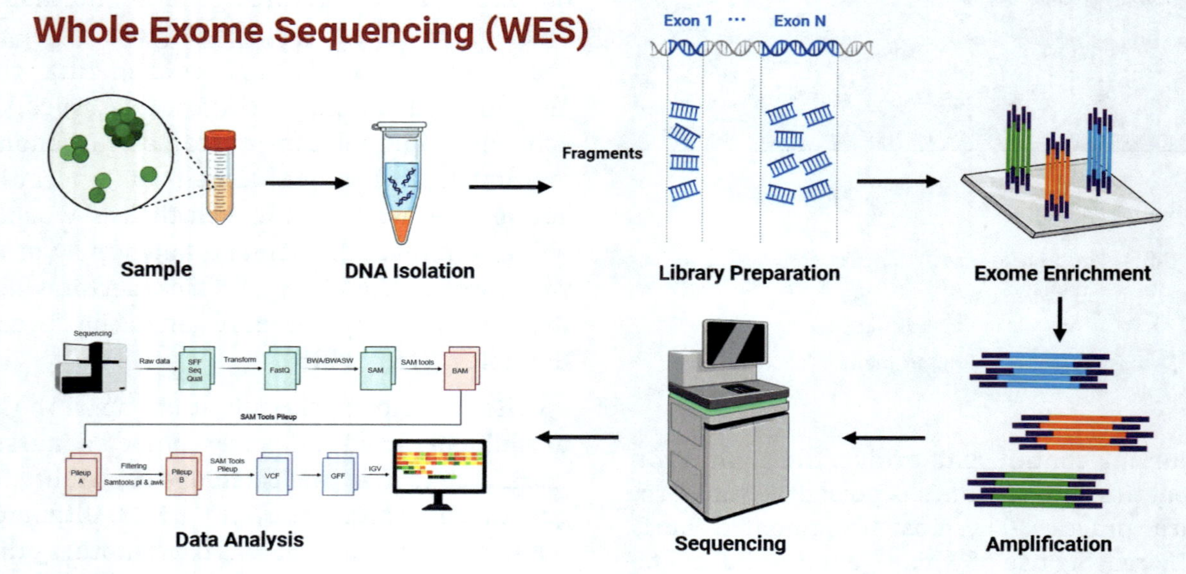

Figure 8.18. Whole-exome-sequencing (WES).

Source: https://microbenotes.com/wp-content/uploads/2024/09/Whole-Exome-Sequencing.jpeg.

8.6.1. Advances In Technology And Their Implications

The rapid evolution of technology has revolutionized fields such as genomics and genetics, thereby reshaping the nursing profession. The technological innovations in these areas allow greater precision in understanding the biological determinants of disease and health. With the use of omics technologies, such as genomics, proteomics, and microbiomics, nursing professionals can acquire comprehensive information regarding the genetic determinants of patient outcomes. The specificity thereof enhances the ability to individualize nursing interventions based on individual patient profiles, further leading to a more tailored mode of care. Incorporation of these innovations into educational curricula is, therefore, of utmost importance; without learning new areas of science, the profession risks being unable to comprehend the significance and implementation of these innovations within everyday practice (Anderson et al., 2015). Thus, nursing education must be modified to include comprehensive training in such technologies, preparing nurses to use genetic information appropriately when making clinical decisions. Historically, nursing education has been hindered by keeping pace with the rapid advancements in scientific technology and healthcare, an endeavor noted by the Council for the Advancement of Nursing Science. The organization's focus on putting the future generation of nursing scientists in developing scientific paradigms is one instance of the necessity to transform curricula. The advancements in genomics and associated sciences have significant implications for patient care and nursing research, so education programs for nursing professionals must become more integrative and interdisciplinary (Conley et al., 2015). With the establishment of a learning culture of continuous acquisition, the nursing profession will be able to develop a workforce that is not only skilled in new technology but also able to adapt to the changing nature of the health field. Thus, the incorporation of these concepts of advanced science into nursing education will assist in the development of competent professionals who contribute meaningfully to health care innovation. As nurses become increasingly involved in precision health initiatives, the relevance of developments in genomics technologies is increasingly evident in practice. The ability to analyze genetic information enables nurses to investigate risk determinants, forecast disease progression, and provide personalized preventive care for individual patients. For instance, understanding a patient's genetic susceptibility to certain diseases may enable early intervention and more effective management strategies. Moreover, genomic data also demand that not only technical competency but also the ability to discuss the very complex issues with patients and families needs to be transmitted in nurses. This dual ability only underscores the necessity of more training in genetics and genomics for nurses, ultimately making them effective advocates for patients in an increasingly biotechnology- and personalized medicine-driven environment. Emphasizing this integration in nursing practice will not only improve patient outcomes but also position nurses as critical members of the multidisciplinary healthcare team.

8.6.2. The Potential for Gene Therapy in Nursing Practice

The incorporation of gene therapy into nursing practice has the greatest potential for tailoring patient care, in concert with the principles of genetics and genomics. As the caregiver of first choice, the nurse is ideally positioned to educate patients and their families about the process of gene therapy, ensuring maximum compliance. Such understanding enables nurses to discuss the scientific principles of gene therapy, for example, targeted gene delivery systems and how these can be employed to treat genetic diseases. By discussing the potential of gene therapy to alter disease at a molecular level, nurses can empower patients to make informed decisions about their treatment. Use of such information not only improves the clinical interactions but also builds a connection that promotes trust among patients and health care providers, an essential component in the quest for ultimate health outcomes for genomic care. The successful implementation of gene therapy into nursing practice is no easy task, however. A gigantic one is the current lack of genomic capability among healthcare professionals. Research has shown that nurses tend to attribute deficiencies in their genomic and genetic education as a hindrance to delivering effective communication to patients regarding gene therapy options. In this regard, Hassen et al. (2020) question how effective models of genomic literacy education can be incorporated into nursing schools. Through such gaps in education, healthcare organizations can enhance the confidence and ability of nurses in delivering patient education about gene therapy. With increasing proficiency in this new field, nurses will be better equipped to understand the complexity of patient care, particularly in genetics, and thus expand patient access to new therapeutics. Furthermore, ethical concerns in gene therapy necessitate a comprehensive approach to nursing practice that integrates ethics, law, and social issues (ELSI). Nurses play a key role in ensuring patients' rights to avoid exacerbating existing inequalities in access to care. The process of informed consent is also more complicated in the context of gene therapy, and nurses should hence facilitate patients through potential risks and benefits through an integrated process. The incorporation of the Healthcare Genetics (HCG) model of practice into nursing, as outlined in Hassen et al. (2020), provides a systematic approach to addressing these ethical issues. Gene therapy as a profession continues to move forward, and nurses are required to remain ahead of these controversies, striking a balance between advancing the field and the ethical demands of nursing practice and cautious patient treatment (Figure 8.19).

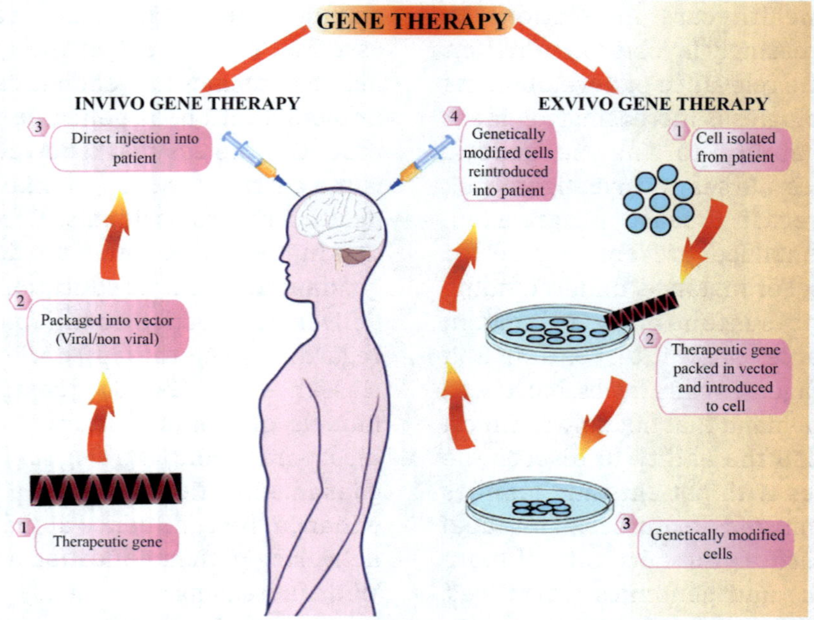

Figure 8.19. Gene therapy: Reshaping the medical future.

Source: https://static.wixstatic.com/media/a902c7_09349abc3a724808b42b17b8e6f52fd8~mv2.png/v1/fill/w_850,h_676,al_c,q_90,enc_auto/a902c7_09349abc3a724808b42b17b8e6f52fd8~mv2.png.

8.6.3. Predictions for the Future of Nursing in Genomics

As the science of genomics continues to advance, the future of nursing care will undoubtedly be shaped by further developments in genetic technology and individualized medicine. Genetic concepts will be an integral part of nursing clinicians' education, enabling them to communicate with patients who have individualized genomic backgrounds effectively. Increasing genetic literacy among nurses will enable them to make informed, evidence-based decisions and communicate effectively with healthcare teams. Nurses will be on the front line of integrating genomic information into treatment plans for patients as healthcare systems begin to implement more genomic medicine. Nurses will also be on the front line of informing patients about their genetic risk, allowing people to understand how their genomic data affects health outcomes. Such forethought will be paramount, particularly with the implementation of predictive genomic technology within the clinical setting, further emphasizing the imperative role that nurses will play in orchestrating the complexities of personalized medicine. In the next decade, the convergence of genomics and nursing practice will also lead to a significant increase in the number of specialists among the nursing demographic. Genetic nurse clinicians with experience of treating patients with genetic disorders will take center stage in genomic care. Organizations will recognize nurse-managed programs specifically dedicated to providing genetic counseling as a top priority, and the emphasis on ongoing education and professional expertise in genetics among nurses will be highlighted. As genetics increasingly becomes an integral part of daily practice, nurses will also function as patient advocates, ensuring fair access to genetic testing and counseling. As direct-to-consumer genetic testing becomes increasingly prevalent, nurses will be crucial in bridging the gap between patients and the nuanced findings generated by genetic testing agencies, thereby facilitating patient-centered care in genomic contexts (Harris et al., 2012). Moreover, the future of genomics nursing will be founded on a greater emphasis on interdisciplinary practice and ethics. The rapid advancement of genomic technology requires collaboration among nurses, geneticists, and other healthcare professionals to deliver patient care comprehensively. The partnership will extend to the management of ethical concerns in genetic information privacy, informed consent, and social life of genetic information. When nurses are confronted with these kinds of complex challenges, they will be compelled to advocate for policies that protect patients' rights and ensure the safe use of genomic data. The nurse's future will not only consist of direct patient care but also research and advocacy, where nurses will be in charge of a healthcare system controlled by genomics. These shifts not only enhance the breadth of the nursing practitioner's function but also underscore the need for ongoing education and transformation to prepare the profession for the future (Aristarán et al., 2016).

Test Your Knowledge

1. In what ways might advances in genomics revolutionize nursing functions in individualized and anticipatory care?
2. What are the new technologies in genetics that nurses must prepare to apply to patient care?

SUMMARY

The practice of integrating genomics and genetics represents a paradigm shift in the healthcare setting. Nurses, as they become more involved with genetic information, have an even better opportunity to treat each patient uniquely by not only curing their patients' disease but also addressing their genetic risk. There must be a revolution in policy-making in nursing and education for nurses so that they are able to interpret genetic data appropriately. Secondly, higher awareness and knowledge levels among nursing practitioners will ultimately translate to improved patient outcomes, with the crucial role that genetics plays in today's nursing practice being highlighted. Geneticists and nursing professionals must collaborate to harness the full potential of genomic information in patient care. In the absence of certified genetic practitioners, who are in short supply, as underscored by current studies, there is an urgent need for nurses to bridge the gap in genetic counseling and interpretation (Bastola et al., 2019). In the process, nurses can initiate conversations about genetic risk and treatment, maximizing patients' knowledge and engagement in their healthcare decisions. On top of that, initiatives toward strengthening genetics education as part of nursing education are necessary to prepare the next generation for this task. Moreover, the cultural context of genetic education, particularly among ethnically diverse communities, cannot be ignored. Efforts like the "Talking Glossary of Genomics Terminology" demonstrate how culturally responsive materials can foster sensitivity and awareness about genomics among groups that are otherwise disconnected from mainstream health discussions (Coe et al., 2012). By promoting inclusiveness and increasing the availability of genetic data, nursing practice can address disparities and empower patients with the appropriate information for informed decision-making. This comprehensive model expands nursing practice and firmly positions genetics within the discipline of integrated patient care in the context of an emerging healthcare environment.

In the emerging context of nursing practice, the integration of genomics and genetics is a key area of concern. Nurses are being asked more frequently to become educated about how genetic knowledge affects patient care, as genetic susceptibilities account for a significant percentage of health outcomes. Curricula are now being reworked to include intensive training in genetic principles, so that nurses are adequately prepared to assume an active role in negotiating genetic risk and intervention with patients. There is also growing emphasis on reviving nursing science education and building the next generation of nurse scientists to be able to utilize the new frontiers of science and technology to thereby enhance the nursing profession's contribution to genomic care, as indicated by the Council for the Advancement of Nursing Science (Conley et al., 2015). These educational milestones are required to build a workforce capable of handling the complexities of genetic information and its related clinical implications. WGS/WES technology also has significant implications for nursing practice. The volume of information produced by genetic sequencing yields important data that can significantly impact patient healthcare decisions. However, the ethics of access and availability to individual genomic information are still controversial issues in the line of work. According to reports by research, although there are numerous sequencing centers where raw data is held in genomic form, there is a vast deficit of routine methods for holding data as well as personal access policies. This inconsistency poses a challenge to nursing professionals, presenting issues in adapting to the evolving regulatory context of genetic data (Blazkova et al., 2020). As such, are cognizant of the ethical concerns regarding access to genomic data since they have a critical role in advocating for patients' rights and ensuring patients are well-informed during decision-making. Lastly, the integration of genomic data into clinical nursing practice fortifies patient-focused care by facilitating the tailoring of interventions. With insight into an individual's genetic makeup, nurses can provide personalized health counseling and management plans tailored to the individual's unique genetic profile. Not only will this improve health outcomes, but it will also enhance patient satisfaction and participation. As genomics nursing is increasingly adopted within the nursing profession, there is a need to ensure that research continues to inform education practices and guidelines in clinical practice. The call by nursing organizations for new models of education reflects the importance of preparing nurses with the skills and knowledge necessary to interpret genetic information appropriately (Conley et al., 2015). Lastly, genomics application in practice is not about data; it is about improving the quality of care and optimizing health outcomes for patients.

KEY TERMS FROM THIS CHAPTER

- Carrier Screening
- DNA (Deoxyribonucleic Acid)
- Ethical, Legal, and Social Implications (ELSI)
- Gene Expression
- Genetic Counseling
- Genome
- Genotype
- Mutation
- Pharmacogenomics
- Chromosomes
- Epigenetics
- Familial Risk Assessment
- Genes
- Genetic Testing
- Genomic Health Promotion
- Hereditary Disorders
- Personalized Care Planning
- Phenotyp

CRITICAL THINKING QUESTIONS

1. **What is the primary function of nurses in genomic medicine?**
   a. Performing genetic surgery
   b. Substituting physicians for genetic counseling
   c. Taking family history and referring patients to testing
   d. Prescribing genetic medication
2. **What is the most appropriate definition of a gene?**
   a. One of the blood cells that has the task of transporting oxygen
   b. A protein-coding DNA sequence
   c. Growth hormone
   d. A virus affecting the health of human beings
3. **What is a pedigree chart used for in genetic nursing?**
   a. Monitoring patterns of blood pressure
   b. Documenting everyday care in nursing
   c. Charting a patient's history of health across generations
   d. Storing laboratory equipment
4. **Which genetic disorder is passed on in an autosomal recessive pattern?**
   a. Huntington's disease
   b. Down syndrome
   c. Cystic fibrosis
   d. Turner syndrome
5. **Why is there a need for nurses to know about genomics in the workplace?**
   a. To carry out laboratory genetic sequencing
   b. To inform patients and refer as appropriate
   c. To develop new genetic technologies
   d. To restrict patient access to genetic testing

Short Answer Questions

1. What is genomics, and how does it differ from genetics?
2. What is the nurse's role within the process of taking a genetic family history?
3. Name two common genetic disorders and describe them briefly.
4. Why do nurses need genetic counseling?
5. What is one of the ethical challenges a nurse might encounter in genomic care?
6. Describe how nurses use pedigree charts in genetic risk stratification and planning care.
7. Describe why genomics must be incorporated into nursing education and practice.
8. Describe the impact of genetic information on individualized medicine and patient outcomes.
9. How must nurses manage patient confidentiality and informed consent for genetic testing?
10. Describe the advantages and disadvantages of using genomic technology in clinical nursing practice.

Answers to Critical Thinking Questions

1. (c) 2. (b) 3. (c) 4. (c) 5. (b)

REFERENCES

1. Laur, C., Ball, L., Ahankari, A., Avdagovska, M., Crowley, J., Deen, D., Douglas, P., Hark, L., Kohlmeier, M., Luzi, L., McCotter, L., Martyn, K., Nowson, C., Wall, C., & Ray, S. (2016). Proceedings of the inaugural International Summit for Medical Nutrition Education and Research. *Public Health*, *140*, 59–67. https://doi.org/10.1016/j.puhe.2016.08.023Alt-White, A. C., Conley, Y. P., Dunbar-Jacob, J., Heitkemper, M. M., et al. (2015). Emerging areas of nursing science and PhD education for the 21st century: Response to commentaries. https://core.ac.uk/download/213079750.pdf (accessed on 28th June 2025).
2. American Nurses Association (ANA), Consensus Panel on Genetic, Battista, R. N., Bellcross, C. A., Burton, H., Cane, P., Cohen, J., Cox, S., et al. (2015). Interventions to improve patient access to and utilization of genetic and genomic counselling services. https://core.ac.uk/download/42138255.pdf (accessed on 28th June 2025).
3. Anderson, C. M., Lyon, D. E., McCarthy, D., Corwin, E. J., Taylor, J. Y., Voss, J., Gregory, K. E., et al. (2015). Educating future nursing scientists: Recommendations for integrating omics content in PhD programs. https://core.ac.uk/download/213074828.pdf (accessed on 28th June 2025).
4. Aristarán, M., Guevara, M. R., Hartmann, D., Hidalgo, C. A., et al. (2016). The research space: Using the career paths of scholars to predict the evolution of the research output of individuals, institutions, and nations. http://arxiv.org/abs/1602.08409 (accessed on 28th June 2025).
5. Baccolini, V., Barnhoorn, F., D'Andrea, E., de Vito, C., et al. (2020). Genomics knowledge and attitudes among European public health professionals: Results of a cross-sectional survey. https://core.ac.uk/download/323191909.pdf (accessed on 28th June 2025).
6. Bastola, K., Kim, K. K., McGrath, S. P., Walton, N., et al. (2019). Are providers prepared for genomic medicine: Interpretation of direct-to-consumer genetic testing (DTC-GT) results and genetic self-efficacy by medical professionals. https://core.ac.uk/download/288432921.pdf (accessed on 28th June 2025).
7. Blazkova, A., Knoppers, B. M., Koesters, R., Markina, A., et al. (2020). Genomic sequencing capacity, data retention, and personal access to raw data in Europe. https://core.ac.uk/download/322827941.pdf (accessed on 28th June 2025).
8. Borry, P., Chokoshvili, D., De Paepe, A., Janssens, S., et al. (2017). Pre- and post-testing counseling considerations for the provision of expanded carrier screening: Exploration of European geneticists' views. https://core.ac.uk/download/84595415.pdf (accessed on 28th June 2025).
9. Burns, H. (2019). The development of hypersensitivity reactions in the pediatric population: A review. https://core.ac.uk/download/213464303.pdf (accessed on 28th June 2025).
10. Burton, H., House of Lords Science and Technology Committee, Human Genomics Strategy Group, Kirk, M., Murphy, M., Nursing and Midwifery Council, Task and Finish Group, et al. (2013). An iterative consensus-building approach to revising a genetics/genomics competency framework for nurse education in the UK. https://core.ac.uk/download/74390356.pdf (accessed on 28th June 2025).
11. Calzone, K., Chiu, P., Dewell, S., Gretchev, I., et al. (2024). Integrating genomics into Canadian oncology nursing policy: Insights from a comparative policy analysis. https://core.ac.uk/download/604541754.pdf (accessed on 28th June 2025).

12. Coe, K., Davies, P., Lane, N., Peters, B., et al. (2012). Talking glossary of genomics terminology: A genomics education module for American Indian communities. https://digitalscholarship.unlv.edu/cgi/viewcontent.cgi?article=1057&context=jhdrp (accessed on 28th June 2025).
13. Conley, Y. P., Dunbar-Jacob, J., Heitkemper, M. M., Henly, S. J., et al. (2015). Integrating emerging areas of nursing science into PhD programs. https://core.ac.uk/download/213079747.pdf (accessed on 28th June 2025).
14. Coutts, A. M. (2013). An overview of coeliac disease: Patterns, causes, symptoms and management. https://core.ac.uk/download/16272080.pdf (accessed on 28th June 2025).
15. Guillory, J. (2022). Genetics and genomics in nursing practice: Assessing barriers, facilitators, and tailoring implementation strategies. https://core.ac.uk/download/543565436.pdf (accessed on 28th June 2025).
16. Harris, A., Kelly, S., & Wyatt, S. (2012). Counseling customers: Emerging roles for genetic counselors in the direct-to-consumer genetic testing market. https://core.ac.uk/download/pdf/11451490.pdf (accessed on 28th June 2025).
17. Hickey, K. T., Housman, D. E., Taylor, J. Y., Wright, F. A., et al. (2017). Genome sequencing technologies and nursing. https://core.ac.uk/download/159108458.pdf (accessed on 28th June 2025).
18. Johnson, N. L. (2013). Genomics and autism spectrum disorder. https://core.ac.uk/download/213064140.pdf (accessed on 28th June 2025).
19. Leblanc, E. M. (2012). Needs analysis of genetics and genomics in communication sciences and its disorders: Evidence for change. https://core.ac.uk/download/161440695.pdf (accessed on 28th June 2025).
20. Linksvayer, T. A., & Mikheyev, A. S. (2015). Genes associated with ant social behavior show distinct transcriptional and evolutionary patterns. https://core.ac.uk/download/194580758.pdf (accessed on 28th June 2025).
21. Norris, A., Trepanier, A., Weber, A., Dierick-van Daele, A. T. M., Zellerino, B., Barnes, C., Cordier, C., et al. (2015). A prospective cohort study assessing clinical referral management & workforce allocation within a UK regional medical genetics service. https://core.ac.uk/download/42137466.pdf (accessed on 28th June 2025).
22. Palomera, G. (2023). Assessing genomic literacy in advanced practice nursing students before and after an intervention. https://core.ac.uk/download/571288557.pdf (accessed on 28th June 2025).
23. Patterson, W. (2022). Genetics and genomics education among physician assistants. https://core.ac.uk/download/539559133.pdf (accessed on 28th June 2025).

PAIN NURSING MANAGEMENT: ASSESSMENT AND INTERVENTIONS

9

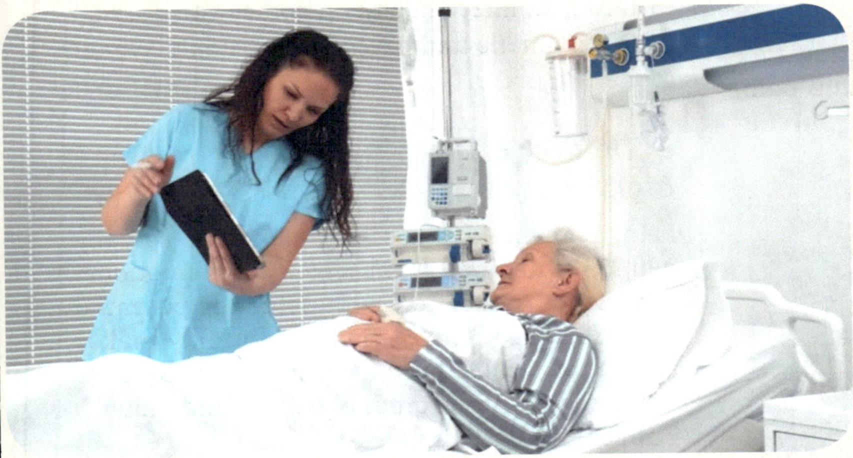

LEARNING OBJECTIVES

After studying this chapter, you will be able to:

1. Understand the pain;
2. Explain the pain assessment techniques
3. Discuss the pharmacological interventions
4. Learn about non-pharmacological interventions
5. Evaluate the patient education and involvement
6. State the challenges in pain management

Introduction

The theory of the management of pain nursing is a critical component of the intersection between the pervasive issues of pain, mental illness, and quality of life among older adults, especially in care home settings. The comorbid association between pain, depression, and anxiety disorders poses significant problems for clinicians, and efforts should be directed towards building a strong assessment strategy to achieve optimal patient outcomes. In nursing facilities, where residents frequently arrive with several chronic illnesses, comprehension of pain management is fundamental. A recent study demonstrated that a significant proportion of nursing home residents—actually, 36% upon admission—are diagnosed with either depression or anxiety disorders, or both, and the complex interplay between these disorders and pain (Hunnicutt et al., 2016). This preliminary review sets the background for exploring successful interventions that can encompass both psychological and physical elements of care.

Besides, qualitative aspects of pain management illuminate the lived experience of nursing home residents. Evidence has been demonstrated that several residents exhibit resistance towards complaining about pain, which they consider an acceptable part of aging. They tend to have poor expectations of medical treatments, founded on fears around pharmacological treatments and also stigmatization of their conditions (Schofield et al., 2006). Not only does this reluctance complicate the process of assessing pain, but it also underscores the need for health professionals to develop a setting that encourages open communication around pain. This is important because it affects nursing interventions that can be employed.

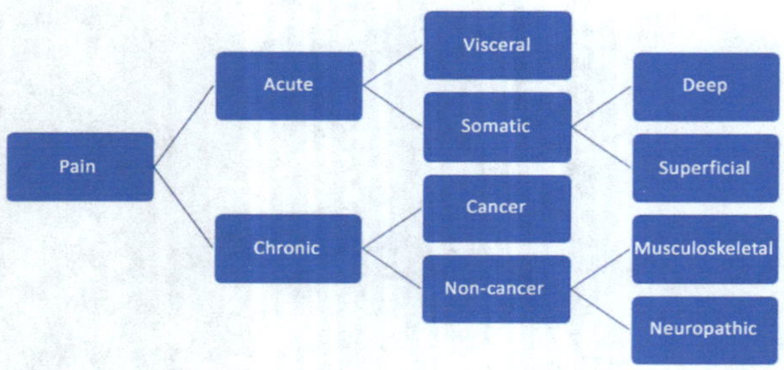

Figure 9.1. Nursing interventions for acute pain management.

Source: https://external-content.duckduckgo.com/iu/?u=https%3A%2F%2Fnursingcecentral.com%2Fwp-content%2Fuploads%2F2021%2F08%2FPain-Classification.jpg&f=1&nofb=1&ipt=d064880864a498282e16c148ccab6474e46fb789f7fc645ad4de25c13c1a8092.

This perspective emphasizes the importance of constructing patient-centered care that incorporates the resident's wishes and takes into account their unique pain experiences. Ultimately, successful pain treatment of nursing home residents requires an intervention strategy for both the pain and its co-morbid psychological conditions. Understanding through resident experiences and practitioner attitudes leads to designing individualized care plans that respond to special needs and personal preferences. The integration of complementary treatments, psychological support, and traditional pain management methods represents a potential avenue for enhancing overall well-being in patients (Schofield et al., 2006). By acknowledging the interdependency among pain, mental health, and patient care modalities, healthcare professionals can establish paths toward maximized health outcomes and develop a more humane and efficient pain management mode (Figure 9.1).

Definition of Pain and Its Significance in Nursing

Pain, a phenomenon of complexity, is actually defined as an unpleasant sensory and emotional experience associated with actual or potential tissue damage. This definition not only makes pain a physical symptom but also a subjective one, and it varies profoundly across individuals. The complexity involved in the process of perceiving pain calls for delicacy in perception during nursing practice. Pain is a significant indicator of health change for which nurses in assessment and intervention need to act. Furthermore, the perception of pain is often the reason patients present to the setting, underscoring the importance of effective pain management practices in the acute care setting. Understanding the multifaceted nature of pain is important for nurses, as it informs their approach to patient-focused care and enhances their ability to manage distressing symptoms in an effective and timely manner. Besides, competent assessment of pain is essential to provide patients with optimal treatment. Competent assessment of pain requires holistic consideration, including not only the biological but also the emotional and psychological dimensions of pain. Various instruments and measures have been employed in evaluating pain intensity, with the patient's subjective report taken into account, which may vary with cultural background and patient pain tolerance. Evidence that patients seek emergency care both for immediate relief and for knowledge of the condition's nature supports the importance of understanding the dimensions. In this situation, nurses must balance pharmacological treatment with other interventions that address patients' diverse needs. This knowledge aligns with the findings of a study, which show that occasionally, patients with pain reject analgesics due to personal beliefs and expectations about their care (Lemow et al., 2009). Pain management assumes an even more critical role in pediatrics due to the particular challenges posed by the varying levels of development and communication abilities of children. Nurses are responsible for identifying and interpreting pain cues among non-verbal patients and adapting interventions as appropriate, which can profoundly influence their overall care outcomes. Pain's acknowledgment extends beyond the individual patient's immediate comfort level; it impacts the children's hospital experience and future impressions of healthcare. For this purpose, the results of pain and sedation projects are utilized to guide specialized training and methodologies, equipping pediatric nurses with the requisite competencies for effective pain management (Latour et al., 2014). By making a conscious decision to opt for whole learning regarding pain and its effect, nurses establish an environment conducive to healing and introduce a more optimistic health care experience for children and their families.

Overview of Pain Management in Healthcare

The healthcare industry's landscape of pain management is a dynamic scene with varied methods aimed at alleviating patient suffering. To effectively manage pain, healthcare providers must adopt a comprehensive approach that encompasses both pharmacological and non-pharmacological management. Pharmacological treatments tend to involve the administration of analgesics, which may range from non-opioid medications, such as acetaminophen and NSAIDs, to the administration of opioids in extreme cases of pain. However, pain control is not just about medicine; it is a holistic process that considers the psychological, emotional, and social dimensions of a patient's experience. Research has shown that ideal pain control requires collaboration among interdisciplinary teams to deliver care in a multidimensional manner, thereby improving patient outcomes and quality of care (Latour et al., 2014). Additionally, advances in pain management practice have also emphasized the importance of evidence-based practice in healthcare settings. An example is the application of Appreciative Inquiry (AI) as a new knowledge translation intervention. In a pediatric academic care setting, AI was highly acceptable and had good fidelity among nurses in relation to pain management practices. The AI intervention introduced improvements by enabling workers to collaborate in developing action plans, thereby emphasizing the practical application of theory in the clinical setting. The models would enable organizations to make systematic improvements in pain assessment and management policies, and thus lead to improved patient satisfaction and outcomes. These kinds of initiatives foster a culture of continuous improvement, as feedback cycles help refine care processes and modify interventions to meet the distinct needs of various patient groups (Challis et al., 2010). Ultimately, optimal pain management in healthcare relies on a long-term commitment to conducting research, educating, and innovating. The integration of effective assessment measures and evidence-based practices is indispensable in addressing the complexity of pain, particularly among high-risk groups such as the elderly and children. Recent research has emphasized the importance of addressing areas such as pain and sedation in nursing research, as it can significantly impact clinical practice. By focusing on pain prevention, education, and the implementation of empirically supported interventions, healthcare systems can better equip their staff to address the challenges of pain management. Collectively, these strategies work to reduce the stigma of pain and provide an environment in which healthcare professionals are more able and willing to advocate on behalf of patients, which ultimately leads to a more compassionate and effective health care system that includes pain relief as a central component of overall health (Latour et al., 2014) (Figure 9.2).

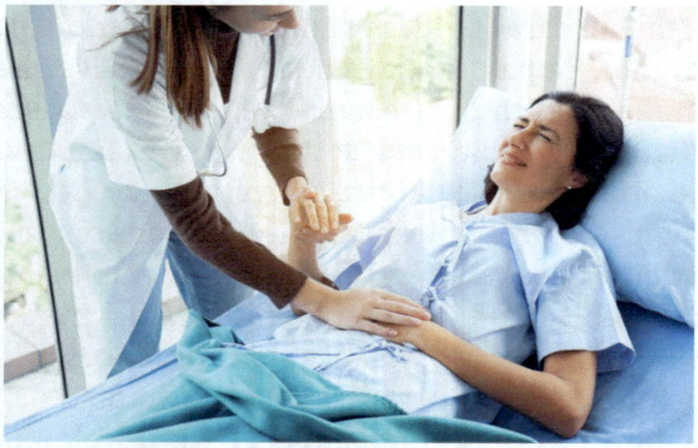

Figure 9.2. Surgical pain.

Source: https://twincitiespainclinic.com/wp-content/uploads/2022/12/Dark-haired-female-wincing-in-pain-while-lying-in-a-hospital-bed-and-being-attended-to-by-a-doctor.jpg.

9.1. Understanding Pain

Learning Outcome

1. Describe the types of pain: acute vs. chronic
2. emphasis on physiological and psychological aspects of pain
3. Pain and Patient Quality of Life Education

One of the main areas of pain management nursing is having an overall understanding of pain in its complex nature. Pain is not only a physical feeling; it is also intertwined with emotional, social, and psychological problems, so that it is challenging to measure and control. The subjective character of pain leads to the fact that all patient experiences are unique, and nurses must take a multifaceted approach to pain assessment. Effective strategies, such as the use of standard pain scales and consideration of a patient's self-reporting, are vital in identifying the severity and impact of pain on their lifestyle. Also, evidence indicates that common barriers such as inadequate communication and lack of appropriate pain assessment are to blame for ineffective pain management practice. Nurses should strive to create a deeper understanding of these complexities in order to provide holistic care and improve outcomes in pain relief within their practice by addressing both the physical and emotional dimensions of pain (Rees et al., 2000). Equally important is the recognition of patients' attitudes and perceptions of pain in various settings, as these determine whether they are ready to verbalize discomfort and seek help. For instance, patients in care homes have been shown to commonly refuse to describe their pain because they appear to have learned to accept that pain is a part of ageing or due to fear of pharmacological treatments. Studies conducted across several care homes discovered that the staff members were eager to assist residents in managing pain but lacked the proper tools and information on pain-control methods (Schofield et al., 2006). Such disconnection not only impacts the quality of pain management provided but also extends the suffering of patients. Thus, establishing an environment where patients are willing and capable of discussing their pain is paramount and requires alteration in both patient and provider attitudes towards pain awareness and management. Finally, the consequences of effective pain management are far-reaching beyond momentary relief and significantly influence a patient's overall quality of life and recovery trajectory. Having empathy for pain as a complex interaction of physical and emotional aspects enables nurses to implement more patient-tailored interventions aimed at addressing the causes of pain. For instance, integrating complementary therapies with pharmacologic therapy might maximize pain relief strategies and ultimately result in improved patient outcomes. Nursing staff education programs with an emphasis on best practice in pain management are imperative, as studies have delineated how enhancing nurses' knowledge equates to enhanced pain assessment and intervention strategies (Rees et al., 2000).

-Through this, developing a culture of learning and adaptation in nursing practice not only contributes to advancing the nursing profession but also facilitates a profound positive change in patient experiences of pain management, and ultimately, provides enhanced health outcomes (Figure 9.3).

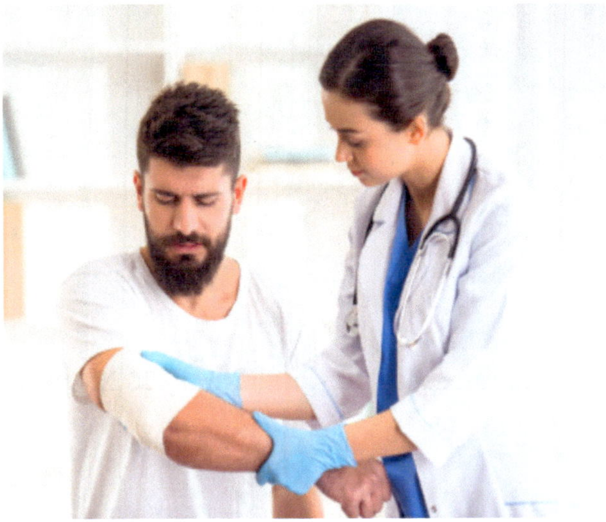

Figure 9.3. Successful at pain assessment nursing.

Source: https://external-content.duckduckgo.com/iu/?u=https%3A%2F%2Fwww.travelnursesource.com%2Fnotes%2Fwp-content%2Fuploads%2Fpain-assessment-nursing.jpg&f=1&nofb=1&ipt=82d529ad90981aea1cc73e10b6279aee6554f03ba57f7e0a17f82321c92e22c8.

9.1.1. Types of Pain: Acute vs. Chronic

It is crucial to understand the difference between chronic and acute pain in pain nursing management, as this knowledge informs both intervention and assessment. Acute pain tends to emerge suddenly and is typically an immediate response to inflammation or tissue damage. It typically resolves after a brief period as the condition improves. Acute pain is a significant warning symptom in a clinical setting, and it is what prompts individuals to seek hospital care. It is typically characterized as having a sharp, stabbing quality, and its treatment may include pharmacologic therapy such as NSAIDs or opioids, depending on the severity. As seen, proper management of acute pain is crucial not only for the patient's comfort but also to prevent the risk of developing chronic pain states that hinder recovery processes (Alexander et al., 2015). Chronic pain, on the other hand, lasts longer than the healing process would dictate, taking months or even years. It can be caused by conditions such as arthritis, fibromyalgia, or neuropathy, and its etiology is also multi-factorial, involving physical, psychological, and social factors. Chronic pain is characterized by its chronicity and may have profound emotional and functional disabilities. Nurses, as members of the health-care team, are mandated to carry out comprehensive assessments that explore the psychosocial dimensions of chronic pain, i.e., how it impinges on patients quality of life. Interventions may involve multidisciplinary treatment that consists of both behavioral interventions and drug management, such as cognitive behavior therapy, to improve coping strategies for pain. The biopsychosocial model is essential in the management of chronic pain and aligns with the current emphasis on developing nursing practice in holistic care (Nurmalia (Editor) et al., 2015). Discussions regarding the distinctions between acute and chronic pain also demand discussion regarding how such pain influences the choice of interventions.

Guidelines for the management of acute pain emphasize quick, effective interventions that induce immediate relief, while chronic pain management might require extensive intervention aligned with the needs of individual patients. Such interventions may vary from drug therapy, physical therapy, to alternative methods such as acupuncture or mindfulness exercises. In addition, the use of prescription drug monitoring programs is critical in controlling opioid use, a determinant that emphasizes the compounded aspect of addressing chronic pain in the presence of the current opioid epidemic. Nurses are key agents in implementing these protocols to ensure patient safety and prevent interference with effective pain relief practices. Lastly, the distinction between acute and chronic pain serves as the basis for total pain nursing management, allowing for individualized assessment and effective interventions to achieve desirable patient outcomes (Alexander et al., 2015) (Figure 9.4).

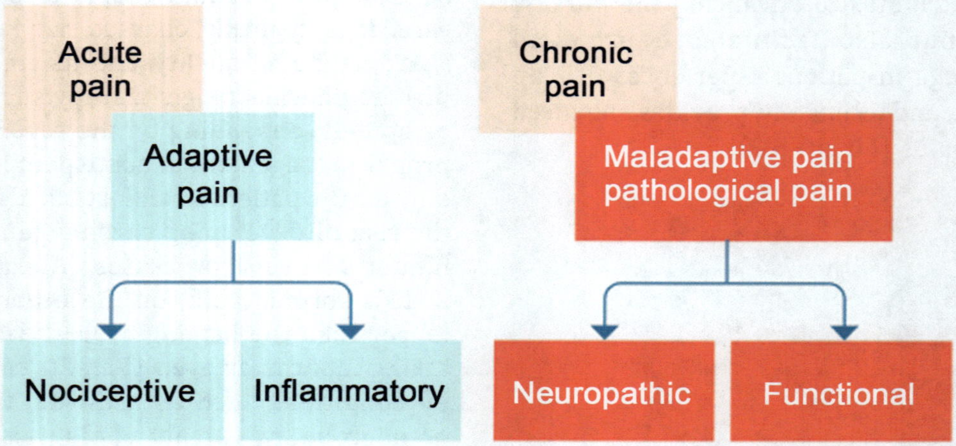

Figure 9.4. Types of pain.

Source: http://www.aaha.org/wp-content/uploads/globalassets/02-guidelines/2022-pain-management/diagram.png.

9.1.2. Physiological and Psychological Aspects of Pain

Understanding the physiological and psychological aspects of pain is crucial for efficient nursing management. Pain is itself a multifaceted sensory event that intertwines physical sensation with emotional reaction, the latter potentially having a disproportionate impact on a patient's general quality of life. Physiologically, pain can trigger several responses from the body, including increased heart rate, fluctuation in blood pressure, and release of stress hormones. Besides impacting the individual's physical status, these responses can also serve to reinforce the pain itself. In nursing practice, knowledge of such physiological changes enables healthcare providers to plan evidence-based interventions that address both the pain and the patient's overall physiological status, thereby limiting the physical burden of pain while establishing an atmosphere conducive to healing. Psychologically, pain has severe consequences that can lead to anxiety, depression, and a diminished quality of life. The emotional aspect of pain will often amplify the physical one, creating a vicious circle of increased suffering. Psychological disturbance as a result of pain can occur in several different ways, ranging from fear of chronicity to body-image issues, especially if pain is linked with visible wounds or bodily changes. As has been noted in recent studies, psychological distress is likely to impede healing significantly, and thus, nursing clinicians must incorporate psychological well-being as an integral aspect of a holistic pain management strategy. Rapport building, the application of mindfulness, and pain education to patients can empower them, enhancing their resilience and coping ability as they progress through the healing process (Edward et al., 2014).

Also, a focus on resilience in pain treatment improves both the psychological and physiological aspects of pain. Research has shown that resilience is more than just a personality trait, as it encompasses behaviors that can be taught and developed to improve patient outcomes. The addition of resilience interventions to pain treatment can lead to improved treatment compliance and coping. Moreover, it has been discovered that the integration of psychological support and physiological interventions can produce synergistic effects, improving the' quality of life for patients who suffer from pain. While existing research has provided the foundation for understanding how these dynamics function, additional studies are needed to investigate the specific clinical benefits of resilience for various pain conditions and to develop tailored interventions based on this concept (Aveyard et al., 2007) (Figure 9.5).

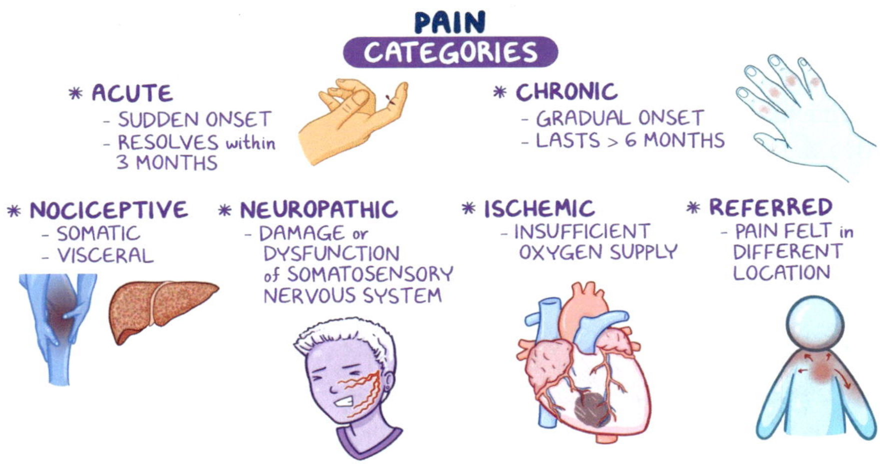

Figure 9.5. Physiological and psychological aspects of pain.

Source: https://d16qt3wv6xm098.cloudfront.net/pmIfFRnDTFOJNj6yYItzx8JAQzWW2wUa/_.jpg.

9.1.3. The Impact of Pain on Patient Quality of Life

Pain is a multifaceted experience that permeates most areas of a patient's life and adversely devastatingly affects quality of life. Chronic pain itself can produce a myriad of physical, emotional, and social challenges. Patients can experience limitations in activities of daily living, meaning even simple tasks become an effort and result in dependency.

This fall is exacerbated if the pain leads to social withdrawal due to patients either being stigmatized or isolated by the condition. Secondly, the chronicity of the pain is known to trigger or increase anxiety and depression, so much so that it creates a feedback loop that worsens suffering (Latour et al., 2014). Understanding the effects of pain on quality of life is therefore essential for healthcare professionals to adopt efficient pain management approaches that target not only the physiological aspects but also the psychological and social aspects of patients' health. Pain management in clinical practice must, therefore, go beyond simple analgesic therapy and adopt a holistic treatment approach. Research highlights the importance of the psychosocial management of pain, pointing to the successful treatment involving education materials and support systems to empower patients (Allison et al., 2018).

Cognitive behavior therapy or mindfulness interventions provide windows of opportunity to teach patients coping skills that decrease the emotional burden of pain. In addition, incorporating multimodal treatment approaches that can include pharmacologic, physical, and adjuvant modalities has the ability to augment patient outcomes powerfully. Not only does this scope of pain consideration attempt to alleviate pain, but it also improves patients' quality of life by cultivating resilience and adaptability towards challenging diagnoses. Finally, healthcare professionals' involvement in promoting improved pain management standards cannot be overstated. Engagement in quality measurement and evidence-based practice leads to better patient outcomes, for example, prioritization of research areas addressing pain in various fields of nursing (Latour et al., 2014). By adopting multidisciplinary team collaborative practices, nurses and healthcare professionals can develop personalized interventions that address specific patient needs. This alliance provides a patient-centered model of care vital for effective pain management with respect to patients' quality of life. As such, recognition and attention to the complex relationship between pain and quality of life remain more vital than ever to facilitate the delivery of effective pain management, improving the quality of patient care in healthcare settings.

Test Your Knowledge

1. What are the principal differences between acute and chronic pain, and how do they affect nursing interventions?
2. How do nurses use pain assessment measures to deal with patients' pain effectively?

9.2. Pain Assessment Techniques

Learning Outcome

1. Explain the subjective assessment: patient self-report
2. Define the observational measures of pain assessment
3. Explain pain scales and assessment tools used

Effective pain assessment is a crucial component of effective pain management in nursing. Nurses employ a range of tools and techniques to assess pain, which is a subjective and multifaceted phenomenon. One of the most widely used methods are self-report scales such as the Numeric Rating Scale (NRS) and the Wong-Baker FACES Pain Rating Scale that allow patients to rate their pain on a quantifiable, observable scale. These measures of testing enable patient-centered interventions, allowing treatment plans to be tailored to individual needs. Also, observational methods can be applied to patients who are unable to report pain through speech, such as infants or intellectually impaired individuals. Through continued pain assessment, nurses can identify alterations and evaluate the efficacy of interventions, gathering valuable information that enhances patient outcomes and satisfaction. For children in pediatric settings, assessment of pain is especially difficult since children lack sufficient descriptive words. Thus, modified assessment techniques are crucial for evaluating pain in pediatric patients. For instance, the use of visual aids, such as charts with illustrations or puppets, can be helpful in the communication process between health professionals and children. Furthermore, integrative approaches that incorporate parental views could improve the accuracy of pain evaluation, as caregivers are known to be intimate observers of their child's behavior and expressions. Evidence-based practice, as described in the literature, suggests that employing a range of strategies can enhance vaccine-related pain assessment in children by mitigating immunization anxiety. Employing broad, multi-dimensional assessment strategies enables nurses to possess more knowledge and decrease pain experiences among their pediatric patients, leading to healthier care experiences. Additionally, ongoing education and training of nursing staff in pain assessment techniques are crucial for facilitating effective pain management practices. There is evidence that indicates that there is a significant disparity between evidence-based pain relief measures and their application in practice (citations such as those by McMurty et al. and Taddio et al. point out the disparity). For example, a course that provided nurses with training in various pain management techniques showed positive outcomes, significantly enhancing the overall patient and caregiver experience during immunization. By fostering an environment where evidence-based practices are regularly updated and integrated into nursing school curricula, healthcare organizations can be assured that they have adequately trained personnel capable of providing high-quality pain assessment and interventions. This emphasis on continuous education not only supports the professional development of nursing staff but also benefits patients as well through the skilled and empathetic alleviation of pain, as evidenced by research (Aveyard et al., 2007; Bears et al., 2023) (Figure 9.6).

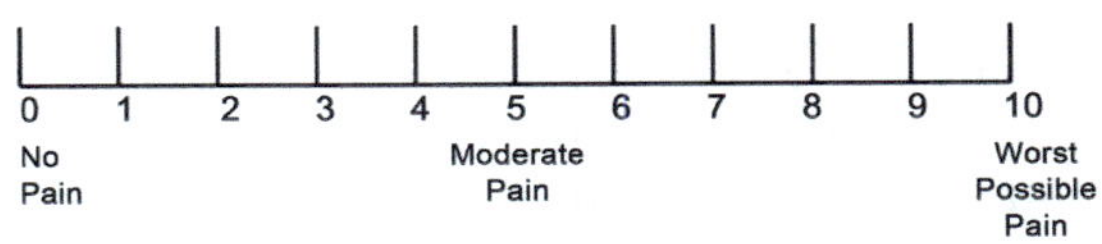

Figure 9.6. Pain assessment techniques.

Source: https://ns-content-service.wkhpe.com/css/images/p3040b.jpg.

9.2.1. Subjective Assessment: Patient Self-Reporting

Subjective assessment through patient self-report is a key component of pain nursing practice because it provides a firsthand account of the pain experience specific to the individual patient. It emphasizes the need for individual perception, which is critical to the capture of the complexity and multidimensionality of pain. Unlike objective instruments, subjective ratings highlight the emotional, psychological, and contextual factors that may accompany a patient's perception of pain. For instance, depression and anxiety can increase pain experience and necessitate that pain management interventions be more complex. By actively engaging with the reporting process, healthcare practitioners can gather helpful information that allows them to tailor chronic pain management strategies to specific patient needs. The self-reporting method, however, is valid and reliable only when the population being assessed has not been affected by cognitive impairment, such as that of dementia. In these cases, patients' ability to accurately report their level of pain may be significantly impaired, which could lead to under-detection of pain and subsequent poor control. This is a consideration that would support employing a variety of assessment instruments designed explicitly for patient groups with cognitive deficits. Yet, while tools can be used to help pain measurement, they cannot be employed to replace the subjective insight provided by patient self-reporting fully. Clinicians need to remain alert and open to the nuances of communication so that patients' experiences are heard and included in care decisions, as evidenced by the need for a balanced assessment strategy. In addition, educational interventions have been demonstrated to increase patient awareness and symptom management of conditions like fatigue and anxiety, particularly among chronic disease patients. For example, education programs on pain and symptom management can empower patients to effectively report their experiences, thus improving the accuracy of self-reporting. Research has shown that the type of educational intervention is capable of enhancing comprehension and adaptation in patients with cancer-related fatigue, which can also lead to improved outcomes in pain assessment and management. These results necessitate an integrative model that incorporates patient education within an integrated pain management program, ultimately leading to greater patient participation and satisfaction in shaping their pain experience (Corbett et al., 2014; Beller et al., 2016) (Figure 9.7).

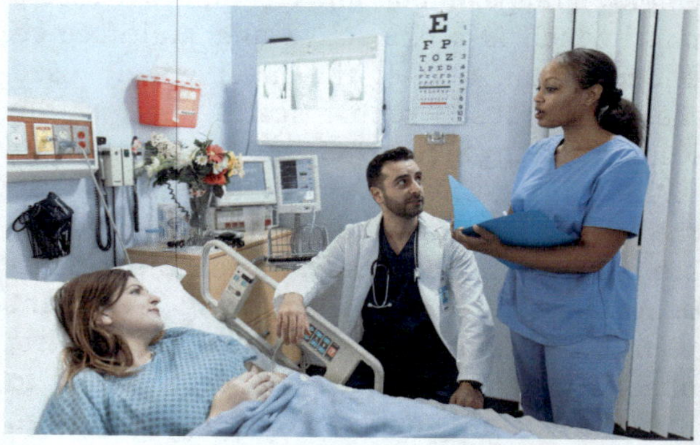

Figure 9.7. Patient self-reporting.

Source: https://www.pcs.ai/hubfs/pexels-rodnae-productions-6129681.jpg.

9.2.2. Objective Assessment: Observational Methods

Observational methods applied to pain assessment are a critical element of objective measurement in nursing management. These approaches focus on direct observation of a patient's behaviors and cues that may indicate the presence and intensity of pain. With the use of observational scales, clinicians can achieve quantifiable data that may be correlated with subjective self-reporting. This type of evidence is extremely valuable in groups who may have difficulty communicating their pain, such as patients with cognitive impairment or dementia. As highlighted in the systematic review submitted by Jones et al. (2019), psychosocial interventions can be enhanced by these observational methods to enhance the effectiveness of pain management. Emphasizing the importance of observational methods even further, nursing education interventions have been shown to have a positive impact on clinical outcomes for acute pain management. A summary of the studies reviewed in Drake et al. (2015) indicated that education regarding observation techniques significantly enhanced the documentation practice of nurses, which is critical for quality pain assessment.

By empowering nurses with the capacity to recognize and respond to observable indicators of pain, health systems can ensure more accurate assessments and timely interventions. This observation suggests that the inclusion of observational practice in nursing education could be adding to an integrated model of pain management, ultimately enhancing the quality of care delivered within health care facilities. Observational assessment also plays a critical role in monitoring patients following intervention. Continuous observation enables nurses to monitor pain management interventions in real-time and adjust treatment accordingly. The ability to observe short-term alterations in patient behaviors, such as body language, facial expressions, and vocalizations, provides helpful information regarding the efficacy of interventions being given. This has been corroborated by studies carried out by Jones et al. (2019), which demonstrated how psychosocial interventions can reduce signs of pain through regular monitoring. Thus, successful pain management also relies not just on the initial assessment but on ongoing monitoring, so interventions remain responsive to the ever-evolving character of patients' experience of pain.

9.2.3. Use of Pain Scales and Assessment Tools

In pain nursing care, the use of pain scales and assessment tools is a critical determinant in measuring the extent to which a patient experiences pain, which can have significant consequences for the patient's overall treatment. They are objective measures that enable the care provider to quantify the extent and character of pain experienced by a patient, allowing for tailored interventions. Frequently employed scales, such as the NRS and the Visual Analog Scale (VAS), quantify the subjective nature of pain into measurable components, such that clinicians are in a position to monitor developments and adjust treatment programs accordingly. The effective use of these tools of measurement is a sign that the multifaceted and individualized experiences of pain are acknowledged, thereby enhancing the patient-centric paradigm demanded by pain management. Additionally, effective pain evaluation extends beyond the use of scales and is complemented by the inclusion of holistic assessment tools that encompass psychosocial variables influencing pain. Tools such as the McGill Pain Questionnaire provide a rich context of interpretation of pain's qualitative aspects, further enhancing the clinician's perception of the patient's experience. The multifactorial etiology of pain demands an assessment that transcends physical measurement; it requires a serious study of the patient's psychological, emotional, and social statuses. This holistic approach aligns with contemporary models of palliative care, which encourage comprehensive assessments to inform the development of individualized care plans, ultimately leading to an improved overall quality of life for individuals presenting with multimodal pain diagnoses (Goodman et al., 2019). Furthermore, the applicability of such measures of assessment may be determined by the clinical and demographic characteristics of the population being assessed. Literature shows that specific demographic parameters, such as gender and age, may have a crucial role in determining pain reporting and sensitivity. For instance, research has shown variability in pain perception and reporting patterns among various age groups, thereby making age-specific assessment tools imperative. Additionally, the incorporation of digital health interventions has opened up a new horizon for enhancing patients' self-management of chronic pain disorders and contributing to the complexities of traditional approaches to assessment (Hartvigsen et al., 2017). In an era of continuous advancements in the specialty of pain management, the development of culturally tailored and universally transferable measures will be essential to address the diverse demands of patients in various global settings (Figure 9.8).

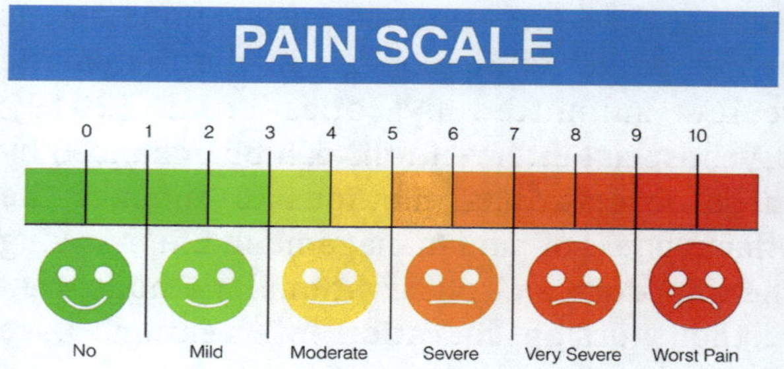

Figure 9.8. Pain scales.

Source: https://www.kauveryhospital.com/blog/wp-content/uploads/2020/09/ThinkstockPhotos-539684888-1280x640-1-1.jpg.

Test Your Knowledge

1. What are the most commonly used pain assessment scales to implement in clinical nursing practice?
2. How does utilizing the PQRST approach contribute to comprehensive pain assessment?

9.3. Pharmacological Interventions

Learning Outcome

1. Discuss the non-opioid analgesics: mechanisms and uses
2. Define the opioid analgesics: advantages and disadvantages
3. Describe the adjuvant medications: role in pain management

Pharmacological interventions are generally accepted as a pillar of pain management in nursing practice, particularly in treating complicated pain syndromes. These therapies primarily include the administration of analgesics, which are classified into three types: non-opioid analgesics, opioid analgesics, and adjuvant medications. Non-opioid analgesics, such as acetaminophen and non-steroidal anti-inflammatory drugs (NSAIDs), are first-line most of the time due to their efficacy in managing pain that is mild or moderate. Opioids, while effective for intense pain, must be taken cautiously due to their potential to create addiction and dangerous side effects. In addition, adjuvant drugs like antidepressants and anticonvulsants may be used to manage neuropathic pain, demonstrating the multidimensional application of pharmacologic interventions in nursing care. Nurses must have comprehensive knowledge of these drug classes because effective pain relief is directly linked to patient satisfaction and outcomes. While pharmacologic interventions are prevalent, some constraints hinder their practical application in pain relief in care centers. Patients in care homes have been found to exhibit reticence to complain about pain as a result of the beliefs these individuals have that it is something which is a natural accompaniment of aging or anxiety about aggressive pharmacologic interventions (Schofield et al., 2006). Furthermore, attitudes among staff are an essential aspect of pain management because healthcare staff are often bound to prioritize pharmacological methods of pain alleviation over the exploration of non-pharmacological interventions. This mindset can create lost opportunities for integrated care, wherein complementary therapies may supplement mainstream pharmacological interventions.

Thus, these barriers—through education and the development of guidelines—will enable a more inclusive approach to pain management, so that both residents' preferences and clinical best practices are respected in care routines. With the evidence claiming the predominance of pharmacological interventions in the treatment of pain among residents, it is imperative to continue exploring other forms of therapy besides conventional drugs. The systematic review regarding the topic indicates a call for non-pharmacological intervention, which is capable of treating pain without the inherent complications of drugs. A few of these alternatives include cognitive-behavioral therapy, physical therapy, and alternative therapies such as acupuncture or mindfulness training (Reid et al., 2006). Incorporating these into pain control regimens not only enhances treatment options but also empowers patients with self-management techniques. Finally, adopting a more holistic approach—balancing drug and non-drug interventions—has the potential to significantly enhance the quality of care provided in the nursing environment, resulting in better outcomes and increased patient satisfaction (Figure 9.9).

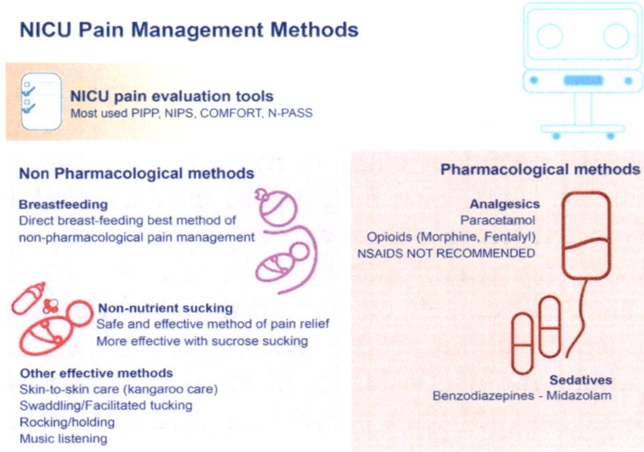

Figure 9.9. Effectiveness of non-pharmacological methods.

Source: https://www.mdpi.com/children/children-09-01568/article_deploy/html/images/children-09-01568-g001.png.

9.3.1. Non-Opioid Analgesics: Mechanisms and Uses

Non-opioid analgesics have emerged as key players in the treatment of pain, particularly as substitutes for opioids in various clinical situations. Their mechanisms of action are pretty distinct from the opioids, since the analgesics primarily act by blocking the synthesis of prostaglandins by COX enzymes. Inhibition of this synthesis leads to decreased inflammation and pain perception suppression. Non-opioid drugs, including NSAIDs and acetaminophen, are used to manage mild to moderate pain, for example, osteoarthritis and postoperative pain. The increasing awareness of side effects caused by opioids has further intensified the need to emphasize the significance of using non-opioids in nursing practice, where appropriate pain management is essential in optimizing patient satisfaction as well as the overall recovery outcomes, hence stressing the need for extensive education and training in their proper usage in nursing programs (Keefe et al., 2025). In the practice of nursing, the use of non-opioid analgesics requires knowledge of their pharmacological profiles and interactions with other drugs. Although the analgesics offer substantial advantages in pain management, they are not risk-free. For example, prolonged NSAID usage may cause gastrointestinal issues, renal toxicity, and heightened cardiovascular risks. Therefore, nurses can play a crucial role in reviewing patient histories and medications to ensure safe and effective utilization. Additionally, education about proper dosages and timing of administration is crucial to maximize the efficacy of such agents while preventing adverse effects.

By combining knowledge of both pharmacodynamics and patient-focused care, nurses can adjust pain control methods most appropriate to individual patient requirements, thereby maximizing the utility of non-opioid analgesics in clinical practice (Keefe et al., 2025). Emerging research shows emerging strategies that further maximize the utility of non-opioid analgesics, including the judicious use of placebos in conjunction with active treatments. Current studies indicate that placebos can prolong analgesic effects after active treatment upon administration and may reduce total drug consumption and associated side effects. This method not only potentially inhibits the dose escalation of painkillers but also promotes less patient reliance on medications, highly relevant in the aftermath of the present opioid crisis. By incorporating such treatment strategies into pain management plans, nurses can optimize treatment plans, ensuring that interventions are both cost-effective and practical. As nurse education continues to evolve, the inclusion of these new concepts in training will enable nurses to tackle the complexities of pain management with confidence, thereby providing an environment conducive to holistic, evidence-based practice (Figure 9.10).

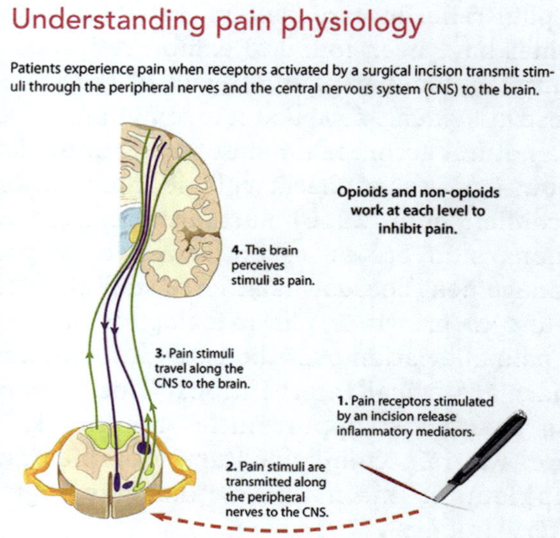

Figure 9.10. Opioid non opioid analgesia surgery.

Source: https://www.myamericannurse.com/wp-content/uploads/2018/05/opioid-non-opioid-analgesia-surgery-understand-pain-physiology.jpg.

9.3.2. Opioid Analgesics: Benefits and Risks

Among the pain relief medications, opioid analgesics are commonly most commended for their effectiveness in relieving moderate to severe pain.

Through the pharmacological effect of opioid interaction on specific receptors within the central nervous system, overall analgesic effects enhance the quality of life of patients with chronic as well as acute pain disorders.

However, while opioid therapy has great benefits, particularly in palliative treatment and in the post-op setting, it is equally necessary to go ahead with their use with caution. The increased incidence of opioid abuse and overdose has produced national guidelines suggesting prudence on the part of healthcare providers, coming to the conclusion that while opioids are effective for pain management, they should nonetheless be prescribed judiciously lest they incur the associated risk (Swezey et al., 2018). As the war on opioid use shifts, the risks of opioid analgesics cannot be overlooked. Perhaps foremost among these is the risk of dependence and the development of tolerance, especially in patients with a history of substance abuse disorders. The public health effects of opioid abuse have prompted calls for a paradigm shift towards nonpharmacologic pain control strategies.

Health care providers are thus encouraged to explore other interventions such as cognitive behavioral therapy, physical therapy, and integrative practices, but with the ability to effectively control levels of pain. An optimum model of care, which maximizes the benefits of opioids against harms, is crucial to guide effective pain management (Bergin et al., 2016).

To address the ongoing issues of opioid abuse, emerging strategies for addressing opioid prescriptions are under study. Best practices established through ongoing studies emphasize a comprehensive approach, including appropriate prescribing habits, patient education, and strict monitoring, to minimize the risk of abuse.

Fostering interprofessional collaboration among healthcare practitioners, regulatory authorities, and patients is also crucial in developing comprehensive management plans that incorporate both pharmacological and non-pharmacological approaches. With the new dynamics in pain management, these results highlight the need to implement efficient interventions alongside being compassionate and patient-centered in caring for patients. Monitoring such dynamics significantly enhances nursing professionalism in pain management (Swezey et al., 2018).

9.3.3. Adjuvant Medications: Role in Pain Management

The multidisciplinary care strategy has increasingly acknowledged the contribution of adjuvant medications in pain management. These medications, including antidepressants, anticonvulsants, and steroids, are not primarily employed as analgesics but have been successful in the management of chronic pain syndromes. For example, tricyclic antidepressants are frequently used in the management of neuropathic pain since they are capable of influencing pain transmission; they essentially alter the perception of pain by the patient (Davis et al., 2020). In addition, anticonvulsants such as gabapentin have been found helpful in relieving pain in postherpetic neuralgia, once again demonstrating the merits of individualized pain treatment modalities. The use of these adjuvant medications as part of treatment plans can enhance outcomes, enhance functionality, and make possible a more comprehensive management of complex pain conditions. Aside from pharmacologic treatment, the psychological and emotional facet of treating pain focuses on the function of adjuvant drugs. Most patients undergoing treatment for chronic pain syndromes also experience different emotional responses, like depression and anxiety, that enhance pain perception. Treatment with antidepressants not only deals with the psychological factors, but it is also two-pronged in action since it alleviates somatic pain symptoms. Studies have indicated that patients who are subjected to an intervention of comprehensive pain management involving adjuvant drugs are satisfied and have a better quality of life (Smith et al., 2021). Therefore, the management of both psychological and physical dimensions of pain in an integrated way can lead to the successful management of pain by nursing. Furthermore, the application of adjuvant medications should be preceded by thorough assessments to monitor their effectiveness and side effects, thereby prioritizing individualized treatment plans. Nurses are responsible for monitoring patient reactions to therapy and adjusting treatment accordingly based on ongoing assessments. For instance, adjustments may be done when side effects occur or when patients report changes in the degree of pain. By utilizing tools such as pain scales and patient-reported outcomes, nurses are able to inform the rest of the healthcare team regarding the efficacy of adjuvant therapies. Such a partnership organization not only enhances patient safety but also ensures that care is provided individually to patients suffering from pain management, thereby optimizing the therapeutic benefit of adjuvant medications in pain nursing management, as supported by the literature (Reynolds et al., 2011; Bear et al., 2015) (Figure 9.11).

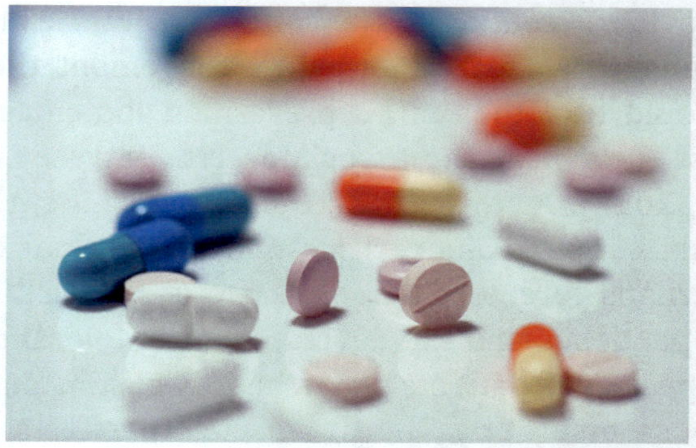

Figure 9.11. Adjuvant analgesics used to treat chronic pain.

Source: https://www.verywellhealth.com/thmb/gNf5p5KxM6utNUyrFMM-m2AiuvU=/2122x1415/filters:fill(87E3EF,1)/GettyImages-476698149-56b2f03b5f9b58def9c9276f.jpg.

Test Your Knowledge

1. What are the considerations nurses need when administering opioids for pain relief?
2. How do the non-opioid analgesics differ in mechanism and use from opioids in nursing care?

9.4. Non-Pharmacological Interventions

Learning Outcome

1. Name the physical therapies: massage, acupuncture, and exercise
2. Define the psychological therapies: cognitive-behavioral therapy and mindfulness
3. Explain the complementary therapies: aromatherapy and music therapy

Within pain nursing, non-pharmacological interventions have emerged as a relevant focus as adjuvants to standard pharmacologic therapies. Healthcare professionals are increasingly realizing that effective pain management involves more than just medication and that a holistic approach to patient care is necessary. A variety of non-pharmacological modalities, such as cognitive-behavioral therapy (CBT), guided imagery, and relaxation techniques, may be especially beneficial in reducing pain. Not only do these techniques address the physical aspects of pain, but also the emotional and psychological, facilitating a more holistic healing environment. Evidence suggests that integrating such interventions into routine pain management practices may enhance patient satisfaction and outcomes, thereby suggesting a paradigm shift in pain nursing management strategies (Reid et al., 2006). Such evidence encourages practitioners to adopt an eclectic approach that acknowledges the interdependence of body and mind in the experience of pain. Moreover, qualitative research reveals a complex relationship between patient experience of pain and response to non-pharmacological interventions. For instance, care home residents will often resist reporting pain, sometimes seeing it as an inevitable aspect of growing older or fearing that doing so will lead to unwelcome drug treatment (Schofield et al., 2006). Awareness of such attitudinal barriers is crucial for nurses intending to establish effective pain management schemes. It emphasizes the need for staff education regarding pain assessment and also promotes complementary therapies as reasonable options. By initiating a system that promotes open discussion of pain, healthcare providers can better tailor their non-pharmacological interventions to specific patient needs, thereby providing overall improved quality of care. Additionally, non-pharmacological approaches must be evidence-based and demonstrate their effectiveness and suitability in specific cases. Studies have identified effective strategies, including complementary therapies such as acupuncture, massage, and music therapy, which have been shown to exhibit a significant reduction in perceived pain among specific patient populations. Nurses with experience in these interventions are better able to educate patients about their potential advantages and relevance, thus involving their patients more actively in their pain management program. Moreover, as Reid et al. (2006) explain, the emphasis placed upon evidence-based practices means that the use of these interventions is not merely new-fangled but also supported by a firm basis of clinical research. This confirms that holistic pain management in nursing extends beyond discrete medical models, ultimately benefiting patients through a multi-component process of understanding their needs and experiences (Figure 9.12).

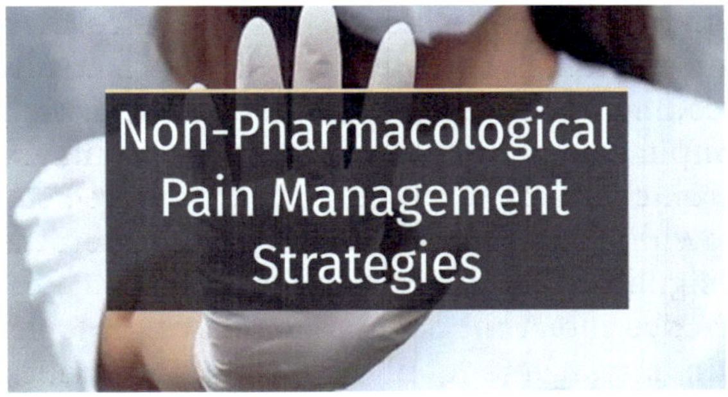

Figure 9.12. Non-pharmacological pain management.

Source: https://i.ytimg.com/vi/StrK-Hv7gPQ/maxresdefault.jpg.

9.4.1. Physical Therapies: Massage, Acupuncture, and Exercise

The integration of physical therapies, specifically massage, acupuncture, and exercise, continues to gain recognition as a viable alternative to orthodox pharmacologic interventions in pain nursing management. In the instance of chronic pain, as is so prevalent among so many veterans, these treatments outside of drugs are full of promise. Massage has been found to induce relaxation, enhance circulation, and soothe tense muscles, potentially leading to a reduction in perceived pain. Furthermore, evidence is available for its use in increasing the quality of life for those with chronic pain disorders. The increasing emphasis on the integration of complementary therapies underlines the virtue of tailoring pain care to the specific needs of individual patients, towards a more holistic style of care, in addition to the appreciation of the shortfall of opioid prescriptions that have increasingly dominated pain care in recent times (Swezey et al., 2018). Acupuncture, another well-known modality for pain relief, establishes its efficacy through the stimulation of specific body points, which produces natural pain-suppressant effects. Studies indicate that the ancient technique can effectively reduce pain levels associated with common illnesses, such as musculoskeletal pain, migraines, and osteoarthritis. With medical recommendations shifting increasingly towards nonpharmacologic approaches in managing chronic pain, the usability of acupuncture keeps growing. A systematic review of the literature designates acupuncture as one of the best-practice interventions for nonpharmacological pain management, highlighting its potential applications across a broad spectrum of patient populations (Anthony et al., 2017). As nurses and healthcare professionals become better educated about these therapies, they become more equipped to implement multidimensional interventions that empower patient autonomy and overall health. Exercise, tailored to the individual's capabilities, is a fundamental intervention in the management of chronic pain.

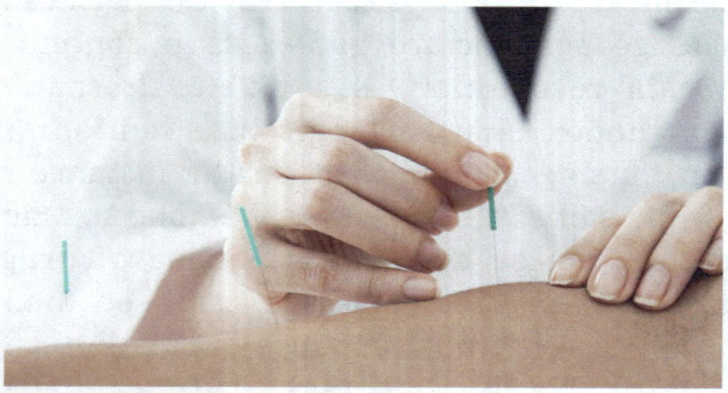

Figure 9.13. Acupuncture: form and function therapy.

Source: https://www.formfunctionpt.com/wp-content/uploads/2020/09/unnamed.png.

Not only does exercise increase physical functioning and flexibility, but it is also essential to the improvement of psychological well-being, which is typically adversely affected by chronic pain. Scientific evidence suggests that exercise reduces pain symptoms and enhances functional independence, ultimately improving overall quality of life. Moreover, the integration of exercise regimens in pain treatment plans can minimize the potential for opioid addiction, aligning with the nation's shift toward nonpharmacological management (Swezey et al., 2018). By creating an integrated knowledge and use of these physical therapy modalities, nursing professionals have the capacity to impact patient outcomes significantly, enabling patients to be a part of their pain management in a beneficial way, as well as minimizing the reliance on medication alone (Figure 9.13).

9.4.2. Psychological Therapies: Cognitive-Behavioral Therapy (CBT) and Mindfulness

Psychological therapies such as CBT and mindfulness are gaining a foothold in pain management, particularly when managing the cognitive-emotional features of chronic pain. CBT is used to alter maladaptive negative cognitions and behavior that act as reinforcement for increased pain perception. By equipping patients with strategies to reinterpret their experience and manage stress, CBT can enhance their coping capacity, possibly reducing the severity of pain and improving quality of life. Evidence has demonstrated that CBT is effective in achieving significant reductions in pain-related distress and disability, which is why it is such a valuable intervention in pain nursing management. Thus, the incorporation of CBT in patient care plans is a multifaceted treatment approach that addresses the psychological dimensions of pain and traditional physical therapies. Another psychological therapy, mindfulness, enables individuals to be more aware of their thoughts, feelings, and bodily sensations without judgment. This therapeutic technique enhances pain coping ability through increased present-moment awareness and acceptance, and thus lessens pain's negative emotional responses. Research has found that mindfulness training can lead to increased pain tolerance and decreased emotional reactivity, making patients more resilient. In pain nursing care, the integration of mindfulness techniques as adjuncts to pharmacological management can provide patients with tangible skills for self-regulation. Interestingly, these nonpharmacological interventions align with the national trend toward greater expectations that healthcare professionals implement holistic pain treatment modalities consistent with best practice recommendations supported by national initiatives (Swezey et al., 2018). The use of psychological treatments like CBT and mindfulness in pain treatment has particularly profound implications for at-risk groups like the elderly and those who have cognitive compromise. A systematic review emphasized the effectiveness of psychosocial interventions in pain management in older adults with dementia and suggested that psychosocial interventions can be a valuable component of a general pain management plan. Psychosocial interventions not only provide a means of pain relief from physical pain but also promote emotional well-being, contributing to an enhanced quality of life. Whereas the health environment gets set for reducing reliance on opioids and increasing utilization of nonpharmacological treatment, the integration of psychological therapies in clinical practice can meet the dual challenge of effective pain management along with the prevention of drug abuse (Jones et al., 2019) (Figure 9.14).

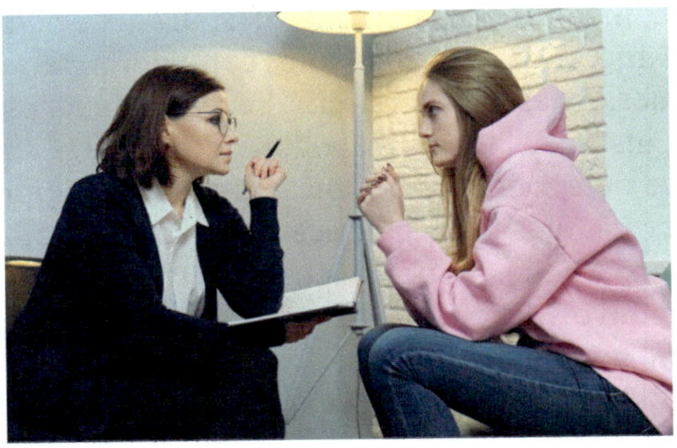

Figure 9.14. Approach to adolescent mental health treatment care.

Source: https://buildbrightcaregroup.com/wp-content/uploads/2025/04/Californias-Leading-Teen-Mental-Health-Program-Build-Bright109.jpg.

9.4.3. Complementary Therapies: Aromatherapy and Music Therapy

The integration of complementary therapies, such as aromatherapy and music therapy, with pain management strategies presents a holistic approach to nursing care. Evidence suggests that they can reduce the perception of pain and enhance patients' quality of life. Aromatherapy, founded on the application of essential oils, has been associated with reduced anxiety and pain, particularly in hospice and palliative care settings. Its ability to promote relaxation can be a blessing to patients with chronic pain. Further, the sensory stimulation provided by aromatic chemicals may activate the brain's inherent systems for producing pain relief. Used as an adjunct to standard pharmacological treatments, aromatherapy can be a vital component of a multifaceted approach to pain management, and its continued investigation in nursing research and practice is recommended (Reid et al., 2006). Music therapy, another therapy option, has also been reported for their therapeutic implications, particularly in pain relief and emotional support among patients. The findings revealed that music listening can alter the subjective experience of pain by distracting and inducing relaxation. Distraction can reduce reliance on analgesic drugs, which is particularly beneficial among populations in which pharmacologic interventions can produce side effects. Within hospice, music therapy has been used to allow patients to release their feelings, which enables them to confront their pain and sorrow. Adding music therapy as a part of standard nursing practice offers nurses a valuable intervention that can improve pain management outcomes, showcasing the potential of patient-centered care. Overall, the inclusion of music therapy enhances the nursing care continuum by targeting physical and emotional dimensions of pain (Ortiz-Cintron et al., 2014). Although they are likely to be of benefit, complementary therapies such as aromatherapy and music therapy are not without their problems when introduced into clinical practice, particularly among a resistant nursing staff who are not formally trained. An interest in them is often evinced, but is later followed by a lack of knowledge or disbelief in their efficacy. Educational programs have emerged as essential to bridging these gaps, as indicated by research to support increased education on complementary and alternative modalities in nursing schools. Incentivizing nurses to incorporate these modalities would not only enhance pain management practices but also align with evolving patient expectations of whole-person care. By fostering an appreciation for a culture that embraces constant education and interprofessional collaboration, the addition of complementary therapies to nursing practice can offer significant improvements in overall pain management (Reid et al., 2006; Ortiz-Cintron et al., 2014).

Test Your Knowledge

1. What are some effective non-pharmacological methods of controlling patient pain?
2. How can patient education enhance the efficacy of non-drug pain relief techniques?

9.5. Patient Education and Involvement

Learning Outcome

1. Describe why patient education is so critical in pain management
2. Clarify what effective strategies are for communicating with the patient
3. Discuss how to encourage patient engagement in their own care

Patient education and activation are paramount in the clinical application of pain nursing management for successful outcomes. Knowing patient preferences and experience inevitably influences pain assessment and management. Engaging patients in communication about their pain is a crucial factor in establishing a team environment that empowers patients to take ownership of the healthcare process. Studies have shown that when patients receive effective education about their illness and treatment options, adherence to the regimen increases significantly. Secondly, patient-focused education helps in the prevention of misconceptions about pain management and eventually leads to better pain control and patient satisfaction with treatment. Apart from enhancing the therapeutic alliance as a preventative measure, this approach also closely aligns with evidence-based practice, whereby the integration of patients' voices into clinical decision-making within pain treatment programs guides practice. Additionally, patient participation is not only about education but also involves an element of shared decision-making that respects and considers patient values. As essential nursing research priorities, for instance, those in pediatric intensive care have determined that decision-making support is crucial in pain management cases (Latour et al., 2014). Patient-centered interventions that involve patients as active participants in pain management plan formulation not only recognize their own experiences but also encourage a sense of ownership of health outcomes. By collaborating with patients to set achievable pain management objectives, care providers can further individualize interventions to meet specific needs and enable a more responsive reaction to care. This interaction provokes ongoing debate on the experience of pain, potentially leading to revisions in care management approaches aimed at optimizing therapeutic impact. A patient-oriented focus on education is crucial in the context of chronic disease, and particularly so for patients laboring under the long-term excesses of disease conditions such as cancer. The National Cancer Survivorship Initiative emphasizes the need for individualized educational resources for survivors dealing with chronic pain and related conditions (Brooks et al., 2014). The initiative reflects a growing recognition that overall pain management is not merely contingent upon clinic therapies, but also on patient empowerment through education, which helps them cope more efficiently with their condition. Through targeted educational interventions, patients can learn self-management techniques, understand when to seek additional medical advice, and identify the importance of mental health in pain management. Therefore, incorporating effective educational components into pain nursing plans establishes a vital support structure, ultimately enhancing coping capacity and quality of life in individuals with chronic pain (Figure 9.15).

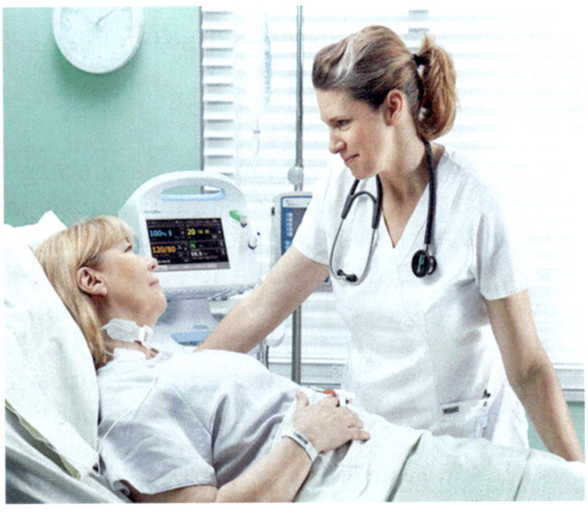

Figure 9.15. Patient education and involvement.

Source: https://www.nursebuff.com/wp-content/uploads/2018/01/surgical-nurse.jpg.

9.5.1. Importance of Educating Patients About Pain Management

Educating patients about pain management is crucial for activating their awareness of treatment options and encouraging their participation in care. Good communication between healthcare providers and patients strongly impacts health outcomes. By informing patients well about nonpharmacological pain treatments, nurses can minimize the misuse of opioid medication. Opioid prescription trends have plagued Oklahoma due to widespread addiction and subsequent deaths from overdoses. In the past, some have responded by presenting a counter-narrative to societal pressures, advocating for responsible use and directing attention toward human factors influencing prescribing practices (Swezey et al., 2018). Nurses can play a key role in empowering patients by educating them about potential avenues of pain relief through targeted education. Also included in the teaching of pain management is the discussion of the psychological aspects that are associated with chronic pain. Patients will display emotional distress, which will complicate the development of pain and hinder recovery. By teaching pain psychology, nurses can help patients develop enhanced coping mechanisms, enabling them to manage their conditions more effectively. When patients understand the intersection of physical and mental well-being, they are more willing to participate in therapeutic interventions. Not only does this enhance their well-being, but it also reduces the likelihood of acute pain developing into chronic pain. Therefore, pain must be addressed on a multi-dimensional scale so that nursing specialists can offer interventions based on precise patient needs while promoting well-being in general. Besides, patient education on pain management has the potential to reduce the expenditure on healthcare through the avoidance of prolonged treatment and hospitalization. In delirium, as well as other conditions, an educated patient is less likely to experience adverse outcomes, leading to shorter hospitalization and reduced healthcare expenditure (Bull et al., 2015). By starting formal educational programs, patients can be assisted by nurses in establishing their risk factors and the indicators of pain management complications. Not only is this proactive approach helpful for patient safety, but it also encourages early intervention in cases of escalating pain or complications. The economic burdens underlie the need for patient education, making it an integral part of nursing care that coordinates clinical practice with patient empowerment and cost-saving healthcare provision (Figure 9.16).

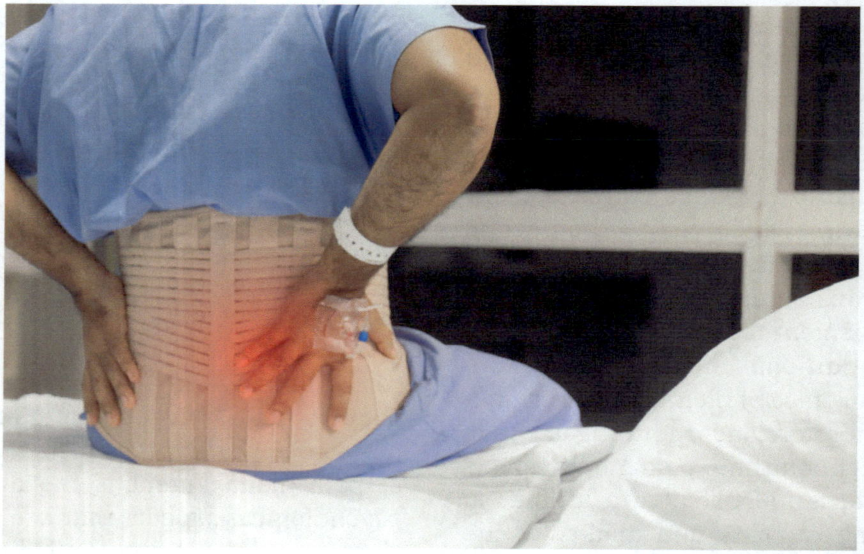

Figure 9.16. Post-surgical pain.

Source: https://www.spinediagnostic.com/wp-content/uploads/2021/08/post-surgical-pain-1.jpg.

9.5.2. Strategies for Effective Communication with Patients

Communication is the backbone of pain management in nursing, particularly in developing a therapeutic relationship between patients and caregivers. Rapport and trust are essential in managing pain because they promote free expression of fears by patients. Active listening techniques, through which nurses demonstrate empathy and acknowledge emotions expressed by the patient, can be utilized. Additionally, open-ended questions ensure that patients give a thorough explanation of their experience of pain so that their concerns and needs are better appreciated. Not only is the observation of pain better validated, but also the patients' feelings of involvement in their pain management plan, building on significant research findings in patients' reluctance to report pain and expectations of relief (Schofield et al., 2006). In addition to verbal communication strategies, nonverbal communication will also be beneficial in patient pain communication. Paying attention to body language, facial expressions, and tone of voice can give a hint at how much pain the patient is experiencing and the patient's emotional status. For instance, the tense posture or scowl of a patient that signals severe pain, even though the patient may not utter a word because they do not want to be perceived as a bother. Nurses must be attuned to these nonverbal communications as they complete the gaps of verbal tests and contribute to an overall picture of the patient's case. Nurses will be able to establish competence in nonverbal communication and become adept at detecting and interpreting pain-based distress, thereby enhancing patient outcomes in pain management (Bunn et al., 2019). In addition, educational programs for enhancing communication skills among nursing staff are essential in maximizing pain management strategies. Skills training on effective patient interaction can help nurses have more effective discussions about pain. Training sessions that involve role-playing and simulated patient interactions should be used to highlight the importance of empathy when evaluating pain. Additionally, promoting interdisciplinarity enhances communication among care teams regarding the treatment of patient pain, ensuring that all practitioners involved share information and are aligned in practice. This inclusive practice is a response to patients' expectations of pain management and enhances the practice-friendly environment of efficient pain treatment practice (Bunn et al., 2019; Schofield et al., 2006) (Figure 9.17).

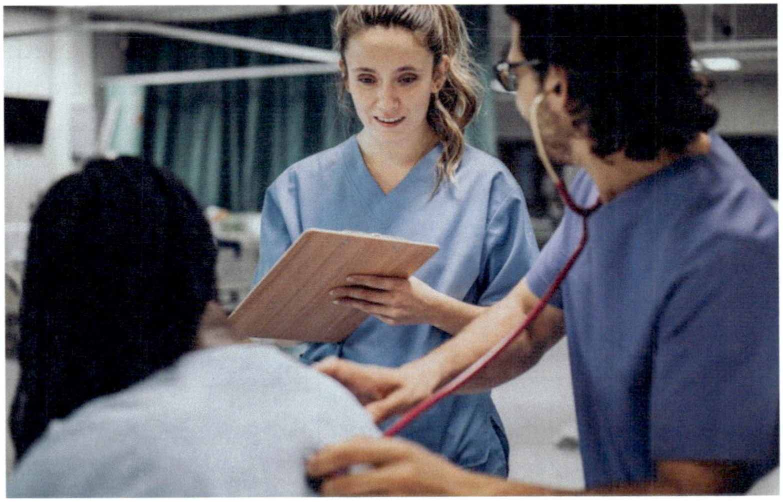

Figure 9.17. Importance of effective communication in nursing.

Source: https://www.masmedicalstaffing.com/wp-content/uploads/2022/01/Importance-of-Effective-Communication-in-NursingFT.jpg.

9.5.3. Encouraging Patient Involvement in Their Own Care

Involving patients in their own care is essential for the best pain management in nursing practice. Enabling patient participation helps build a sense of control, which in turn enhances their understanding of pain and facilitates self-management of care. Such collaborative care enables not only patient empowerment but also individualized interventions tailored to their preferences and experiences with pain.

Research has indicated that when patients are included in decision-making processes concerning their treatment interventions, e.g., selecting preferred modes of pain relief, there is an increased perception of satisfaction and adherence to the regimen prescribed. Also, through patient involvement, healthcare professionals can obtain valuable information regarding the individual pain profiles of patients, and through this, improved assessment and intervention strategies suiting the patient's culture as well as context of living. Secondly, educating the patient is at the core of motivating their involvement in care. It can range from familiarity with the physiological processes responsible for pain to awareness of the potential side effects of interventions. Through controlled educational interventions and discourses that involve information provision, patients are equipped with the knowledge necessary to make informed decisions about their care. It is essential to implement multi-faceted interventions, according to studies of effective delirium prevention and practice in dementia care, which demonstrate that partnership models of staff, patient, and family work contribute to patient-centered care and outcomes. The integration of these ideals into pain management plans enables nursing professionals to effectively enhance patients' confidence in their ability to manage pain, thereby facilitating an active and motivated approach to their own health. Significantly, it involves not only effective communication but also the establishment of trust between patients and medical practitioners. Nurses should listen to and validate patients' concerns in establishing a therapeutic relationship that fosters open communication. The therapeutic relationship is critical when addressing pain management preferences and collaborating on treatment objectives. In addition, overcoming potential obstacles—such as myths about pain treatment or the complexity of healthcare systems—is required to promote increased patient involvement. Changes in nursing practice and systems, with the application of guidelines such as those employed in delirium prevention research, can facilitate more effective implementation of patient-centered care. This, in turn, yields improved outcomes, highlighting the inherent value of engaging in supportive activities for active patient participation in pain management programs (Edlund et al., 2013; Bunn et al., 2019).

Test Your Knowledge

1. Why is patient education so vital to effective pain management?
2. How can nurses facilitate patient involvement in creating an individualized pain management plan?

9.6. Challenges in Pain Management

Learning Outcome

1. Explain the challenges to effective pain management in nursing
2. Outline the ethical aspects of pain management
3. Identify the role of cultural differences in pain

The multifaceted nature of pain presents several challenges in its effective management, particularly within clinical settings. Pain not only represents a physiological condition but also emotional, psychological, and social aspects, thus complicating the assessment process. This multidimensionality necessitates that nurses employ comprehensive and multi-dimensional assessment instruments to develop an informed base of knowledge of a patient's individual pain experience. Furthermore, differences in pain perception among patients due to cultural, emotional, and particular considerations can lead to underreporting or miscommunication of pain levels and thus render treatment decisions even more difficult. Resolution of such problems requires a nuanced understanding of the patient's history, along with the use of various assessment techniques beyond simple pain scales. The integration of individualized approaches is necessary to tailor intervention strategies that are sufficient and appropriate responses to the patient's pain experience. Apart from issues in assessment, logistical considerations typically present barriers to the implementation of effective pain management strategies. Clinicians often face challenges such as limited resources, staff shortages, and a lack of time, which restrict their ability to properly evaluate and manage pain. Such barriers risk augmenting the already high levels of stress and anxiety among patients, forming a vicious cycle of poor pain control and heightened distress.

Embracing new approaches, such as Appreciative Inquiry (AI), has the potential to facilitate more effective pain management practice through stronger teamwork between the nursing staff. From the findings of an AI intervention in a pediatric surgery ward, the intervention increased engagement and developed action plans for improved quality in pain assessment documentation, demonstrating its ability to address systemic problems in pain management (Challis et al., 2010). Additionally, the beliefs and attitudes of patients regarding pain perception and control should be explored, as these are likely to impact the outcomes of treatment.

Stigmatization of chronic pain disorders tends to render patients stigmatized, thus leading to poor control of pain. Nurses play a significant role in being patient advocates, but may also have prejudices against which their judgments for controlling pain are made. These deep-seated attitudes must be overcome through ongoing education and training on current best practices and patient-focused strategies. The AI project reported on in Challis et al. (2010) found that removing barriers to implementation, such as change overload and lack of structured follow-up, is required to make pain management practices possible and clinically relevant. Highlighting the importance of ongoing improvement of nursing practice will eventually enhance the quality of care provided to patients with pain (Figure 9.18).

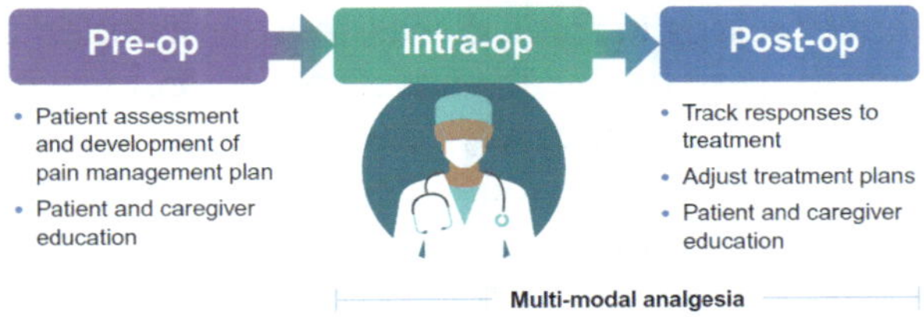

Figure 9.18. Pain management in surgery clinical module.

Source: https://alosahealth.org/wp-content/uploads/2022/11/Screen-Shot-2022-11-02-at-9.29.26-AM.png.

9.6.1. Barriers to Effective Pain Management in Nursing

A range of barriers, from institutional systemic barriers in healthcare to nurse-specific issues often hinders effective pain management nursing. A primary concern relates to the inconsistent use of tools for pain assessment, which may lead to an error in evaluating the patient's pain level. Nurses may lack adequate training in assessing pain, and thus, subjective indicators are used more frequently than objective ones. Additionally, organizational policies may not support active pain management actions due to concern about related side effects or addiction. This generates a culture of fear among nurses, in which they do not want to prescribe opioids or other potent analgesics, thereby compromising patient care. Moreover, the stigma that is attached to pain management, particularly in drug-abusing populations, can create fear among nurses and also patients, exacerbating the situation and leading to under-treatment of pain. No other factor is more significant in the minds of nurses' barriers to successful pain management than the role of communication.

Poor communication between health care providers, patients, and caregivers can limit the delivery of comprehensive pain management interventions. For the majority of instances, nurses will most likely be overwhelmed or unsupported and hence restrict themselves from engaging in frank discussions with patients regarding pain experiences and outcomes of preference. Additionally, effective information sharing with informal caregivers is crucial because they ultimately become an integral part of pain control. As stated, caregivers recognize that it is crucial to possess knowledge of pain management guidelines; however, when this knowledge is lacking or inadequate, it leads to inequalities in treatment and understanding, which ultimately affect patients' capacity to manage their pain appropriately (Owens et al., 2008). Hence, enhancing communication frameworks between nursing practices is essential in dismantling the barriers. Another critical barrier to successful pain management among nurses is a lack of ongoing education and training in current pain management standards and best practices. Ongoing professional learning in healthcare is necessary, particularly in a practice as complex and dynamic as pain management. Without access to new findings and evidence-based practices, nurses can be left with outdated information and practices, which can limit their capacity to provide the best possible care. Furthermore, as delineated in the present literature, the need for capacity building of nurses in pharmacological and non-pharmacological pain management is of extreme priority. Advanced educational interventions are necessary to close knowledge gaps for newer pain management interventions, facilitating more competent nursing practice (Bunn et al., 2019). Through prioritizing education, the healthcare system is able to empower nurses with the competency to break through barriers and enhance the quality of life for patients through effective pain management.

9.6.2. Ethical Considerations in Pain Management

Ethics of pain management continue to be central to nursing practice because they have a direct bearing on patient care and outcomes. Nurses are confronted with complicated dilemmas in the relief of pain, especially among vulnerable groups such as the elderly and the sick. The text of beneficence—do what is best for the patient—is compelling health professionals to control pain effectively but at no risk of harming the patient, e.g., drug addiction or opioid drug toxicities. In addition, ethical questions are most likely to develop when patients hold opposing beliefs regarding pain experience and management, and as such, patients' beliefs and decisions are needed. With increasing ageing populations and forecasted spectacular growth in dementia sufferers by 2050, the question of pain management in an ethical yet effective way grows more significant in the terminal care of such patients. It marks out areas where practice deviates from guidelines (Ballard et al., 2006). As part of managing pain, informed consent is a crucial factor in ensuring ethical practices. Patients should be educated on the options available for pain management, the risks and benefits of interventions, and other relevant information. Informed patients then become self-empowered to make decisions themselves, especially whether or not analgesics such as opioids are appropriate. With severe dementia or cognitive impairment, the problem is complex because the patient cannot be involved in the decision-making process. In this case, the nurses have an ethical responsibility to advocate for the comfort of patients while balancing the need to ensure effective communication with caregivers and family members. Establishing mechanisms that enable the incorporation of both patients' and families' values when making decisions on pain management ensures patient-centered care, thereby upholding ethical standards and improving the quality of care during life-threatening health events (Plante et al., 2018).

In addition, ethical aspects of managing pain extend beyond individual patients to include society at large. The different impacts of chronic pain on disadvantaged populations raise underlying questions of the fairness of access to care in medicine and the equality of pain treatment. For example, research has proven that patients with low health care access or low socioeconomic status are not well treated for pain. This inconsistency not only provokes bodily discomfort but can actually foster a cycle of avoidance of healthcare services for further deterioration of their conditions. Ethical practice as a nurse frames advocacy against such inconsistencies and demands a policy that promotes equality in terms of accessing pain management services. Apart from that, constant education of healthcare professionals regarding implicit biases will minimize inappropriate pain management, ensuring that all patients receive equal treatment regardless of their background (Ballard et al., 2006). A model of ethically managing pain, therefore, must take into account both unique patient needs as well as larger system problems that affect the provision of pain care (Figure 9.19).

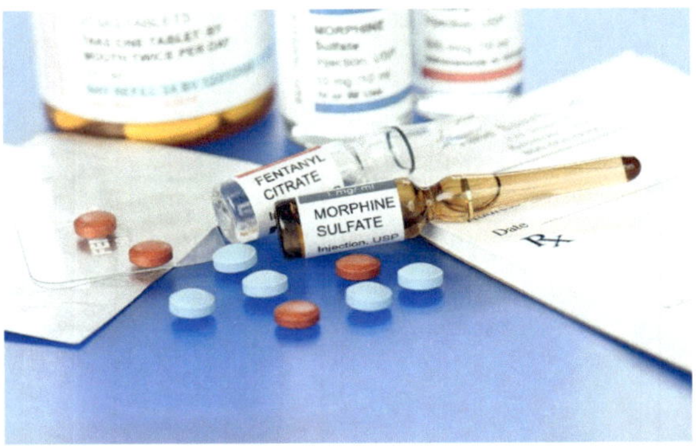

Figure 9.19. Barriers to effective pain management in senior care.

Source: https://www.drjimcollins.com/wp-content/uploads/2020/02/2020-03-30-Barriers-to-Effective-Pain-Management-in-Senior-Care-770x500.jpg.

9.6.3. The Role of Cultural Differences in Pain Perception

Cultural differences play a significant contribution to pain perception, influencing how individuals experience and express pain. Various cultures perceive and conceptualize pain differently, and this is reflected in variations in interpretation and treatment. For instance, pain can be interpreted as a test of endurance or punishment within certain societies, where individuals endure in silence so that they won't demand it be removed. Others could suffer pain in words and discover that the experience of such words is to receive assistance and sympathy. These cultural frameworks not only shape the experience of emotional pain but also openness to medical intervention, directly affecting nursing assessments and interventions. Sensitivity to these cultural differences is required for those healthcare professionals interested in delivering culturally sensitive care that respects and honors patients' personal attitudes towards pain. Effective nursing management of pain needs sensitivity to how cultural origin can influence patients' attitudes towards pain and their expectations of what outcomes from treatment should be. Evidence suggests that patients from different cultural backgrounds may vary in their experience of both the intensity of pain and the success of treatments in reducing it. For instance, studies have highlighted that certain groups of individuals doubt the pharmacological strategy and thus prefer to select alternative interventions or believe that holistic or spiritual interventions are essential in providing relief from pain (Schofield et al., 2006). Beliefs and knowledge among caregivers also significantly influence this in multicultural populations. The need for increased training of health care professionals in the realm of these cultural differences is underscored by the need to practice effective communication, which can serve to close gaps between clinical practice and patient expectations. Moreover, the interaction between patients and healthcare professionals is often influenced by cultural factors, which can either reinforce or complicate pain management techniques. Cultural beliefs contribute to the misinterpretation of pain behavior and to health professionals' inability to assess accurately, leading to suboptimal treatment. For example, non-treatment or inappropriately treated illnesses have ensued from failure to report pain in some patients due to cultural shame of weakness (Owens et al., 2008). In contrast, however, policies of effective communication that respect culture can develop an environment in which patients are empowered to explain their experience of pain. Thus, the application of cultural competence to pain nursing management is critical to the development of evidence-based, patient-centered interventions that enhance patient outcomes without insensitivities to their culture (Figure 9.20).

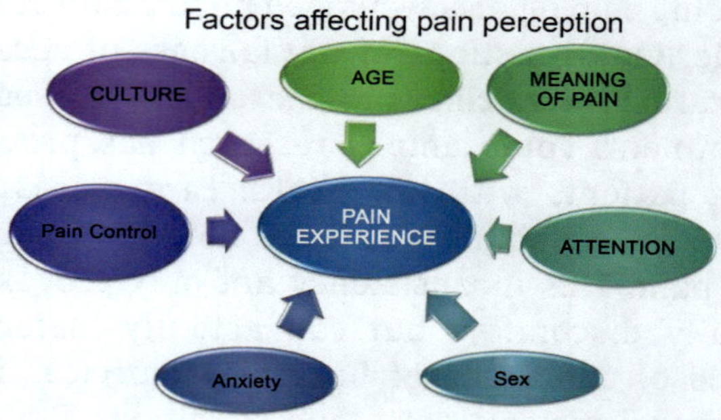

Figure 9.20. Pain perception.

Source: https://i.pinimg.com/originals/8a/b9/e1/8ab9e19e1c6674c2d9387b34dd375f8d.jpg.

Test Your Knowledge

1. What are common issues that nurses have in assessing and managing patient pain effectively?
2. How do misconceptions regarding pain medications affect pain management outcomes?

SUMMARY

Pain management for nursing is an interdisciplinary issue that requires an integrative and holistic approach. The assessment phase is the foundation of pain management, where practitioners can evaluate the intensity and nature of a patient's pain. As recent studies have indicated, optimal pain management practices can significantly contribute to enhanced patient outcomes, particularly in the acute care environment where timely intervention is crucial. Nurses are uniquely positioned not only to assess pain but also to implement specific interventions. Results derived from employing Mediawati et al. (2023) indicate that the application of non-pharmacological treatments such as relaxation and music therapy alongside pharmacological treatments will see significant improvement in pain severity and hence supplement the ultimate goal of alleviating suffering. Additionally, employing education interventions as a means to eradicate myths surrounding pain treatment is crucial in enhancing the nurse's ability to deliver care. As identified in Alexander et al.'s (2016) research, overcoming challenges means proper pain management by offering specific education programs, which empower nurses to raise their knowledge concerning opioid therapy and the sensitivity of evaluating pain. Such results are directly applicable to better patient care and the necessity for nurses to be active participants in their professional advancement. These training programs not only equip the nursing staff with competencies but also help instill a learning culture that is essential for maintaining the evolving nature of pain management. Pain nursing management is not so much about symptomatic relief of bodily pain, but more about developing a holistic framework that's accountable for the general welfare of patients. Effective pain management is not just the consideration and intervention measures identified, but also the psychological and emotional dimensions of patient care. Through the incorporation of holistic assessment procedures, evidence-based treatment approaches, and ongoing education, nurses play a significant role in determining the quality of care offered to patients with pain. The evidence from Alexander et al. (2016) and Mediawati et al. (2023) demonstrates the applicability of a systematized pain nursing management system, designed to ultimately achieve patient dignity, comfort, and quality of life throughout the healthcare continuum.

In pursuing the complexities in pain nursing management, the relationship between psychological determinants and postoperative pain presents a significant area of focus. Studies have again and again shown high levels of anxiety among patients undergoing surgery that can have adverse effects on their postoperative course and pain experience. Research in the environment of a gynecologic operating room implied that preoperative, as well as postoperative, anxiety was significantly connected to increased postoperative pain. More specifically, high trait anxiety individuals were most at risk of increased distress on hospital admission. This means that management of anxiety with targeted interventions is essential in pain management strategies, as not only does it alleviate immediate psychological distress, but it can also potentially decrease the intensity of pain experienced postoperatively (Abbott et al., 2006). Furthermore, nursing interventions cannot be overstated in improving patient outcomes. Nursing courses can respond to the personal requirements of the patients, primarily cancer survivors undergoing rehabilitation of their experience. Systematic review evidence indicates that interventions like these lead to improved quality of life across various domains, including cognitive and social functions. Specifically, increased satisfaction in managing fatigue and emotional functioning was observed in recipients of nurse care, suggesting the value of tailored support in cancer therapy survival. Findings brought together in several trials indicated that the practice of innovative nursing is to blame for alleviating chronic pain and fatigue among cancer survivors, which are two of the most prevalent problems they face following cancer, thus acting as a significant guide to patient care improvement (Berg et al., 2019). Finally, the incorporation of anxiety management skills in nursing practice related to pain is necessary to optimize patient experience. As seen through recent studies, it is crucial in the creation of successful nursing interventions to know the very factors that cause preoperative anxiety to be heightened or lessened. Not only do specially focused interventions, such as providing information, alleviate patients' concerns, but they are also a central determinant of good operating room results. Consequently, incorporating patient experience and feedback into care plans has the potential for making pain management measures more contextual and relevant to the specific needs of individual patients. From this integrated perspective, nurses' emphasis on states of mind and pain must be continued so that interventions can effectively be tailored to enhance patient care (Abbott et al., 2006).

KEY TERMS FROM THIS CHAPTER

- Acute Pain
- Analgesics
- Chronic Pain
- Neuropathic Pain
- Non-Pharmacological Interventions
- Pain Assessment
- Pain Scale
- Pharmacological Management
- Adjuvant Therapy
- Chronic conditions
- Multimodal Pain Management
- Nociceptive Pain
- Opioids
- Pain nursing management
- Patient-Controlled Analgesia (PCA)
- PQRST Method

CRITICAL THINKING QUESTIONS

1. **How is a patient's pain optimally assessed?**
   a. By observing the face
   b. By taking vital signs
   c. By having the patient rate his/her pain using a pain scale
   d. Waiting for the patient to request pain medication
2. **What is the most common adult pain assessment tool?**
   a. FLACC scale
   b. Wong-Baker Faces scale
   c. Numeric Rating Scale (NRS)
   d. CRIES scale
3. **Which of the following is a non-pharmacologic pain management intervention?**
   a. Morphine injection
   b. Acetaminophen administration
   c. Cold or heat therapy
   d. NSAID prescription
4. **What is the nurse's first responsibility when a patient reports pain?**
   a. Ignore if vitals are fine
   b. Only administer medication as ordered
   c. Assume the patient and take additional assessment
   d. Refer the patient to a psychologist
5. **What type of pain is described as shooting, tingling, or burning and typically associated with nerve damage?**
   a. Nociceptive pain
   b. Somatic pain
   c. Visceral pain
   d. Neuropathic pain

Short Answer Questions

1. What two non-pharmacological approaches are utilized in pain management?
2. Why would a re-evaluation of pain after an intervention be indicated?
3. What is the acronym PQRST when used in the assessment of pain?
4. What is the nurse's role in an effective pain assessment and documentation process?
5. Compare and contrast nociceptive and neuropathic pain and their corresponding nursing interventions.
6. Define psychological and cultural variables that can affect a patient's perception and reporting of pain.
7. Create a nursing care plan for a postoperative client with severe-to-moderate pain.
8. Describe the benefits and liabilities of opioid use in pain management and the nurse's role in managing their effects.

Answers to Critical Thinking Questions

1. (c) 2. (c) 3. (c) 4. (c) 5. (d)

REFERENCES

1. Carr, E., Brockbank, K., Allen, S., & Strike, P. (2006). Patterns and frequency of anxiety in women undergoing gynaecological surgery. *Journal of Clinical Nursing, 15*(3), 341–352. https://doi.org/10.1111/j.1365-2702.2006.01285.xAlexander, G. C., & Frattaroli, S. (2015). The prescription opioid epidemic: An evidence-based approach. https://core.ac.uk/download/75783788.pdf (accessed on 28th June 2025).
2. Alexander, S. (2016). A project to improve nurses' knowledge of, and attitudes towards, pain management at end of life. https://core.ac.uk/download/77511392.pdf (accessed on 28th June 2025).
3. Allison, M., Beloat, A., Daugherty, S., Hanson-Abromeit, D., et al. (2018). Reporting quality of music intervention research in healthcare: A systematic review. https://core.ac.uk/download/227054380.pdf (accessed on 28th June 2025).
4. Anthony, Y. L. (2017). Appraisal of nonpharmacological chronic pain management. https://core.ac.uk/download/147837998.pdf (accessed on 28th June 2025).
5. Aprilyadi, N., Aprilio, R., Martalina, W., Zuraidah, Z., & Wibowo, W. D. A. (2024). Application of foot massage therapy to reduce pain scale of elderly with rheumatoid arthritis. *Healthcare in Low-Resource Settings.* https://www.semanticscholar.org/paper/2caff76cd10d3013b82ac31e79c99786cf773400 (accessed on 28th June 2025).
6. Asian American Pacific Islander Nurses Association. (2016). Proceedings of the 2015 Asian American/Pacific Islander Nurses Association conference: Biological measures: A role in nursing self-management research. https://digitalscholarship.unlv.edu/cgi/viewcontent.cgi?article=1017&context=apin (accessed on 28th June 2025).
7. Aveyard, B., Schofield, P., & Smith, P. (2007). Developing annotated bibliographies: A tool for education, collaboration and research development. https://core.ac.uk/download/177011.pdf (accessed on 28th June 2025).
8. Ballard, C., Daley, S., Hughes, J., Keady, J., et al. (2006). End-of-life care and dementia. https://core.ac.uk/download/4145979.pdf (accessed on 28th June 2025).
9. Bear, H., Elswick, R. K., Kelley, D., Lyon, D., et al. (2015). Randomized sham-controlled trial of cranial microcurrent stimulation for symptoms of depression, anxiety, pain, fatigue and sleep disturbances in women receiving chemotherapy for early-stage breast cancer. https://core.ac.uk/download/84402734.pdf (accessed on 28th June 2025).
10. Beller, E. M., Bennett, S., Delaney, C., Haines, K., et al. (2016). Educational interventions for the management of cancer-related fatigue in adults. https://core.ac.uk/download/196601432.pdf (accessed on 28th June 2025).
11. Berg, M., Bulsara, M., Monterosso, L., Platt, V., et al. (2019). Systematic review and meta-analysis of patient reported outcomes for nurse-led models of survivorship care for adult cancer patients. https://core.ac.uk/download/213607897.pdf (accessed on 28th June 2025).
12. Bergin, M., Norman, I. J., Parry, C. D., van Hout, M. C., et al. (2016). Best practices and innovations for managing codeine misuse and dependence. https://core.ac.uk/download/132282006.pdf (accessed on 28th June 2025).

13. Brooks, J., Featherstone, V. A., King, N., Topping, A., et al. (2014). Supporting people with active and advanced disease: A rapid review of the evidence. https://core.ac.uk/download/19780349.pdf (accessed on 28th June 2025).

14. Bull, M. J. (2015). Managing delirium in hospitalized older adults. https://core.ac.uk/download/213076068.pdf (accessed on 28th June 2025).

15. Bunn, F., Goodman, C., & Handley, M. (2019). Supporting general hospital staff to provide dementia-sensitive care: A realist evaluation. https://core.ac.uk/download/287581550.pdf (accessed on 28th June 2025).

16. Challis, A., Franke, A., Kitson, A., Kitson, A., Twycross, A., Stevens, B., Carter, C., et al. (2010). Process evaluation of appreciative inquiry to translate pain management evidence into pediatric nursing practice. https://core.ac.uk/download/45680.pdf (accessed on 28th June 2025).

17. Colloca, L., DeGrazia, D., & Enck, P. (2016). Relieving pain using dose-extending placebos. https://core.ac.uk/download/131209441.pdf (accessed on 28th June 2025).

18. Corbett, A., Liberati, A., Hurley, A. C., Long, A. F., Jordan, A. I., Cook, A. K. R., American Geriatrics Society (AGS) Panel on Persistent Pain in Older Persons, et al. (2014). Pain assessment for people with dementia: A systematic review of systematic reviews of pain assessment tools. https://core.ac.uk/download/29019170.pdf (accessed on 28th June 2025).

19. Drake, G. F. (2015). Barriers and potential solutions to effective pain management on a gastro-intestinal ward: An action research study in a university hospital. https://core.ac.uk/download/79496357.pdf (accessed on 28th June 2025).

20. Edlund, A., McIntyre, A., Powell, A. E., May, C., May, C., Lukas, C. V., Kiely, D. K., et al. (2013). Developing and implementing an integrated delirium prevention system of care: A theory-driven, participatory research study. https://core.ac.uk/download/19595465.pdf (accessed on 28th June 2025).

21. Edward, K. L., & Ousey, K. (2014). Exploring resilience when living with a wound—An integrative literature review. https://core.ac.uk/download/30729891.pdf (accessed on 28th June 2025).

22. Garvey, L., Hamadeh, S., & Willetts, G. (2024). Pain management interventions of the non-communicating patient in intensive care: What works for whom and why? A rapid realist reviews. https://core.ac.uk/download/619431112.pdf (accessed on 28th June 2025).

23. Goodman, C., Cohen, J., De Koning, J., Sampson, E. L., Higginson, I., Robinson, L., Murtagh, F., et al. (2019). A systematic review and critical appraisal of quality indicators to assess optimal palliative care for older people with dementia. https://core.ac.uk/download/287581642.pdf (accessed on 28th June 2025).

24. Hartvigsen, J., Kjær, P., Mair, F. S., McCallum, M., et al. (2017). Digital support interventions for the self-management of low back pain: A systematic review. https://core.ac.uk/download/80697442.pdf (accessed on 28th June 2025).

25. Hunnicutt, J. N., Lapane, K. L., & Ulbricht, C. M. (2016). Triad of suffering: Pain, depression, and anxiety among newly admitted nursing homes residents. https://core.ac.uk/download/56530130.pdf (accessed on 28th June 2025).

26. Jones, C., Moyle, W., Pu, L., Todorovic, M., et al. (2019). Psychosocial interventions for pain management in older adults with dementia: A systematic review of randomized controlled trials. https://core.ac.uk/download/196606964.pdf (accessed on 28th June 2025).
27. Keefe, G. (2025). The development and evaluation of a computer-based resource to enhance the education of pre-registration nursing students regarding knowledge and attitudes towards pain management. https://core.ac.uk/download/33570891.pdf (accessed on 28th June 2025).
28. Latour, J. M., Tume, L. N., van den Hoogen, A., Wielenga, J., et al. (2014). An electronic Delphi study to establish pediatric intensive care nursing research priorities in twenty European countries. https://core.ac.uk/download/42136644.pdf (accessed on 28th June 2025).
29. Lemow, J. J. (2009). Patients' attitudes to analgesics and expectations of emergency care: A thesis presented in partial fulfilment of the requirements for the degree of Master of Arts in Psychology at Massey University, Palmerston North, New Zealand. https://core.ac.uk/download/157568891.pdf (accessed on 28th June 2025).
30. Mediawati, A. S., Rohmania, C., & Setyorini, D. (2023). Manajemen asuhan keperawatan pada Ny.M dengan masalah nyeri akut post sectio caesarea. https://core.ac.uk/download/587868379.pdf (accessed on 28th June 2025).
31. Nurmalia, D., Padmasari, S., Rokhana, N., Utami, S., et al. (2015). *Proceeding: 3rd Java International Nursing Conference 2015 "Harmony of Caring and Healing Inquiry for Holistic Nursing Practice; Enhancing Quality of Care," Semarang, 20–21 August 2015*. https://core.ac.uk/download/76930906.pdf (accessed on 28th June 2025).
32. Ortiz-Cintron, H. (2014). Use of complementary and alternative therapies: A pilot survey. https://core.ac.uk/download/236292416.pdf (accessed on 28th June 2025).
33. Owens, A., Docherty, A., Gagnon, P., House of Commons, Hughes, P. M., Williams, J., Asadi-Lari, M., et al. (2008). Knowledge and information needs of informal caregivers in palliative care: A qualitative systematic review. https://core.ac.uk/download/49252.pdf (accessed on 28th June 2025).
34. Plante, S. (2018). An inpatient rehabilitation interprofessional care pathway for traumatic hip fracture: A pilot quality improvement project. https://core.ac.uk/download/215520988.pdf (accessed on 28th June 2025).
35. Rees, N. W. (2000). Nursing management of postoperative pain: Perceived care and actual practice. https://core.ac.uk/download/195631910.pdf (accessed on 28th June 2025).
36. Rehan, H., Asghar, M., Geetha, K. D., Zameer, A., & Sambreen, Z. (2024). Nursing perspective on pain management. *I-Manager's Journal on Nursing*. https://www.semanticscholar.org/paper/476ec43ae82bd45b39d05818b942702bf9963d1f (accessed on 28th June 2025).
37. Reid, D. M., & Schofield, P. (2006). The assessment and management of pain in older people: A systematic review of the literature. https://core.ac.uk/download/177013.pdf (accessed on 28th June 2025).
38. Reynolds, H. K. (2011). Palliative nursing care in pediatric oncology. https://core.ac.uk/download/58824032.pdf (accessed on 28th June 2025).

FLUID, ELECTROLYTE, AND ACID-BASE BALANCE IN NURSING PRACTICE

10

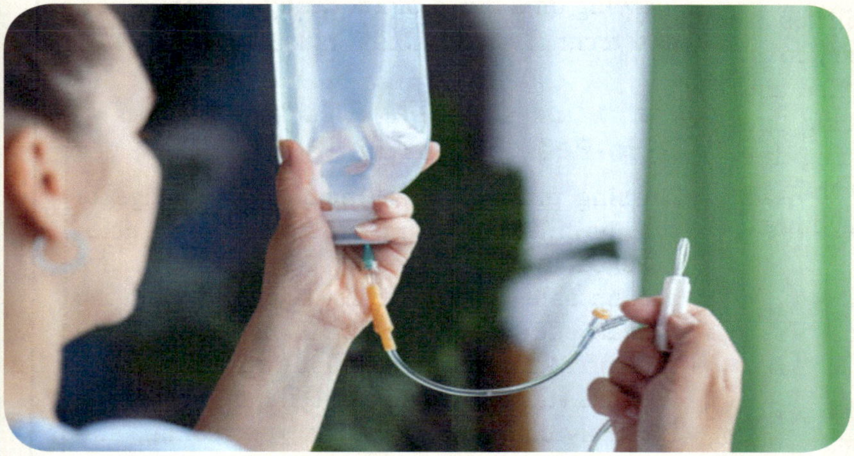

LEARNING OBJECTIVES

After studying this chapter, you will be able to:

1. Understand the anatomy of kidney function
2. Describe mechanisms of reabsorption
3. Discuss renal physiology secretion
4. Emphasize the regulation of fluid balance
5. Learn electrolyte balance
6. Evaluate acid-base homeostasis
7. Mention the renal function pathophysiologye

Introduction

Practice in nursing is significantly dependent on fluid, electrolyte, and acid-base balance, with major implications for patient health outcomes. These balances must be maintained to ensure physiological homeostasis; any imbalance can lead to significant complications. Nurses stand at the center of patient care and must measure these critical parameters daily. This necessitates a comprehensive understanding of fluid dynamics, electrolyte functions, and acid-base homeostasis, particularly in vulnerable populations such as neonates. As the healthcare environment continues to evolve, the roles of evidence-based practices in sustaining these balances cannot be overstated. Intelligence derived from ongoing research forms the template from which nursing professionals can assess and intervene adequately in acute and chronic conditions to deliver optimal care to patients. New challenges in managing fluid and electrolyte imbalances arise from varying patient conditions, necessitating individualized treatment. A case in point is preterm babies, who are particularly vulnerable to fluid balance derangement due to their immature physiology. Preterm infants born at less than 29 weeks of gestation often rely on parenteral nutrition to achieve adequate macronutrient levels, as recommended by contemporary studies (Dinerstein et al., 2011). The targeting of personalized nutritional interventions is critical, as they directly influence growth and subsequent developmental outcomes. Ignoring such nuances can exacerbate conditions for neurocognitive disabilities in high-risk populations. Nurses, in turn, must be specially educated with the expertise and skills to implement effective monitoring and therapeutic interventions, highlighting the importance of ongoing education and training in fluid, electrolyte, and acid-base management.

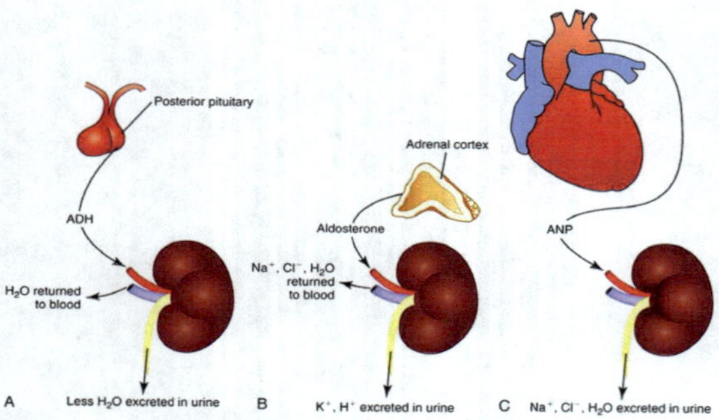

Figure 10.1. Fluid, electrolyte, and acid-base balance.

Source: https://nursekey.com/wp-content/uploads/2016/11/F000418f041-006ac-9780323079334.jpg.

Additionally, technological and monitoring system innovations are also revolutionizing nurses' handling of fluid and electrolyte balance in clinical settings. The next-generation multiparametric monitoring systems enable clinicians to monitor and treat these physiological parameters more deeply (N/A). The technology partially overcomes the shortcomings of traditional monitoring, particularly in complex cases such as neonatal and adult blood gas monitoring. As these technologies become integrated into practice, they streamline clinical decision-making and improve patient outcomes. Understanding and utilizing such innovations in conjunction with a basic knowledge of fluid and electrolyte dynamics enables nurses to master the complexities of patient care. Lastly, proficiency in managing fluid, electrolyte, and acid-base balance is central to nursing practice, drawing on a blend of knowledge, competence, and technological skills (Figure 10.1).

Definition of Fluid, Electrolyte, and Acid-Base Balance

Nursing practice must include knowledge of the definition of fluid, electrolyte, and acid-base balance because these components are accountable for maintaining homeostasis in the human body. Fluid balance is all about having the correct control of the body's water supply, which is vital in maintaining cellular functioning. Electrolytes, such as sodium, potassium, and calcium, are ions that carry a charge and are involved in various physiological processes, including the contraction of muscles and the transmission of nerve impulses. Acid-base balance involves regulating pH levels within the body, specifically controlling the concentration of hydrogen ions, which in turn affects metabolic and respiratory functions. When any of these balance systems is disrupted, it can lead to serious health consequences, highlighting the importance of close monitoring and intervention actions of nursing care (Andruskiw et al., 1961). Fluid, electrolyte, and acid-base balance are interrelated in such a way that each one affects the others. For instance, fluid status imbalance can affect electrolyte levels, and vice versa. Hypervolemia, or fluid overload, has the effect of diluting electrolytes in the blood, thereby creating hyponatremia, a condition characterized by low sodium levels. Conversely, dehydration may lead to hypernatremia, an elevated sodium content in the serum. Acid-base balance crosses over with these constituents as well; for example, metabolic acidosis may ensue when there is excessive bicarbonate loss through fluid loss, which poses a complicated clinical picture for health professionals to deal with. Nurses find knowing about such interdependencies significant to make patient care plans based on accurate assessments and interventions tailored to the return of balance (Fox et al., 2019). In clinical practice, nurses apply their understanding of fluid, electrolyte, and acid-base balance to guide treatment decisions and maximize patient outcomes. This type of understanding is applied in the interpretation of laboratory values, the assessment of vital signs, and the monitoring of patient symptoms. For instance, ailments such as kidney disease or heart failure would necessitate fluid limitation and careful regulation of electrolyte intake to prevent complications. The nurses are also responsible for educating patients on the importance of adhering to prescribed diet adjustments and medication regimens, as understanding that such interventions have a critical impact on their fluid and electrolyte balance is essential. Lastly, a full comprehension of these fundamental principles enables nurses to deliver efficient patient care and ensure healing while minimizing the risk of adverse effects in various healthcare settings (Andruskiw et al., 1961).

Importance in Nursing Practice

Inclusion of fluid, electrolyte, and acid-base balance in clinical nursing is crucial to ensure patient safety and facilitate optimal recovery. Nurses are pivotal in the monitoring and assessment of patients' hydration status and electrolyte levels, crucial for numerous physiological processes like nerve conduction, muscle contraction, and even metabolism. Failure to maintain these balances can cause serious complications, including hypernatremia, which is an ailment responsible for increased morbidity and mortality in human and veterinary medicine. The development of hypernatremia in dogs and cats, although infrequent, has been documented with a 20.6% case fatality rate in dogs and 28.1% in cats, indicating that healthcare practitioners should immediately identify and effectively treat fluid imbalances (Epstein et al., 2015). Such statistical evidence highlights the importance of nurses being properly informed and skilled in detecting and intervening early. The importance of formal support tools, such as symptom lists, in nursing care cannot be overstated, particularly in postoperative management involving fluid and electrolyte balance. Research has demonstrated that when surgical nurses employed a checklist of precise symptoms and reactions to fluid and electrolyte balance, their detection and response to these symptoms were significantly improved. This finding demonstrates that structure-directed clinical practice patterns can lead to improved nursing outcomes and ultimately, better patient care. Nurses were more effective at identifying signs of imbalance and intervening appropriately, which resulted in measurable improvements in patient reactions (Walkingshaw et al., 2008). As such, the use of these kinds of tools must be a standard of best practice within nursing education and continuing professional education. Moreover, nurses' role in fluid and electrolyte balance is more than just identification. It encompasses the collaboration of health professionals to formulate a comprehensive care plan tailored to the patient's needs. Efficient management encompasses not just the assessment of physiological readings by the nurses but also the interpretation of laboratory tests and responding to symptoms promptly. Interdisciplinary communication enhances the ability to resolve complicated cases efficiently, where disturbances in electrolytes might be indicative of metabolic derangements. As direct caregivers, nurses are responsible for advocating evidence-based practices, utilizing assessment tools, and engaging in ongoing education to meet the demands of maintaining fluid, electrolyte, and acid-base balance. Such a holistic strategy is essential for delivering quality care and minimizing potential complications, highlighting the nurses' pivotal role in effective health management practice (Figure 10.2).

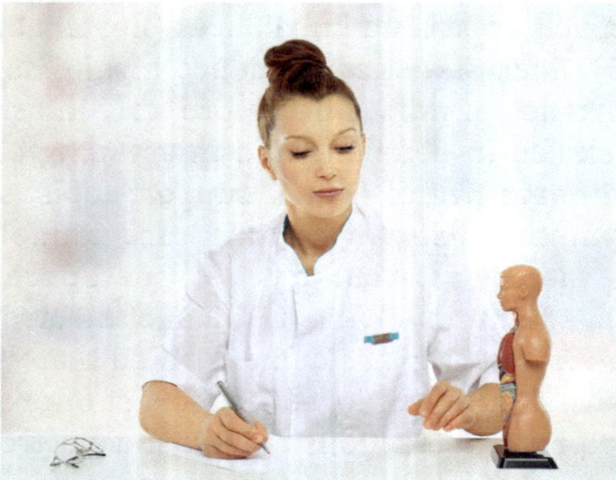

Figure 10.2. Nursing practice.

Source: https://img.freepik.com/premium-photo/doctor-his-office-waiting-patient-skin-model-human-body-model-dermatology-cosmetology_979672-1679.jpg?ga=GA1.1.594720847.1750063652&semt=ais_hybrid&w=740.

10.1. The Role of Fluids in the Body

Learning Outcome

1. Describe the types of body fluids
2. Highlight body fluid functions in body processes
3. Discover how an imbalance of fluids affects health

Body fluid function is pivotal in maintaining overall body health and physiological processes. Body fluids constitute a large percentage of body weight, mainly in the cells (intracellular fluid) and between the cells and organs (extracellular fluid). These compartments act synergistically to facilitate the transport of nutrients, regulate temperature, and maintain metabolic function. During clinical practice, understanding fluid balance is crucial, as derangements may underlie various clinical syndromes, such as dehydration or fluid overload. Furthermore, early assessment of fluid balance supports nurses in developing effective care plans that address the individual needs of patients, particularly among vulnerable groups such as the elderly, where dehydration appears to be prevalent, costly, and associated with unfavorable outcomes. In summary, vigilant appreciation of fluid dynamics is the foundation for successful patient management in acute and chronic care environments (Lacey et al., 2019). Electrolytes, or ions in body fluids, play a significant role in fluid balance and are critical to muscle and nerve function, nerve conduction, and acid-base balance. Balance between the electrolytes and the fluid is crucial; for instance, sodium helps to regulate extracellular fluid volume and osmotic pressure, while potassium is required for intracellular processes. Electrolyte level changes can lead to extreme physiological responses, from cardiac rhythm changes to alterations in muscle contractions. Nurses should therefore have a solid background in electrolyte management to identify potential imbalances that can compromise a patient's health. Understanding the significance of these ions, their sources, and functions is crucial in clinical practice nursing, particularly when monitoring patients at risk of electrolyte imbalance, such as those undergoing extended fluid shifts during illness or surgery (Goswami, 2017). The importance of acid-base balance through adequate fluid intake cannot be overstated. The body's pH levels are kept tightly regulated, as even minor fluctuations can have drastic effects on health. Body fluids function as buffers that neutralize acids and bases and maintain the internal environment stable and required for enzymatic activity and metabolic reactions. Clinically, assessing a patient's hydration status can provide helpful information about their acid-base balance. For instance, diarrhea-evoked abnormalities, such as metabolic acidosis or alkalosis, may be influenced by factors like vomiting or diarrhea-induced fluid loss, which exacerbate the clinical condition. As medical caregivers, nurses are tasked with implementing interventions that will reestablish fluid and electrolyte balance, thus optimal metabolic process function. Lastly, understanding the intricate interrelationship between acid-base balance, fluids, and electrolytes is crucial for effective nursing practice as well as promoting patient well-being (Goswami, 2017; Lacey et al., 2019) (Figure 10.3).

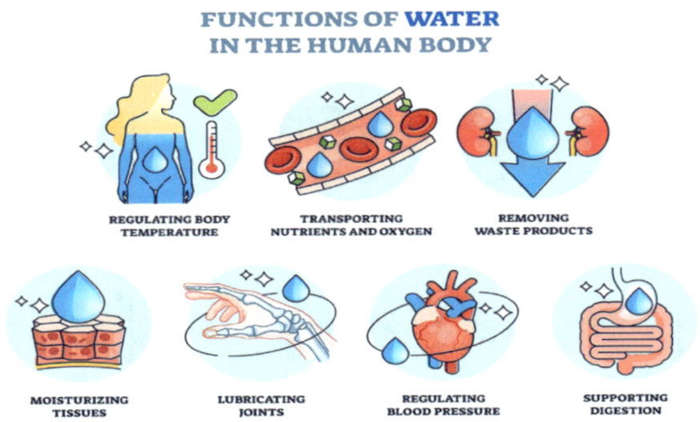

Figure 10.3. Functions of water in human body and drinking benefits.

Source: https://vectormine.b-cdn.net/wp-content/uploads/functions_of_water_in_the_human_body_outline_diagram-1.jpg.

10.1.1. Types of Body Fluids

Understanding various types of body fluids is essential for nursing practice, particularly the management of fluid, electrolyte, and acid-base balance. Body fluids are classified into two broad categories: intracellular fluid (ICF) and extracellular fluid (ECF). The ECF constitutes about one-third of the body fluids and is subdivided into interstitial fluid and plasma. Interstitial fluid fills the spaces within cells, where nutrients and waste are exchanged, while plasma is the fluid component of blood that transports cells, nutrients, and electrolytes throughout the body. To the ICF, however, which makes up the remaining two-thirds of body fluid and resides inside cells to facilitate maintenance of cellular function and metabolic processes, the different compositions of the fluids underscore the necessity to balance nutrients and electrolytes, and this is most important in health and disease. The structure of body fluids themselves extends further; they are also at the heart of homeostatic control and the maintenance of physiological processes. Water, as the largest and most significant component of body fluids, serves as a medium for biochemical reactions, heat regulation, and transport of essential substances. Electrolytes such as sodium, potassium, and calcium are present in solution in the body's fluids and play crucial roles in muscle contraction, nerve transmission, and maintaining hydration status. In practice, an understanding of alterations in body fluid compartments enables nurses to make informed decisions in patient management. For example, electrolyte disturbance may represent overhydration or dehydration and require manipulations to correct these states. It is especially crucial in some populations, such as preterm infants, whose development and growth heavily rely on the regulation of body fluids, as described through evidence of the importance of individualized fluid management (Dinerstein et al., 2011). Acid-base balance is another essential aspect related to body fluids, which describes the interdependence of fluid regulation and metabolic processes. The body maintains a tightly regulated pH level, and the bicarbonate and carbonic acid buffering system plays a decisive role in ensuring this balance. An effective balance between acids and bases is essential to enzyme function, respiratory processes, and overall metabolic stability. And of course, fluctuations from the normal range of pH do have dangerous clinical effects, such as acidosis or alkalosis. Nurses therefore need to continually monitor fluid status and electrolyte levels to prevent or correct such imbalances. Adherence to standardized protocols in fluid therapy, especially for vulnerable populations like neonates, can go a long way in enhancing patient outcomes, as studies of the impact of optimized parenteral nutrition (Andruskiw et al., 1961) have shown. This comprehensive picture of body fluids is essential for the effective delivery of nursing care and the overall management of the patient (Figure 10.4).

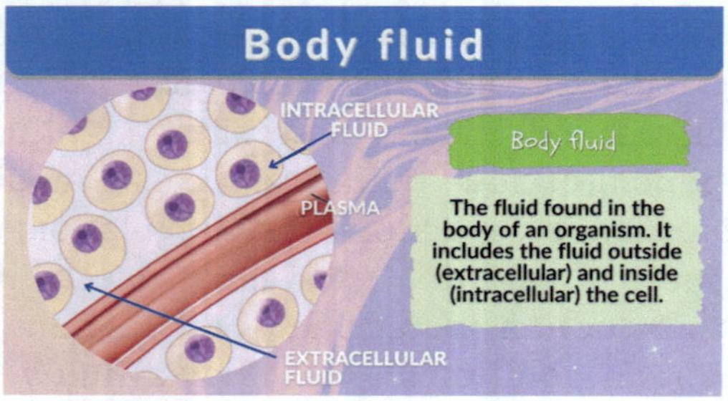

Figure 10.4. Types of body fluids.

Source: https://www.biologyonline.com/wp-content/uploads/2019/10/body-fluid-definition-and-examples.jpg.

10.1.2. Functions of Fluids in Physiological Processes

The human body relies upon a highly controlled system of fluids to ensure essential physiological processes. The different fluids serve more than one function, including the transport of nutrients, the regulation of body temperature, and the removal of waste, all of which are necessary for maintaining homeostasis. Blood, comprising approximately 55% plasma fluid, is responsible for transporting oxygen, nutrients, hormones, and waste products to and from the cells. In this instance, the effectiveness of fluid transport directly influences metabolic effectiveness as well as overall cellular health. As the International Classification for Nursing Practice shows, understanding the mechanisms that regulate fluid balance is paramount, especially in the care of patients with chronic diseases that may alter fluid dynamics, such as cardiac or renal disease (Camacho et al., 2021). Also essential is the electrolyte composition of the fluid, which has a direct impact on the electrolytic balance necessary for good muscle function and nerve conduction. Electrolytes such as sodium, potassium, and calcium in body fluids are crucial for conducting electrical impulses, thereby facilitating muscular contraction and regulating heart rhythms. Derangement in these electrolytes is most likely to result in serious complications, such as arrhythmia or muscle weakness. With the evolution of nursing practice, there is an increased focus on the necessity of general education in physiology, particularly in fluid and electrolyte management (Chandler et al., 2020).

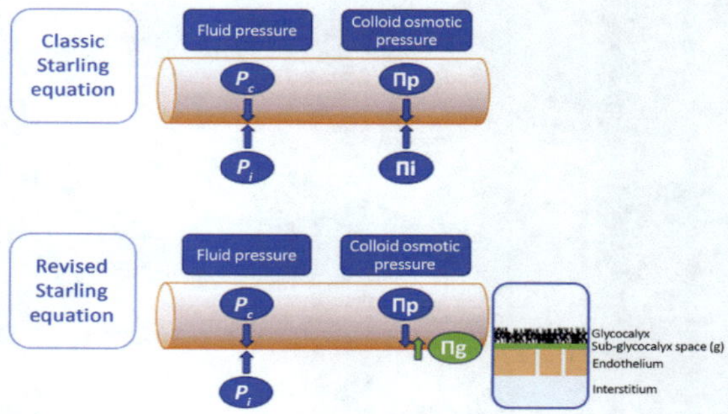

Figure 10.5. Functions of fluids in physiological processes.

Source: https://ars.els-cdn.com/content/image/1-s2.0-S0007091217540714-gr2.jpg.

This information enables nurses to make informed clinical decisions that promote patient stability and healing, as a key highlighting element of fluid functions towards optimal care provision. The acid-base balance of body fluids is another important aspect of physiological stability. The body is capable of operating within a narrow range of pH, with any derangement prone to inducing acidosis or alkalosis, which can significantly impair organ function and lead to systemic complications. Body fluids, such as blood and interstitial fluid, transport buffers that help maintain acid-base balance by neutralizing excess bases or acids. Understanding the acid-base dynamic is essential for nurses, particularly for patient populations at risk of developing respiratory or metabolic disturbance. Ongoing monitoring and management of fluid volumes and compositions enable health professionals to intervene early in the development of imbalances, thereby providing optimal results for patients. These liquid functions not only mold near-term physiological responses but also play a significant role in guiding nursing activities and promoting well-being in various healthcare settings (Figure 10.5).

10.1.3. Impact of Fluid Imbalance on Health

Fluid balance is crucial for maintaining homeostasis in the human body and affects both cellular function and overall health. Fluid imbalance can occur in various ways, and clinically, it can manifest as either fluid overload or dehydration. Dehydration is the result of inadequate fluid intake or excessive fluid loss, with consequent hypernatremia and associated signs, such as confusion and decreased urine output. Conversely, fluid overload typically results in states like hyponatremia or congestive heart failure, and the resulting symptoms include edema, hypertension, and respiratory compromise. Fluid and electrolyte levels at optimal levels are significant because profound disturbances of sodium, in particular, have been associated with increased morbidity and mortality and are substantial markers of patient prognosis across all clinical contexts (Bajantri et al., 2018). Through clinical practice, it is essential to closely scrutinize these imbalances in order to reverse their effects on the patient's health. The role of critical care nursing in managing fluid imbalances cannot be overstated. Nurses play a pivotal role in implementing intervention protocols to ensure accurate fluid and electrolyte management, a crucial factor in the treatment of hospitalized patients. For instance, in the management of total parenteral nutrition (TPN) among critically ill patients, adherence to prescribed nursing protocols significantly improves patient outcomes. Research shows that compliance with TPN protocols strictly can decrease complications related to fluid imbalance, resulting in reduced morbidity and shorter hospital stays (Abdelal et al., 2019). This highlights the necessity for specialized knowledge in fluid management among nurses, enabling them to recognize and rectify imbalances before they develop into full-scale, life-threatening issues. Educational courses designed to enhance nurses' knowledge of fluid and electrolyte imbalances are crucial for optimizing clinical practice. Comprehensive training for detecting and treating these imbalances equips nurses with the skills to identify risk factors and utilize successful treatments. Because imbalances in fluids and electrolytes can impact patient outcomes, nurses must possess the ability to make accurate assessments, formulate effective care plans, and revise interventions accordingly based on emerging clinical data. Through the acquisition of a solid foundation in fluid management, nurses become highly valuable in reducing patient complications caused by imbalances, resulting in enhanced health outcomes and promoting a culture of safety in healthcare environments (Bajantri et al., 2018). The impact of fluid imbalance is thus not only confined to individual health but has broader effects on healthcare quality and efficiency in general.

Test Your Knowledge

1. In what ways do body fluids help to maintain homeostasis and normal cellular function?
2. How do fluids help in regulating body temperature, pH , and the transport of nutrients?

10.2. Electrolytes and Their Functions

Learning Outcome

1. Define the key electrolytes present in the human body
2. Define the role played by electrolytes in cell function
3. Describe the impact of electrolyte imbalance

Electrolytes, or minerals that dissociate to ions in solution, are essential for most physiological processes. These positively charged ions, including sodium, potassium, calcium, and chloride, play a crucial role in maintaining homeostasis within the body. They serve primarily to maintain fluid balance, transmit nerve impulses, and facilitate muscle contraction. For instance, sodium and potassium are essential for generating electrical signals that enable neurons to communicate with one another, and calcium is used for muscle fibers to contract effectively. Nurses, as healthcare providers, need to understand these roles to identify electrolyte imbalances that may result in serious clinical manifestations, such as arrhythmias or muscle weakness, highlighting the necessity of regular monitoring in patient management (Andruskiw et al., 1961). Electrolyte balance is highly interconnected with fluid status in the body, where water movement relies upon osmotic gradients determined by the concentration of electrolytes. For example, in dehydration, the body experiences changes in electrolyte balance that can potentially lead to adverse health effects. Electrolyte function is involved in osmotically regulating pressure, which affects the retention or excretion of fluids in tissues. Nursing practice involves assessing hydration status and understanding how electrolyte imbalance can cause or develop as a result of dehydration. Through the incorporation of electrolyte monitoring into routine assessments, nurses can develop interventions tailored to promoting proper hydration and overall patient safety. Maintaining such a balance is key to preventing resulting complications as a consequence of disruptions to the body's systemic relationships (Miller et al., 2017). Beyond immediate physiological effect, the implications of electrolyte management have a considerable influence on determining patient outcomes in a number of clinical settings. In elderly adults, for instance, the risk of dehydration and electrolyte imbalance that can ensue is significantly magnified due to physiological compromise and frequent inadequate fluid intake. For the nurse, recognizing that caregivers play a crucial role in maintaining hydration is essential, particularly in light of nursing interventions.

Active hydration protocols should be applied, along with caretaker education, to prevent dehydration-related complications. Moreover, recognition of how cooperating medical conditions alter electrolyte needs guides clinical decision-making regarding treatment planning. By highlighting the interrelationship between fluid management and electrolyte function, nurses can further enhance the quality of care, resulting in improved patient health and recovery (Miller et al., 2017) (Figure 10.6).

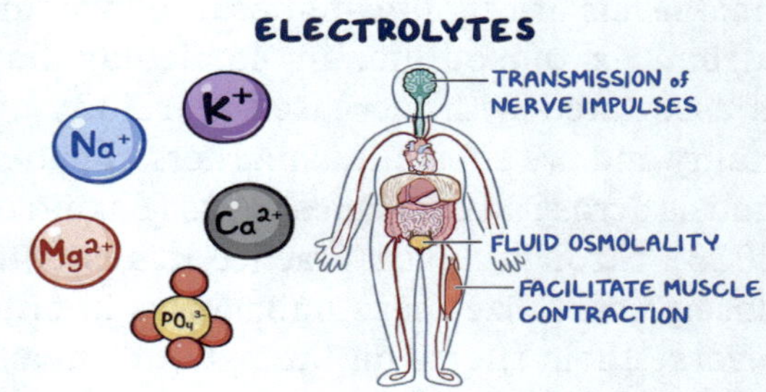

Figure 10.6. Electrolytes and their functions.

Source: https://d16qt3wv6xm098.cloudfront.net/VYMhVKlIRqKrvW1SlPIvdcH3TWa_-zhw/_.jpg.

10.2.1. Key Electrolytes in the Human Body

Electrolytes are crucial ions in the human body responsible for maintaining fluid balance, transmitting nerve impulses, and regulating muscle function. The chief electrolytes employed are potassium, sodium, chloride, magnesium, calcium, and bicarbonate. Sodium is the chief extracellular electrolyte, playing a vital role in maintaining osmotic pressure and water retention, while potassium is the chief intracellular electrolyte, utilized for nerve transmission and muscle contraction. Imbalance in these electrolytes would lead to significant clinical effects, such as cardiac disease or hypertension. Therefore, tracking and sustaining electrolytes during nursing practice, particularly in vulnerable populations such as the elderly or those with intensive medical cases, is crucial. Also worthy of emphasis is the contribution of bicarbonate to acid-base balance. As a critical buffer, it ensures the blood remains within a very narrow range most suitable for physiologic functions. Kidneys and lungs play pivotal roles in regulating bicarbonate; any defect can lead to metabolic or respiratory acidosis/alkalosis. Nursing assessment generally involves assessing arterial blood gases (ABGs) to determine acid-base status, allowing for early interventions to be initiated. Here, the knowledge of bicarbonate levels and homeostasis as a whole is essential for nurses, who should be able to recognize the beginning of electrolyte imbalance as part of integral patient care. Moreover, control of electrolytes is most relevant to specific clinical conditions. For instance, dehydration can severely disrupt electrolyte homeostasis and lead to symptoms such as confusion, muscle weakness, and an increased risk of falls (Miller et al., 2017). Clinical evidence demonstrates that effective hydration processes significantly improve patient outcomes, requiring nurses to employ proactive hydration strategies. In addition, observation for electrolyte imbalance such as hyperkalemia or hyponatremia may be necessary for chemotherapy patients because these may complicate recovery and treatment (Bambaci et al., 2016). Consequently, a proper comprehension of the roles played by electrolytes and an application of appropriate monitoring practices are essential skills for nurses while attempting to achieve fluid, electrolyte, and acid-base balance in clinical practice (Figure 10.7).

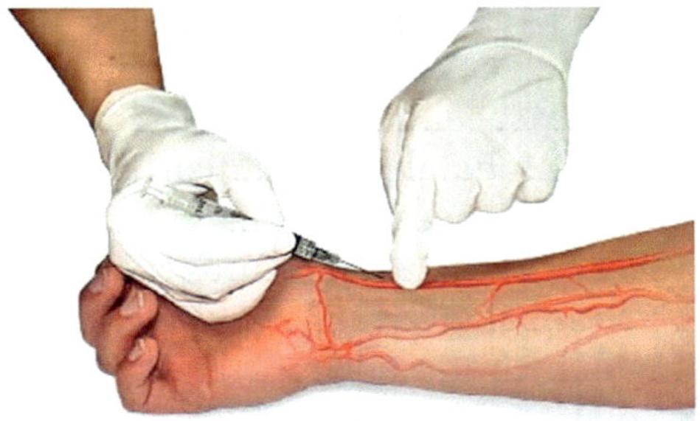

After a pulse is found, a blood sample is taken from the artery

Figure 10.7. Arterial-blood-gas (ABG)-analysis.

Source: https://www.rnpedia.com/wp-content/uploads/2014/12/Arterial-Blood-Gas-Analysis-1.jpg.

10.2.2. Role of Electrolytes in Cellular Function

Electrolytes are essentials in maintaining cellular function, as they allow for a number of physiological processes critical to cellular homeostasis. These charged ions, including sodium, potassium, calcium, and chloride, are involved in various cellular functions, such as maintaining membrane potential, facilitating nutrient transport, and transmitting nerve impulses. Sodium and potassium gradients across the cell membrane, for instance, are central to the generation of action potentials in muscle cells and neurons. This balance, also referred to as the sodium-potassium pump, highlights the importance of electrolytes in converting electrical messages that are essential for communication and coordination in biological processes.

Disturbance in these electrolyte levels could lead to severe pathological states, altering cellular function and disrupting physiological processes. Thus, the role played by nursing professionals in monitoring and regulating electrolyte levels cannot be overstated, particularly in acute care environments where sudden changes may occur. Furthermore, electrolyte interaction and fluid balance are core to cellular function and overall homeostasis. Electrolytes control osmotic pressure and, consequently, intracellular as opposed to extracellular water distribution. Not only does this balance establish cell volume, but it also influences the removal of nutrients and wastes. Changes in fluid levels due to electrolyte imbalance can lead to complications, including dehydration, edema, and disturbances in electrolyte balance, which can manifest in a variety of clinical presentations. For the nurse's practice, evaluation of a patient's fluid and electrolyte balance is key to preventing and managing complications. With the application of evidence-based practice, nurses can identify vulnerable patients, for instance, those undergoing conditioning regimens for stem cell transplants, to intervene early and reduce the risk of electrolyte imbalance-related adverse events (Bambaci et al., 2016). In addition to maintaining fluid and electrolyte balance, the application of electrolytes in acid-base balance is crucial for sustaining cellular function. The pH of the body's fluids is closely regulated by bicarbonate, carbonic acid, and other electrolytes, particularly sodium and potassium. Acid-base balance may be disrupted due to several factors, including respiratory disease, metabolic derangements, or renal failure. These derangements can exert profound effects on cell enzymes and metabolic function with life-threatening implications. Nurses play a key role in monitoring patients' acid-base status from lab findings, clinical assessments, and prompt interventions. For instance, in the application of induced hypothermia for treating cerebral injury, it is essential to maintain electrolyte and acid-base balance to sustain neuronal function and promote recovery, as noted in recent therapeutic modality research (Zimmerman et al., 2011). Thus, understanding of the intricate function of electrolytes is vital to nurses engaged in fluid, electrolyte, and acid-base balance management (Figure 10.8).

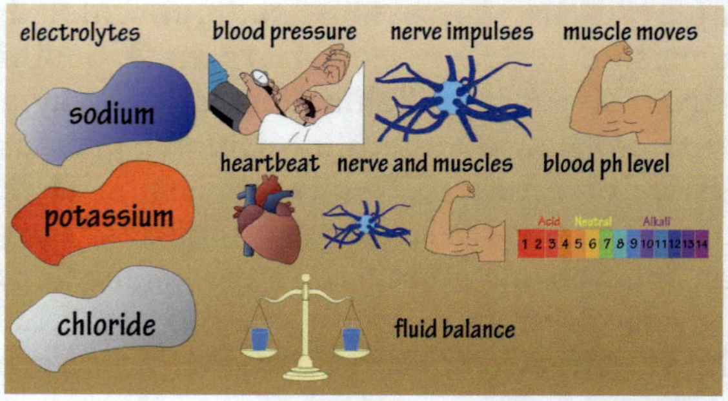

Figure 10.8. Role of electrolytes in cellular function.

Source: https://i.ytimg.com/vi/4CKATVXoepQ/maxresdefault.jpg.

10.2.3. Consequences of Electrolyte Imbalances

Electrolyte imbalance can have profound physiological effects and influence a wide range of body functions. For instance, disparity in sodium levels—either hypernatremia or hyponatremia—can compromise fluid balance and osmotic pressure and lead to cellular malfunction and neurological abnormalities. Vicinal individuals can present with anything from confusion and seizures to extreme lethargy and coma, thereby complicating the clinical presentation appreciably. Serum sodium is a crucial parameter to monitor in nursing practice, especially in acute care, where prompt assessment and intervention can significantly prevent untoward consequences. In reality, correction of sodium derangements should be done with care, as overspill with abrupt changes has been linked to osmotic demyelination syndrome, indicating the need for strict adherence to clinical guidelines. These considerations underscore the critical intersection between electrolyte management and patient safety in nursing practice (Bhengu et al., 2017). Potassium derangements are also necessary, with both hyperkalemia and hypokalemia carrying disastrous implications for cardiac function. Hyperkalemia can lead to lethal arrhythmias, which can result in cardiac arrest if untreated. Hypokalemia may lead to muscle weakness and respiratory failure by causing impaired neuromuscular transmission. In ICU patients, there is a requirement for continuous monitoring of electrolytes, particularly in those with concomitant diseases, such as chronic renal disease, or in patients on certain medications, including diuretics. Studies have reported an extensive occurrence of electrolyte derangements in ICUs; for example, research has established that hyperkalemia is associated with high mortality rates, which calls for active nursing management in balancing potassium levels to prevent complications (Sheyo et al., 2019). This highlights the importance of nurses being well-versed in identifying and managing these imbalances promptly and accurately. In addition, the combined effect of electrolyte imbalances can exacerbate comorbid diseases, making it more challenging to manage patients in general. Chronic disease patients, such as those suffering from kidney disease or heart failure, are particularly at risk from the effects of a less closely regulated electrolyte balance. The role of nursing extends beyond the immediate patient care in the acute environment; dietetic restriction, fluid status, and drug therapy are also addressed by the healthcare team to provide support for treatment compliance. Evidence shows that dietary and fluid restriction non-adherence is highly prevalent among patients with chronic kidney disease, highlighting nurses' educator and advocate role. Thus, understanding the impact of electrolyte imbalance cannot be separated from enhancing patient self-management strategies, ultimately resulting in improved health outcomes and a better quality of life for patients who experience these problems during their healthcare journeys (Bhengu et al., 2017).

Test Your Knowledge

1. What are the principal roles of sodium, potassium, and calcium in the body?
2. How do imbalances of critical electrolytes affect neuromuscular and cardiac function?

10.3. Acid-Base Homeostasis

Learning Outcome

1. Explain the importance of acid-base balance
2. Define acid-base regulation mechanisms
3. Explain clinical manifest

Acid-base homeostasis is a critical physiological process that maintains the balance of hydrogen ions (H^+) in the body to allow for optimal cellular function. This is a complex regulation, as small alterations in pH can lead to severe health issues. The body has various mechanisms, primarily the kidneys, lungs, and buffer systems, for maintaining a balance of acid and base. The kidneys regulate bicarbonate (HCO_3^-) and H^+ excretion, and the lungs regulate carbon dioxide (CO_2) levels via breathing, thereby controlling carbonic acid production. Understanding these mechanisms is essential to healthcare professionals as incorrect regulation can lead to conditions such as acidosis or alkalosis, which can be detrimental to patient outcomes. Thus, nursing practice must encompass a clear understanding of these principles to provide effective patient care and rapidly and accurately restore imbalances. Effective nursing practice in the environment of acid-base homeostasis requires clinicians to possess an acute appreciation of the signs and symptoms of imbalance. Empirical findings have shown that awareness and recognition of such symptoms significantly enhance patient care. Specifically, nurses who utilize checklists or symptom-identification tools demonstrate superior abilities in recognizing pertinent signs of fluid and electrolyte imbalance, which result in timely interventions. This is particularly vital in postoperative cases, where patients are at a higher risk of developing acid-base imbalances. Furthermore, the distinction between metabolic and respiratory imbalances enables nurses to implement pertinent nursing interventions based on actual assessments. According to recent studies, there is a clear correlation between the use of structured tools and enhanced patient care, suggesting that in-service education and training of nurses in these critical areas are essential (Walkingshaw et al., 2008). Furthermore, the importance of establishing a solid foundation of knowledge of fluid, electrolyte, and acid-base management cannot be overemphasized. Nurses need to be updated with evidence-based knowledge to manage and attend to fluid balance effectively. Research has revealed that fluid intake and output measurement is not consistently satisfactory among most nursing professionals, which is a crucial foundation for patient safety and effective care (Shepley et al., 2007). The ongoing evolution of medical science necessitates that nurse education involves intensive training in fluid and electrolyte management, thereby enhancing nurses' ability to provide quality care. Professional courses, such as in-service training and workshops, must be structured in a way that bridges the gaps in nursing knowledge, enabling each practitioner to manage issues related to acid-base homeostasis and thereby drastically enhance patient outcomes (Figure 10.9).

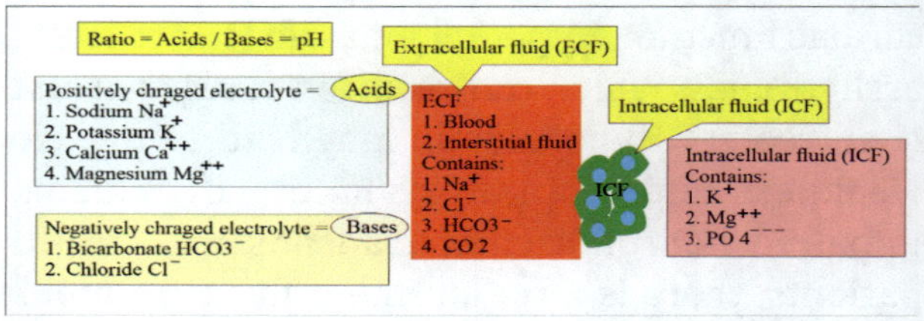

Figure 10.9. Acid base balance straight a nursing.

Source: https://www.labpedia.net/wp-content/uploads/2021/03/Acid-base-definition.jpg.

10.3.1. Definition and Importance of Acid-Base Balance

Acid-base balance is a major concept in human physiology that explains the control of hydrogen ion concentration in the body's fluids, which is essential for maintaining the body in homeostasis. pH of the arterial blood is strictly controlled between 7.35 and 7.45, and variations thereof have serious health consequences. The body utilizes different mechanisms to maintain such a balance, ranging from physiological buffers, the respiratory mechanism, and renal action. Buffers such as bicarbonate and proteins respond quickly to neutralize added base or acid, whereas respiratory regulation occurs through the control of carbon dioxide concentration by the respiratory process. Renal function maintains acid-base balance by excreting hydrogen ions and reabsorbing bicarbonate, thereby offering long-term stability of blood pH. Nurses find it highly significant to understand these processes, as they immediately impact patient treatment and the provision of care for conditions such as metabolic acidosis or alkalosis. The significance of maintaining acid-base balance cannot be overstated, as it is crucial to enzymatic activity, oxygen transport, and overall cellular function.

Acid-base disturbances may be caused by many different physiological conditions, such as respiratory disease, kidney disorders, or excessive metabolic production, and can result in potentially life-threatening complications. For example, respiratory acidosis can present in the patient with chronic obstructive pulmonary disease (COPD), and metabolic acidosis can result from diabetic ketoacidosis or renal insufficiency.

Being able to identify such disturbances and responding appropriately is crucial for nursing practice. Nurses will often perform assessments and follow laboratory results, such as ABG levels, to evaluate a patient's acid-base status and determine intervention. As nurses intervene to correct these imbalances, this health deterioration can be prevented, and recovery facilitated. Within clinical nursing practice, knowledge and evaluation of acid-base balance are not only essential for monitoring the patient, but also for creating appropriate treatment regimens.

Educating the patient and their family about the importance of acid-base balance encourages a team healthcare process. For example, during the management of a patient with critical metabolic acidosis, the nurse interventions that can be done include administration of therapy with bicarbonate or altering intake to reduce acid load. Also, for critically ill patients, constant monitoring and early intervention prevent severe complications caused by imbalances. Thus, the role of the nurse extends beyond simple evaluation; it also encompasses patient education, advocacy, and the application of evidence-based practice to achieve improved patient outcomes. As part of a multi-dimensional approach to fluid, electrolyte, and acid-base balance, nurses must be vigilant and current with the latest guidelines in this vital component of patient care (Haworth et al., 2017; Halvorsen et al., 2022).

10.3.2. Mechanisms of Acid-Base Regulation

Acid-base regulation mechanisms play a crucial role in maintaining homeostasis in the human body, particularly in nursing practice. The body gains one of its primary mechanisms of acid-base balance through the use of buffering systems such as bicarbonate, phosphate, and protein buffers. The buffers gain their purpose either by donating or accepting hydrogen ions (H^+) to minimize pH level changes. The bicarbonate buffer system, for instance, plays a critical role in maintaining a serum pH within a good range of 7.35–7.45. Nurses should be aware of these buffering systems, as they provide essential information regarding patients' care, especially in emergency conditions where the acid-base status may change rapidly, requiring instant and professional intervention to restore balance. Furthermore, the respiratory system is also vital in acid-base balance via regulation of CO_2 levels. Through respiration, the body can remove CO_2, a metabolic waste that, when its levels build up, can lead to respiratory acidosis. Conversely, increased respiratory rate can lead to respiratory alkalosis via decreasing CO_2 levels. Monitoring the respiratory function of patients in nursing care is crucial, as alterations in breathing rates directly impact acid-base balance. Some examples are those patients with COPD or under mechanical ventilation, where there is a requirement for serious assessment of respiratory status to prevent potential derangement of acid-base homeostasis. Detection of these respiratory contributions enables nurses to intervene appropriately and at the correct time whenever necessary, thereby enhancing patient outcomes in critical care settings. Lastly, renal processes also regulate acid-base balance by primarily functioning through the reabsorption and excretion of H^+ ions and HCO_3^-. When regulating long-term acid-base balance, the kidneys absorb or excrete these ions according to the body's needs. In the midst of an acute disease or recovery from surgery, where extensive fluid and electrolyte management is required, the nurse's understanding of renal physiology is invaluable. For example, in patients presenting with metabolic acidosis, kidney compensation may not be sufficient; therefore, it is essential to administer adequate fluid and electrolyte replacement. A significant knowledge shortfall has been identified among nursing staff regarding the fundamental principles of fluid balance, and there is a strong emphasis on the importance of ongoing education in these concepts to facilitate holistic nursing care (Shepley et al., 2007). Thus, a general understanding of renal considerations in acid-base balance is crucial for optimizing nursing practice and enhancing patient care outcomes in the healthcare environment (Figure 10.10).

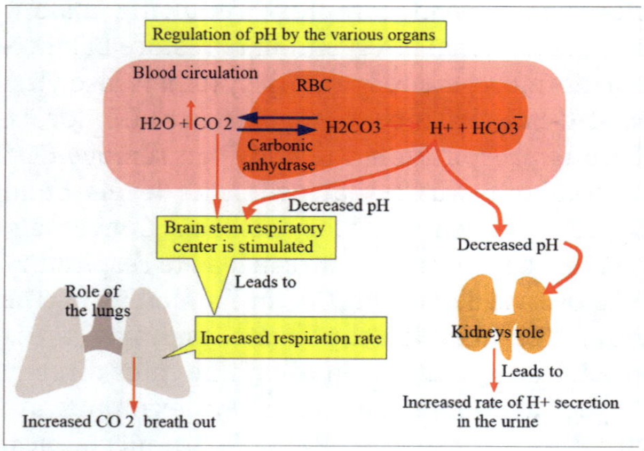

Figure 10.10. Acid base pH control.

Source: https://labpedia.net/wp-content/uploads/2020/04/acid-base-ph-control.jpg.

10.3.3. Clinical Implications of Acid-Base Disturbances

Disturbances in acid-base are a key topic in nursing practice, particularly due to the grave clinical relevance to patient care. Nursing professionals should have a broad knowledge of metabolic and respiratory acidosis and alkalosis, as imbalances can lead to serious physiological disturbances. For example, respiratory acidosis typically arises due to causes such as COPD or overdose of sedative medication, producing excess amounts of carbon dioxide and low pH. Metabolic acidosis, however, may arise due to causes such as renal failure or extensive diarrhea, lowering bicarbonate concentrations. Detection of such disturbances would typically rely on arterial blood gas analysis, meaning nurses must be taught to intervene and interpret the results.

The development of these skills, as research recommends, can yield dividends in terms of patient outcomes by enabling the timely detection and management of acid-base imbalance symptoms (Walkingshaw et al., 2008). The importance of acid-base disturbances extends beyond the context of acute clinical presentations, as they carry implications that can profoundly impact the balance of treatment and recovery. In ischemic strokes, for instance, acid-base status regulation influences neurological recovery. Furthermore, research indicates that variations in venous blood gases, electrolytes, and pH can potentially be used to predict the volume of infarction and death (Martha et al., 2019). For this purpose, nurses are tasked with monitoring these parameters and responding quickly to deviations from the norm. Nursing protocols must prioritize routine checks for patients with pre-existing respiratory or renal diseases.

Being able to mitigate risks associated with such disturbances by ensuring an active monitoring process for acid-base balance through nurses can enhance patient safety as well as recovery chances. Furthermore, the treatment modalities applied to correct acid-base dysequilibrations must be tailored according to the clinical context. In acidosis, treatment may include the administration of bicarbonate or elimination of carbon dioxide through respiratory assistance. For alkalosis, repletion of electrolytes, e.g., potassium, would generally be necessary. Blending educational content and clinical guidelines that define symptoms and interventions for various acid-base disturbances is integral to nursing practice. Systematic approaches, such as the use of symptom checklists, are supported by studies as significantly enhancing nurses' proficiency in identifying and treating imbalances (Walkingshaw et al., 2008). Accordingly, the application of standard protocols in the education of nursing and clinical practices is capable of empowering nurses to apply a holistic approach in taking care of patients fluid, electrolyte, and acid-base balance successfully and on time.

Test Your Knowledge

1. What are the mechanisms the body uses to maintain acid-base balance within the normal range of pH?
2. How do nurses recognize and respond to signs and symptoms of metabolic or respiratory acidosis and alkalosis?

10.4. Assessment of Fluid and Electrolyte Status

Learning Outcome

1. Identify methods for evaluating fluid balance
2. Define laboratory tests for electrolyte level
3. Describe signs of imbalance

Careful assessment of fluid and electrolyte status is crucial in nursing, particularly in those at risk for imbalance due to most medical illnesses. This assessment typically entails the measurement of history, physical evidence on examination, and lab work to determine the patient's fluid and electrolyte needs. Effective monitoring of these parameters is crucial for preventing complications arising from either deficit or excess. For instance, nursing practice requires constant monitoring of vital signs, intake, and output, and dehydration or overhydration. The nurses are supposed to be able to read abnormal lab results that reveal the patient's electrolyte status, further guiding interventions such as fluid resuscitation or diuretic therapy. These routine assessments enable proactive handling of the patient's condition and provide a tailored approach to treatment, ensuring patient safety and therapeutic efficacy. Multiparametric monitoring systems promise to play a crucial role in assessing fluid and electrolyte status. Technologies involving current transducers allow for multiple physiological parameters to be tracked simultaneously, which gives the nurse enhanced ability to achieve a clear picture of a patient's fluid status. Such sophisticated monitoring can be applied in a variety of clinical contexts, ranging from intrapartum patient management to neonatal and adult blood gas analysis, as highlighted by new evidence. Implementation of the systems into practice increases not only the accuracy of assessments but also allows for timely interventions. Proper know-how of the technologies will enable nurses to react quickly to modifications in fluid and electrolyte status, improving patient outcomes and the quality of care (N/A). The guidelines developed for fluid and electrolyte management also provide valuable information to nursing practitioners involved in dialysis and related therapies. As specified in current clinical guidelines, dialysis efficacy may significantly differ between patients with certain strategies necessary to maximize fluid removal and electrolyte management (Fox et al., 2019). For instance, monitoring the adequacy of dialysis sessions, dialysate composition adjustments, and anticoagulation strategies is an important aspect in caring for patients undergoing dialysis. Nurses, being well-versed in such guidelines, can thus work in harmony with patients to tailor treatment plans according to individual needs, ensuring that fluid and electrolyte management adheres to best practice and maximizes the delivery of high-quality care. Moreover, emphasizing patient involvement in the process not only enhances nursing practice but also benefits patient compliance with treatment protocols (Figure 10.11).

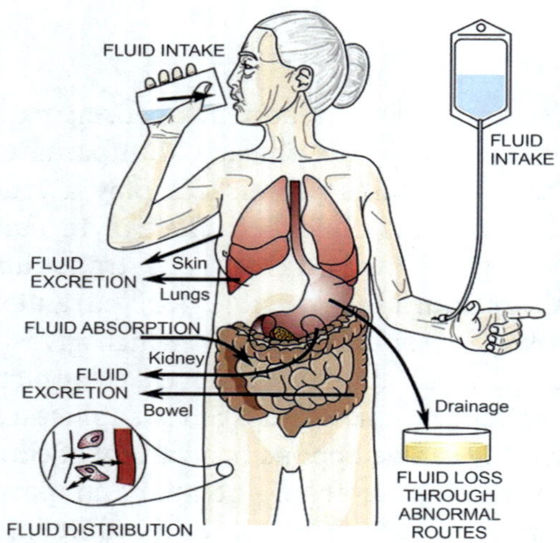

Figure 10.11. Assessment of fluid and electrolyte status.

Source: https://basicmedicalkey.com/wp-content/uploads/2016/09/F000243f24-03-9781455726509.jpg.

10.4.1. Methods for Evaluating Fluid Balance

Assessment of fluid balance is crucial for achieving optimal patient outcomes in clinical practice, particularly in nursing care, where attention to the patient's fluid, electrolyte, and acid-base balance is essential. There are many methods employed in fluid balance assessment, including daily patient weighing, which provides valuable information on fluid changes in the body. Through monitoring of weight fluctuations, nurses can identify unexplained fluid retention, weight gain, or unexplained dehydration-weight loss. Additionally, accurate intake and output (I&O) record systems become a mainstay in evaluating fluid balance, including all fluids consumed and removed. These methods require not only the easier detection of imbalances but also guide nurses' decisions in patient-specific care, allowing for the alteration of fluid and nutrition administration according to the results of real-time measurements. Beyond traditional methods, newer methods also play an important role in the measurement of fluid balance. For instance, bioelectrical impedance analysis (BIA) is an available option that estimates body compartments for water and fat without invasive quantification. This method is particularly valuable in cases of compromised or incorrect clinical assessment, such as in the obese or in critically ill patients. Furthermore, a multiparametric monitoring system with various available transducers can provide comprehensive information about a patient's fluid and electrolyte state. This new method not only optimizes the precision of fluid balance measurement but also has significant implications for assessing patients' overall well-being and metabolic activity in real time. These methods give nursing professionals greater insight to guarantee complex patient-centered tactics for fluid management. A critical element of fluid balance measurement is the application of laboratory tests, specifically blood gas and electrolyte analysis. These are utilized to determine not only fluid volumes but also the amount of significant electrolytes in the blood that might exhibit underlying pathophysiology. Abnormal bicarbonate, potassium, and sodium levels can not only indicate dysregulation of fluid balance but also signify the presence of complications that must be corrected immediately. An increased understanding of the dynamic relationship between fluid status and electrolyte status enables nursing practitioners to design interventions tailored to patients' unique needs, particularly for vulnerable populations such as newborns or patients with chronic illnesses. This convergence of clinical knowledge and technological advancements underscores the pivotal role of continuous and multifaceted evaluations in managing fluid balance, as reaffirmed by recent research and developments in the field (Dinerstein et al., 2011; N/A, 2025) (Figure 10.12).

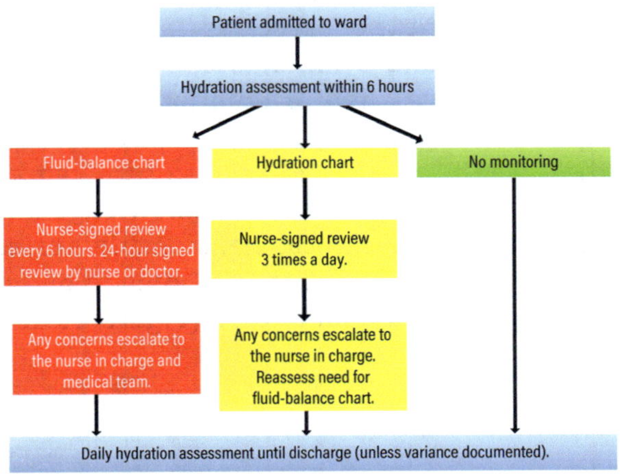

Figure 10.12. Assessing and documenting fluid balance.

Source: https://d1ipglwbj780rd.cloudfront.net/rcni/static/journals/ns/aop/ns.2016.e10432/graphic/ns.2016.e10432_0002.jpg.

10.4.2. Laboratory Tests for Electrolyte Levels

Laboratory tests to screen for electrolyte levels are essential in nursing practice and for maintaining fluid and electrolyte balance. Electrolytes, such as sodium, potassium, calcium, and bicarbonate, play fundamental roles in physiologic processes, including muscle contraction, nerve conduction, and acid-base balance. Continuous monitoring of these electrolyte levels allows practitioners to detect imbalances that may lead to serious complications. For instance, hyponatremia, a condition of lowered sodium levels, may cause neurological abnormalities, while precipitating catastrophic cardiac events due to hyperkalemia. Thus, accurate laboratory analysis and early interpretation of the tests are crucial to successful patient management, particularly in acute situations where immediate interventions may avert unfavorable outcomes. Moreover, electrolyte testing is vital for monitoring some clinical conditions, such as diabetic ketoacidosis (DKA), which is a significant nursing concern. DKA patients can have critical electrolyte imbalances, the most common of which is increased potassium, which requires intense and emergent nursing care. Laboratory tests provide immediate feedback that directs treatment interventions for restoring these levels to normal and establishing homeostasis. Through the evaluation of acid-base status and detection of metabolic derangements, clinicians are in a position to administer targeted interventions that reverse both the original hyperglycemia and related electrolyte imbalances, thereby reducing complications associated with the condition. Electrolytic evaluation is therefore an integral part of the care plan for patients with profound metabolic derangements, such as those in DKA (Bartosiak et al., 2019). Also, monitoring of electrolytes during acute medical events, such as ischemic stroke, emphasizes the importance of laboratory tests within nursing. Research finds that changes in electrolyte levels are reflective of patient outcomes following such events. For example, changes in bicarbonate and ionized calcium levels during initial presentation are reflective of potential infarct sizes and mortality. It is only through understanding these interrelationships that nurses can order patient assessment and intervention effectively, allowing for faster and more informed interventions to take place. In this case, the laboratory test plays a role greater than mere diagnosis; it becomes a cornerstone of patient management guidelines, with the goal of optimizing recovery and minimizing complications in critical care settings (Martha et al., 2019).

10.4.3. Clinical Signs of Imbalance

The clinical manifestations of fluid and electrolyte imbalance are significant indicators that should be recognized by nurses for the provision of appropriate care. Fluid and electrolyte imbalance tends to occur through a range of symptoms, including alterations in vital signs, changes in mental status, and bodily signs such as edema or dehydration. Dehydration, for instance, can be demonstrated by dry mucous membranes and reduced skin turgor, while hypervolemia can cause shortness of breath and elevated blood pressure. Moreover, electrolyte imbalance, for example, hypernatremia or hypokalemia, may lead to more severe outcomes, including neurological and cardiovascular diseases. Nurses' capability to identify these signs significantly influences patient care quality and the need for intervention. It has been suggested that evidence indicates improvement in nurses' capacity to recognize and treat these imbalances when a list of possible signs and symptoms is provided (Walkingshaw et al., 2008). It is crucial in the clinical setting to identify disturbances in electrolytes early, particularly in high-risk patient populations, such as those with diabetes or renal failure. Diabetic ketoacidosis patients, for example, typically present with clinical manifestations of derangement of metabolism, such as breath smelling of fruit, tachypnea, and polydipsia. There is a critical need for continuous monitoring and observation of these signs for effective intervention and management. Nursing practice, therefore, needs to include a sharp sense of potential complications associated with such imbalances. Failure to identify clinical signs can lead to delayed treatment, worsening the patient's condition. As witnessed by studies, possessing a clear guide for symptom identification significantly enhances a nurses observing ability and decision-making ability in treating fluid and electrolyte imbalances (Bartosiak et al., 2019). Lastly, the importance of clinical signs of imbalance to practice cannot be overestimated. Not only are these signs pointers to patients' current health status, but also determine the nursing intervention needed in restoring homeostasis. Educating nursing staff on the correlation between observed clinical signs and the underlying physiological derangements is essential to support improved patient outcomes. Evidence suggests that using lists or classification systems that highlight specific signs and symptoms can help nurses clearly improve their evaluation skills and interventions (Walkingshaw et al., 2008). In a setting where timely and precise care can be a matter of life and death, the knowledge and detection of these clinical signs enable nurses to respond quickly, ultimately leading to better patient safety and quality care (Figure 10.13).

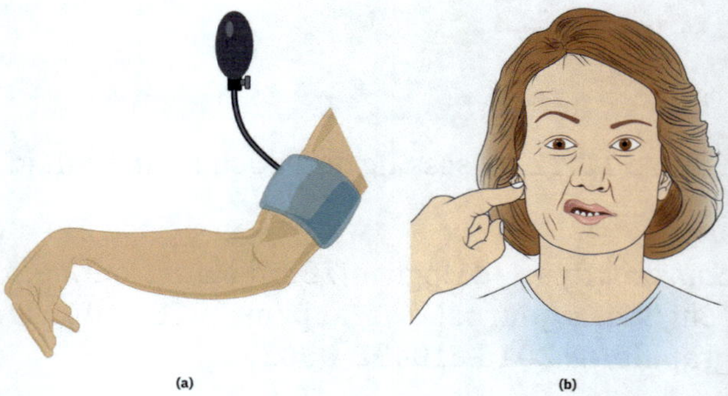

Figure 10.13. Clinical signs of imbalance for nursing.

Source: https://med.libretexts.org/@api/deki/files/68658/d69b4e7316833db6365e61459889ffde9a02d915?revision=1.

Test Your Knowledge

1. What are the clinical signs and symptoms of fluid volume deficit or excess in a patient?
2. Which laboratory values are most essential to assess electrolyte imbalances in nursing practice?

10.5. Nursing Interventions for Fluid and Electrolyte Imbalance

Learning Outcome

1. Describe strategies for fluid replacement
2. Define the administration of electrolytes
3. Discuss monitoring and adjusting treatment plans

Management of fluid and electrolyte balance is a cornerstone of nursing practice, emphasizing the importance of practical assessment and early intervention. When patients indicate an imbalance, such as dehydration or overhydration, the nurse's role in monitoring vital signs, daily weights, and intake/output becomes a matter of extreme priority. Research has indicated that nurses employing a systematic approach, such as symptom checklists, significantly enhance their ability to detect such imbalances. Support is evidenced in the research findings that surgical nurses with a standard list of symptoms recognized and treated fluid and electrolyte status more accurately than those without these resources (Walkingshaw et al., 2008). Hence, the provision of practical aids to nurses has the benefit of not only making their clinical decision-making easier but also of enhancing the quality of patient care, enabling timely and appropriate interventions to be delivered. An understanding of the underlying pathophysiology of these imbalances must underpin effective execution of fluid and electrolyte balance nursing interventions. For instance, conditions such as heart failure or renal dysfunction can precipitate radical shifts in the dynamics of fluid that need close observation and intravenous fluid, electrolyte, or diuretic therapy as appropriate. Nurses are centrally engaged in forming part of multidisciplinary teams to formulate treatment strategies that suit the particular needs of individual patients. Furthermore, the application of critical thinking, as well as clinical judgment, in the two cases is essential for achieving successful outcomes (Quandt et al., 2022). The application of comprehensive evaluations, including physical exams and lab values, enables nurses to make proper decisions, thereby optimizing fluid and electrolyte management in patients with various medical conditions. In addition to direct clinical management, education measures are a crucial part of nursing practice in the context of fluid and electrolyte imbalance.

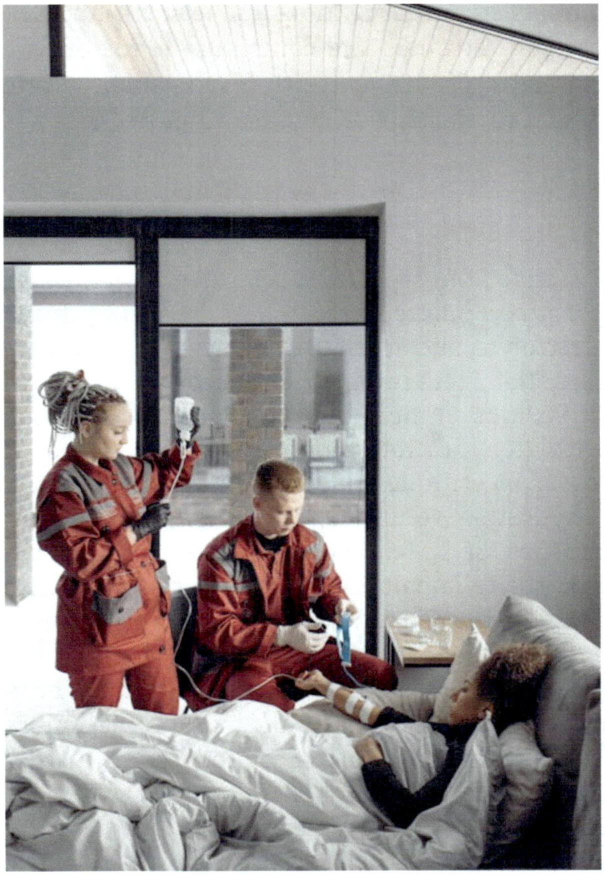

Figure 10.14. Nursing interventions for fluid and electrolyte imbalance.

Source: https://images.pexels.com/photos/6753441/pexels-photo-6753441.jpeg.

Education of patients about changes in diet, symptoms of balance disorders, and compliance with treatment regimens is part of the nurses' function. Effective education promotes active involvement in patients' health care, and hospitalization rates due to complications of balance may be reduced. Furthermore, nursing staff continuing education programs, workshops, and case studies increase their skills in fluid and electrolyte management and assist in fostering a culture of continuous improvement in healthcare settings. Through the integration of clinical competencies with educational programs, nursing staff interventions can lead to improved patient outcomes and contribute to fostering a culture of proactive health management within fluid and electrolyte balance (Figure 10.14).

10.5.1. Strategies for Fluid Replacement

Effective fluid replacement strategies in nursing practice, particularly when handling fluid, electrolyte, and acid-base balance responses, are essential. Fluid replacement becomes necessary in various clinical scenarios, including those with dehydration, renal failure, or acute GI losses. A critique based on evidence from oral rehydration solutions, intravenous fluids, and the use of specialized preparations to treat electrolyte imbalances is necessary to optimize patient outcomes. By identifying patient-specific needs based on consideration of the patient's age, existing conditions, and severity of fluid loss, nurses can tailor fluid replacement therapy that is safe and effective. The use of isotonic fluids for initial resuscitation with later adjustment based on monitoring parameters is a practice recommended within acute settings. When selecting appropriate fluids to replace, medical professionals must first identify the type of fluid loss and its quantity. In patients with acute kidney injury (AKI), as indicated in research examining Sustained Low Efficiency Daily Dialysis (SLEDD) and SLEDD-f strategies, fluid balance monitoring is crucial to prevent both fluid overload and deficit complications (Wahab et al., 2015). The choice between crystalloids and colloids impacts not only short-term resuscitation but also long-term renal and acid-base status. Moreover, adherence to guidelines, which emphasize individualized care and evidence-based practice, assists nurses in taking effective decisions regarding fluid replacement modalities (Fox et al., 2019). Ultimately, a comprehensive strategy that incorporates patient assessment, fluid selection, and ongoing evaluation will facilitate effective fluid management. Nurses play a pivotal role in educating patients and healthcare teams regarding the importance of maintaining fluid balance through proper replacement strategies. This didactic aspect is not technically restricted to direct patient care, as nurses commonly work in conjunction with interdisciplinary teams designing guidelines and protocols standardizing fluid replacement in numerous varied clinical settings. Monitoring serum electrolytes and renal function regularly, for example, can detect abnormalities in acid-base balance early on, allowing for timely intervention.

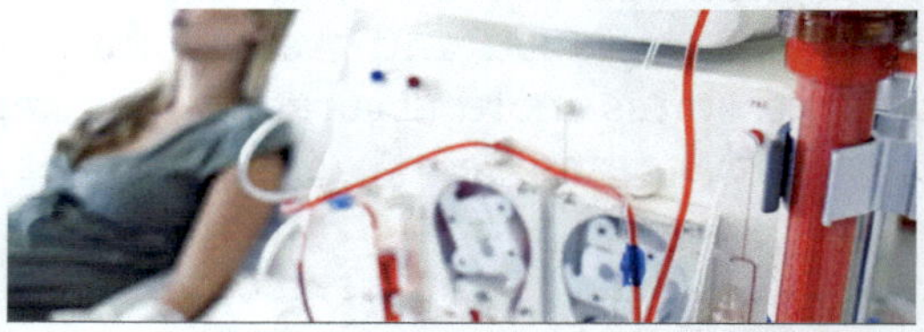

Figure 10.15. Sustained low efficiency daily dialysis (SLEDD).

Source: https://external-content.duckduckgo.com/iu/?u=https%3A%2F%2Fckbirlahospitals.com%2Frbh%2Fuploadedfiles%2Fgallery%2F1679562983_Sustained-low-efficiency.webp&f=1&nofb=1&ipt=c0250da060104473a2f415b46ae10cea9dd1dd0cd1c4ee9074137e0c4b8e73f3.

Additionally, the application of technology, such as electronic health records, can enhance communication and patient care by tracking fluid input and output. Through the establishment of a culture of continuous learning and best-practice implementation, nursing providers can make a substantial contribution to patient outcomes related to fluid and electrolyte balance, thereby supporting the integral relationship between effective fluid replacement techniques and overall well-being (Figure 10.15).

10.5.2. Administration of Electrolytes

Administration of electrolytes forms an integral part of fluid and electrolyte management in the nursing care process. Maintaining proper electrolyte balance is crucial for most of the body's physiological functions, including nerve conduction, muscle contraction, and acid-base balance. Nurses play an essential role in maintaining patients' electrolyte balances, identifying any abnormalities, and implementing necessary interventions. Understanding the physiological actions of primary electrolytes, such as sodium, potassium, calcium, and magnesium, enables clinicians to intervene appropriately. For example, hypokalemia will lead to cardiac arrhythmias, and immediate administration of potassium is required. Dinerstein et al. (2011) point out that optimal delivery of macronutrients, including electrolytes, is of essential importance to patient outcome, particularly in vulnerable individuals such as premature infants, where imbalance has long-term effects. In the hospital setting, the routes of administration for electrolytes tend to vary based on patient status and urgency. Oral rehydration is typically used in cases of mild dehydration or depletion among patients. However, when there is a critical status, intravenous (IV) delivery comes into play to compensate for electrolyte balance appropriately. This is particularly crucial in intensive care units, where restoration of electrolytes promptly is crucial for hemodynamic stabilization. The decision to use the appropriate electrolyte solutions, such as normal saline or lactated Ringer's, is predicated on the specific clinical situation, including systemic illnesses and the patient's individual requirements. Moreover, continuous monitoring must be performed while it is being administered to avoid complications, such as phlebitis or fluid overload, which may jeopardize patient safety and recovery. N/A (2025) supports the idea of the development of monitoring technologies for fostering patient safety in the application of electrolytes as well as following best practices. Patient education about the necessity of maintaining adequate electrolyte levels also increases nursing practice. Food sources of required electrolytes, such as fruits and vegetables for potassium and milk for calcium, should be discussed with patients during patient education by nurses.

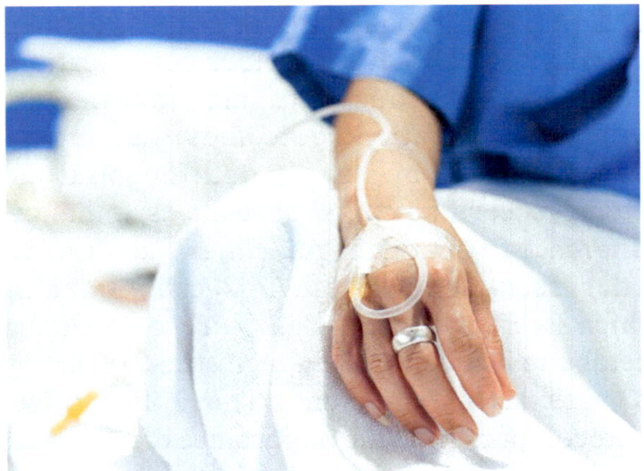

Figure 10.16. Electrolyte balance.

Source: https://external-content.duckduckgo.com/iu/?u=https%3A%2F%2Fimages.wisegeek.com%2Fpatient-receiving-iv.jpg&f=1&nofb=1&ipt=9e304dbc15a4b83ddbdbd6d02cd1b7e8b76e8ad6c6c7efd9d37dd5222bb23d5d.

This anticipatory approach not only helps directly with the management of electrolyte balance but also gives patients the capacity to become responsible for their own well-being. Understanding when to seek medical attention—such as recognizing symptoms of imbalance, including confusion or muscle cramping—helps to enhance patient involvement and compliance with therapy. Briefly, electrolyte therapy is a comprehensive procedure that involves precise evaluation, early intervention, and patient education to ensure the optimal health status in nursing care (Figure 10.16).

10.5.3. Monitoring and Adjusting Treatment Plans

Effective monitoring and adjustment of treatment plans in nursing practice are crucial to maintaining fluid, electrolyte, and acid-base balance. Ongoing monitoring of a patient's status enables nurses to recognize any deviation from expected outcomes and adjust interventions accordingly. For instance, in diabetic emergencies such as DKA or hyperosmolar hyperglycemic state (HHS), early adjustment of the treatment regimen is able to avoid serious complications. Standardized order sets are justified, as evidenced by patient outcomes that include reduced length of stay in both hospital and intensive care settings, as well as enhanced adherence to treatment guidelines. Standardized order sets facilitate quick decision-making, which is crucial when high glucose levels and metabolic acidosis pose a significant challenge to patient management. These formalized protocols underline the importance of systematic surveillance for making timely adjustments to therapeutic interventions (Gort et al., 2020). With geriatric patients, hydration and nutritional status surveillance is especially important because they both present with dehydration and malnutrition, which only serves to increase the complexity of their clinical profile. Through systematic assessment of hydration status and food intake, nurses can modify interventions better to suit the unique needs of this groupto suit the unique needs of this group better. Evidence suggests that comprehensive screening for low intake dehydration and malnutrition is necessary, and the call is being made for individualized strategies to be developed to enhance nutritional care. In addition to dietary modification education, practical interventions such as individualized counseling and oral supplements are also recommended (Beck et al., 2019). Implementing these approaches not only guarantees an optimal clinical result but also enhances the quality of life of elderly patients, illustrating the pivotal importance of ongoing evaluation in treatment planning. In addition, the multidimensional nature of care necessitates collaboration among diverse healthcare providers on multiple levels to monitor and adjust treatment regimens accordingly. Interdisciplinary interaction among physicians, dietitians, and nurses provides a comprehensive approach to all facets of a patient's fluid, electrolyte, and acid-base balance simultaneously. There are regular interdisciplinary meetings that facilitate timely discussions on patient progress, allowing for quick readjustments of treatment procedures when necessary. Team collaboration is especially significant in those cases where patients have more than one problem, such as obesity or chronic illnesses from electrolyte imbalance. By collaborating with various professionals, nursing practice can optimize care delivery to ensure interventions are maintained for preventing and managing dehydration or imbalances, thereby enhancing patient outcomes in diverse healthcare settings (Beck et al., 2019).

Test Your Knowledge

1. What are some of the nursing interventions that are essential when caring for a patient with hyponatremia or hyperkalemia?
2. How do nurses individualize fluid and electrolyte replacement based on a patient's presentation and lab results?

10.6. Patient Education and Management

Learning Outcome

1. Discuss the importance of patient education in fluid intake
2. Define diet-related components of electrolyte balance
3. List patient self-monitoring strategies

Effective patient education is a cornerstone of nursing practice, particularly in managing fluid, electrolyte, and acid-base balance. Nursing personnel and patients must understand complicated mechanisms governing these physiological processes. Nurses play a key role in bridging the gap between complex medical concepts and patient comprehension. Through the proper application of educational approaches tailored to specific patient needs, nurses are capable of making significant contributions to patient engagement and compliance. This venture not only allows patients to control their health independently but also decreases complication rates resulting from imbalances. Moreover, by encouraging open communication, nurses can help minimize patients' misconceptions and anxieties about their treatment regimens, leading to improved overall health outcomes. Patient management is a multidimensional process that entails education, assessment, and intervention practices to correct fluid, electrolyte, and acid-base imbalances. Holistic assessment by healthcare practitioners enables the identification of risk factors and symptoms associated with imbalances, which are crucial for introducing timely interventions. Education about potential balance indicators, such as fluid retention or electrolyte imbalance, is essential in enabling patients to recognize when to access assistance. Additionally, a multidisciplinary team approach can optimize patient management. Multidisciplinary collaboration by engaging a team ensures that education is not just directed at patients but also at their families, providing optimal support for patients addressing complex health issues. Ultimately, effective patient management relies on the coordination of information and resources, enabling patients to be active participants in their own care. Application of formalized teaching programs is beneficial in allowing the patients to grasp the disease and balance the fluid, electrolyte, and acid-base levels. Such programs should be evidence-based and incorporate monitoring of patient learning and accommodation. For instance, ongoing monitoring of patient progress can provide vital information about the effectiveness of educational interventions, allowing for individualized modifications as needed. Moreover, new learning materials, such as visual aids or computer-based systems, can facilitate better comprehension by those patients with varying literacy levels. Furthermore, knowledge of patient heterogeneity guides culturally responsive care, further augmenting the education process. Lastly, patient education and management responsibility lead to enhanced clinical outcomes, as well as unite healthcare professionals and patients to foster an improved overall healthcare experience (Schneider et al., 2021; Halvorsen et al., 2022) (Figure 10.17).

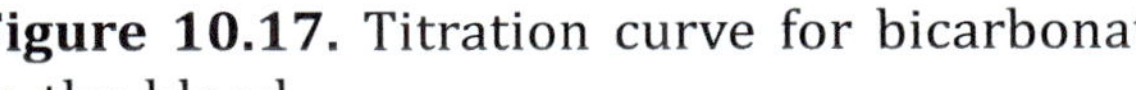

Figure 10.17. Titration curve for bicarbonate in the blood.

Source: https://cdn.lecturio.com/assets/Titration-curve-for-bicarbonate-in-the-blood.jpg.

10.6.1. Importance of Educating Patients on Fluid Intake

Education of patients regarding fluid intake is a significant aspect of nursing care related to fluid, electrolyte, and acid-base balance. Proper hydration is essential for maintaining homeostasis, regulating cardiovascular function, and facilitating metabolic processes. Educating patients about their own daily fluid requirements helps prevent dehydration and its related complications. Such an educational initiative should not only focus on the quantity of fluid consumption but also on the quality of fluid sources, as certain fluids can induce unplanned electrolyte imbalances. Growing health awareness of individual fluid requirements as a function of age, sex, activity, and illness empowers the patient to become an active health care provider for themselves, with long-term health outcome benefits. Secondly, patient education regarding the signs and symptoms of fluid imbalance more suitably prepares patients to monitor themselves and adequately manage their hydration needs. With greater awareness of how excessive fluid loss or retention will affect their health, patients are motivated to seek help where necessary. For instance, diseases like heart failure or kidney dysfunction require utmost monitoring of fluid intake and output. Instructing patients to recognize signs of swelling, excessive thirst, or changes in urination will also minimize the risk of complications. Nurse education interventions can facilitate the learning necessary for patients to develop healthy behaviors, enabling them to make informed decisions about hydration. Awareness of the evolving guidelines regarding fluid management necessitates nursing practice to remain current and adaptive. Recent research and expert recommendations offer valuable insights into the optimal fluid replacement solutions, particularly in healthcare settings where fluid status is crucial. The European Resuscitation Council Guidelines of 2021 exemplify such a commitment to evidence-based practice, with an integrative consideration of fluid management during resuscitation activities, among others (Perkins et al., 2021). Educational comprehensiveness ensures that patients are not just passive recipients of care but active partners who have the knowledge to advocate for their own health. Such holism solidified nursing's role in facilitating optimal fluid intake and, in turn, improving health outcomes, which aligns with broader goals for patient well-being and quality care (Figure 10.18).

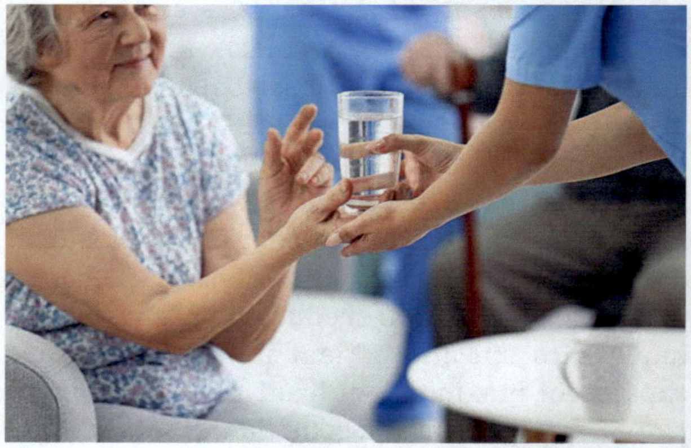

Figure 10.18. Importance of educating patients on fluid intake.

Source: https://ausmed-images.s3-ap-southeast-2.amazonaws.com/ausmed.com/ausmed-articles/20200518_body_3.jpg.

10.6.2. Dietary Considerations for Electrolyte Balance

Electrolyte balance is essential for overall health, especially in nursing, where patient care requires an integrated understanding of dietary aspects. These include sodium, potassium, calcium, and magnesium, which play important roles in body functions such as muscle contraction, nerve conduction, and fluid balance. A diet lacking in these critical minerals can result in imbalances that are expressed as symptoms from fatigue to life-threatening cardiac arrhythmias. Thus, it is crucial that healthcare professionals assess patients' dietary intake and establish guidelines for supplementing them with an adequate amount of electrolytes. Specifically, dietary guidance should consider age, preexisting medical conditions, and dietary limitations to provide targeted interventions that address patient-specific needs while maintaining optimal electrolyte balance in the body. From a nursing perspective, knowledge of particular dietary sources of electrolytes maximizes the potential to instruct patients on how to maintain balance. For example, potassium-rich foods like bananas, oranges, and spinach help counteract the effects of sodium on blood pressure, thereby reducing the risk of hypertension. In contrast, foods high in sodium can worsen fluid retention and cardiovascular stress, making it imperative to approach diet counseling with caution. Additionally, practical education on hydration can avoid dehydration, which is a serious threat to older adults and those with chronic conditions, who also suffer from malnutrition due to poor intake of nutrients. Since dehydration can impair kidney function and upset electrolyte balance, nursing practice should promote routine screening and proactive education on fluid and food intake to maximize patient outcomes, emphasizing the need for a holistic approach to nutrition and hydration within healthcare settings. Electrolyte imbalances can also result from medical conditions, and consideration of diet becomes increasingly important in some patient populations. For instance, patients with chronic kidney disease (CKD) have to follow certain electrolyte-restricted diets to control their condition successfully. The guidelines emphasize reducing potassium and phosphorus while maintaining adequate calcium levels. Research emphasizes dietary management as a means of preventing dehydration and malnutrition, particularly among elderly individuals who may be reluctant to make dietary adjustments due to established eating habits or educational deficits regarding the consequences of their eating habits (Beck et al., 2019). Recognizing these nutritional complexities enables nurses to broker conversations with healthcare providers, teaching patients and families how to follow dietary guidelines while optimizing fluid and electrolyte balance, ultimately resulting in improved clinical outcomes and a greater quality of life for at-risk populations.

10.6.3. Self-Monitoring Techniques for Patients

Self-monitoring methods should be used by patients who are regulating their fluid, electrolyte, and acid-base balance, particularly in illnesses such as renal failure or during stem cell transplantation. Through active participation in self-monitoring, patients can better understand their health and make informed decisions about their management. Daily monitoring of intake and output of fluids, for example, enables patients to recognize any deviations from their intended regimen. This proactive strategy is essential, as excessive fluid retention or loss may result in serious complications, such as veno-occlusive disease (VOD), significantly affecting the outcome of survival after transplantation (Bambaci et al., 2016). In addition, self-monitoring promotes a sense of control among patients, increasing compliance with medical advice and allowing them to discuss concerning developments in their condition in a timely manner with healthcare professionals. Integrating mobile technology has further enhanced self-monitoring functions in patients, especially those undergoing treatments such as hemodialysis. Personalized mobile phone short message service systems provide patients with crucial diet-related information and assistance, enabling compliance with complex nutritional diets essential for maintaining fluid and electrolyte balance. The KIDNEYTEXT intervention, for instance, provides personalized messaging that supports both renal dietary advice and overall health guideline recommendations, encouraging improved lifestyle habits (Brown et al., 2019). Through the reinforcement of education with advanced technology, healthcare professionals can significantly enhance patient participation in their care. This combined effort not only encourages awareness but also bridges the gap between clinical advice and patients' everyday habits, ultimately leading to improved health outcomes. Optimal self-monitoring involves both comprehension and action based on feedback from one's health data. Patients must be taught to recognize signs of electrolyte imbalance, such as muscle weakness, fatigue, or altered mental status, which facilitates early intervention. Frequent consultation with healthcare providers is essential, as it enables adjustments to diet, medication, or fluid intake based on self-monitored data. Nursing practice is also an essential aspect in preparing patients for the skills and knowledge required for successful self-monitoring. An organized program, such as training sessions, coupled with follow-up evaluations, can make patients feel empowered and able to care for their health, thus reducing the occurrence of complications and improving the quality of life while they undergo the challenges of their medical conditions (Figure 10.19).

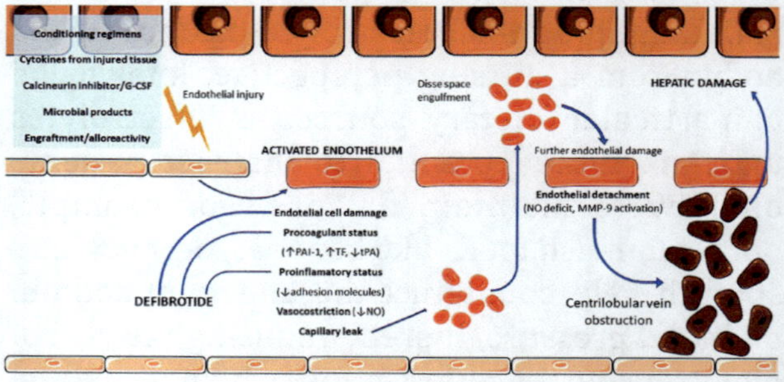

Figure 10.19. Diagnosis and treatment of veno-occlusive disease (VOD).

Source: https://www.frontiersin.org/files/Articles/495243/fimmu-11-00489-HTML/image_m/fimmu-11-00489-g001.jpg.

Test Your Knowledge

1. What are the most essential details nurses should inform patients about preventing fluid and electrolyte imbalance in the home setting?
2. How can nurses empower patients to monitor and manage their fluid and electrolyte status in chronic disease?

SUMMARY

The critical role that fluid, electrolyte, and acid-base balance plays in nursing practice, especially in the acute care environment. Given that imbalances in these regions have the potential to cause serious complications, nurses need to have a comprehensive knowledge of the physiological processes that regulate these balances. Many patients, particularly those in intensive care, will come with multifaceted histories and comorbidities that require careful evaluation and intervention. Through an understanding of the basic principles of fluid and electrolyte management, nurses can apply evidence-based interventions to ensure patient safety and optimal recovery outcomes. The application of systematic evaluations and timely interventions remains critical in reducing risks of imbalances, ultimately promoting improved quality of care in hospital environments. Additionally, the role of nursing interventions in managing fluid and electrolyte imbalances cannot be overstated. Proper nursing training and education on these aspects are paramount in developing a workforce that can handle the intricacies exhibited by patients. The results of several studies reveal that nursing interventions are not only comprehensive but also well-aligned with established clinical practices, thereby substantiating their relevance. In particular, the identification of commonly used interventions in intensive care units illustrates the complexity involved in upholding homeostasis. The association of nursing care prescriptions and the Nursing Interventions Classification (NIC) underscores nursing professionals' commitment to upholding standards that reflect the magnitude and complexity of patient needs, ultimately leading to enhanced health outcomes (Barros et al., 2010). In summary, the interaction between fluid, electrolyte, and acid-base balance requires an assertive and informed nursing practice. Through ongoing education and practice of clinical best practices, nurses can overcome challenges associated with patient care. Specifically, the occurrence of severe imbalances, as observed in morbidity-related studies involving humans and animals, underscores the importance of intensive monitoring and intervention measures (Epstein et al., 2015). As the practice of nursing evolves, placing these aspects at the forefront of nursing education and lifelong learning will guarantee an adequately prepared workforce able to meet the needs of contemporary healthcare settings. Ultimately, the future of nursing practice hinges on maintaining a steadfast commitment to these fundamental principles, thereby ensuring the safety of patients in critical care and beyond.

Within nursing practice, understanding the significance of fluid, electrolyte, and acid-base balance is crucial to providing proper patient care. This trio of measures affects physiological processes at all levels, particularly in susceptible patients, such as premature infants. Infants born before 29 weeks gestation risk neurocognitive disabilities that the nature of early nutritional intake and subsequent growth trends may significantly impact. In fact, failure to grow after birth has been attributed to poor nutrition, underscoring the importance for nurses to closely monitor and regulate fluid and electrolyte balance. A concern is that inadequate macronutrient intake may hinder optimal head growth velocity in these infants, which is crucial for their future neurodevelopmental status (Dinerstein et al., 2011). Therefore, providing proper nutrition to patients under close observation and supervision becomes crucial in nursing. Additionally, the role of nurses in detecting signs of fluid and electrolyte imbalance should not be overstated. Studies have shown that nurses with a checklist of possible symptoms report significantly better detection of such clinical signs than when no such resources are available. This highlights the need for ongoing education and the implementation of tools that enhance the observational skills of nursing staff. The inclusion of symptom lists or guidelines as part of nursing practice not only improves the identification of imbalances but also with more action taken on identifying these symptoms. By promoting a systematic process for symptom identification, nursing practice can enhance patient safety and improve outcomes (Walkingshaw et al., 2008). Preparation and knowledge play a crucial role in a nurse's ability to maintain balance, underscoring the importance of ongoing professional development. Finally, adequate fluid, electrolyte, and acid-base balance control in nursing practice requires a multifaceted solution that integrates both theory and applied skills. Evidence-based recommendations must be implemented to harmonize care practices and ensure that patients receive the right interventions. Furthermore, the evaluation and adjustment of parenteral nutrition protocols, as suggested by research, can significantly improve patient outcomes, especially for critically ill patients. Nurses' capacity to initiate well-formulated nutritional schedules might prevent some of the risks posed by inadequate dietary status and improper fluid balance. As nursing education moves forward, it is crucial to instill these ideas deeply into the curriculum, thus making future nurses focus on fluid and electrolyte balance as a foundation of patient care in their practice (Walkingshaw et al., 2008; Dinerstein et al., 2011).

KEY TERMS FROM THIS CHAPTER

- Acid-Base Balance
- Arterial Blood Gas (ABG) Analysis
- Bicarbonate (HCO_3^-)
- Calcium (Ca^{2+})
- Chloride (Cl^-)
- Diffusion
- Electrolytes
- Fluid Volume Deficit
- Fluid Volume Excess
- Homeostasis
- Hypervolemia
- Intravenous (IV) Fluid Therapy
- Magnesium (Mg^{2+})
- Metabolic Alkalosis
- Osmosis
- Respiratory Acidosis
- Sodium (Na^+)
- Potassium (K^+)

CRITICAL THINKING QUESTIONS

1. **Which electrolyte is most critical for cardiac function?**
   a. Sodium
   b. Potassium
   c. Calcium
   d. Chloride
2. **A patient with vomiting and diarrhea is at risk for which type of fluid imbalance?**
   a. Fluid overload
   b. Hypovolemia
   c. Hypernatremia
   d. Hypokalemia
3. **What is the normal pH range of arterial blood?**
   a. 6.8–7.0
   b. 7.35–7.45
   c. 7.50–7.60
   d. 7.25–7.30
4. **Which acid-base imbalance is associated with rapid, deep breathing (Kussmaul respirations)?**
   a. Metabolic alkalosis
   b. Respiratory alkalosis
   c. Metabolic acidosis
   d. Respiratory acidosis
5. **Which of the following signs is most characteristic of hyponatremia?**
   a. Hypertension and dry skin
   b. Confusion and muscle cramps
   c. Fever and tachycardia
   d. Increased thirst and dry mucous membranes

SHORT ANSWER QUESTIONS

1. What are two leading reasons for electrolyte imbalances in hospitalized patients?
2. Define hypokalemia and identify two frequent symptoms.
3. What is the role of the kidneys in acid-base balance?
4. Provide two indications of fluid volume deficit (dehydration).
5. What is the normal value for serum sodium and why is it significant?
6. Describe the process a nurse must follow when conducting an assessment of a patient for fluid and electrolyte imbalance.
7. Discuss causes, clinical presentation, and nursing management of hypernatremia.
8. Describe compensatory mechanisms of the body in response to metabolic acidosis.
9. Contrast and compare respiratory acidosis and respiratory alkalosis, such as causes and nursing interventions.
10. Outline the importance of fluid and electrolyte monitoring in elderly patients and those with chronic illnesses.

Answers to Critical Thinking Questions

1. (b) 2. (b) 3. (b) 4. (c) 5. (b)

REFERENCES

1. Ab Wahab, M. N. A. (2015). A pilot randomized controlled trial comparing the outcome of sustained low efficiency daily dialysis (SLEDD) with sustained low efficiency daily diafiltration (SLEDD-F) in critical care patients with acute kidney injury. https://core.ac.uk/download/154383245.pdf (accessed on 28th June 2025).
2. Mahgoub, A. A., Abdelhafez, N. G. E., & Abdelal, E. (2019). Effect of implementing total Parenteral Nutrition nursing guidelines on adult critically ill patients' outcomes. *Journal of Health Medicine and Nursing*. https://doi.org/10.7176/jhmn/61-04Adams, S., American Society for Parenteral and Enteral Nutrition, Ayers, P., Boullata, J., et al. (2014). A.S.P.E.N. parenteral nutrition safety consensus recommendations. https://core.ac.uk/download/62428919.pdf (accessed on 28th June 2025).
3. Andruskiw, O., & Battick, B. L. B. (1961). Identification of nursing problems of maintenance of oxygen supply and fluid and electrolyte balance. https://open.bu.edu/bitstream/2144/25622/1/Andruskiw_Olga_et_al_1961_web.pdf (accessed on 28th June 2025).
4. Bajantri, B., Diaz-Fuentes, G., & Venkatram, S. (2018). Fluids and sodium imbalance: Clinical implications. https://core.ac.uk/download/322438480.pdf (accessed on 28th June 2025).
5. Bambaci, M., Banfi, M., Bonifazi, F., BOTTI, G., et al. (2016). Veno-occlusive disease nurse management: Development of a dynamic monitoring tool by the GITMO nursing group. https://core.ac.uk/download/54013988.pdf (accessed on 28th June 2025).
6. Barros, A. L. B. L. de, Echer, I. C., Gutiérrez, M. G. R. de, Lucena, A. F., et al. (2010). Intervenções de enfermagem utilizadas na prática clínica de uma unidade de terapia intensiva. https://core.ac.uk/download/37709325.pdf (accessed on 28th June 2025).
7. Bartosiak, E., Czykieta, I., Jankowska-Polańska, B., & Tylak, K., et al. (2019). Patient with diabetic ketoacidosis. https://core.ac.uk/download/587243063.pdf (accessed on 28th June 2025).
8. Beck, A. M., Bischoff, S. C., Cederholm, T., Cruz-Jentoft, A. J., et al. (2019). *ESPEN Guideline on Clinical Nutrition and Hydration in Geriatrics*. https://core.ac.uk/download/159073557.pdf (accessed on 28th June 2025).
9. Berman, A., Dwyer, T., Erb, G. L., Hales, M., et al. (2015). *Kozier and Erb's Fundamentals of Nursing* [3rd Australian edition]. https://core.ac.uk/download/303778222.pdf (accessed on 28th June 2025).
10. Bhengu, B., Chironda, G., & Manwere, A. (2017). Adherence of adult chronic kidney disease patients with regard to their dialysis, medication, dietary and fluid restriction. https://core.ac.uk/download/478463593.pdf (accessed on 28th June 2025).
11. Brown, M., Campbell, K. L., Chow, C., Craig, J., et al. (2019). Targeted, structured text messaging to improve dietary and lifestyle behaviors for people on maintenance haemodialysis (KIDNEYTEXT): Study protocol for a randomized controlled trial. https://core.ac.uk/download/323229018.pdf (accessed on 28th June 2025).
12. Cafferty, P., Casagrand, J., Co, E., Flemming, J., et al. (2023). Creating the HAPS physiology learning outcomes: Terminology, eponyms, inclusive language, core concepts, and skills. https://core.ac.uk/download/590971416.pdf (accessed on 28th June 2025).

13. Camacho, A. C. L. F., da Silva, R. A. R., de Menezes, H. F., Ferreira, G. M., et al. (2021). Validez de diagnósticos de enfermería para personas en condiciones renales crónicas en tratamiento conservador. https://core.ac.uk/download/481367571.pdf (accessed on 28th June 2025).
14. Chandler, C., Connolly, S., Davies, C., Finn, G. M., et al. (2020). Designing and developing core physiology learning outcomes for pre-registration nursing education curriculum. https://core.ac.uk/download/520513595.pdf (accessed on 28th June 2025).
15. Dinerstein, A., Grover, A., Ogilvy-Stuart, A., Riskin, A., Dusick, A. M., Hart, A., Koletzko, B., et al. (2011). SCAMP: Standardized, concentrated, additional macronutrients, parenteral nutrition in very preterm infants: A phase IV randomized, controlled exploratory study of macronutrient intake, growth and other aspects of neonatal care. https://core.ac.uk/download/1557189.pdf (accessed on 28th June 2025).
16. Epstein, S. E., Hopper, K., & Ueda, Y. (2015). Incidence, severity and prognosis associated with hypernatremia in dogs and cats. https://core.ac.uk/download/323071592.pdf (accessed on 28th June 2025).
17. Fox, A. R. N., Ashby, D., Borman, N., Burton, J., et al. (2019). Renal Association Clinical Practice Guideline on haemodialysis. https://core.ac.uk/download/287582168.pdf (accessed on 28th June 2025).
18. Gort, S. (2020). Effectiveness of order sets in the management of diabetic ketoacidosis and hyperosmolar hyperglycemia. https://core.ac.uk/download/328112832.pdf (accessed on 28th June 2025).
19. Goswami, N. (2017). Falls and fall-prevention in older persons: Geriatrics meets spaceflight! *Frontiers in Physiology, 8*. https://doi.org/10.3389/fphys.2017.00603 (accessed on 28th June 2025).
20. Halvorsen, S., Mehilli, J., Cassese, S., Hall, T. S., et al. (2022). 2022 ESC guidelines on cardiovascular assessment and management of patients undergoing non-cardiac surgery. *European Heart Journal, 43*, 3826–3924. https://doi.org/10.1093/eurheartj/ehac270 (accessed on 28th June 2025).
21. Haworth, C., Banks, J., Capstick, T., Fisher, A. J., et al. (2017). British Thoracic Society guidelines for the management of non-tuberculous mycobacterial pulmonary disease (NTM-PD). *Thorax, 72*, ii1–ii64. https://doi.org/10.1136/thoraxjnl-2017-210927 (accessed on 28th June 2025).
22. Lacey, J., Corbett, J., Forni, L. G., Hooper, L., et al. (2019). A multidisciplinary consensus on dehydration: Definitions, diagnostic methods and clinical implications. *Annals of Medicine, 51*, 232–251. https://doi.org/10.1080/07853890.2019.1628352 (accessed on 28th June 2025).
23. Martha, S. R. (2019). Neurochemical factors associated with the initial pathophysiological reaction to large vessel occlusion stroke. https://core.ac.uk/download/232598167.pdf (accessed on 28th June 2025).
24. Miller, C. G. (2017). Dehydration in nursing home residents: A meta-analysis of causes of dehydration, implications, and those most at risk. https://core.ac.uk/download/84674618.pdf (accessed on 28th June 2025).
25. Perkins, G. D., Gräsner, J. T., Semeraro, F., Olasveengen, T. M., et al. (2021). European Resuscitation Council guidelines 2021: Executive summary. *Resuscitation, 161*, 1–60. https://doi.org/10.1016/j.resuscitation.2021.02.003 (accessed on 28th June 2025).

26. Quandt, M. (2022). Critical care nursing: A case study compilation and analysis. https://core.ac.uk/download/554922664.pdf (accessed on 28th June 2025).
27. Schneider, B. J., Naidoo, J., Santomasso, B., Lacchetti, C., et al. (2021). Management of immune-related adverse events in patients treated with immune checkpoint inhibitor therapy: ASCO guideline update. *Journal of Clinical Oncology, 39*, 4073–4126. https://doi.org/10.1200/jco.21.01440 (accessed on 28th June 2025).
28. Shepley, E. F. (2007). MS. https://core.ac.uk/download/276267856.pdf (accessed on 28th June 2025).
29. Sheyo, N. (2019). Changes in selected electrolytes in adult intensive care patients at the University Teaching Hospital, Lusaka, Zambia. https://core.ac.uk/download/618068766.pdf (accessed on 28th June 2025).
30. Walkingshaw, C. L. (2008). MS. https://core.ac.uk/download/276270396.pdf (accessed on 28th June 2025).
31. Zimmerman, A. D. (2011). Nursing interventions in the care of patients undergoing induced hypothermia. https://core.ac.uk/download/236291505.pdf (accessed on 28th June 2025).

SHOCK, SEPSIS, AND MULTIPLE ORGAN DYSFUNCTION SYNDROME IN NURSING

11

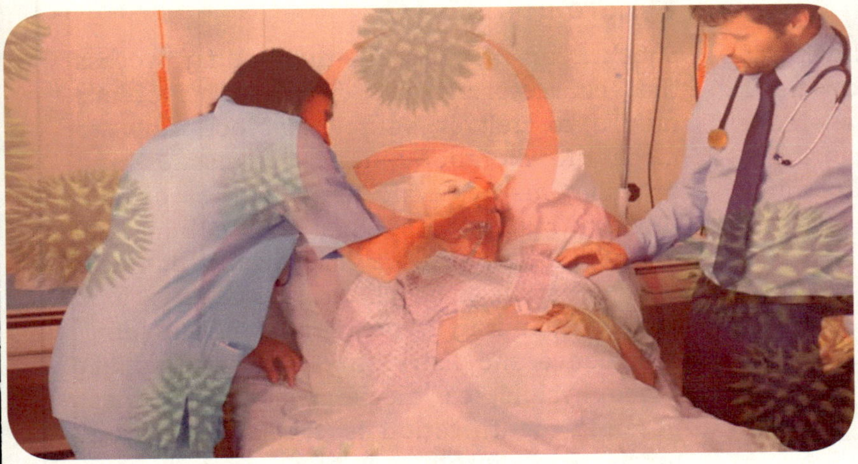

LEARNING OBJECTIVES

After studying this chapter, you will be able to:

1. Define the shock in nursing
2. Describe sepsis in nursing
3. Discuss the association between sepsis and shock
4. Highlight multiple organ dysfunction syndrome (MODS)
5. Understand nursing assessment and interventions
6. Assess the difficulties in nursing care

Introduction

The syndrome of shock, sepsis, and multiple organ dysfunction syndrome (MODS) is a complex nursing problem dominated by complex pathophysiological responses that require an intuitive understanding and timely management. Shock is essentially a state of inadequate tissue perfusion and oxygenation, which, if not addressed, can lead to the induction of sepsis—a systemic inflammatory response syndrome to infections that can result in disastrous organ failure. The frequency of such diseases highlights that early identification and treatment should be given, since mortality would very much escalate when these syndromes are left to follow their own course unchecked. Nursing professionals play a critical role in identifying early signs and implementing appropriate therapeutic interventions, an aspect that highlights the influence of clinical practice on outcomes in intensive care units. Sepsis and MODS can be caused by a wide range of precipitating factors, making them hard to diagnose and manage. For instance, postoperative morbidity, particularly that related to peritonitis, has been shown prospectively to increase morbidity and mortality in surgical patient populations. As per studies, patients who show signs of postoperative peritonitis usually exhibit mild local symptoms along with systemic complications such as respiratory failure and cardiovascular insufficiency that aggravate overall health status (Droniak et al., 2019). The multifaceted interaction among the operative variables and the body's reaction to sepsis necessitates nursing personnel to remain vigilant with regard to trends towards decline, as delayed treatment profoundly alters patient trajectories. A complicated knowledge of acute lung injury and acute respiratory distress syndrome (ARDS) likewise illustrates the necessity of nursing management of sepsis and MODS.

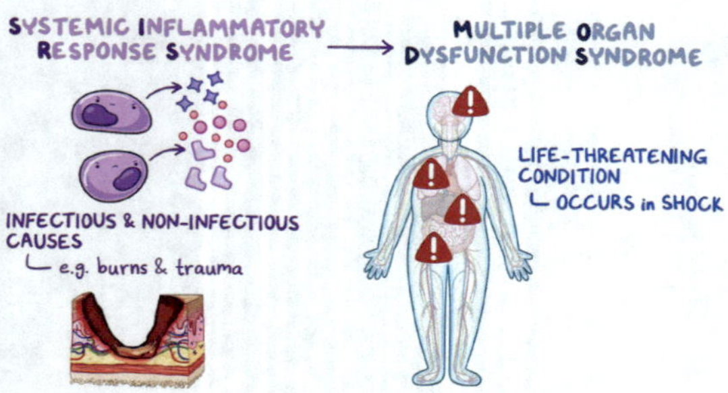

Figure 11.1. Multiple organ dysfunction syndrome (MODS).

Source: https://d16qt3wv6xm098.cloudfront.net/Ar165wAxTa_tJSrKME4j7OglQVSIRAql/_.jpg.

This information is essential when the diverse presentation and course of these conditions are considered. Literatures indicate that acute respiratory failure complicating ARDS can involve multiple organ systems and that there is a higher mortality that is proportional to the number of organs that have failed (Chimbira et al., 2001). This synergy leads to the value of holistic nursing practice, one that encompasses active monitoring, early intervention, and interprofessional collaboration to maximize patient outcomes. Through diligent assessment and implementation of sophisticated care methods, nurses can become a leading force in guiding recovery processes for patients with shock, sepsis, and MODS (Figure 11.1).

Definition of Shock, Sepsis, and Multiple Organ Dysfunction Syndrome (MODS)

Shock is an instantly life-threatening process that characterizes the circulatory system's failure to deliver sufficient blood flow to meet the metabolic needs of tissues and organs. This systemic deficiency of oxygen delivery results in cellular dysfunction and, if uncorrected, causes irreparable damage. Categorization of shock encompasses various forms, including hypovolemic, cardiogenic, obstructive, and distributive, each with distinct pathophysiological mechanisms. The earliest possible identification is crucial to prevent further complications, as these patients often present with significant physiological instability that can become life-threatening. It is an essential for clinicians, particularly nurses, to gain a comprehensive understanding of clinical signs of shock in order to facilitate timely interventions that promote patient recovery and prevent the risk of deterioration (Day et al., 2013). Sepsis, dangerous, hazardous, and potentially fatal consequence of infection, results when the body's reaction to infection creates a system of inflammation. This out-of-control response can also lead to MODS, where two or more organ systems fail, significantly increasing the mortality risk. Early detection of sepsis relies on recognizing clinical indicators, such as fever, tachycardia, and changes in mental status, which necessitate treatment. According to recent studies, early therapeutic interventions, including antibiotic administration and fluid resuscitation, are crucial in effectively treating sepsis. The severity of sepsis increases the necessity for nursing practitioners to gain experience with its progression and various scoring systems that seek to stratify its seriousness. CURB65 scoring, initially used in the assessment of pneumonia, can also provide valuable information when managing sepsis and is a good predictor of mortality in patients (Davey et al., 2014). MODS is the extreme state of a runaway systemic inflammatory response, typically following extreme sepsis or trauma. It is critically important for medical professionals, particularly nurses, to understand the interaction between MODS and sepsis, as clinical outcomes are influenced by the rapid assessment of the patient. MODS can occur through the sequential action of sepsis, with the result being rearranged blood circulation, tissue hypoxia, and secondary organ failure. Presentation clinically can be varied among patients, and the typical signs are respiratory compromise, hepatic dysfunction, and renal dysfunction. Since nurses are at the core of evaluating and caring for patients with MODS, their ability to recognize early signs of deteriorating function is crucial for initiating interventions aimed at re-establishing homeostasis. With the high mortality rate of MODS, integrating knowledge of its pathophysiology into nursing practice is essential to promote survival and the quality of care provided (Day et al., 2013) (Figure 11.2).

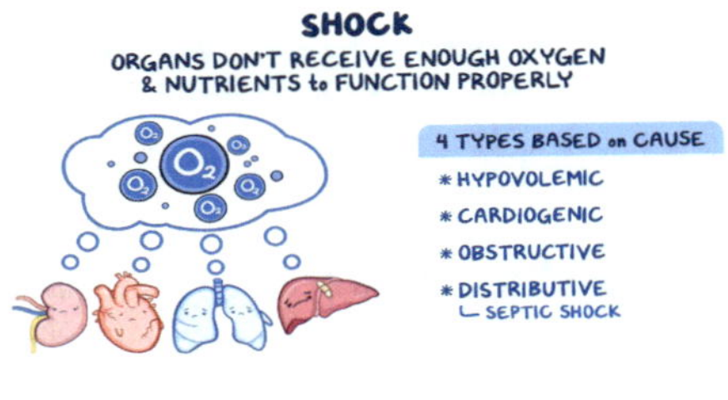

Figure 11.2. Shock.

Source: https://www.osmosis.org/_next/image?url=https%3A%2F%2Fd16qt3wv6xm098.cloudfront.net%2FMIxr4cLrSS6W99ynTOhl_d0ORyi7YM6F%2F_.jpg&w=3840&q=75.

Importance of Understanding These Conditions in Nursing

It is essential that nursing practitioners be aware of the complexities of shock, sepsis, and MODS due to the emergent character of these conditions for patient management. Nurses are often at the frontline of patient inspection and intervention, and their familiarity with the syndromes is therefore priceless. The ability to recognize early warning signs of shock or sepsis can have a life-changing effect on patient outcomes because timely intervention can reduce morbidity and mortality of these conditions. Furthermore, the addition of high-fidelity simulation (HFS) and reflection with guidance in nursing education, as discussed in research, points to the importance of equipping nurses with effective practical skills in the recognition and management of these life-threatening illnesses (Loving et al., 2010). Therefore, having a firm grasp of these concepts enables nurses to deliver evidence-based, timely care, ultimately enhancing the level of care provided in the acute environment. Additionally, the far-reaching consequences of shock, sepsis, and MODS extend far beyond the immediate clinical reaction, necessitating an extensive patient education plan and long-term recovery plan. Nursing professionals are not only asked to contend with the physiological aspects but also with the social and psychological aspects of patient care in such important health episodes. Nurses should be aware that conditions such as postoperative peritonitis could quickly deteriorate. Nurses must facilitate discussions with patients and their relatives about potential outcomes, therapy options, and rehabilitation processes (Droniak et al., 2019). Through establishing a comprehensive understanding of these conditions, nurses are better equipped to support patients throughout the complexities of treatment and recovery, as well as in navigating their healthcare needs. Such an interdisciplinary approach helps in reducing patients' and families' feelings of helplessness and anxiety during such difficult periods. The importance of a strong foundation in understanding shock, sepsis, and MODS necessitates ongoing education in nursing practice. Professional continued education in workshops, simulation, and interprofessional is expanding nurses' capacity to treat these conditions in a successful way as they are in a state of change. This dynamic knowledge is especially relevant considering new healthcare trends that need to incorporate new technology and treatment processes. With complication rates as high as they are for diseases like postoperative peritonitis, as evidenced by recent studies, it is imperative that nursing schools also prioritize improving accordingly (Droniak et al., 2019). By embracing a commitment to continued learning and a willingness to innovate, nurses can enhance their proficiency and ultimately be more responsible for achieving better patient outcomes and safety, thereby building a culture of excellence in nursing practice.

11.1. Understanding Shock

Learning Outcome

1. Describe the shock classification: hypovolemic, cardiogenic, distributive, and obstructive.
2. Highlight the pathophysiology of shock and the consequences it has on the body;
3. Learn clinical manifestations of shock.

Nursing experts need to understand shock as it is a significant part of sepsis and multiple organ dysfunction syndrome (MODS). Shock is the underperfusion of tissues that leads to cellular dysfunction and eventually organ failure. Various mechanisms will be responsible for shock, e.g., hypovolemic, cardiogenic, distributive, and obstructive. All shock categories necessitate individualized nursing care interventions to achieve hemodynamic stability. Hypovolemic shock, for instance, generally ensues after significant loss of fluid and thus needs immediate fluid resuscitation to counteract the deficit. Appreciation of the etiology of shock facilitates timely and effective intervention, subsequently leading to enhanced patient outcomes in critical care. The balance between shock and sepsis serves as a poignant reminder of the vital importance of early identification and management in critical care nursing. Sepsis, as a systemic inflammatory response to infection, can evolve into septic shock if it is not treated early. The inflammatory response manifests as widespread vasodilation and increased vascular permeability that exacerbates hypotension and tissue hypoperfusion.

As emphasized in the Surviving Sepsis Campaign, early treatment and aggressive resuscitation protocols have a catastrophic impact on the mortality of septic shock. Evidence-based standards are essential for nursing care, enabling patients to receive interventions and monitoring that effectively counteract the effects of sepsis and shock (Alhazzani et al., 2017). Nurses can forego care and plead on behalf of their patients without delay, being privy to these facts. Finally, MODS often arises as a complication of sepsis and shock and adds to the burden of healthcare providers. Local infection progressing to systemic dissemination may challenge the body's hemostatic capacity and organ function. Literature indicates that MODS patients have a significantly higher mortality rate; therefore, close monitoring and supportive care are recommended. For example, patients with acute respiratory distress syndrome (ARDS), which is a form of MODS, are characterized by a dramatic decline in survival rates, especially when combined with an increased rate of organ failure (Chimbira et al., 2001). Understanding the interaction between shock, sepsis, and MODS is an essential part of nursing professionals ' practice because it is the foundation for taking proactive management strategies in order to reverse the severe effects of these interrelated clinical conditions (Figure 11.3).

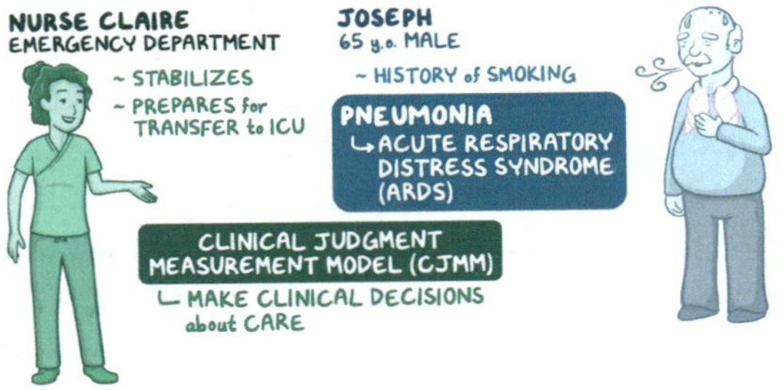

Figure 11.3. Acute respiratory distress syndrome (ARDS).

Source: https://www.osmosis.org/_next/image?url=https%3A%2F%2Fd16qt3wv6xm098.cloudfront.net%2FCSwj-J7iShmCbooXx0kI8gHPT8GlnK4n%2F_.jpg&w=3840&q=75.

11.1.1. Types of Shock: Hypovolemic, Cardiogenic, Distributive, and Obstructive

The mechanism of shock is multifactorial and can be categorized into several distinct types, each with its own diverse pathophysiological mechanisms. Hypovolemic shock is most broadly characterized by the acute reduction in circulating blood volume, typically resulting from trauma, hemorrhage, or severe dehydration.

This condition leads to inadequate perfusion of the vital organs and can cause pronounced and instantaneous effects if not addressed promptly. Clinical evidence implicates hypovolemic shock in a large proportion of pediatric emergency admissions, accounting for approximately 41.97% of the reported cases in research comparing pediatric shocks (Vijayamohan et al., 2011). Effective identification and immediate fluid resuscitation are key elements of nursing care that aim to counteract hypovolemic shock, emphasizing the nurse's role in early action. Cardiogenic shock, on the other hand, arises when the heart fails to circulate blood efficiently, due either to myocardial infarction or acute heart failure. Cardiac output falls short, leading to compromised tissue perfusion and multi-organ failure.

In pediatric patients, cardiogenic shock can be precipitated by congenital heart abnormalities or myocarditis, highlighting the diverse etiologies of cardiogenic shock. Evidence in the recent past has shown that death due to cardiogenic shock may reach up to 31.0%, with powerful implications for nursing care planning and intervention decision-making (Nisha et al., 2018). Close hemodynamic monitoring and the use of supportive measures, such as inotropic agents, are essential for nursing personnel to render the involved patients stable. The unique nature of cardiogenic shock requires individualized nursing assessments for cardiac stability and organ function. Distributive shock encompasses a range of conditions characterized by abnormal vasodilation, resulting in relative hypovolemia despite normal or increased overall blood volume.

Septic shock is one such category that is most commonly triggered by severe infections that result in systemic inflammatory response syndromes. Distributive shock presents unique challenges to nursing staff since, in addition to quick diagnosis, it also requires effective control of fluid resuscitation and, if necessary, vasopressor therapy. Recent studies emphasize the fact that septic shock represents an eminent segment of the causes of shock, with mortality being as high as 66.7% as reflected through the studies on pediatric patients (Nisha et al., 2018). This highlights the importance of treating septic shock early to avoid the development of multi-organ dysfunction syndrome. Nurses play a central role in observing the subtle nuances of distributive shock and integrating cross-disciplinary treatment to optimize patient outcomes, cementing their core position on the healthcare team (Figure 11.4).

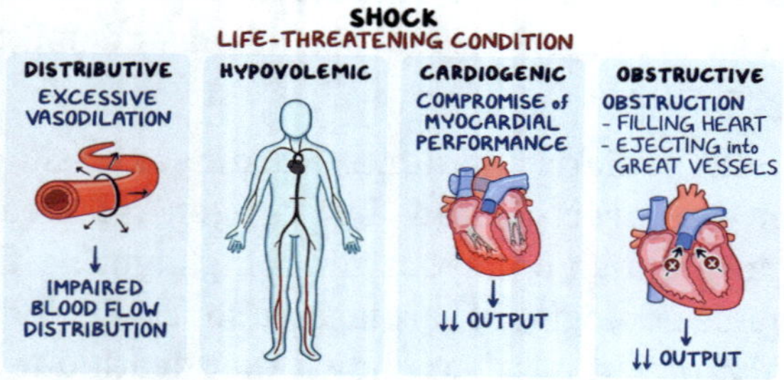

Figure 11.4. Types of shock.

Source: https://d16qt3wv6xm098.cloudfront.net/34saqA2CSvaePIbD9wjgxSMlRqCLD8M0/_.jpg.

11.1.2. Pathophysiology of Shock and Its Effects on the Body

The pathophysiology of shock is a complex interplay between body responses initiated as a consequence of impaired perfusion of organs and tissues, leading to cellular impairment. Various reasons, including hypovolemia, cardiogenic failure, or vasodilation secondary to overwhelming infections may trigger this state. The initial response of the body is to compensate for deficient blood flow through mechanisms such as tachycardia and peripheral vasoconstriction. If homeostasis is not preserved, compensatory mechanisms are overwhelmed, and tissue hypoxia and metabolic acidosis ensue. This progresses to the development of MODS, where vital organs such as the kidneys, liver, and lungs fail more and more, significantly enhancing patient morbidity and mortality in clinical situations. In shock, the systemic inflammatory response syndrome (SIRS) is of particular importance because it often reflects the progression from compensatory mechanisms to overt shock. Research indicates that the trend in clinical parameters of SIRS, such as temperature, respiratory rate, and heart rate, is crucial in identifying the onset of sepsis and its subsequent consequences. The study emphasized that the increase in these parameters post-surgery may indicate an early inflammatory process that requires careful monitoring. Early diagnosis and management of potential sepsis in patients, especially those undergoing high-risk interventions, are essential since they can influence outcomes, such as prolonged hospital stays and high mortality rates, as determined in research settings such as the one at the Haukeland University hospital (Eriksson et al., 2016).

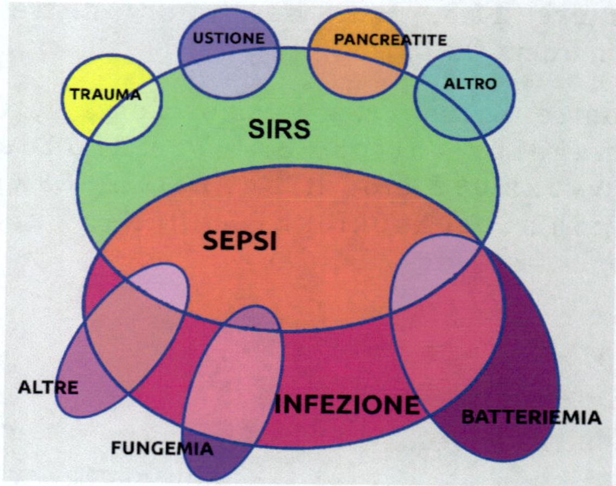

Figure 11.5. Systemic inflammatory response syndrome.

Source: https://upload.wikimedia.org/wikipedia/commons/thumb/c/cf/Sepsi-SIRS.png/1200px-Sepsi-SIRS.png.

Moreover, the presence of comorbid diseases, such as diabetes mellitus, complicates the pathophysiology of shock. Diabetic patients have a higher risk of developing acute illness, and this can lead to sudden increases in blood glucose levels, making sepsis and shock treatment procedures more complex. Increased blood glucose levels are associated with higher mortality and hospitalization rates. Evidence underlines the importance of glucose control in the blood in order to improve outcomes in septic patients, and this is also consonant with the Surviving Sepsis Campaign's recommendations in keeping levels below 180 mg/dl across diabetic or nondiabetic patients (Cardoso et al., 2016). The fundamental knowledge of such pathophysiologic relationships will support nursing personnel in employing evidence-based practices to early detect and intervene in shock, facilitating improved patient outcomes (Figure 11.5).

11.1.3. Clinical Signs and Symptoms of Shock

Clinical symptoms and signs of shock are essential indicators that need immediate identification and management in nursing. Some of the common presentations include hypotension, tachycardia, and tachypnea, which can be variable in severity depending on the cause of shock. For instance, during hypovolemic shock, reduced cardiac output results from blood loss, leading to ensuing hypotension, a consistent sign of reduced tissue perfusion. Compensatory tachycardia often accompanies hypotension as the body's attempt to counteract reduced blood volume through increased cardiac output. In addition, altered mental status may also ensue, manifesting as a lack of adequate cerebral perfusion. Early detection of these signs is essential, as they not only facilitate diagnosis of the cause of shock but also inform proper nursing measures that can arrest further deterioration of the patient's status. At advanced stages of shock, other clinical features may emerge, underscoring the importance of close monitoring. Such patients may exhibit evidence of tissue hypoxia, such as cyanosis or pallor, indicating a lack of adequate delivery of oxygen to peripheral tissues. Moreover, the skin assessment can produce cool, wet extremities due to vasoconstriction since the body redistributes the blood flow to the core organs. Vital signs also play a critical role in assessing shock states; for example, increased breathing rates can present as the body attempts to compensate for metabolic acidosis, which is caused by inadequate oxygenation. Observation of these presentations in the clinic is crucial, as they provide key clues to medical personnel about the patient's hemodynamic status and overall prognosis. Clinical vigilance is especially vital in cases of shock coinciding with sepsis, where other signs, such as fever and flushing, may exacerbate the clinical presentation. The interactions between shock and MODS introduce complexities in the clinical presentation. Shock is often a precursor to MODS, as inadequate perfusion can lead to cell injury and organ failure. Signs of MODS may evolve stepwise in an orderly manner, beginning with mild dysfunction of one organ system and eventually extending to multiple systems, and leading to a cascade of signs, making diagnosis and treatment more complex. For instance, renal failure can present as oliguria or anuria, while liver dysfunction can lead to jaundice and coagulopathy. In the field of nursing, understanding the changes is highly essential; timely detection of such trends can inform interventions and improve patient outcomes. Last but not least, clinical presentations of shock provide a critical reference guide for nursing assessments, underscoring the need for regular education and sensitivity in managing such life-threatening conditions effectively (Day et al., 2013; Droniak et al., 2019).

Test Your Knowledge

1. What are the early signs and symptoms of shock that can be instantly identified by nurses?
2. How is nursing care associated with the pathophysiology of different types of shock?

11.2. Sepsis: An Overview

Learning Outcome

1. Explain sepsis classification
2. Define risk factors and high-risk populations in sepsis
3. Explain the immune response in sepsis

Sepsis is a severe and potentially fatal condition that results from the body's response to an infection, causing a systemic inflammatory response. A systemic inflammatory response can trigger various physiological changes, including alterations in blood flow, inflammatory marker levels, and organ function. Innate immune response, though vital in defense against infections, can go awry, leading to a chain reaction that can lead to septic shock and MODS. The clinical course of sepsis is very inconstant, typically beginning with specific nonspecific findings, including fever, tachycardia, and altered mental status. Early detection of these findings is of utmost importance for proper treatment because delayed detection can significantly increase morbidity and mortality due to sepsis. Sepsis is managed in a multi-component fashion in a clinical setting, depending on early diagnosis and early therapy. This typically involves the use of the Surviving Sepsis Campaign guidelines, which focus on early fluid resuscitation, prompt administration of broad-spectrum antibiotics, and regular measurement of vital signs. Particularly, nursing care makes a great contribution to the early detection of sepsis through thorough assessment and the utilization of standardized screening tools. Additionally, the use of technology, specifically high-fidelity simulation (HFS), has been demonstrated to enhance the clinical judgment of nursing students in managing critical cases by facilitating reflective learning through live debriefing and review of simulated clinical cases that replicate sepsis management (Loving et al., 2010). Although there has been some advancement in sepsis care, postoperative peritonitis (PP) shows the challenge healthcare practitioners still face. Studies have shown a high mortality rate with PP, particularly for patients having abdominal surgery, where risk factors are the systemic inflammatory pathways that lead to cardiovascular and respiratory collapse (Droniak et al., 2019). In addition, managing the problems of sepsis thus entails not only early detection and therapy but also careful postoperative monitoring to prevent risks of secondary infection and organ failure. Overall, the interplay between prompt nursing interventions and the advanced understanding of sepsis pathophysiology provides the basis for improving patient outcomes in critical care settings (Figure 11.6).

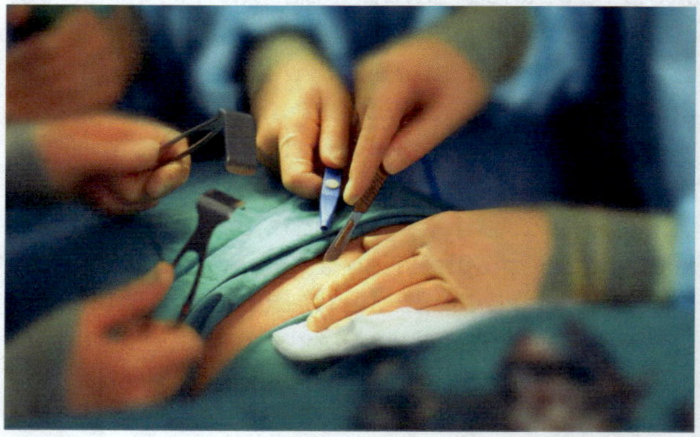

Figure 11.6. Septic shock: Causes, signs, and diagnosis.

Source: https://www.verywellhealth.com/thmb/9ftpxMTNhZSOf9E4EiSru7AMlVc=/1500x0/filters:no_upscale():max_bytes(150000):strip_icc()/stk16511hsd-56a912605f9b58b7d0f7da97.JPG.

11.2.1. Definition and Classification of Sepsis

Understanding the definition and classification of sepsis is crucial in nursing practice, as its impact on patient outcomes is particularly far-reaching. Sepsis is a condition characterized by organ dysfunction resulting from a dysregulated host response to infection. The illness is heterogeneous and therefore presents with significant variability in clinical presentation and course. Classification of sepsis is essential for effective diagnosis and management, as it informs clinical decision-making. The most widely used classification system categorizes sepsis into three categories: sepsis, severe sepsis, and septic shock. These stages are a continuum, with sepsis being a body-wide response to infection, severe sepsis being organ dysfunction, and septic shock being persistent hypotension and a high likelihood of mortality. Nursing staff should be able to understand these stages in assessing and managing critically ill patients with sepsis. Due to advancements in medical technology and machine learning algorithms over the last few years, it is now possible to diagnose and manage sepsis more effectively. For instance, a randomized controlled trial revealed that the application of a sepsis prediction system utilizing machine learning resulted in a significantly shorter average length of hospital stay and lower in-hospital mortality rates. The study found that the application of predictive systems helped healthcare teams implement the right interventions and improve patient outcomes, resulting in a statistically significant decrease in mortality compared to traditional monitoring. These gains underscore the importance of integrating technology into nursing interventions with an emphasis on greater education and training for nurses in the management of sepsis. This innovation not only enables early detection but also empowers nursing professionals to respond effectively to evolving sepsis challenges (Barton et al., 2017). In addition, the public health importance of sepsis necessitates proper knowledge of its prevalence and risk factors, including the distinction between hospital-acquired and community-onset forms. The heterogeneity of sepsis presents challenges that require rigorous research to elucidate its epidemiology and etiology. A systematic review on this topic would assess current studies to elucidate the salient factors contributing to the two types of sepsis, thereby informing healthcare policies and clinical practice guidelines. With a comprehensive understanding of risk factors, nurse practitioners can effectively contribute to public health measures aimed at early detection and prevention. By promoting sepsis awareness in the general public and correcting early diagnosis, the nurses can play a key role in reducing the incidence and associated health burden of sepsis (McCarthy et al., 2015).

11.2.2. Risk Factors and Populations at Higher Risk

When in shock, sepsis, or MODS, it is essential to identify the risk factors in order to manage and treat patients efficiently. Age is also a significant risk factor, particularly in older individuals, who have a significantly higher risk of mortality following sepsis. According to statistics, patients over the age of 80 years have an odds ratio for increased mortality over patients younger than 60 years of 5.79, demonstrating the vulnerability of this group. Besides age, emergency admissions have also had three times the risk of death, which underlines the need for early diagnosis and management of sepsis. The above statistics underscore the significance of healthcare professionals adopting intensive assessment strategies, particularly in emergency care units, where timely management can significantly impact patient outcomes in the event of sepsis, as well as the onset of MODS (Davey et al., 2014). Additionally, the ward a patient is in may also be linked to whether they will experience sepsis and complications. According to studies, patients in surgical or orthopedic wards have lower mortality rates compared to those in medical wards, presenting an interesting challenge for healthcare planners. This disparity may be attributed to variations in the underlying health conditions, the complexity of surgical procedures, or the level of care and monitoring. For instance, patients in elective procedure wards can have a heterogeneous risk profile compared to their acute medical emergency peers. As these ward amenities play a significant role in determining patient outcomes, doctors and nurses should be keenly aware of how sepsis care is influenced by environmental determinants and ensure that adequate support and resources are proportionately aligned (Davey et al., 2014). In infants and children, some pathological conditions critically escalate the risk of ARDS and acute lung injury (ALI) and complicate management further in vulnerable populations. Incidence of ALI and ARDS may be quite variable, with mortality reaching as high as 90%. In one study, for example, of an 85 population of pediatric patients that were being investigated, there was a staggering 14.3% mortality among those who developed ARDS, marking the severity of these conditions. Moreover, the median number of organs that failed in non-survivors was significantly higher, suggesting a direct correlation between the failure of multiple organs and death rates among pediatric sepsis. Nursing practitioners should be aware of these dynamics, particularly those related to respiratory failure and prognosis, as timely interventions can significantly impact the outcome for this high-risk population (Figure 11.7).

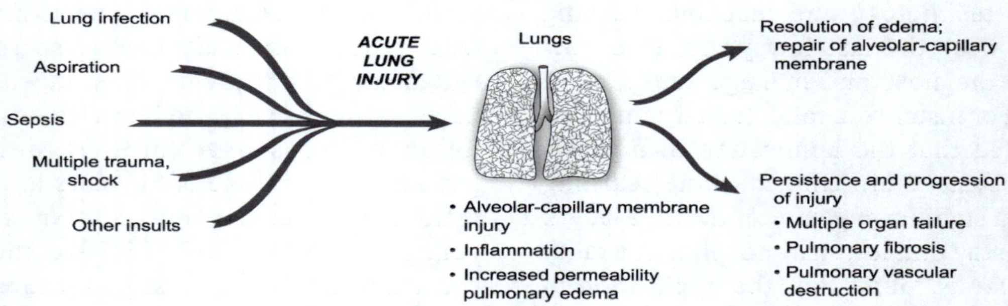

Figure 11.7. Acute lung injury (ALI).

Source: https://www.liebertpub.com/cms/10.1089/jamp.2009.0775/asset/images/large/figure2.jpeg.

11.2.3. The Role of the Immune Response in Sepsis

The immune response is a key player in sepsis pathophysiology, a double-edged sword in the battle to clear infection, but also causing extensive tissue damage. In sepsis, the host immune system reacts to infection by generating pro-inflammatory cytokines and mediators that attempt to kill the invading organisms. However, an unchecked and overexaggerated immune response can result in systemic inflammation, which subsequently leads to MODS. This is a constant equilibrium between and adequate clearance of pathogens and protection against overwhelming the inflammatory response, since the latter could enhance morbidity and mortality among the respective patients, whereas the former guards the body against infection. This immunoreactive response dynamics is necessary in guiding nursing practice towards better sepsis and complication management. Among the various pathways involved in sepsis, the concept of SIRS is a crucial clinical determinant for early identification. Assessment of key parameters such as respiratory rate, heart rate, body temperature, and C-reactive protein (CRP) level provides valuable information on the development of inflammatory processes. Research has established that the trend of these clinical markers can predict the onset of postoperative sepsis, particularly in high-risk surgical patients (Eriksson et al., 2016). By recognizing these parameters as indicators of immune system dysregulation, nurses can implement early interventions to mitigate the risk of sepsis, ultimately promoting improved patient outcomes. Therefore, a nuanced understanding of the immune response and careful monitoring of critical signs vastly enhance sepsis diagnosis and management in clinical practice. Interactions between the immune response and outcomes in sepsis are also evident in how inflammatory mediators influence the recovery process. The study of trauma patients has demonstrated that severe trauma results in elevated levels of inflammatory markers that may predict adverse outcomes, including prolonged intensive care unit stay and greater MOD scores (Abboud et al., 2019). The findings suggest the importance of an adaptive immune response, where well-controlled inflammation facilitates healing. In contrast, uncontrolled inflammation exacerbates tissue injury and prolongs the recovery process. In practice within nursing, recognition and knowledge of the components of the immune response not only aid in monitoring the course of sepsis but also direct treatment modalities that can make recovery for the patient possible. By applying this understanding in practice, nurses play a central role in caring for sepsis and mitigating its potentially disastrous impact.

Test Your Knowledge

1. What are the most significant clinical determinants in sepsis recognition in a patient?
2. Why is early detection and intervention critical in the management of sepsis?

11.3. The Connection between Sepsis and Shock

Learning Outcome

1. Explain how sepsis leads to numerous forms of shock
2. Define sepsis to the progression of septic shock
3. Explain the clinical significance to nursing practice

The relationship between shock and sepsis is complicated and needs to be understood in nursing care. Sepsis is a severe disease resulting from the host's response to infection, leading to a systemic inflammatory response and potential organ dysfunction. The inflammation can extend to septic shock, characterized by profound hypotension and impaired tissue perfusion despite fluid resuscitation. Sepsis that progresses to shock impairs the body's critical organs, which increases the risk of MODS. As circulating inflammatory mediators accumulate, they become potent enough to overcome the body's compensation mechanisms and generate an expanding gap between oxygen supply and demand. This evolution must be closely monitored and early identified by nurses to determine the transition from sepsis into shock, thereby decreasing morbidity and mortality rates for these lethal processes. Familiarity with the pathophysiology of septic shock is a prerequisite to effective nursing intervention. Septic shock results when sepsis causes intense vasodilation and heightened vascular permeability, which decreases blood pressure and can cause organ failure. Clinical presentations can range from altered mental status to tachycardia and an elevated lactate level, both of which can suggest poor perfusion. As described in the present literature, various organ support therapies, such as renal replacement therapy and methods of blood purification, have been used more and more frequently in patients with sepsis for the management of organ dysfunction. Sound fluid management and the prompt administration of vasopressors are necessary nursing measures that can reverse the fatal effects of shock. Interdisciplinary approaches, with emphasis on the focal role of nursing in the early identification and timely intervention, are paramount in the improvement of patients with sepsis and shock outcomes. Additionally, the link between septic shock and multiple organ dysfunction highlights the need for intensive nursing monitoring and intervention strategies. The evolution of MODS in patients with sepsis happens more quickly as the case progresses to shock, making the clinical picture even more complex. The data indicate that the severity of organ failure correlates with the overall mortality of the patient in sepsis, and, hence, early detection and treatment are vital components of nursing interventions. Nurses must have an excellent understanding of the physiological changes that occur during septic shock and their consequences on respiratory and cardiovascular functions. In particular, the management of acute lung injury in septic shock is one example of specialized nursing treatment, which has been supported by studies that reported a high level of failure among non-survivors in ventilation interventions. Active nursing intervention will make a significant difference in the progression of sepsis and shock, resulting in better patient outcomes (Chimbira et al., 2001; Bagshaw et al., 2016) (Figure 11.8).

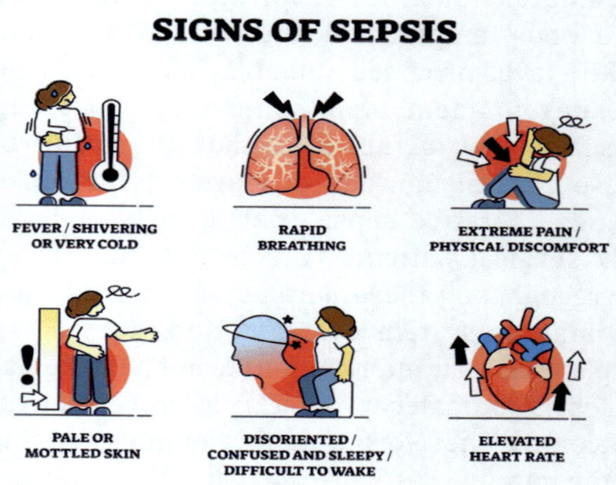

Figure 11.8. Sepsis symptoms and treatment.

Source: https://www.homed.gr/wp-content/uploads/SIGNS-OF-SEPSIS-TREATMEANTS-DIAGNOSIS-DOCTORS-EXPERTS-HOMED-1-1.jpg.

11.3.1. How Sepsis Leads to Different Types of Shock

It is essential to understand how sepsis leads to different forms of shock in order to provide effective nursing care, as this brings to the nurse's attention the most significant pathophysiological changes occurring in the body. Sepsis, being a systemic inflammatory response to infection, essentially interferes with hemodynamic stability and can lead to different forms of shock, particularly septic shock, hypovolemic shock, and cardiogenic shock. In septic shock, the inflammatory mediator release systemically provokes vasodilation in the vascular bed, compromising systemic vascular resistance and adequate perfusion. Vascular tone abnormality results in underperfusion, leading eventually to tissue ischemia and organ dysfunction. The severity of sepsis determines the course leading to shock, underscoring the importance of early detection and intervention in optimizing patient outcomes (Loving et al., 2010). In addition to septic shock, the progression of sepsis is also potentially accountable for cardiogenic and hypovolemic shock. Hypovolemic shock can result as a secondary consequence of fluid loss due to capillary leak in the context of severe sepsis. Interstitial migration of fluid creates relative hypovolemia, resulting in impaired circulating blood volume and, consequently, reduced cardiac output. Maintaining adequate fluid status in these patients becomes crucial, highlighting the importance of judicious fluid resuscitation in clinical practice. In contrast, cardiogenic shock in septic patients occurs through myocardial depression secondary to the pathologic levels of circulating cytokines. This shift in cardiac contractility has the potential to cause severe reductions in blood pressure and organ perfusion, necessitating a stepwise system of monitoring and treatment in the critical care environment (Day et al., 2013). The complexity of how sepsis can translate into all types of shock reflects the importance of having nursing staff fully understand the mechanisms behind such events. Early identification of the kind of shock is crucial, as each type requires distinct therapeutic interventions. For instance, septic shock patients need aggressive fluid resuscitation and vasopressor therapy, while cardiogenic shock patients may need inotropic therapy for enhanced cardiac output. Moreover, the potential shift from sepsis to shock may also result in MODS, making patient management more challenging. The detection of initial signs of sepsis and the use of evidence-based practice are extremely important for nursing professionals to prevent shock and MODS development, thereby improving patients' prognoses in this pathophysiological care environment (Loving et al., 2010).

11.3.2. The Progression from Sepsis to Septic Shock

The progression of sepsis to septic shock is a critical problem within the nursing practice, which is a crucial escalation of the severity of a patient's condition. Sepsis tends to arise as a response to infection that causes a systemic inflammatory reaction that can result in severe impairment of organs. If sepsis is not quickly identified and treated, the compensatory mechanisms of the body give way to septic shock, where hypotension and inadequate perfusion to end organs are observed despite adequate fluid resuscitation. According to available literature, sepsis occurs frequently among hospitalized patients and is frequently the proximate cause of death, emphasizing awareness of this pathway in clinical settings (Anderson et al., 2019). Nurses play a crucial role in monitoring signs of deterioration, as timely action significantly impacts patient outcomes. With septic shock, resultant circulatory collapse leads to further dysregulation of metabolic activities and oxygen delivery, ultimately to MODS. The condition generally develops through overt clinical presentation by means of altered mentation, renal insufficiency, and respiratory distress. It has been proven that optimal sepsis management leads to reduced hospitalizations and in-hospital mortality (Barton et al., 2017). Therefore, not only does nursing intervention target immediate treatment, but it also focuses on ongoing assessment and execution of the sepsis protocol. Effective nursing practice requires vigilance and evidence-based practice adherence to prevent the sepsis-to-septic shock transition to enable timely intervention that improves prognoses in this high-risk population of patients. The importance of sepsis to septic shock transition is not limited to single-patient outcomes but has significant implications for healthcare systems generally. As a leading cause of in-hospital mortality, sepsis puts enormous resource burdens on healthcare facilities, calling for effective models of care that focus on rapid identification and treatment. Nurses can facilitate prevention and early intervention by understanding the pathophysiological changes that occur during this progression. Additionally, fostering interprofessional collaboration among healthcare providers can help enhance the efficacy of sepsis management guidelines and improve patient outcomes. As hospital settings become increasingly inclined towards employing machine learning algorithms and predictive monitoring systems, the future for nursing will further expand its scope, putting nurses at the forefront of reducing sepsis morbidity and mortality in practice (Barton et al., 2017) (Figure 11.9).

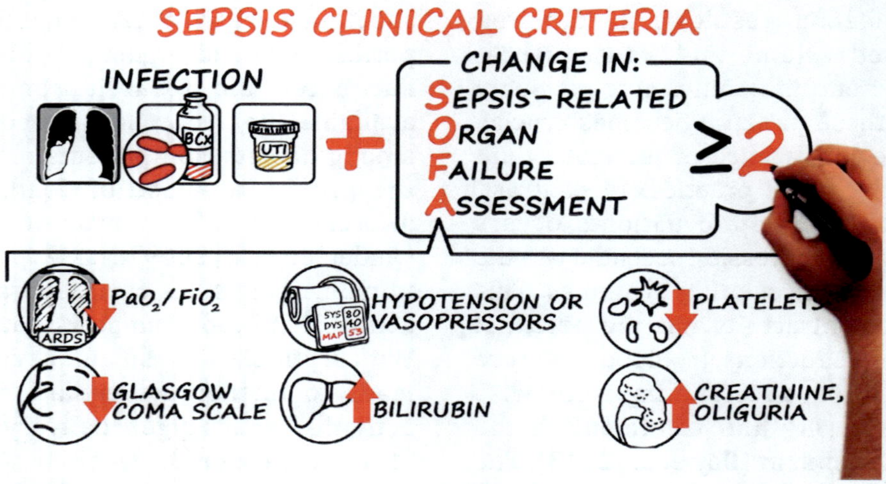

Figure 11.9. Progression from sepsis to septic shock.

Source: https://i.pinimg.com/originals/c1/b4/f6/c1b4f6cd1cfb1a0646579f163fb62f82.jpg.

11.3.3. Clinical Implications for Nursing Practice

The nursing role in the management of shock, sepsis, and MODS is multifaceted and critically important to patient outcomes. Nurses are often the initial responders and typically have the greatest contact with patients in critical care settings, making them critical to the early detection of sepsis and associated syndromes. Recognition of subtle alterations in patient status, such as changes in vital signs or alterations in mental status, enables nurses to initiate protocols for rapid assessment that can lead to timely interventions. The implications for nursing practice include the administration of therapeutic measures according to established guidelines, such as those outlined in the Surviving Sepsis Campaign, with aggressive resuscitation and protocol-driven care (Conboy et al., 1995). Thus, ongoing training and education in identifying and managing sepsis are critical components for enhancing nursing practice and ultimately maximizing patient survival. Nurses also need to ensure effective interdisciplinary communication in case of sepsis and MODS. The nature of working under these conditions necessitates a cooperative effort among healthcare professionals, including physicians, pharmacists, and respiratory therapists. Nurses play a critical role in bridging the communication gap and ensuring that significant updates related to patient status are conveyed in a timely and effective manner. In addition to that, involvement in multidisciplinary rounds allows nurses to present their observations on patients and possibly influence clinical decisions. Such practice in teamwork ensures an integrative approach that is consonant with evidence-based guidelines, reaffirming the significance of the nurse's role as a component member of the health team in the management of shock and sepsis patients (Conboy et al., 1995). Facilitation of such collaborative practices directly impacts the quality of patient care provided to patients with life-threatening diseases. Patient education is also a vital aspect of nursing practice when handling shock, sepsis, and MODS. Nurses are responsible for communicating important information to patients and their families, thereby closing the gap between patient understanding and clinical knowledge. This involves describing what sepsis is, why it is critical to follow through with treatment schedules, and alerting patients to symptoms that indicate an immediate need for medical intervention. Providing this education empowers patients and families, while also building adherence to follow-through care, which is paramount in preventing recurrence and complications. Furthermore, incorporating evidence-based practices within educational programs further emphasizes the significance of proactive care. Through involvement in patient and family education, nurses play a crucial role in ensuring that treatment extends beyond the hospital into the home and community, thereby establishing a continuum of care that promotes recovery and reduces the risks of sepsis and MODS (Alhazzani et al., 2017).

Test Your Knowledge

1. How does septic shock evolve from sepsis, and what are the pathophysiologic changes on which it depends?
2. What are the highest-priority nursing needs for the care of a patient with sepsis evolving to septic shock?

11.4. Multiple Organ Dysfunction Syndrome (MODS)

Learning Outcome

1. Identify the diagnostic criteria for MODS
2. Define the typical organs of MODS
3. Describe the pathophysiological mechanisms of MODS

MODS is a highly challenging condition to modern medical practice, typically presenting as a consequence of one of numerous types of severe insult such as shock and sepsis. Clinically, the condition is characterized by the sequential failure of two or more organ systems, which necessitates interventions early enough to prevent further decline and mortality. Pathophysiologic processes in MODS are multifactorial, involving systemic inflammation, microbial translocation, and metabolic changes that amplify organ dysfunction. It is also notable that early diagnosis and treatment remain essential for optimal patient outcomes. Since nurses are typically the first point of contact in patient care, their ability to detect the prodrome of MODS significantly influences treatment protocols and subsequent recovery rates among critically ill patients. The interaction between MODS and sepsis is particularly fascinating, as sepsis is often a precipitating cause for multi-organ failure to follow. Literature indicates that the septic patient may develop many complications, such as cardiovascular, respiratory, and renal instability, all the characteristics of MODS (Loving et al., 2010). Recent studies confirm that enhanced inflammatory reactions and the subsequent release of pro-inflammatory cytokines can lead to a cascade effect, destabilizing hemodynamics and tissue oxygenation supply. Thus, sepsis can be effectively treated at the outset by appropriate nursing interventions. Early diagnosis and management interventions, such as fluid resuscitation and antibiotic treatment, can halt the progression towards MODS and improve the patient's overall prognosis. Nursing care for MODS patients involves a comprehensive approach that incorporates continuous observation, patient education, and multidisciplinary collaboration. Nurses play an essentialrole in the implementation of evidence-based practices, which helps reduce the risk of organ dysfunction. For instance, placing more emphasis on fluid management and early assessment can aid in detecting alterations in organ function (Droniak et al., 2019). Moreover, high-fidelity simulation training allows nursing staff to practice critical thinking and clinical judgment abilities under simulated conditions. It not only prepares them for actual clinical issues but also gives a solid foundation for rendering quality patient care in complex cases of MODS. The integration of advanced nursing techniques is necessary to achieve optimal results in patients experiencing the widespread consequences of MODS (Figure 11.10).

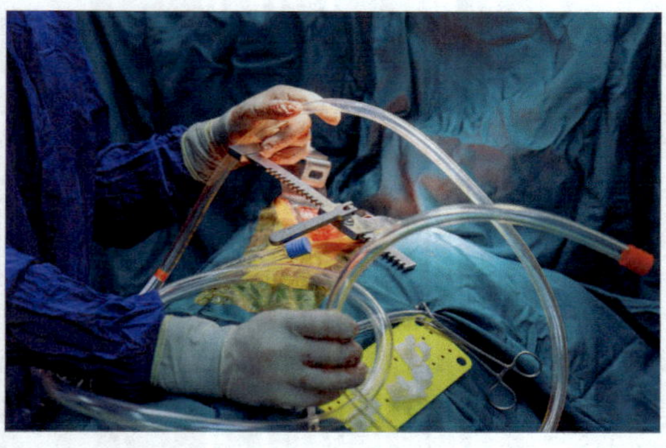

Figure 11.10. Cardiothoracic surgery.

Source: https://blog.amopportunities.org/wp-content/uploads/2023/02/iStock-1169181489-1200x800.jpg.

11.4.1. Definition and Criteria for Diagnosing Multiple Organ Dysfunction Syndrome (MODS)

MODS refers to the failure of two or more organ systems in a progressive manner due to an uncontrolled systemic inflammatory response to extreme infection or trauma. MODS usually occurs as a sequel to sepsis, but it may also result from trauma, burns, pancreatitis, and other life-threatening events. The pathophysiology of MODS involves a complex interaction of inflammatory mediators, cellular injury, and impaired microcirculatory perfusion, ultimately leading to organ failure. Clinically, the early recognition of MODS is vital because it typically represents a terminal process that significantly impacts patient outcome. Thus, healthcare professionals and nurses should be vigilant for signs indicative of the development of this syndrome, particularly in those at risk who are located in intensive care units or following significant surgery. MODS diagnostic criteria are founded on clinical observation and evidence-based practice and focus on the inclusion of greater than one system to represent a patient's physiological status. The SOFA score is an illustration of a measure that evaluates function in six organ systems, including the respiratory, coagulation, liver, cardiovascular, renal, and neurological systems. It evaluates patients over time, with an increased SOFA score indicating worsening organ function. Studies show that alterations in the vital signs, such as tachycardia, hypotension, and alterations in the level of consciousness, are the critical parameters utilized in detecting the onset of organ dysfunction. Furthermore, laboratory results showing elevated levels of abnormal liver enzymes or elevated creatinine levels can also be used to confirm MODS. Continuous monitoring of the criteria is crucial to ensure that medical treatment is initiated and the survival of patients in critical care is optimized. Research highlights the importance of early detection and management of MODS to achieve better patient outcomes. Various studies have shown that understanding organ function dynamics can guide physicians in introducing timely interventions, thereby avoiding further organ failure. For instance, a prospective observational study found that initial physiological instability is significantly linked with subsequent complications, such as MODS (Day et al., 2013). Conversely, postoperative conditions can also complicate the clinical picture, as postoperative sepsis is often challenging to differentiate from the inflammatory response to surgery (Eriksson et al., 2016). While medical professionals continue to advance diagnostic definitions and assessment tools for MODS, the inclusion of SIRS parameters and continuous monitoring of clinical and laboratory markers will be essential in detecting MODS at an early stage and improving patient care (Figure 11.11).

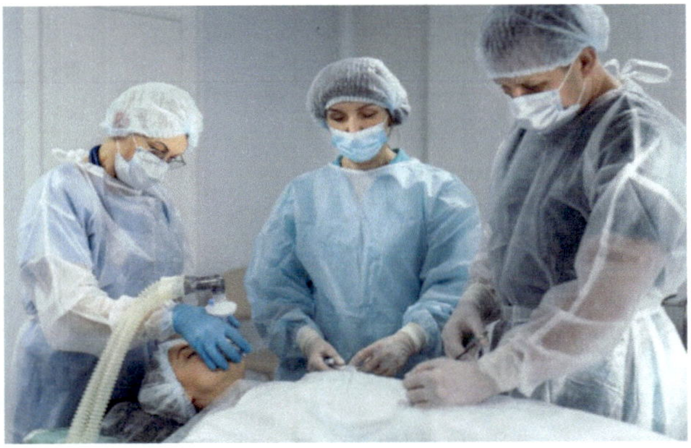

Figure 11.11. Sequential organ failure assessment (SOFA).

Source: https://img.freepik.com/free-photo/medical-team-with-patient-operator-room_23-2149372309.jpg?ga=GA1.1.892546656.1750072108&semt=ais_hybrid&w=740.

11.4.2. Common Organs Affected by Multiple Organ Dysfunction Syndrome (MODS)

MODS is characterized by the simultaneous dysfunction of two or more organ systems, typically in critically ill patients following a generalized inflammatory response. Of the most frequently involved organs, the lungs, kidneys, liver, and cardiovascular system are most commonly affected. Pulmonary dysfunction often constitutes the initial presentation, with ARDS being one of the significant complications. ARDS is the result of an inflammatory cascade with resultant alveolar-capillary membrane permeability, leading to pulmonary edema and impaired gas exchange. This negative pulmonary condition can quickly deteriorate to a critical situation. Therefore meticulous monitoring and proper intervention by nursing staff is necessary to recognize early respiratory distress in patients with possible MODS (Elfeky et al., 2013). The renal system also becomes a victim of MODS effects, typically through acute kidney injury (AKI), which makes it complicated to present clinically among critically ill patients. The pathophysiology of AKI in this context is usually related to impaired renal perfusion and ischemia as a result of shock or sepsis, which is prevalent in most cases of MODS. Increased creatinine and blood urea nitrogen levels are indicative of compromised renal function, making fluid management plans, which are frequently employed during nursing interventions, more complicated. Additionally, electrolyte disturbances are also frequent among the patient population, exacerbating treatment protocols. Detection of these alterations promptly is essential because preventive measures can prevent irreversible kidney damage and improve global patient outcomes (Eriksson et al., 2016). Hepatic failure is also a critical element of MODS, most often due to systemic inflammatory responses, hypoperfusion, and direct bacterial translocation, especially sepsis-associated. The liver plays a crucial role in metabolism, detoxification, and protein synthesis; therefore, failure can significantly impair healing. Clinically, increased liver enzymes and jaundice are typically presented, indicating hepatocyte injury and impaired hepatic synthesis. Nursing professionals take the lead in monitoring the development of these changes, initiating appropriate pharmacological treatment, and establishing nutritional support tailored to preserve hepatic function. Concurrently, cardiovascular instability, as expressed by hypotension or cardiovascular collapse, also commonly develops with MODS syndrome, necessitating close cardiovascular monitoring and potential interventions to restore patient hemodynamics (Elfeky et al., 2013).

11.4.3. The Pathophysiological Mechanisms Behind Multiple Organ Dysfunction Syndrome (MODS)

The pathophysiologic processes of MODS are multifaceted and predominantly result from an overactive inflammatory response to a primary infection, trauma, or ischemia. In the case of shock or sepsis, the body releases a cascade of pro-inflammatory cytokines, inducing a condition of systemic inflammation.

The process can disrupt normal hemodynamics, leading to microcirculatory failure and tissue non-perfusion. Therefore, this oxygen delivery failure initiates cell injury and evokes further inflammatory responses, creating a vicious cycle that promotes organ dysfunction at an accelerated rate. As the inflammation persists, the body is more likely to transition from hyperinflammation to an immunosuppressive response, impairing the immune system's capacity to combat infection, thereby providing a platform for secondary infections that can further complicate the clinical picture.

Early detection of these processes is crucial for treatment and improved patient outcomes. Perhaps the most aspect of MODS is the persistent inflammation it entails, which can create a self-perpetuating cycle of organ dysfunction that has a profound impact on patient recovery. Persistent Inflammation, Immunosuppression, and Catabolism Syndrome (PICS) is a useful model for conceptualizing this process. PICS evolves through the production of hypercatabolism and immunosuppression, and both of these conditions can result in recurrent infection as well as metabolic derangement. Persistent inflammation not only affects the immune system but also alters bone marrow function and causes sarcopenia, which is an overwhelming force for the frailty that occurs in critically ill patients.

The most crucial interaction is between the chronic inflammation and resulting immunosuppression, which creates a situation in which once-manageable infections can become unbearable complications that overwhelm already diseased organ systems. Sustaining this delicate balance remains challenging in clinical circumstances.

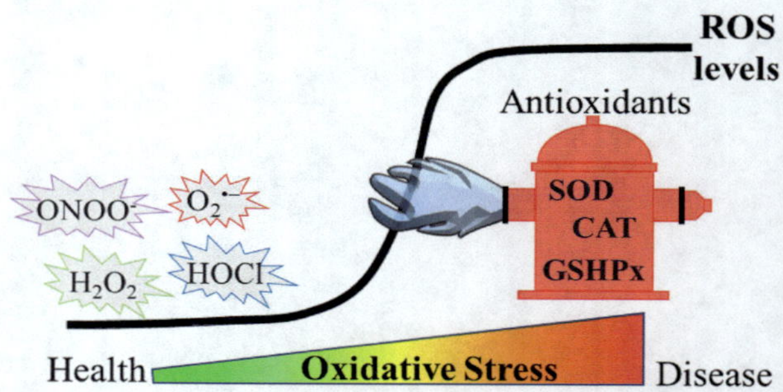

Figure 11.12. Oxidative stress in age-related neurodegenerative diseases.

Source: https://www.mdpi.com/antioxidants/antioxidants-12-00131/article_deploy/html/images/antioxidants-12-00131-g001.png.

MODS's complexity warrants the employment of a holistic management technique based on an understanding of its pathophysiology.

As MODS is a heterogeneous syndrome, there is a need for a multimodal approach tailored to counteract a specific component of the syndrome. Recent evidence suggests that therapies targeting immune homeostasis, such as the infusion of interleukin receptor antagonists or antioxidants to prevent oxidative stress, may offer potential benefits. Moreover, nutritional interventions for blocking the onset of PICS, including ketogenic dieting and probiotics administration, must also be researched further. Furthermore, there is a need for consensus on what defines the PICS definition and treatment approach to guide research directions. By expanding our understanding of the pathophysiologic mechanisms of MODS, healthcare professionals will be better equipped to treat this multifaceted syndrome, ultimately leading to improved patient outcomes in this growing clinical problem (Figure 11.12).

Test Your Knowledge

1. What are the common causes and early warning signs of MODS in critically ill patients?
2. How must nurses order care to support organ function and prevent progression of MODS?

11.5. Nursing Assessment and Interventions

Learning Outcome

1. Explain the key assessment techniques for shock and sepsis detection
2. Define nursing interventions in managing patients in shock
3. Discuss monitoring and support of organ function

Nursing assessment continues to be a cornerstone in the management of patients with shock, sepsis, or MODS. The interrelated dynamic between these conditions necessitates a holistic approach that is different from the traditional method. Nurses must utilize cutting-edge technology, including high-fidelity simulation and guided reflection tasks, to refine their clinical judgment and decision-making skills. The limitations of conventional hands-on training have been addressed by introducing state-of-the-art educational technologies, promoting a more secure understanding of patient needs in life-or-death scenarios. Through the administration of evidence-based assessment protocols, nurses can precisely identify the early warning signs of deterioration, thereby permitting timely and effective interventions that are essential in averting adverse patient outcomes and mortality due to these complex syndromes (Loving et al., 2010). Utilization of specific nursing interventions is also significant in the care of shock and sepsis patients. These interventions typically involve the administration of IV fluids, monitoring of vital signs, and the implementation of infection control practices. A recent study indicates the complexity of postoperative peritonitis, a formidable complication that can ensue, causing sepsis and organ failure. Nurses are at the forefront of detecting the minute hints of development, which sometimes may not be visible, and thus emphasize the need for vigilant observation and immediate intervention. Interventions should further involve coordination with multidisciplinary teams to streamline care pathways, offering holistic treatment tailored to presentations of individual patients (Droniak et al., 2019). These coordinated approaches have the capacity to enhance rates of recovery while restricting complications radically. In addition to assessment and intervention, education and practice transformation based on changing evidence form another core part of nursing care. Ongoing professional education enables nurses to stay current with the latest diagnostic technologies and treatment guidelines relevant to shock and sepsis. Simulation training and scenario debriefing enable nursing staff to practice skills while considering real-world applications. These training opportunities are particularly beneficial due to the high-stakes environments in which nurses must practice. By fostering an education and reflection culture, healthcare organizations can train their nursing staff to become meaningful contributors to sepsis and MODS management, thereby delivering improved patient outcomes and reducing healthcare-associated complications (Loving et al., 2010) (Figure 11.13).

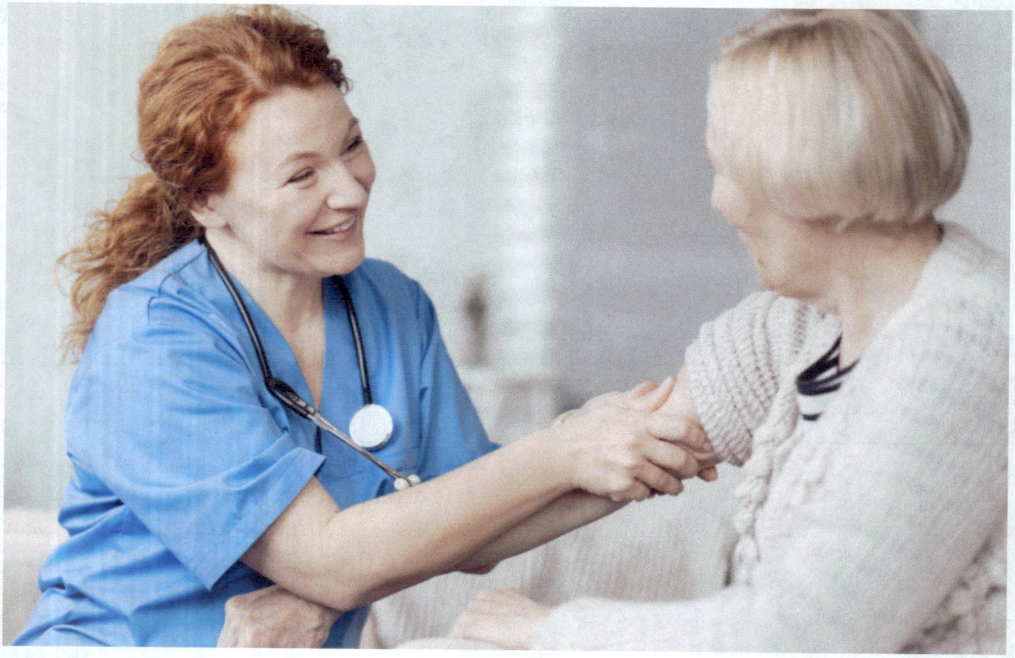

Figure 11.13. Nursing assessment.

Source: https://www.keithrn.com/nurse/wp-content/uploads/2021/09/nurse-with-senior-woman.jpeg.

11.5.1. Key Assessment Techniques for Identifying Shock and Sepsis

Key methods of assessment are crucial in identifying shock and sepsis, as they have the potential to develop into MODS if not identified early. Comprehensive clinical assessment is one of the primary methods, wherein vital parameters such as blood pressure, heart rate, and respiratory rate are monitored. Identification of early hypotension or tachycardia can be an indicator of shock. Moreover, the use of specific scoring systems, such as the SOFA score, allows nurses to quantify the degree of organ dysfunction and assess sepsis severity. These measurement methods are prioritized by formal protocols, which indicate early intervention in patients suspected of having sepsis, thereby enhancing patient outcomes through early nursing intervention and resource allocation (Vijayamohan et al., 2011). Laboratory tests play a vital role in diagnosing shock and sepsis, as they provide objective evidence of deranged physiological functions. Notably, markers such as lactate concentration, complete blood cell count, and blood cultures are crucial for assessing the severity of infection and the body's response. Elevated lactate levels, for instance, signal tissue hypoperfusion, in accordance with clinical trial results that identify their utility in stratifying risk (Chimbira et al., 2001). Blood cultures not only confirm infection but also guide appropriate targeted antibiotic therapy, which is valuable for the best care. The integration of laboratory findings into a comprehensive assessment model allows nursing professionals to intervene promptly that can significantly reduce mortality and morbidity associated with sepsis and shock. Moreover, continuous monitoring of patients and reassessment are crucial components of effective nursing care for vulnerable patients with shock and sepsis. Continuous vital sign monitoring technology can help facilitate the early detection of deteriorating trends, enabling a rapid response. Moreover, the incorporation of early warning systems can enhance situational awareness among nurses, such that changes in the status of a patient are responded to promptly. Educational programs focused on recognizing the subtle signs and symptoms of sepsis can improve the nursing staff's ability to provide high-quality care. Individually, these assessment techniques and integration into practice give a proactive approach to the management of shock and sepsis, eventually leading to improved patient outcomes and reduced incidence of MODS (Vijayamohan et al., 2011) (Figure 11.14).

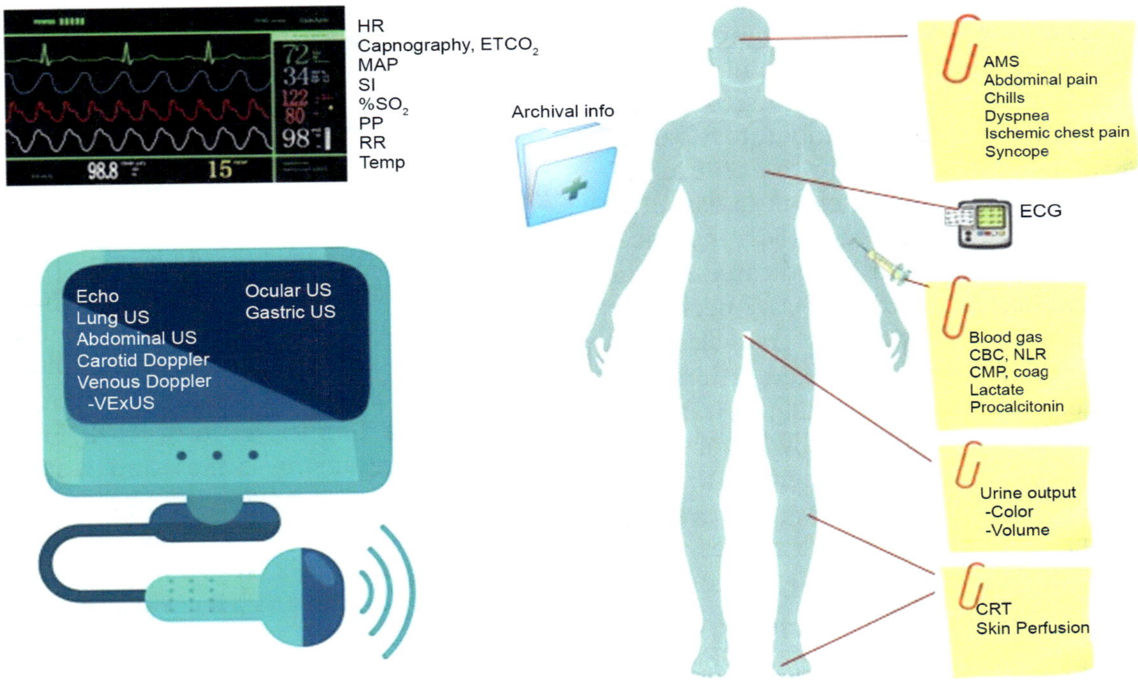

Figure 11.14. The realm of tissue perfusion: systemic hypoperfusion and congestion.

Source: https://external-content.duckduckgo.com/iu/?u=https%3A%2F%2Frecapem.com%2Fwp-content%2Fuploads%2F2023%2F02%2Fshock-evaluation.png&f=1&nofb=1&ipt=be2b65d6e9989ca7ac7633a7551603aedec3761c60d557ab27cf790081fc5943.

11.5.2. Nursing Interventions for Managing Patients in Shock

Shocked patients must be handled urgently and systematically by nursing staff to stabilize the patient's condition and prevent further complications. Initial assessments should initially seek clinical signs of shock like hypotension, changed mental status, and deranged skin perfusion. Proper management relies on the prompt application of fluid resuscitation to reverse hypovolemia, particularly in septic shock where fluid redistribution is extreme. Additionally, nurses must closely monitor vital signs to assess the effectiveness of interventions and detect any worsening of patients' conditions. Further, the application of evidence-based clinical guidelines, such as those implemented by the Surviving Sepsis Campaign, provides a structured framework for nursing care, such as risk assessment and the potential complications of shock (Abele-Horn et al., 2011). In addition to fluid resuscitation, nursing practice should involve careful observation of laboratory values such as lactate level to guide the efficacy of therapy. Pathophysiology of shock is essential in the customization of care. For instance, vasopressor support might be indicated if fluid resuscitation fails to restore effective perfusion pressures and cardiac function. Nurses also play a role in checking that these medications are administered correctly and checking their impact on hemodynamic stability. Equally important is control of possible sources of infection through appropriate administration of antibiotics and rigorous infection prevention strategies, since infection is a familiar lead-in to septic shock and tends to worsen patient outcomes (Huffer et al., 2017). This multidimensional approach emphasizes the role of nurses in using clinical judgment to manage complex cases of shock. Supportive care is a critical component of nursing intervention in patients with shock. This encompasses proper nourishment, as the body must replenish its energy to recover from the metabolic cost of shock. A thoughtful assessment of the nutritional requirements of the patients, along with the use of enteral or parenteral nutrition regimens, can significantly influence the healing process. Patient comfort and safety through proper pain control and prevention, such as skin care to prevent pressure ulcers, are also of primary concern. Education of patients and their families is also an essential part of nursing care, ensuring they are aware of their condition and the interventions being performed. Holistic nursing management, as evidenced by research, not only addresses immediate physiological issues but also involves planning for the patient's long-term recovery (Abele-Horn et al., 2011). Such comprehensive intervention approaches are strictly necessary for optimizing outcomes in patients affected by shock.

11.5.3. Strategies for Monitoring and Supporting Organ Function

Good monitoring and management of organ function are key components of patient management for those who are experiencing shock, sepsis, and MODS. Monitoring vital signs, such as heart rate, blood pressure, respiratory rate, and temperature, regularly is very important information that can indicate the status of organ function. Others, like some specialized parameters like urine output, serum lactate levels, and the ratio of PaO2/FiO2, are critical in measuring kidney and respiratory function, respectively. For example, decreased urine output may reflect renal impairment, while changes in PaO2/FiO2 values reflect acute respiratory distress. These variables enable medical personnel to identify deteriorating trends early and implement the appropriate interventions, ultimately improving patient outcomes in critical care settings, particularly for patients with sepsis and MODS complications (Chimbira et al., 2001). Apart from regular vital sign checks, the application of sophisticated monitoring equipment can greatly assist in preserving organ function. Equipment such as continuous cardiac output monitors and invasive blood pressure monitoring equipment can provide instant feedback regarding a patient's hemodynamics, allowing for early interventions. For instance, the detection of septic shock in its initial stages by hemodynamic instability would call for immediate fluid resuscitation and the start of vasopressor therapy, crucial components in the recovery of organ perfusion. Furthermore, the application of protocols that guide nursing interventions according to these advanced monitoring data guarantees a uniform care approach. As emphasized in expert guidelines, supportive care encompasses not only technical surveillance but also holistic care, including nutrition management and preventive strategies for nosocomial infections (Abele-Horn et al., 2011). Nursing staff work together to actively monitor and support organ function in the critically ill patient. Careful communication among team members guarantees an integrated approach to responding to patient status changes and coordinating treatment plans in accordance with those responses. Nurses are often the first to notice clinical deterioration, which enables them to advocate for early intervention. Moreover, ongoing education about assessing and managing organ dysfunction, as outlined in the Surviving Sepsis Campaign guidelines, enhances nurses' proficiency in caring for complex cases of sepsis and MODS. Continuing education and hiring in the nursing field have a significant influence on survival rates and patient care overall, demonstrating the gravity of skilled nursing in the treatment of such potentially fatal illnesses (Abele-Horn et al., 2011) (Figure 11.15).

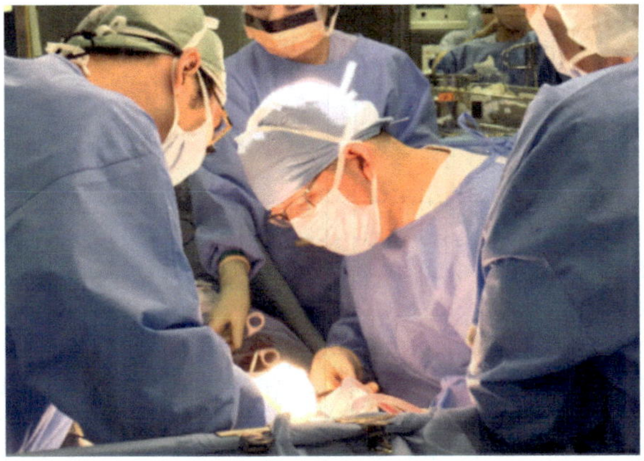

Figure 11.15. Artificial organ and transplantation surgery.

Source: https://external-content.duckduckgo.com/iu/?u=https%3A%2F%2Fwww.h.u-tokyo.ac.jp%2Fenglish%2Fcenters-services%2Fclinical-divisions%2Fartificial-organ-and-transplantation-surgery%2F_icsFiles%2Fafieldfile%2F2022%2F03%2F15%2Fartificialorgantransplantation.jpg&f=1&nofb=1&ipt=a8ddb70f89ae66943e54418cba92fed77a63d5ede47e33be19cac0889babc934.

Test Your Knowledge

1. What findings from an assessment aid nurses in identifying the onset and progression of MODS?
2. What are essential nursing interventions to aid patients with compromised organ systems in MODS?

11.6. Challenges in Nursing Care

Learning Outcome

1. Describe the challenges to early recognition and management of shock and sepsis
2. Define the ethics of managing MODS patients
3. Describe the importance of interdisciplinary care

The challenges in nursing care play an essential role in managing life-threatening conditions such as shock, sepsis, and MODS. One of the highly recognized problems is the general scarcity of nursing practitioners that overworks healthcare systems and compromises the quality of patient care. There exist numerous studies that indicate astronomical death rates caused by medical mistakes, emphasizing the necessity of resolving the workforce problem in nursing (Loving et al., 2010). This shortage affects not only the number of hands in patient care but also puts significant pressure on available staff, leading to burnout and decreased job satisfaction. Subsequently, nurses may find it challenging to deliver the quality of attention and skill required for the effective management of complex patients, such as those with sepsis, which necessitates prompt and accurate intervention. One of the other significant problems nurses face is navigating the subtlety of clinical judgment amid shifting guidelines for treatment and best practices. As treatment models for chronic conditions, such as sepsis, continue to evolve, nurses must stay current with new evidence-based practice guidelines (Alhazzani et al., 2017). This type of continuing education is particularly crucial in acute care settings, where precise interventions have direct implications for patient outcomes. Nurses also need to demonstrate proficiency in employing more advanced technologies and simulation-based education in practice, a requirement that can even further complicate their ability to provide care. The disparity in accessing educational materials can exacerbate these issues, rendering certain nurses unable to respond to the complexities of care necessary for shock patients or septic patients. In addition to problems in workforce and clinical knowledge, communication remains an essential element in shaping nursing care in life-threatening conditions. Effective communication in a timely and accurate manner among the interprofessional team is required to coordinate the handling of sepsis and MODS. Ineffective communication or delayed exchange of information through high-stress environments, common in acute care settings, is significantly responsible for patient safety and treatment outcomes. Furthermore, the necessity of family involvement in care procedures presents an additional challenge, as nurses must balance the need to educate families with the urgency of stabilizing critically ill patients. Such complexity highlights the multidimensionality of nursing issues in high-stakes settings, underscoring the need for systemic reform and increased support in responding effectively to shock, sepsis, and MODS (Figure 11.16).

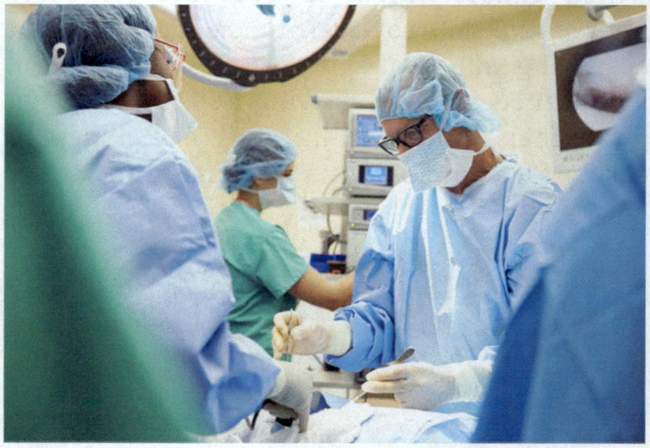

Figure 11.16. Nurse practitioners can 'transform' surgical departments.

Source: https://cdn.ps.emap.com/wp-content/uploads/sites/3/2017/03/ING_17215_10757.jpg.

11.6.1. Barriers to Early Recognition and Treatment of Shock and Sepsis

Early treatment and recognition of shock and sepsis for patients are the major drivers for improving outcomes, but several barriers are involved in the processes within healthcare organizations. One of them is the lack of standardized assessment protocols at various healthcare facilities. The lack of standardized guidelines will render it difficult for healthcare professionals to detect the initial signs of sepsis and shock. This inconsistency will lead to a delay in initiating treatment, thereby deteriorating the patient's status. Furthermore, the embedded variability in training and expertise among staff members about identifying sepsis will render monitoring ineffective. A greater focused effort at education in nursing programs and continued professional development is necessary in order to move beyond these deficits and create a greater level of care. Closing educational gaps in the nursing workforce is essential to creating a more educated workforce capable of identifying these life-threatening conditions. Intricate interprofessional communication dynamics that exist within the acute care setting represent another barrier that is essential. Effective communication is essential to interdisciplinary practice in patient care, but existing hierarchies and departmental silos may hinder timely communication between healthcare workers. For instance, the nurse's alarm regarding a patient's worsening status may not effectively reach the attending physician, leading to delays in indicated interventions. Such a lack of timely communication has the potential to significantly impact patient outcomes, particularly in cases of shock and sepsis, where minutes matter in the delivery of life-saving interventions. The adoption of formalized communication tools, such as SBAR (Situation, Background, Assessment, Recommendation), can facilitate more effective and clearer exchanges of information between team members, ultimately resulting in improved identification and treatment of critical conditions. Finally, the systemic problem of staffing deficits and high patient-to-nurse ratios makes it difficult to identify and intervene early for shock and sepsis. Fatigued nursing personnel might not possess the ability to conduct thorough assessments and provide the necessary critical care for at-risk patients. Nursing staff being in such high demand can lead to failure in monitoring significant vital signs or status changes for emergent sepsis. In addition, studies indicate that the training and education of nurses in sepsis care is not uniform, indicating a demand for improvement in the system's healthcare practice and training. Enhancing support and training among staff can allow nurses to recognize pivotal conditions more accurately, which in turn can optimize the timely provision of necessary treatment and minimize the risk of patient adverse outcomes (Loving et al. 2010; Abele-Horn et al., 2011) (Figure 11.17).

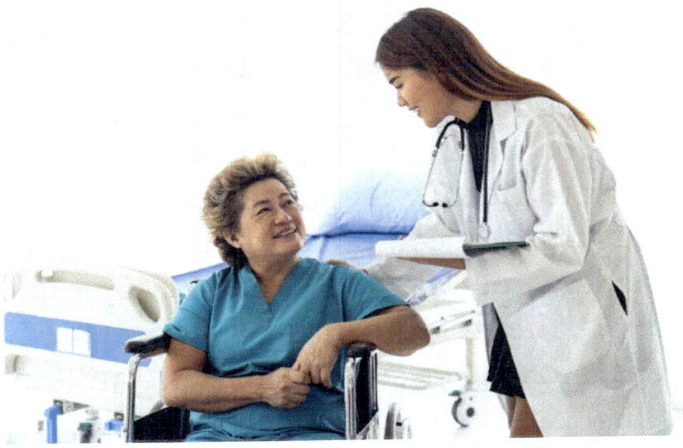

Figure 11.17. SBAR (Situation, Background, Assessment, Recommendation).

Source: https://blog.hostalky.com/wp-content/uploads/2024/11/image-6-1024x683.jpeg.

11.6.2. Ethical Considerations in Managing Patients with Multiple Organ Dysfunction Syndrome (MODS)

Ethical problems in treating MODS patients are complex and dominated by the complexity of the condition. As MODS often arises from septic shock and widespread infections, treatment demands that clinicians balance between injurious treatment protocols and the prognosis and quality of life of the patient. The ethical principle of beneficence mandates clinicians and nurses to do the best for the patient's interest. But when there is forceful resuscitation and extensive organ support systems involved, the likelihood of suffering and compromised quality of life raises significant ethical issues. As proposed by Castillo et al. (2023), gaps in sepsis education in nursing can hinder proper management. Therefore, the importance of ongoing education comes into play to ensure that ethical values are incorporated into clinical practices, which consequently affect patient care in MODS cases. Apart from beneficence, the principle of autonomy also stands vital in the ethical care of MODS patients. The patients might not be able to make sound decisions due to the severity of their condition and how rapidly sepsis converts into multiple organ failure. In such situations, medical professionals must conduct surrogate decision-making or advance care planning consultations as appropriate. Acknowledging patient values and preferences can complicate treatment plans. For example, as Cardoso et al. (2016) explain, diabetic patients presenting with sepsis may conceptualize aggressive treatment differently in the light of their comorbid conditions. Thus, healthcare professionals should practice within the ethical sphere with cultural sensitivity and consciousness in relation to patient circumstances to optimize care and uphold patients' rights to participate in decision-making. Ultimately, resource distribution becomes a pressing ethical issue in the treatment of MODS. The increasing number of septic states places greater demands on healthcare systems, particularly in terms of intensive care bed capacity. The ethical dilemma arises when there is a need to triage, as some patients are likely to require life-sustaining therapies, while others will not benefit—leaving the difficult work of patient equity and justice. Nurses as first-line providers advocate on behalf of patients' interests and may be confronted with ethical dilemmas when prioritizing treatments according to clinical outcomes or perceived quality of life. In working overcome these challenges effectively, interdisciplinary collaboration is essential, with open communication regarding available resources and treatment goals, in a manner that allows each patient's case to be analyzed from an overall ethical standpoint tailored to their unique needs and circumstances (Figure 11.18).

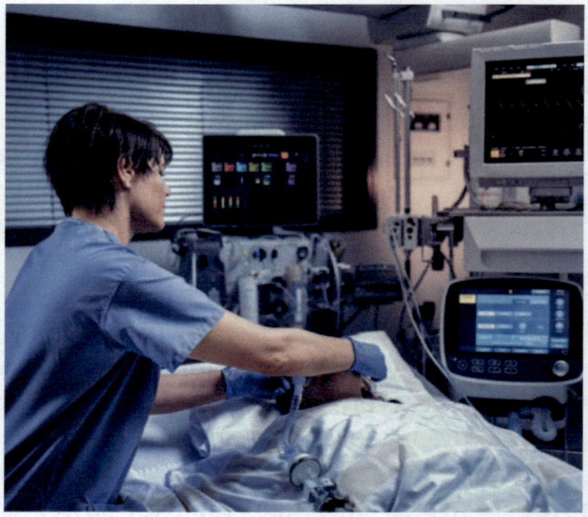

Figure 11.18. Extensive organ support systems.

Source: https://acutetherapies.baxter.com/sites/g/files/ebysai3966/files/2022-04/Nurse_helping_patient_hospitalbed.jpeg.

11.6.3. The Importance of Interdisciplinary Collaboration in Care

Interdisciplinary collaboration is crucial in nursing care, particularly in managing complex conditions such as shock, sepsis, and MODS. Effective communication and collaboration among health care professionals will have a profound impact on patient outcomes. For instance, nurses, doctors, pharmacists, and other experts can collaborate to create comprehensive care plans, which can leverage fragmented knowledge to identify and manage complications more effectively. This collaborative approach not only increases the responsiveness of interventions but also creates an ethos of shared responsibility, which is so vital in high-stakes environments such as emergency departments. Without such interprofessional teamwork, key gaps in sepsis treatment protocols might lead to increased mortality rates and longer hospital durations, as evidenced by recent quality improvement projects aimed at enhancing compliance with sepsis protocols in the nursing setting (Castillo et al., 2023). Interdisciplinary practice integration can be exemplified through the integration of strategies like nurse-initiated sepsis screening tools. Studies have shown that such teamwork allows nurses to become actively involved in the timely detection and treatment of deteriorating signs, thereby increasing the possibility of patient recovery (Biju et al., 2021). For instance, when nurses utilize screening instruments integrated within electronic health records (EHR), they are able to assess sepsis symptoms in patients quickly. This prompt response is crucial, as timely intervention can be the key to complete recovery versus the development of severe sepsis or MODS. Therefore, engaging nurses in the development and refinement of these instruments ensures that they are practical and effective in clinical practice, creating a system in which interprofessional teamwork is key to delivering high-quality patient care. Additionally, promoting interprofessional collaboration minimizes the risk of burnout among healthcare professionals. If the roles of a multi-disciplinary care team are clearly defined, individuals can alleviate the workload of demanding caseloads and make difficult decisions. This division, in turn, enhances the efficiency of care while enhancing the job satisfaction of team members, creating an improved support environment for work. Shared learning sessions for managing sepsis and recurrent education programs may address knowledge gaps, as suggested by reports revealing the need for ongoing staff training to improve protocol compliance in emergency departments (Castillo et al., 2023). Lastly, the importance of interdisciplinary collaboration in nursing extends beyond its direct impact on patient outcomes; it has strong effects throughout healthcare systems, affecting provider well-being, team performance, and the continuous optimization of patient-focused strategies in the challenging environments of shock and sepsis care.

Test Your Knowledge

1. What are the biggest challenges for nurses in coordinating care for MODS patients in intensive care units?
2. How can ethical considerations be weighed against life-supporting interventions in the end-of-life care of MODS patients?

SUMMARY

Shock, sepsis, and MODS are hard-to-treat conditions. It needs a good understanding of the pathophysiology involved. Effective nursing interventions are essential in the detection and management of complications of these life-threatening conditions. It is believed that timely recognition of sepsis, with appropriate fluid resuscitation and immediate antibiotic administration, is essential in improving patient outcomes. As shown in some studies, death due to inadequately treated postoperative conditions, such as peritonitis, can be dramatic, showing the urgency required in nursing interventions. Thus, an aggressive approach with early evaluation and management can significantly undermine the progression of sepsis to MODS, ultimately saving the lives of more patients (Droniak et al., 2019). The dynamic character of managing shock and sepsis patients requires nurses to be more vigilant and adaptable in the care approach. The dynamic nature of diseases affecting multiple organ systems requires healthcare workers to employ continuous monitoring and reassessment approaches. As suggested by the retrospective analysis of acute lung injury, a primary concern should be the early detection of perturbations in respiratory and cardiovascular functions, so that preemptive measures can be implemented, thereby avoiding systemic worsening. Recognition of the interplay among organ failures is crucial; therefore, an up-to-date integration of evidence-based clinical interventions into nursing practice is necessary to optimize patient recovery mechanisms within critical care settings (Chimbira et al., 2001). Lastly, integrating nursing competencies with ongoing research and evidence-based practice standards is crucial in addressing the complex dimensions of shock, sepsis, and MODS. Continuing upgraded education in nursing of such life-threatening ailments will empower professionals with information to make impactful decisions in high-stakes settings. Through multimodal assessment and intervention frameworks, nurses can significantly influence patient management outcomes. The healthcare team cooperation, coupled with a commitment to lifelong learning, emphasizes the key position of nursing in combating life-threatening infection. Intensive care strategies that incorporate psychological support and family involvement can further enhance the patient care process, facilitating an integrated treatment and recovery approach, which is essential in contemporary nursing practice (Chimbira et al., 2001; Droniak et al., 2019).

The interaction between shock, sepsis, and MODS calls for their significance in nursing practice and patient outcomes. Shock, characterized by inadequate tissue perfusion and resulting in tissue hypoxia, may trigger systemic inflammatory responses. On the other hand, sepsis, an extreme response to infection, frequently leads to similar catastrophic perfusion-related complications. As nurses, knowledge of the pathophysiologic basis of such conditions is imperative to enable early intervention and optimal care for patients. Successful management involves keen observation and aggressive response measures to avert further progression to MODS, a life-threatening condition in which several organ systems collapse due to persistent insult and failure of compensation. In the patient care environment, the application of HFS in nursing education is a breakthrough in how nurses are trained to manage such complex cases. As put forth, traditional education in clinical judgment has proven wanting in equipping nurses to handle the real-life challenges of shock and sepsis management. Through reflective practice and guided debriefing after HFS sessions, students develop procedural skills and clinical reasoning. The integration of technology in education can enhance nursing curricula to equip students for the acute and unexpected presentation of MODS, with resultant enhanced patient outcomes (Loving et al., 2010). The severity of ALI and ARDS in the

MODS context further highlights the worth of nursing interventions. Studies have indicated that ALI and ARDS are prevalent illnesses with very high morbidity and mortality and pose a challenge in managing septic patients. Recognition of physiological markers such as the PaO2/FiO2 ratio enables nurses to assess the severity of respiratory distress and implement resultant interventions promptly. Active nursing interventions, including vigilant monitoring, early detection of clinical deterioration, and the application of evidence-based therapy, have significant implications for influencing patient survival outcomes. Additionally, the understanding of the relationship between organ failure and patient mortality emphasizes the importance of holistic nursing approaches that not only respond to urgent clinical demands but also facilitate extended recovery (Chimbira et al., 2001).

KEY TERMS FROM THIS CHAPTER

- Anaphylactic Shock
- Critical Care Nursing Interventions
- Early Goal-Directed Therapy (EGDT)
- Hypovolemic Shock
- Mean Arterial Pressure (MAP)
- Neurogenic Shock
- Perfusion
- Septic Shock
- Shock
- Tissue Hypoxia
- Cardiogenic Shock
- Distributive Shock
- Hemodynamic Monitoring
- Lactic Acidosis
- Multiple Organ Dysfunction Syndrome (MODS)
- Oxygen Delivery (DO_2)
- Sepsis
- Severe Sepsis
- Systemic Inflammatory Response Syndrome (SIRS)
- Vasopressors

CRITICAL THINKING QUESTIONS

1. **Which of the following is the first clinical sign of shock?**
   a. Low blood pressure
   b. Cyanosis
   c. Tachycardia
   d. Coma
2. **Which type of shock is caused by a severe allergic reaction?**
   a. Hypovolemic shock
   b. Cardiogenic shock
   c. Anaphylactic shock
   d. Septic shock
3. **What is the most critical nursing action in the early management of sepsis?**
   a. Administering sedatives
   b. Delaying antibiotics until cultures return
   c. Early identification and prompt initiation of antibiotics
   d. Waiting for physician's instructions
4. **What is a key characteristic of Multiple Organ Dysfunction Syndrome (MODS)?**
   a. A single organ failure with full recovery
   b. Progressive failure of two or more organ systems
   c. Only cardiac and respiratory involvement
   d. Localized infection without systemic effects
5. **Which lab value is most commonly elevated in septic shock?**
   a. Hemoglobin
   b. Serum calcium
   c. Lactate
   d. Sodium

Short Answer Questions

1. Define shock and give two major categories.
2. What is the leading cause of septic shock?
3. Give two early signs and symptoms of shock to be measured by the nurse.
4. What is the function of fluid resuscitation in the management of hypovolemic shock?
5. List two organs commonly affected in Multiple Organ Dysfunction Syndrome (MODS).
6. Describe the pathophysiology of septic shock and systemic response to infection.
7. Describe the nursing interventions and priorities in the care of a cardiogenic shock patient.
8. Describe how sepsis can cause MODS and how its early detection will hinder complications.

Answers to Critical Thinking Questions

1. (c) 2. (c) 3. (c) 4. (b) 5. (c)

REFERENCES

1. Almahmoud, K., Abboud, A., Namas, R. A., Zamora, R., Sperry, J., Peitzman, A. B., Truitt, M. S., Gaski, G. E., McKinley, T. O., Billiar, T. R., & Vodovotz, Y. (2019). Computational evidence for an early, amplified systemic inflammation program in polytrauma patients with severe extremity injuries. *PLoS ONE, 14*(6), e0217577. https://doi.org/10.1371/journal.pone.0217577Abele-Horn, A., Abidia, A., Ahrens, A., Aiken, L., et al. (2011). Nursing considerations to complement the Surviving Sepsis Campaign guidelines. https://core.ac.uk/download/20540080.pdf (accessed on 28th June 2025).
2. Alhazzani, W., Angus, D. C., Annane, D., Antonelli, M., et al. (2017). Surviving Sepsis Campaign: International guidelines for management of sepsis and septic shock: 2016. https://core.ac.uk/download/286716214.pdf (accessed on 28th June 2025).
3. Anderson, D. J., Dantes, R. B., Epstein, L., Hamad, Y., et al. (2019). Prevalence, underlying causes, and preventability of sepsis-associated mortality in US acute care hospitals. https://core.ac.uk/download/288812794.pdf (accessed on 28th June 2025).
4. Bagshaw, S. M., Balducci, A., Baldwin, I., Barbarigo, L., et al. (2016). Nomenclature for renal replacement therapy and blood purification techniques in critically ill patients: Practical applications. https://core.ac.uk/download/153365476.pdf (accessed on 28th June 2025).
5. Barton, C. W., Das, R., Feldman, M. D., Mataraso, S., et al. (2017). Effect of a machine learning-based severe sepsis prediction algorithm on patient survival and hospital length of stay: A randomized clinical trial. https://core.ac.uk/download/323074084.pdf (accessed on 28th June 2025).
6. Biju, R. (2021). Early identification of sepsis: A nurse driven protocol to reduce morbidity, mortality and hospital costs. https://core.ac.uk/download/401856742.pdf (accessed on 28th June 2025).
7. Cardoso, K. (2016). Effects of hyperglycemia on adults hospitalized with sepsis. https://core.ac.uk/download/232660687.pdf (accessed on 28th June 2025).
8. Castillo, O. J. (2023). Optimizing sepsis management through enhanced protocol compliance in the emergency department. https://core.ac.uk/download/596873148.pdf (accessed on 28th June 2025).
9. Chadda, K. R., & Puthucheary, Z. (2024). Persistent inflammation, immunosuppression, and catabolism syndrome (PICS): A review of definitions, potential therapies, and research priorities. https://core.ac.uk/download/603253990.pdf (accessed on 28th June 2025).
10. Chimbira, W., Crawford, H., Gupta, S., Legg, J., et al. (2001). Acute lung injury in paediatric intensive care: Course and outcome. https://core.ac.uk/download/pdf/8715345.pdf (accessed on 28th June 2025).
11. Conboy, K., DiPiro, J. T., Duffy, L. C., Grasela, D. M., et al. (1995). Sepsis syndrome and associated sequelae in patients at high risk for Gram-negative sepsis. https://deepblue.lib.umich.edu/bitstream/2027.42/90154/1/j.1875-9114.1995.tb04333.x.pdf (accessed on 28th June 2025).
12. Davey, P. G., Evans, J. M. M., Guthrie, B., Marwick, C. A., et al. (2014). Identifying which septic patients have increased mortality risk using severity scores: A cohort study. https://core.ac.uk/download/30660276.pdf (accessed on 28th June 2025).

13. Day, D. E. (2013). Determining predictors of underlying etiology and clinical deterioration in patients with physiologic instability in the emergency department. https://open.bu.edu/bitstream/2144/12083/6/Day_Danielle_2013_nosig_nocv.pdf (accessed on 28th June 2025).
14. Docking, R., Kinsella, J., Moss, L., Sim, M., et al. (2012). An investigation into the effects of commencing hemodialysis in the critically ill. https://core.ac.uk/download/1439066.pdf (accessed on 28th June 2025).
15. Droniak, M. (2019). Management of postoperative peritonitis in low-resources services. https://core.ac.uk/download/301580706.pdf (accessed on 28th June 2025).
16. Elfeky, A., Mohammed, H., & Morsy, F. A. E. Y. M. (2013). Factors predisposing to organ(s) dysfunction among critically ill adult patients at a selected university hospital in Egypt. https://core.ac.uk/download/234686829.pdf (accessed on 28th June 2025).
17. Eriksson, L. (2016). Postoperative sepsis in an upper gastrointestinal surgical ward. https://core.ac.uk/download/43561672.pdf (accessed on 28th June 2025).
18. Gupta, E., Saxena, J., Kumar, S., Sharma, U., Rastogi, S., Srivastava, V. K., Kaushik, S., et al. (2023). Fast track diagnostic tools for clinical management of sepsis: Paradigm shift from conventional to advanced methods. *Diagnostics, 13*, 277–277. https://doi.org/10.3390/diagnostics13020277 (accessed on 28th June 2025).
19. Hamilton, R. (2015). The pathophysiology of sepsis. https://core.ac.uk/download/144427957.pdf (accessed on 28th June 2025).
20. Hanna, R., Dalvi, S., Sălăgean, T., Pop, I., Bordea, I. R., & Benedicenti, S. (2021). Understanding COVID-19 pandemic: Molecular mechanisms and potential therapeutic strategies. An evidence-based review. *Journal of Inflammation Research, 14*, 13–56. https://doi.org/10.2147/jir.s282213 (accessed on 28th June 2025).
21. Huffer, K. (2017). Improving new graduate critical care nurse practitioner knowledge and retention using a dedicated orientation and mentoring program. https://core.ac.uk/download/217321337.pdf (accessed on 28th June 2025).
22. Loving, G., McPherson, M. A., & Shortridge, A. (2010). Using web-based reflection with video to enhance high fidelity undergraduate nursing clinical skills education.
23. McCarthy, N. D., Royle, P., & Tsertsvadze, A. (2015). Community-onset sepsis and its public health burden: Protocol of a systematic review. https://core.ac.uk/download/42617129.pdf (accessed on 28th June 2025).
24. Nisha, R. (2018). Clinical profile etiology risk factors and outcome of children with shock in PICU in a tertiary care hospital. https://core.ac.uk/download/235668829.pdf (accessed on 28th June 2025).
25. Vijayamohan, V. K. (2011). Clinical profile of shock in children in a tertiary care hospital, Madurai. https://core.ac.uk/download/235666362.pdf (accessed on 28th June 2025).

CANCER NURSING: PRINCIPLES OF ONCOLOGIC MANAGEMENT

12

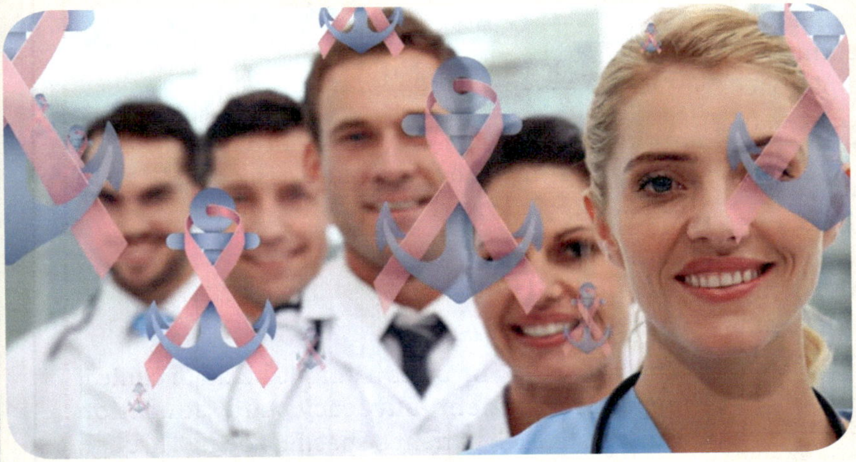

LEARNING OBJECTIVES

After studying this chapter, you will be able to:

1. Understand the cancer
2. Clearly define the role of the cancer nurse
3. Describe the assessment and diagnosis of oncologic management
4. Focus on treatment modalities in oncologic management
5. Learn about psychosocial considerations in cancer nursing
6. Evaluate the ethical and legal issues in oncology

Introduction

Cancer nursing is a vital specialty in the comprehensive management of cancer patients. By providing holistic care that addresses both physical and psychological concerns, cancer nurses become advocates, educators, and caregivers. With cancer increasingly becoming an illness of elderly individuals, healthcare providers will need to adapt their approaches to address the unique requirements of geriatric patients. To obtain optimal results, there must be a sound understanding of the concepts of oncologic care, such as knowledge of the cancers, their treatments, and the potential side effects of the treatments. This overall understanding is not only necessary for patient care but also for ensuring effective interdisciplinary collaboration between health professionals treating cancer patients, thereby enhancing the quality of care administered to patients diagnosed with cancer. One of the most important characteristics of cancer nursing is emphasis on individualized assessment of patients, particularly in oncogeriatric patients.

According to new research, inappropriately low rates of use for comprehensive pre-surgical geriatric assessment have been an ongoing challenge in optimal management of older patients with cancer. By incorporating intensive assessments with the Frailty Index and other relevant measures, practitioners are able to stratify patients more efficiently based on risk and thereby make improved treatment choices and results. The proposed educational interventions focus on reinforcing the skill set of future oncology nurses and clinicians, enabling them to conduct thorough geriatric assessments. As cancer treatment evolves toward a patient-centered model, the integration of these assessments will not only decrease risk but also enable clinicians to meet the changing needs of an increasingly aging patient population, as reported in the literature (Lampugnale et al., 2017). Furthermore, rigorous training in the principles of geriatric oncology will be crucial in educating the next generation of healthcare providers. Educational programs in oncologic care and cancer nursing principles should prioritize geriatric assessment frameworks and tools, enabling clinicians to detect and address age-related factors that impact cancer therapy. This forward-thinking approach will not only enhance the clinical competency of oncology practitioners but also prepare them to address the complexities involved with caring for older cancer patients. The increased prevalence of cancer among older adults requires collaborative efforts in sensitizing practitioners towards optimal management strategies in this population, thus improving treatment experiences and outcomes. These efforts can bridge the existing gaps in the care of oncologic patients, corroborating the need for additional training and education to maximize care and address the specific needs of oncogeriatric patients, as discussed in the literature (N/A, 2005) (Figure 12.1).

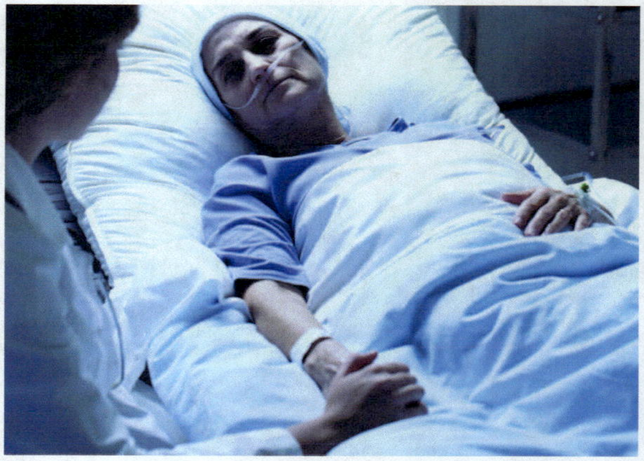

Figure 12.1. Oncology nursing.

Source: https://www.myamericannurse.com/wp-content/uploads/2020/01/an1-Oncology-1219.jpg.

Definition and Scope of Cancer Nursing

Cancer nursing involves a unique blend of clinical expertise, patient advocacy, and education tailored to each patient's specific needs. Through the process of holistic assessment, cancer nurses play a central role in the resolution of the complex physical and emotional issues affecting patients throughout the cancer trajectory. This profession not only requires a sound understanding of cancer biology and treatment methods but also the skill in psychosocial support techniques and communication. Cancer nurses are pivotal intermediaries between patients and multidisciplinary teams, ensuring that patients receive personalized care tailored to their individual needs and preferences. Therefore, the field of cancer nursing extends beyond mere clinical management; it encompasses holistic approaches that acknowledge the multifaceted nature of disease, as well as the importance of patient and family quality of life. Key to cancer nursing is the integration of palliative care principles into patient management. Palliative care, which is often misconstrued as equivalent to end-of-life care, is actually directed towards enhancing the quality of life for patients at any stage of their disease, including those undergoing curative therapy. The cancer nurses, therefore, must be adequately educated on palliative care interventions to effectively address pain, psychosocial distress, and advanced care planning. This is particularly critical, as healthcare reform initiatives, such as the Patient Protection and Affordable Care Act, have recognized the necessity for coordinated care—allowing patients to receive both curative and palliative treatments simultaneously (Cerminara et al., 2011). Unfortunately, potential regulatory obstacles, such as the additional requirement imposed on hospice recertification of care, can complicate cancer nurses' ability to offer uninterrupted palliative care (Cerminara et al., 2011). Hence, it is the responsibility of nursing practice and education to adapt to these shifting standards in order to maintain the effectiveness and pervasiveness of care to cancer patients. Cancer nursing also encompasses the critical mandate of educating cancer patients and their families about cancer, its treatment, and accessible resources. Education is also key to enabling patients to be involved, hence enhancing treatment adherence and outcomes. Cancer nurses allow this through the imparting of information on a wide spectrum of issues, such as the nature of the diagnosis, extent of potential treatments, and side effects. Additionally, they help families navigate the complexity of healthcare systems, which can be overwhelming at such a difficult time. In communicating information to patients and their families, cancer nursing fosters a culture of collaboration and teamwork, thereby significantly enhancing the patient's experience. Accordingly, the definition and boundaries of cancer nursing are invariably entangled with the issue of advocacy, which remains a key aspect of enhancing patient experience and care management in oncological settings (Figure 12.2).

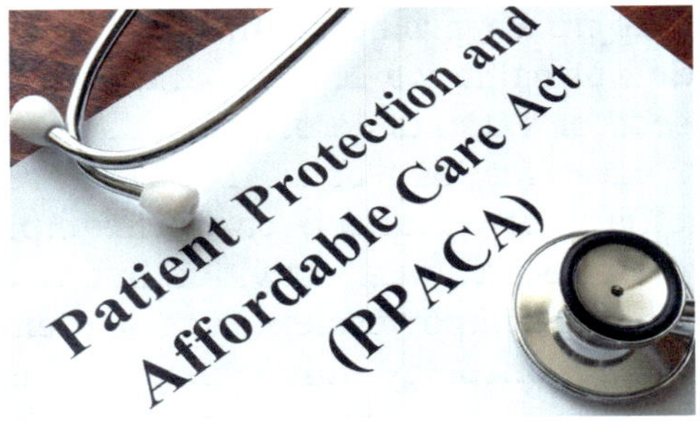

Figure 12.2. Patient Protection and Affordable Care Act.

Source: https://www.cbiz.com/wp-content/uploads/insights-ppaca.jpg.

Importance of Specialized Care in Oncology

In oncology, the relevance of specialist care is particularly important due to the complexity and heterogeneity of cancer as a disease. Conventional treatments, as effective as they are for some cancers, do not necessarily meet the specific requirements and symptoms that the individual patient is facing. This variation underscores the importance of expert oncology nurses who are trained to deliver personalized care tailored to each patient's unique profile, thereby enhancing outcomes and patient satisfaction. Since clinical advances are advancing at a rapid rate, oncology nursing clinicians must remain current with changing treatment modalities and approaches to cancer management so that care integrates physical symptom control with psychosocial issues and offers holistic care. The integration of expert oncology care also allows for the inevitable transition from curative to palliative care. As individuals live with cancer, the timing and how palliative care is provided have a significant influence on quality of life. Evidence indicates that early integration of palliative care alongside routine oncology care significantly improves health-related quality of life outcomes for patients with advanced cancer, but the practice remains underutilized. Oncology nurses are well-positioned to advocate for this approach, promoting the need for earlier initiation of palliative services and addressing the needs of patients across various stages of cancer care (Rughani et al., 2022). Moreover, the activity of advanced care encompasses not only direct clinical activities but also the education and empowerment of the patient and their family. Oncology nurses play a vital role in providing support by educating patients on treatment modalities, side effects, and self-care measures, thereby promoting informed decision-making. Such an educational component can help minimize anxiety and enhance patient participation in the treatment process, fostering a collaborative partnership among healthcare professionals and patients. Essential, advanced oncology nursing not only addresses biological therapies but also emphasizes emotional and psychological therapy as integral aspects, which will eventually culminate in a more empathetic and effective model of oncolytic management (N/A, 2005).

12.1. Understanding Cancer

Learning Outcome

1. Identify the category and classification of cancer
2. Tackle the pathophysiology of the development of cancer
3. Comprehend risk factors and the prevention of the development of cancer

Cancer requires an integrated approach to understanding not only the biological basis of neoplastic disease but also the social, cultural, and psychological factors that influence patient care and outcomes. Cancer arises through a cascade of genetic mutations and alterations that permit the cells to proliferate unrestrained. These can be due to a range of causes, including environmental exposures, lifestyle choices, and inherited genetic vulnerabilities. A key component of oncologic care is understanding these factors and incorporating them into tailored treatment plans that address the unique needs of each patient. Additionally, variation in the incidence of cancer and cancer types among populations also underscores the necessity for worldwide consideration in the development of effective nursing interventions and practices to address cancer (Are et al., 2016). In oncologic nursing, the understanding of the complexities of cancer not only enhances the quality of care but also highlights the need for continuous education among healthcare professionals. With global cancer statistics indicating trend-breaking increments in the incidence rate, it becomes absolutely imperative to establish standardized models of schooling for oncology nursing (Are et al., 2016). For instance, the development of a global surgical oncology curriculum aims to produce a sufficiently trained workforce capable of addressing various oncological needs in different regions. The curriculum is predicated on the realization that local variations in training may be necessary to accommodate local conditions, but that essential competencies necessary to provide effective cancer care need to be consistent. Thus, this effort serves as the essential stepping stone towards harmonizing the treatment of cancer and encouraging cooperation between oncology professionals globally. In addition, the communication between medical practitioners and patients has a significant impact on cancer management. This includes not only communicating medical details but also comprehending patients' emotional and psychological reactions to their condition and treatment. Cancer nursing involves patient advocacy, facilitation of support systems, and active patient involvement in care planning, which can enhance treatment plan compliance and outcomes. The incorporation of the patient-centered approach has also been shown to decrease anxiety levels and empower patients with a cancer diagnosis. Thus, oncology nurses must not only be clinically skilled but also have outstanding interpersonal skills to cover the intricate relationships inherent in cancer care.

In addressing both the medical and emotional components of cancer care, oncology nursing holds potential to be at the center of quality of life improvement for cancer patients and to facilitate them to live with their cancers (Are et al., 2016) (Figure 12.3).

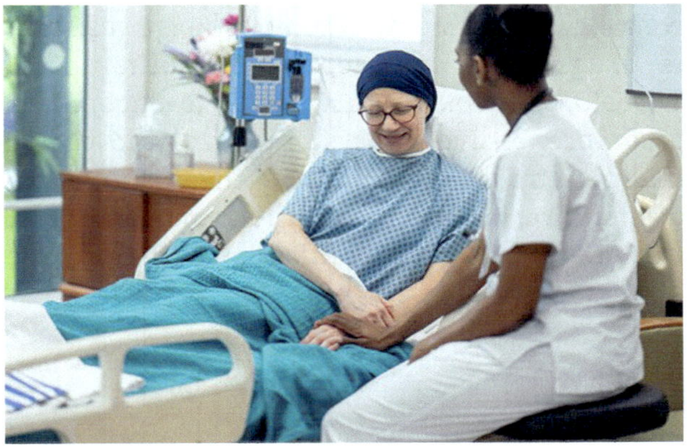

Figure 12.3. Cancer nursing workforce.

Source: https://dm1zcrsul8wju.cloudfront.net/sites/rcn_nspace/files/styles/tile_image/public/Article-images/199131/67496.jpeg?itok=lt6L9HA7.

12.1.1. Types of Cancer and Their Classifications

Cancer is a heterogeneous group of diseases characterized by the loss of control over normal cell growth and the ability to metastasize to other locations in the body. Cancers are difficult to classify and are generally organized based on tissue of origin, histologic characteristics, and genetics.

For instance, carcinomas originate from epithelial tissue, which constitutes the body's surface and lines its cavities, while sarcomas arise from connective tissues, such as bone and muscle. Hematological malignancies such as lymphoma and leukemia arise from blood-forming tissues and affect the immune system. This heterogeneity not only determines the treatment type but also governs the nursing care required, as different cancers will necessitate different management strategies depending on their biological behavior and the patient's prognosis. Apart from histologic classification, cancers are also divided based on their stage and grade. The staging process assesses the extent of cancer spread within the body, using systems such as the TNM classification system, which integrates tumor size, lymph node status, and metastasis detection. Grading, however, examines the extent of cancer cell abnormality, an indicator of the aggressiveness with which the cancer will develop. Oncology nurses need to understand these classifications because they have immediate implications for clinical decision-making and treatment planning. As an example, the plan of care for a patient will be vastly different depending upon whether they have localized stage I breast cancer or stage IV disease, highlighting the significance of proper classification in oncologic care (Beauchemin et al., 2019). The nursing workload required for the treatment of different cancers is significant and varies depending on disease classification, along with distinctive requirements for patients. Research has shown that the Nursing Activities Score (NAS) is highly correlated with the amount of care required by patients undergoing palliative care, indicating a strong relationship between nursing workload and patient performance status (Fuly et al., 2016). Oncology nursing is not just the administration of medication and symptom tracking, but also emotional support and teaching of patients and families with complex decisions regarding treatment. With the advancement of technologies and therapies, nurses play a crucial role in integrating these new developments into patient care. The understanding of the classification of cancer allows nursing professionals to develop their interventions to meet every specific type of cancer, both their physical and psychological issues (Figure 12.4).

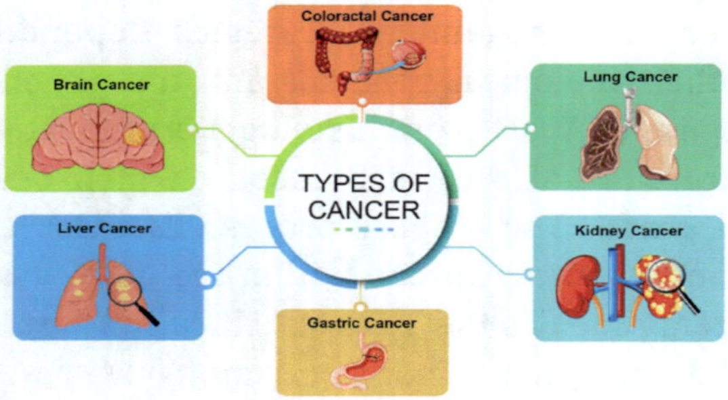

Figure 12.4. Types of cancer.

Source: https://media.geeksforgeeks.org/wp-content/uploads/20240207122109/Types-of-cancer.png.

12.1.2. Pathophysiology of Cancer Development

The pathophysiology of cancerogenesis is intricately linked to a cascade of genetic and epigenetic changes that lead to the uncontrolled growth of cells. Somatic cell DNA mutations can result in the activation of oncogenes or the inactivation of tumor suppressor genes. These changes can be caused by a variety of external events, such as carcinogens, tobacco smoke, and ultraviolet light, or by events that are intrinsic to cellular function, such as mistakes in DNA synthesis. With the accumulation of changes, they can disrupt normal cellular functions such as apoptosis and cell cycle control, resulting in a malignant phenotype characterized by abnormal growth and resistance to cell death. Understanding these underlying changes is crucial for cancer nursing professionals, as they must assess how these pathophysiological characteristics influence treatment and patient management (Lampugnane et al., 2017). In addition to genetic mutation, cancer is also influenced by the tumor microenvironment, which is formed by host stromal cells, immune cells, and extracellular matrix elements. This microenvironment can also promote tumor growth through complex signal networks that allow for the process of angiogenesis, or the formation of new blood vessels. The microenvironment of the tumor can also contribute to tumor heterogeneity, where heterogeneous cells within a single tumor exhibit different genetic and phenotypic features. This cellular heterogeneity can complicate treatment, as some cells are resistant to drugs when targeted against other cells. Therefore, oncologic care needs to encompass a comprehensive understanding of the tumor microenvironment, enabling the formulation of effective interventions, the management of side effects, and the identification of therapeutic targets (N/A, 2003).

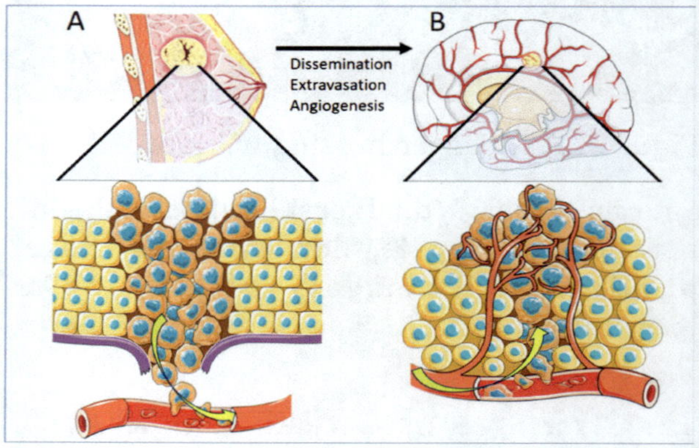

Figure 12.5. Pathophysiology of cancer spread for breast cancer.

Source: https://www.researchgate.net/publication/360226653/figure/fig1/AS:1152771722100737@1651853604152/Pathophysiology-of-cancer-spread-for-breast-cancer-A-Dissemination-of-breast-cancer.jpg.

While the complexity of cancer pathophysiology is intimidating, it also underscores the necessity of individualized oncologic care. By recognizing the novel molecular pathways and microenvironmental determinants that lead to cancer, nurses are better positioned to optimize patient outcomes. In addition, multidisciplinary management, which incorporates oncologists, pathologists, and surgeons, is crucial for the accurate treatment of malignancies. With advancing cancer research, keeping pace with innovative therapies targeting specific molecular pathways will improve the skills of nurses in coping with the complexity of patient care. With this comprehensive understanding of pathophysiologic processes, nurses can tailor individualized treatment protocols for each patient based on the specific characteristics of their cancer (Lampugnane et al., 2017) (Figure 12.5).

12.1.3. Risk Factors and Prevention Strategies

Identifying risk factors for cancer is crucial in oncologic management for effective prevention strategies. Intrinsic factors, including susceptibility due to genetic factors, age, and hormonal influences, can significantly increase susceptibility to certain cancers. Extrinsic factors, which encompass environmental exposures, lifestyle, and socio-economic status, also play a significant role in cancer risk. For instance, lifestyle issues such as smoking, alcohol consumption, and physical inactivity are known carcinogens for which preventive measures are readily available. By implementing a public health model that emphasizes education and awareness, healthcare workers can utilize evidence-based practices to mitigate these risk factors, thereby improving patients' overall health status and reducing cancer incidence. In cancer therapy, the role of successful contraception and family planning cannot be overemphasized, especially in young women receiving oncologic treatment. An unplanned pregnancy during cancer therapy is dangerous to both the patient and fetus and warrants proactive prevention. Unfortunately, recent practices show an alarming deficit in contraception screening and referral by oncologic practitioners that results in poor patient counseling on this essential issue. They are more interested in diagnosing the already existing pregnancies rather than preventing them, so this shows the need for systemic changes in cancer care protocols. By enhancing interdisciplinary coordination and incorporating education materials on contraception, the providers can deliver all-encompassing care that addresses both reproductive and physical needs of cancer patients, hence improving patient education and decision-making (Lindsay et al., 2018). In addition to caring for the reproductive health of patients, initiating risk stratification for the growing number of oncogeriatric patients should also be considered. A greater number of cancer diagnoses accompanies the growing population of elderly people, and this is an indication of the need for individually tailored treatment approaches that address the unique challenges of geriatric patients. A proper pre-surgical geriatric assessment is crucial for identifying underlying conditions that may increase surgical risks. However, the low number of full evaluations reflects systemic barriers within the healthcare system, primarily due to the prolonged nature of these evaluations. By emphasizing the necessity of geriatric assessments in oncology education programs and designing novel educational interventions for physicians, it is possible to enhance knowledge of the determinants of postoperative outcomes, thereby optimizing oncologic care for older individuals (Lampugnane et al., 2017).

Test Your Knowledge

1. What are the fundamental distinctions between cancer and benign tumors in terms of growth and expansion?
2. What is the function of genetic mutations in tumor formation and the advancement of cancer?

12.2. Role of the Cancer Nurse

Learning Outcome

1. Explain the role in patient care
2. Establish the importance of patient education and advocacy
3. Talk about the working with inter-disciplinary teams in cancer nurse

The role of the cancer nurse is multifaceted, encompassing not only clinical responsibilities but also the crucial task of supporting the emotional well-being of patients and their families. Cancer nurses have a key role to play in the delivery of treatments such as chemotherapy, as well as the management of the side effects of such therapies. This responsibility is critical, as a lack of confidence in chemotherapy administration has been noted among oncology nursing staff working in low-volume practices, leading to anxiety about handling oncologic care effectively (Littlepage et al., 2020). Their education fills gaps in patient care by ensuring that the individual can handle the complexities of their regimen while dealing with the psychological and emotional concerns that accompany a diagnosis of cancer, thus underscoring the value of ongoing education and support in this area. In addition to treatment provision and emotional support, cancer nurses are extremely valuable for the provision of promoting palliative care, namely that with the patient with advanced illness. Epidemiology demonstrates that, although palliative care has been shown to improve the quality of life in cancer patients, its integration into treatment remains suboptimal (Rughani et al., 2022). Oncology nurses, having undergone specialized training, are better equipped to promote the early integration of palliative care with traditional curative therapies. This twofold practice not only addresses cancer's physicality but also psychological distress, consequently improving the cancer patient and their family's care process. In providing support for this twofold practice, cancer nurses facilitate a team culture that values holistic patient care in a responsive approach for clinical need and quality of life. Moreover, the ongoing refinement of competency programs explicitly tailored for oncologic nursing is essential to enhance the competence of cancer nurses, ultimately impacting patient outcomes. According to research, incorporating web-based education with simulation-based training can significantly enhance the confidence and competency of nurses in delivering oncologic care (Littlepage et al., 2020). Through continuous learning and competency validation, oncology nurses can ensure they are up to date with the best practices in oncology management. This is particularly critical considering the rapid pace at which the oncology area evolves with new treatments and technological advancements. Creating an educational culture within healthcare settings will not only enable nurses but makealso create an optimally trained workforce better equipped to meet the demands of cancer treatment, with a beneficial impact on patient outcomes and the overall efficacy of oncologic therapy (Figure 12.6).

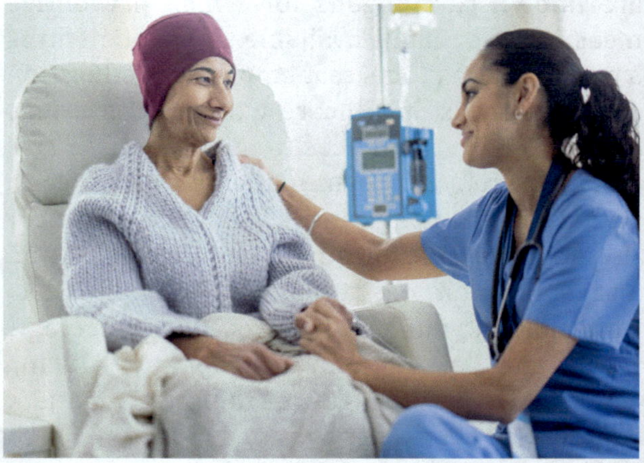

Figure 12.6. Role of the cancer nurse.

Source: https://ce.mayo.edu/sites/default/files/media/2023-04/Oncology%20curriculum.jpg.

12.2.1. Responsibilities in Patient Care

In cancer nursing, the role in patient care extends beyond clinical management to encompass holistic assessment tailored to the individualized needs of each patient. Due to an aging population, cancer incidence rises, especially among older adults who tend to have other comorbidities and psychosocial problems. One of the most essential elements of quality care for this population is to conduct comprehensive geriatric evaluations to properly assess their unique health status and the risks associated with surgery. Although the value of such assessment has been well established, it is underutilized in practice because of the time pressures experienced by healthcare providers. Delays in such risk stratifications can lead to poorer treatment outcomes, underscoring the importance of oncologists and nurses prioritizing these evaluations in managing oncogeriatric patients to enhance the overall quality of treatment delivered (Lampugnane et al., 2017). Moreover, the evolution of oncology nursing roles also signifies a greater emphasis on comprehensive patient care and efficient resource utilization. One such new model is the Advanced Breast Cancer Clinical Nurse (ABCCN), a good representation of this trend. The ABCCN specializes in coordinating the numerous services required by the patient during the course of treatment, thus having an even flow of psychosocial and clinical care. This role is vital as it not only observes the delivery of care but also comforts patients' emotional and pragmatic needs, particularly for those dealing with late-stage breast cancer. By equipping nurses with the competencies necessary to navigate complex healthcare systems, the ABCCN optimizes available resources and achieves a more integrated patient experience, thereby significantly enhancing the quality of oncologic care (Colomer et al., 2016). Apart from specialized tasks, cancer nursing responsibilities entail collaboration in multidisciplinary teams. Good communication among medical practitioners is necessary to ensure patients are adequately covered and ongoingly attended to throughout treatment regimens. This collaboration involves sharing relevant information on treatment options, managing side effects, and addressing patients' issues and preferences. This interprofessional cooperation fosters a supportive environment that encourages healthcare professionals to develop effective, personalized care plans. Additionally, patient involvement in care decisions promotes patient autonomy and adherence to treatment regimens. Nurses must remain adaptable in the ever-changing environment of cancer care, actively participating in the development and implementation of care plans that focus on patient wellness and the optimal use of healthcare resources (Figure 12.7).

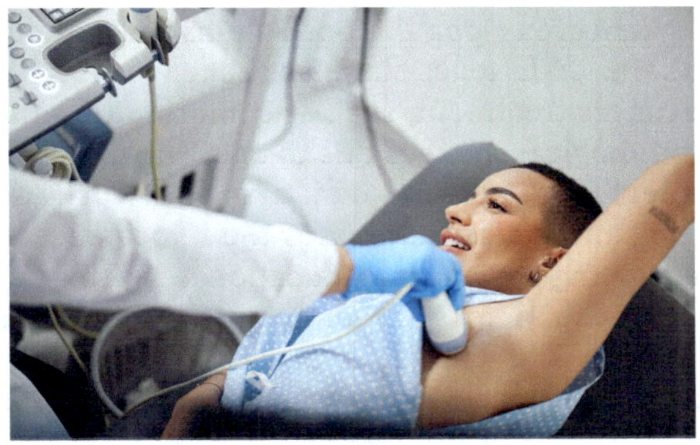

Figure 12.7. Advanced breast cancer clinical nurse (ABCCN).

Source: https://images.ctfassets.net/yixw23k2v6vo/30NHTut39moHdzIA1lafCo/43e49825b4b66e683c9d902912ce0b06/GettyImages-1394005533-3000x2000.jpg.

12.2.2. Importance of Patient Education and Advocacy

The significance of patient education and advocacy in cancer nursing cannot be overstressed, as it has an important role to play in improving the outcomes of patients and improving the general care experience. Patient empowerment through knowledge helps them make informed decisions regarding their treatment choices, thereby enhancing therapy compliance and levels of satisfaction with care. In environments where oncologic patients require immediate nursing attention, it is the common complaint to hear that nurses lack confidence in chemotherapy administration and care, emphasizing the need for comprehensive educational programs. By applying specific educational interventions, as outlined in Littlepage et al. (2020), health professionals can enhance their skill level and deliver more competent care, thereby improving the culture of safety and efficacy in the treatment of cancer patients. In addition to building self-assurance among nurses, patient education is also essential in addressing the unique requirements of particular groups among the cancerous population. For instance, older patients experience singular challenges related to cancer treatment, such as comorbidities and physiological changes due to age. The initiative undertaken by the Canadian Network on Aging and Cancer addresses the importance of developing specialized educational approaches that respond to such singular challenges, as elaborated in Alibhai et al. (2017). Advocacy for both of these groups calls for the creation of a coordinated network of cooperation that prioritizes research and education in geriatric oncology, thereby empowering healthcare providers to overcome age-related barriers and deliver optimal patient care. Furthermore, optimal patient advocacy extends beyond education, promoting institutional reform that enables greater access to information and treatment modalities. This requires a multidisciplinary approach, involving medical professionals from various disciplines to establish a robust patient care system. Through the intervention of barriers existing in current oncologic care, such as inadequate educational resources, as noted in Littlepage et al. (2020), patient advocacy programs can help fill gaps in care and enhance the quality of care offered. Lastly, the development of a setting where patient education and advocacy are the focal points not only optimizes nursing staff's expertise and capabilities but also prepares patients to become active participants in their own healthcare journey, with beneficial impacts on their end outcomes (Figure 12.8).

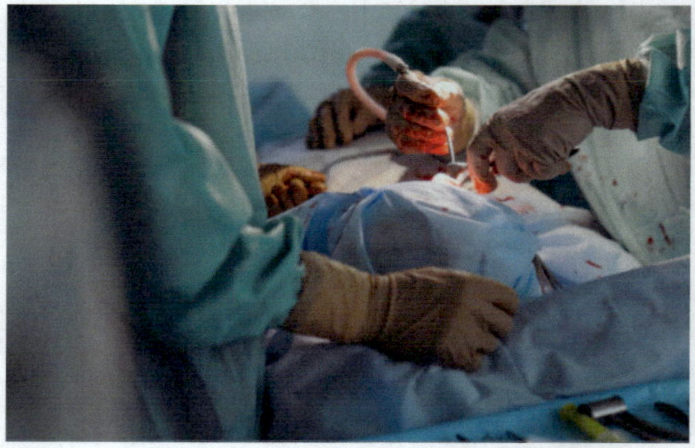

Figure 12.8. New partnership between the Canadian network for international surgery.

Source: https://external-content.duckduckgo.com/iu/?u=https%3A%2F%2Fimages.squarespace-cdn.com%2Fcontent%2Fv1%2F5c838b3aab1a621eed7c5c41%2F1578991272931-PKSWE97ZXOP8O5PS3G91%2Fimage-asset.jpeg&f=1&nofb=1&ipt=3eb4535dbe6c135d1704cb22bcafd6195e6b370b7b950172f1e7d5d65acbc00c.

12.2.3. Collaboration with Interdisciplinary Teams

Successful multidisciplinary team collaboration is the foundation for effective cancer nursing and is essential for achieving optimal patient outcomes. The complexity of cancer care necessitates that healthcare professionals from various disciplines, including oncologists, nurses, pharmacists, social workers, and nutritionists, pool their particular skill sets. The aggregate knowledge facilitates comprehensive patient assessment and individualized care plans that address the multifaceted needs of patients undergoing cancer treatment. Interdisciplinary collaboration also enhances communication between team members, resulting in prompt intervention and optimal support to patients as they navigate the physical and psychological dimensions of their diagnoses. Empirical research evidence supports the notion that interprofessional collaboration can lead to enhanced patient satisfaction and improved overall health outcomes, suggesting a need for optimally coordinated teamwork in oncologic nursing settings. In addition, the adoption of formal interdisciplinary rounds has been shown to increase teamwork and patient care on oncology wards. During these rounds, team members come together to discuss patient progress, share information, and make action plans according to the specific needs of individual patients. This approach not only promotes a teamwork approach but also keeps everyone on the same page regarding treatment plans and patient progress. Moreover, through soliciting input from all parties, including nursing staff members who often interact directly with patients, multidisciplinary groups can facilitate a broader view of patient care dynamics. By prioritizing this collaborative practice, oncology teams not only feel more confident and effective in their practice but can also potentially contribute to lower rates of readmission and improved long-term health outcomes for patients, as indicated in ongoing research on care models within oncologic nursing (Littlepage et al., 2020). Despite the apparent advantages of interdisciplinary collaboration within oncology treatment, there continue to be hurdles in entirely creating these teams within clinical settings. Many nurses lack confidence and competency in delivering nuanced oncologic treatments due to inadequate training and support, which can disrupt smooth collaboration. This can be primarily observed in facilities where patient volumes are low, making it challenging to maintain consistent competencies in oncologic nursing care (Littlepage et al., 2020). Fill these knowledge gaps, and it becomes feasible to consider facility-based competency programs involving new models of training. Web-based learning systems and simulation training can enable nurses to acquire the training and skillset necessary to be effective participants in interprofessional teams, ultimately gaining confidence in providing safe and effective care. With the evolution of healthcare systems, establishing a culture of teamwork will be instrumental in overcoming challenges to efficient oncology nursing management.

Test Your Knowledge

1. What are the primary roles of cancer nurses in providing holistic care across the cancer care continuum?
2. How do cancer nurses address patients and their families' emotional, physical, and educational needs throughout treatment?

12.3. Assessment and Diagnosis

Learning Outcome

1. Explain the comprehensive patient assessment practices in cancer care
2. Set up the diagnostic tests and how they are applicable in cancer care
3. Describe the significance of early detection in the outcomes of treatment in cancer care

An effective assessment and diagnosis process is at the forefront of successful oncologic practice, particularly in oncology nursing. As the population ages, there is ongoing expansion that adds to the occurrence of cancer diagnosis in the elderly, hence the demand for an individualized approach to care. Cancer treatment teams must adopt an integrated assessment protocol that addresses not just physical but also psychosocial aspects, thereby enhancing patient quality of life. Completion of a pre-surgical geriatric assessment is an optimal model, as it reveals important factors such as frailty, social support, and nutritional status that are necessary to forecast risk and tailor interventions. While the importance has been acknowledged by health professionals, many oncogeriatric patients are not assessed holistically, highlighting an existing gap that needs to be addressed to attain the maximum benefit of therapy (Lampugnane et al., 2017). The inclusion of an evidence-based, structured assessment protocol can maximize oncology nursing diagnostic accuracy. Variations in surgical oncology training and practice highlight the need for a unified framework that enhances identification and management processes while being sensitive to regional differences. A global curriculum developed by renowned professional organizations aims to establish crucial standards in surgical oncology training, which, when applied to the nursing framework, can enhance oncology nurses' assessment abilities. Through adherence to these global standards for nursing practice, professionals of cancer care can better equip themselves to perform thorough assessments that inform diagnosis and subsequent treatment planning. Collaboration is critical, as it not only ensures practice consistency but also enables evidence-based practice by nurses, ultimately improving patient outcomes and satisfaction (Are et al., 2016). Additionally, the continuous evolution of assessment tools is crucial in responding to the dynamic nature of oncologic practice.

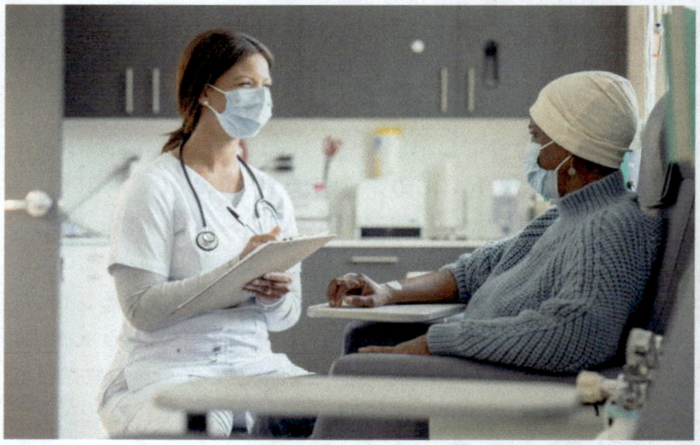

Figure 12.9. Assessment and diagnosis in oncology nursing.

Source: https://simplenursing.com/wp-content/uploads/2023/04/iStock-1384528169-1024x683.jpg.

The developments so far indicate that holism, which integrates physical, emotional, and social well-being, can significantly contribute to diagnostic accuracy and management effectiveness. Telehealth, for instance, has been established as an effective means of conducting patient assessments, particularly during the pandemic when in-person encounters were minimized. Use of technology to engage patients in their own health assessment not only allows for greater access but also for more intense monitoring of future symptomatology. Additionally, interdisciplinary communication among oncology nurses, physicians, and allied healthcare professionals can create a more complete picture of patient needs and encourage earlier interventions. Lastly, having the assessment and diagnosis process proceed is essential in providing world-class, patient-centered care in oncology nursing, which yields improved management interventions and patient results (Figure 12.9).

12.3.1. Comprehensive Patient Assessment Techniques

In the context of oncologic care, integrated patient assessment methods play a pivotal role in successful nursing practice. Integrated patient assessment methods not only enable the detection of cancer symptoms but also enable the healthcare providers to keep an eye on a balanced perception of the patient's experience. Through the systematic use of evaluative procedures, healthcare professionals can collect factual data regarding a patient's physical, emotional, and psychosocial aspects. This extensive assessment is significant since it paves the way for personalized treatment protocols that address not only the physiological aftermath of cancer but also the psychological consequences that accompany it. With an increasing focus on individualized care in cancer nursing, incorporating extensive assessment practices is a crucial step toward achieving optimal outcomes for patients and enhancing their quality of life. At the forefront of successful cancer control is the implementation of non-pharmacological interventions to manage symptoms such as pain and dyspnea. The interventions, including psycho-emotional counseling, hypnosis, and relaxation therapy, underscore the importance of multimodal intervention in the relief of oncologic symptoms. Specifically, systematic assessment has been deemed the gold standard in developing effective ways to manage symptoms. By applying non-pharmacological interventions in conjunction with traditional treatments, health professionals can maximize the health benefits for patients. This complete assessment, besides giving the health professionals the information about the physical symptoms, also documents the emotional and psychological stressors to which patients are subjected so that, through more focused and efficient intervention, these can be addressed as per their individual requirements (Fonseca et al., 2017). Moreover, the value of an organized assessment protocol is highlighted in current guidelines and literature, reaffirming that comprehensive assessments of patients must encompass a range of factors. The Oncology Nursing Society, among other top organizations, advocates for a standardized approach to measuring the needs of cancer patients across various environments (Fonseca et al., 2017). These protocols enable practitioners to recognize and systematically refer to issues that arise due to cancer or its treatment, such as pain control, nutrition, and psychosocial support. In the application of complete assessment approaches, nurses not only shed light on the patient's complex clinical presentation but also construct more effective therapeutic relationships by being in a position to appreciate the multidimensional character of cancer care. This improvement in patient-centered communication actually increases compliance and satisfaction with the overall treatment process.

12.3.2. Diagnostic Tools and Their Significance

The function of diagnostic equipment in oncology is becoming more crucial with the population trend shifting towards an aging population with increased cancer susceptibility. More specifically, geriatric-specific diagnostic assessments are crucial to the success of oncologic care. Geriatric assessment implementation is essential, as it enables providers to more accurately identify the unique risks and needs of older patients. Unfortunately, despite their known importance to healthcare providers, their use in practice remains limited. Time constraints generally prevent providers from conducting these time-increased assessments. Hence, enhancing educational programs to increase awareness and geriatric assessment training can increase utilization, ultimately leading to better surgical results and fewer morbidities among oncogeriatric patients (Lampugnani et al., 2017). Apart from geriatric assessment, the use of novel diagnostic technology is transforming cancer care. From imaging equipment to biomarker testing, the technology enables oncologists to develop highly individualized treatment plans for patients. For instance, molecular diagnostic advances enable the identification of tumor markers specific to a patient's type of cancer, upon which treatment would be based. Because patients' reactions to treatments can be highly inconsistent, precision medicine facilitated by such diagnostic tools becomes necessary to maximize outcomes. Additionally, real-time data obtained through diagnostic technologies provide ongoing evaluation of treatment response, allowing timely adjustment of management regimens as needed (Copeland et al., 2018). Finally, training and education of future healthcare professionals must be provided to enable the maximum utilization of these diagnostic technologies. Inclusion of geriatric and precision medicine elements in medical school curricula can ensure that future clinicians are sufficiently equipped with training on the latest diagnostic technologies and their relevance in oncology. It's not just about training them to apply these tools operationally but also about instilling in them an appreciation for the context within which they are used. By enhancing the confidence and competence of medical students through targeted educational interventions, we can improve the quality of oncogeriatric patient care. Ultimately, by integrating advanced diagnostic practices with targeted educational initiatives, we can enhance cancer management across the entire spectrum of patient populations, particularly among the elderly (Lampugnale et al., 2017).

12.3.3. Importance of Early Detection in Treatment Outcomes

The importance of early detection in cancer treatment outcomes cannot be overemphasized since it plays a direct role in patient survival rates and the possibility of curative interventions. Studies time and again prove that cancers diagnosed at an early stage tend to have a considerably better prognosis than those diagnosed at a later stage. For instance, if breast cancer is detected while in its localized state, the five-year survival rate is up to 99% (American Cancer Society, 2020). Such a stark contrast in outcomes is a testament to the power of regular surveillance and screening in spurring the early detection of cancers. Moreover, nursing experts make an essential contribution to patients' education on cancer signs and symptoms, such that active health behaviors and early consultation with clinicians and diagnostic tests are more likely. Cancer nursing professionals not only arrange screenings but also help develop targeted mechanisms for follow-up that enhance early detection activities. For example, the application of risk assessment forms and assessment of family history can lead to individually tailored screening recommendations, thereby improving the likelihood of cancers being diagnosed at an earlier stage. Such preventive measures, supported by evidence-based interventions, reduce the number of late-stage diagnoses and potentially intensive treatment modalities. The application of technology to the surveillance of high-risk populations plays a crucial role as well; technological innovations, such as cell phone health applications and telehealth visits, can facilitate enhanced access to screening services, allowing for early detection in various patient populations. Through the support of such interventions, oncology nursing can improve patient outcomes and overall care considerably. In addition, the uses of early-stage cancer detection extend beyond individualized patient treatment to encompass broader public health objectives. An education-encouraging awareness strategy can serve to reduce overall cancer death rates through routine screening promotion. Targeted programs addressing underserved populations, typically disproportionately affected with late-stage diagnosis, are a public benefit of early detection programs. Investigation of the underlying determinants, like socioeconomic status, education, and availability of healthcare facilities, illustrates how these factors impact screening practices and resultant treatment outcomes. As evidence suggests, redressal of these inequalities not only helps targeted individuals but also improves the resilience of community health in general. Thus, early detection serves as a cornerstone in oncologic care, emphasizing the importance of an integrated approach towards improved individual and population health outcomes (N/A, 2003, 2005) (Figure 12.10).

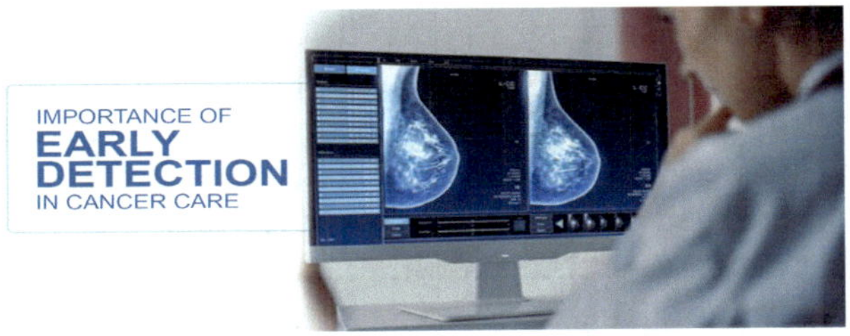

Figure 12.10. Importance-of-early-detection-in-cancer-care.

Source: https://www.kokilabenhospital.com/blog/wp-content/uploads/2023/02/Importance-of-early-detection-in-cancer-care--768x314.jpg.

Test Your Knowledge

1. What key assessments do nurses perform to support early detection and staging of cancer?
2. How do diagnostic imaging, biopsy, and tumor markers influence nursing care planning?

12.4. Treatment Modalities

Learning Outcome

1. Identify the chemotherapy, radiation, and surgery
2. Establish the emerging therapies and clinical trial
3. Explain the palliative care and symptom management

The therapeutic modalities of oncologic therapy encompass a broad range of techniques aimed at combating the unique characteristics of each patient's tumor, as well as the patient's overall health status. Surgical intervention is still a source of cancer therapy, particularly for solid tumors, as it allows direct removal of tumor tissue. However, surgical oncology training varies across the globe, thereby influencing availability and quality of surgical cancer care across populations globally. Having a global curriculum in surgical oncology aims to establish core standards for surgical training, enabling physicians to acquire the necessary knowledge and skills in managing the growing global cancer burden. This is a modular and flexible curriculum designed to meet the unique needs of various regions, thereby enhancing the capacity of the surgical oncology workforce to deliver responsive care within the local environment (Are et al., 2016). In addition to surgery, other treatment options for cancer, such as chemotherapy, radiotherapy, and immunotherapy, have revolutionized cancer treatment to ensure more targeted and effective treatments. Chemotherapy is inherently a systemic modality, trying to eradicate cancer cells that have spread from the primary location, with radiation localizing control. More recent advances in immunotherapy, involving the use of the body's immune response to target the cancer, have created additional opportunities for treatment. The integration of these modalities must be founded on patient-specific factors, particularly in the elderly, where inherent health status can influence the complication of treatment programs.

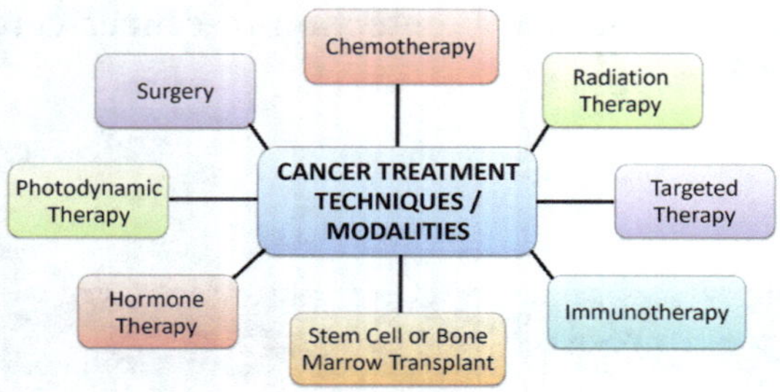

Figure 12.11. Cancer treatment modalities.

Source: https://prinsli.com/wp-content/uploads/2022/04/cancer-treatment-techniques-or-cancer-treatment-modalities.png.

Initiating treatment with comprehensive geriatric assessments preceding it is critical, as it enables practitioners to tailor therapies according to patients' capacities and preferences, thereby optimizing benefits while minimizing adverse effects (Lampugnale et al., 2017). Finally, the multimodal cancer treatment must involve a supportive care modality that addresses the whole spectrum of patients' needs during their treatment journey. This entails the control of physical symptoms such as pain and nausea, and psychological support to help deal with the psychological impact of cancer. Interdisciplinary care among oncology nurses, social workers, and palliative care specialists is essential in the overall management of cancer patients. Such collaboration helps ensure that treatment is not only disease-oriented but also intended to enhance patients' quality of life. Individualized, patient-centered care strategies are essential for addressing the challenges of cancer treatment, emphasizing the need for a holistic approach that combines curative and palliative components in oncologic care (Figure 12.11).

12.4.1. Overview of Chemotherapy, Radiation, and Surgery

The three principal treatment modalities in oncologic management of cancer patients are chemotherapy, radiation, and surgery. All of these approaches are designed to target cancer in its unique way, often in conjunction with each other, to achieve the best therapeutic effects. Chemotherapy involves the use of cytotoxic agents to destroy or inhibit the growth of fast-growing cancer cells. This method is particularly beneficial for cancers that are systemically disseminated, in that it can be used to treat them beyond the localized area. Surgery, on the other hand, involves the physical removal of the tumor and adjacent tissue with the aim of complete resection of neoplastic cells. Radiation therapy, on the other hand, uses high-energy particles or waves to damage the DNA of cancer cells, preventing them from dividing. Both the choice and combinations of these treatments are tailored based on tumor type, extent, and patient-specific factors, highlighting the complexity of oncologic management. The use of these modalities requires a multidisciplinary approach with coordinated care and ongoing communication among healthcare providers. An example is that practice in surgical oncology not only requires excellent technical skills but also an understanding of how surgery is integrated into overall treatment regimens, such as chemotherapy and radiation. Implementing global standards for surgical oncology training may enhance the proficiency of healthcare professionals and ultimately lead to improved cancer patient outcomes worldwide (Are et al., 2016). Quality indicators also need to be continuously monitored to ensure that all modalities are compliant with the set clinical guidelines, thereby optimizing patient care. As multidisciplinary teams assess individual patient needs, they can plan overall treatment plans that ensure effective management of oncology, leading ultimately to improved survival as well as better quality of life. For specific examples such as breast cancer, overall treatment involves not only surgical therapy but also adjuvant therapy which improves recovery and lowers recurrence risk. Institutions, such as breast units, have established that an end-to-end approach significantly improves patient care outcomes (Assaf et al., 2016). T

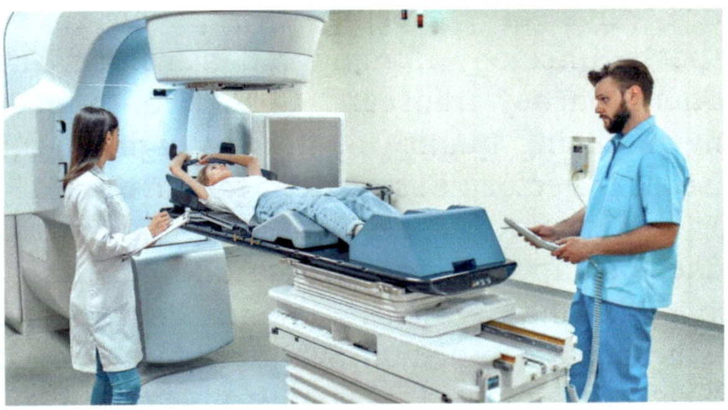

Figure 12.12. Difference between chemotherapy and radiation.

Source: https://external-content.duckduckgo.com/iu/?u=https%3A%2F%2Fwww.medicine.com%2Fcms%2Fimg%2Ffeatured%2FRadiation-therapy-iStock-1311263618.jpg&f=1&nofb=1&ipt=9afc8494a037e36a9f0aa65ede51b41531814d9731e4e87aee05d3c42f90701a.

hese specialty units monitor process and performance indicators with certainty that the entire spectrum of care for patients, including surgical intervention to postoperative recovery, is subject to high standards of quality. This multimodal process allows for optimal planning of therapy based on real-life outcomes, making it essential that clinicians remain current with new oncologic therapies. Ultimately, the integration of chemotherapy, radiation, and surgery underscores the potential for individualized, positive cancer care as outlined by patient status (Figure 12.12).

12.4.2. Emerging Therapies and Clinical Trials

The practice of oncology is evolving at an unmatched rate, driven by novel treatments and clinical trials that will enhance treatment efficacy and patient outcomes. Immunotherapy, precision medicine, and targeted therapies are new treatments that utilize advancements in genetics and molecular biology to administer therapies tailored to the unique characteristics of each cancer. These therapy approaches have been phenomenal in managing various cancers and minimizing side effects associated with traditional treatments like chemotherapy. By individualizing treatment protocols, oncology nurses remain pivotal in monitoring patient responses and managing side effects, thereby ensuring that patients are engaged and informed throughout their care. With an enhanced need for sophisticated oncology therapies, the role of clinical trials becomes even more critical, providing valuable platforms to evaluate the latest interventions and their impact in diverse groups. Clinical trials are the foundation of creating and using new cancer therapies, allowing scientists to study them for safety and efficacy before they can be used extensively. In this setting, the interaction of the healthcare team members, researchers, and nurses is essential, enabling data collection, patient safety monitoring, and adherence to protocols. Nurses involved in clinical trials not only provide physical and emotional care to patients but also serve as patient advocates, ensuring that participants are informed of the potential consequences of their involvement. Trials typically involve several phases, all crucial to evaluating the promise of drugs and optimizing best practices for administration and management. Greater insight and engagement in these trials are a step toward more dynamic and evidence-based practices in oncology, generating an environment in which new therapies can be considered as part of comprehensive cancer care. Comprehensive cancer programs are required to integrate emerging therapies and clinical trials into oncologic management. These programs prioritize not only the implementation of novel treatment modalities but also integrative care aimed at fulfilling the diverse needs of cancer patients. An effectively structured program facilitates interdisciplinary practice, bringing together oncology nurses, oncologists, and researchers who are passionate about improving patient care through innovative approaches. By establishing best practices in clinical trials and new therapies, integrated cancer care centers empower practitioners to navigate the complexities of modern oncology with confidence. This innovation wave, embedded within the integrated care scope, aims to optimize the quality of life and overall survival rates of cancer patients. With regard to a systematic approach, the value of such cancer programs is also enhanced by their ability to address problems in both low- and high-income nations, ultimately resulting in optimized cancer management globally, as advanced by N/A (2001, 2005) (Figure 12.13).

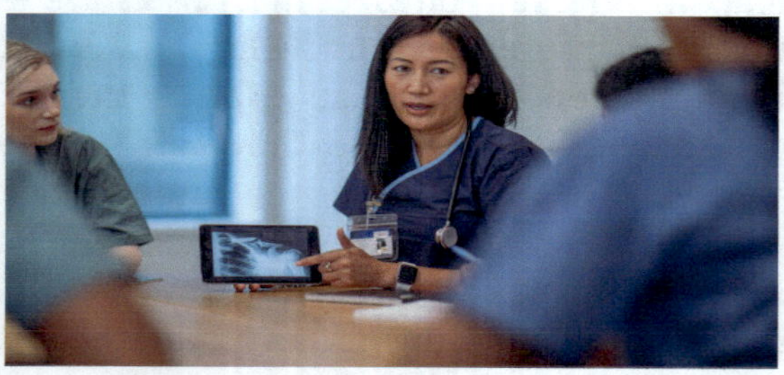

Figure 12.13. Multiple myeloma clinical trials and emerging therapies.

Source: https://themmrf.org/wp-content/uploads/2023/04/trials-hero.png.

12.4.3. Palliative Care and Symptom Management

Palliative care is a significant area of improving the well-being and quality of life of patients when they are facing advanced illness in the discipline of cancer nursing. Historically, palliative care was considered solely as an end-of-life service. Notwithstanding this, newer studies show the critical value of earlier integration of palliative care alongside standard oncologic therapy, as such treatment has been shown to improve health-related quality-of-life indicators in advanced cancer patients highly. Oncology nurses, by virtue of their first-point of contact with patients and their families, are in an optimal position to facilitate this integration, thereby fostering an environment that prioritizes comprehensive symptom control and integrative patient care (Rughani et al., 2022). Treating both physical suffering and psychosocial aspects, oncology nursing can transform the patient journey, transcending survival to focus on enhancing quality of life throughout the disease trajectory. Best patient care in oncology services is based on successful symptom control. Cancer symptoms are diverse and can range from pain and tiredness to mental distress and disturbances of nutrition. Symptom control must be multi-oriented, integrating pharmacologic treatment with supportive therapies, patient education, and family support. Nurses play a crucial role in this process, as they are typically the first to identify symptoms and initiate the relevant interventions (Rughani et al., 2022). Research evidence is that by implementing evidence-based guidelines to control symptoms, oncology nurses can tailor their interventions to individual patients' needs, thereby improving treatment adherence and patient satisfaction. Moreover, discussing patients' symptom experiences can empower them in such a way that care plans are more personalized and grounded in their values and preferences, as well as their understanding of the complexity of their illness. Introducing palliative care principles into oncology practice should also be cognizant of the educational model transferred to healthcare professionals. Developing a global curriculum that includes necessary palliative care competencies in oncologic education will be crucial for establishing a well-trained nursing workforce. Such a curriculum will need to address the diverse and multifaceted competencies to provide symptom management and care for the patients across various sociocultural settings.

Thus, an aspirational curriculum can serve as a common platform for the education of surgical oncologists and oncology nurses worldwide, thereby providing universality to the quality of care offered to cancer patients. By acquiring critical thinking, communication, and patient-centered care skills, nursing education can well equip practitioners to manage the psychological and physiological needs of patients, ultimately leading to improved patient outcomes through quality integration of palliative care (Figure 12.14).

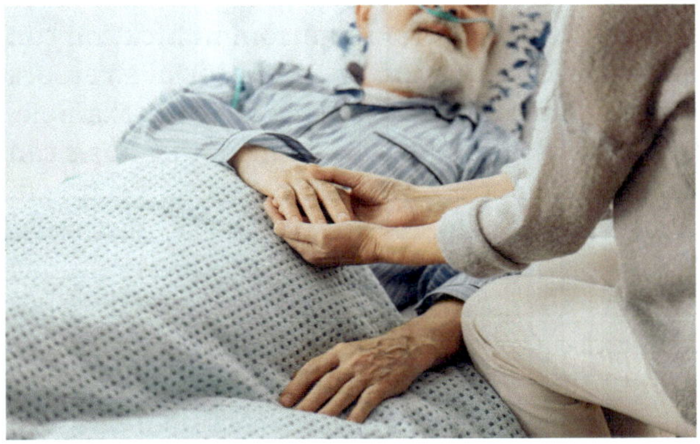

Figure 12.14. Palliative care.

Source: https://planwellguide.com/wp-content/uploads/2022/12/AdobeStock_392089525-2048x1366.jpeg.

Test Your Knowledge

1. What are the main forms of cancer treatment modalities, and how do they vary in mechanism and application?
2. How can nurses ensure the management of side effects and the care of patients undergoing chemotherapy, radiation, or surgery?

12.5. Psychosocial Considerations

Learning Outcome

1. Describe the impact of cancer diagnosis on mental health
2. Define support systems for patients and families
3. Discuss the coping strategies and resources

It is essential to know the psychosocial problems of cancer nursing to provide ideal oncologic care. Cancer patients tend to have a complex interaction of emotional, psychological, and social issues along with their symptoms. The may be anxiety and depression, to isolation and role impairments in social functioning. All such psychosocial problems can significantly impair the patient's adherence to therapy, the quality of their health-related life, and their coping ability. For example, studies have shown that addressing these factors in the early stages of treatment can improve patient outcomes and satisfaction. By integrating comprehensive psychosocial assessments into practice, oncology nurses can better identify the distinct needs of their patients, enabling care to be tailored not only to address the physical, but also the emotional, aspects with a more holistic approach to cancer care. Integrating psychosocial support into cancer care requires a multidisciplinary approach and coordination among oncology nurses, social workers, psychologists, and other healthcare providers. Team communication can enhance identification of psychosocial stressors that are the sources of patient care. For example, the psychological effect of a cancer diagnosis can render patients less compliant towards treatment, which may interfere with recovery outcomes. The implementation of supportive interventions such as counseling and peer groups can both alleviate distress and foster resilience. Moreover, the unique needs of different populations must be appreciated. An international surgical oncology curriculum emphasizes that care must be individualized to account for sociocultural variability, which can significantly impact psychological functioning (Are et al., 2016). In doing so, health professionals can create a supportive environment that recognizes and respects the individual experiences of patients undergoing cancer therapy. A second key region of psychosocial considerations is the integration of palliative care at the beginning stages of cancer treatment. Research has shown that the early integration of palliative care can significantly improve the quality of life in patients by addressing physical issues as well as psychosocial challenges that arise as they progress with cancer (Rughani et al., 2022). Oncology nurses play a pivotal role in advocating for such integration, ensuring that patients receive comprehensive care that encompasses both curative and palliative interventions. By talking over the topic of palliative care with patients, nurses are able to de-mystify the perception of this newfound treatment and invite patients to receive the emotional and psychological care that they need. This initiative reduces the anxiety associated with prognosis and decision-making regarding treatment, thereby empowering patients to make informed treatment decisions.

12.5.1. Impact of Cancer Diagnosis on Mental Health

The cancer diagnosis is also accompanied by profound psychological problems extending well beyond the disease's clinical presentation. Individuals with a cancer diagnosis exhibit very generalized emotional responses, including fear, worry, and depression. These psychological states are usually induced by unpredictable prognosis, physical problems during treatment, and changes in identity associated with a severe illness. Research has established that psychological impairment is most extreme among the elderly, who not only experience death but may also incur additional vulnerabilities of prior illness or social isolation. In a population that is becoming progressively older, as cancer incidence increases with age, there is an urgent need to incorporate the provision of mental health assistance into the treatment regimen of healthcare practitioners. Addressing these emotional needs is crucial in promoting the overall well-being and quality of life of patients throughout their oncologic journey (Lampugnani et al., 2017). Furthermore, the psychological impact of cancer may lead to complications that may hinder treatment and recovery. Anxious or depressed patients may have lower response to medical advice, reduced adherence to supportive care, and poorer overall health outcomes. This calls for a holistic approach to nursing cancer with an emphasis on mental health screening as early as when the patient is diagnosed. Utilizing geriatric assessments tailored for oncologic care can determine patients who are at risk of developing adverse mental health conditions and subsequently can receive interventions promptly. Utilizing tools such as the Geriatric Depression Screening Scale and the Frailty Index can provide valuable information regarding a patient's emotional well-being, facilitating more tailored care. These assessments are not just preventive but can contribute significantly to better treatment outcomes by promoting a favorable environment for the patient (Lampugnale et al., 2017). Last but not least, enhancing the mental well-being of cancer patients requires an interdisciplinary approach among oncologists, nurses, and mental health experts. An integrated cancer care plan shall comprise psychological support services to facilitate normalization of mental health discussion among oncology units. As different cultural and social environments can influence the perception of cancer and mental illness, nursing staff must be culturally sensitive in their practice. As cancer incidence continues to increase globally, the need to address mental health as part of an integrated package of cancer care rises. The implementation of standardized guidelines that incorporate mental health services can ensure that all patients are receiving the complete treatment they need, irrespective of their geographical or sociocultural location (Figure 12.15).

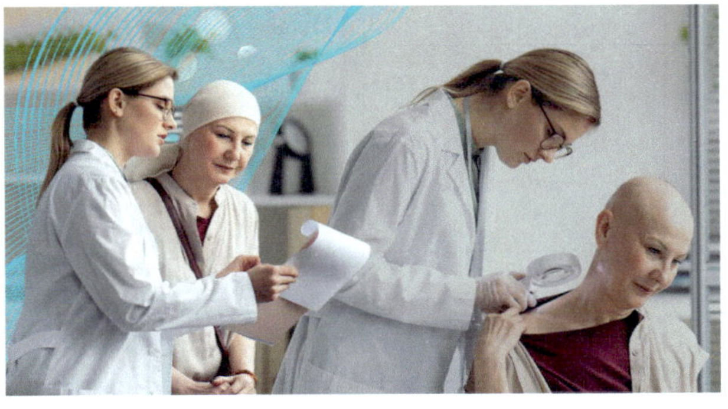

Figure 12.15. The psychological impact of a cancer diagnosis.

Source: https://healthgroovy.com/wp-content/uploads/2023/10/psychological-impact-of-a-cancer-diagnosis.webp.

12.5.2. Support Systems for Patients and Families

The multidimensional nature of cancer therapy necessitates the integration of robust support systems for patients and their' families. These systems consist of an array of resources, including psychological counseling, social services, and community support groups, which are crucial when coping with the emotional and practical challenges faced by a cancer diagnosis. Effectively designed support systems not only equip the patient with the capacity to cope with the disease itself, but also serve as a pool of support for family members who are typically no less distressed. Family participation in the decision-making has been seen to enhance patients' emotional coping, subsequently enhancing treatment adherence and overall satisfaction with the care process. In this case, education on family role dynamics and the importance of comprehensive education regarding cancer can lead to more effective support systems that foster teamwork and better outcomes for all parties involved. Additionally, the role of professional healthcare experts in establishing these support groups cannot be overstated. Oncologists, nurses, and allied healthcare experts are a key component in ascertaining the personal needs of patients, as well as their family members, and guiding them through the challenging waters of cancer treatment. By taking a holistic approach that encompasses the physical, psychological, and social needs of care, health workers can tailor their interventions to most suit the unique needs of each patient. Standardised tools, such as the comprehensive geriatric assessment in older cancer patients, can also further individualize support given, so that care providers can determine key considerations like social support and mental status, which need to be addressed (Lampugnane et al., 2017). Personalised care contributes to creating supportive environments that facilitate healing and emotional well-being. Ultimately, interdisciplinary cooperation emerges as a vital approach to enhancing support mechanisms in oncology nursing. Engaging a range of specialists, including social workers, dietitians, and mental health practitioners, facilitates a multi-faceted response to care for patients. Such partnerships can facilitate workshops, educational programs, and outreach initiatives for communities, empowering patients and families with the information and tools needed to navigate the complexities of cancer therapy. The development of community-based support systems and coalitions can also serve to alleviate emotional burdens from families, ensuring they are not left to face this challenging endeavor alone. As evidenced by global models, such as the development of a modular curriculum for training surgical oncologists, the emphasis on models of collaborative care becomes instrumental in effectively empowering health systems to combat the growing burden of cancer (Are et al., 2016). It is through concerted efforts that robust support systems are fostered, bringing hope and healing to lives touched by cancer (Figure 12.16).

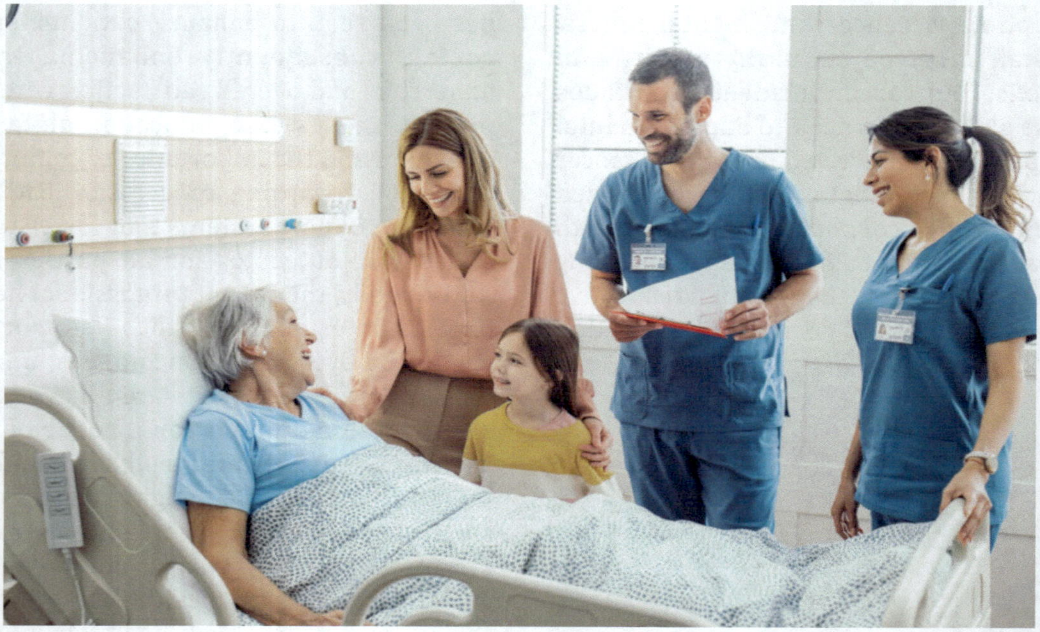

Figure 12.16. Importance of social support in helping patients with cancer deal with change.

Source: https://www.oncologynurseadvisor.com/wp-content/uploads/sites/13/2024/05/elderly-female-patient-nurses-family_G_1392605531.jpg.

12.5.3. Coping Strategies and Resources Available

Coping mechanisms are of most significant importance in the case of cancer, affecting psychological health as much as the quality of life. Patients have been reported to employ diverse coping strategies when faced with the emotional and physical distress of diagnosis and treatment. Patients' active problem-solving, seeking social support, and employing emotion-focused strategies, such as acceptance or positive reinterpretation of their circumstances, are common active coping strategies. The diversity of coping strategies among patients legitimates the existence of heterogeneity in coping strategies, which suggests that individuals may respond diversely to the same stressor, indicating that they should be approached individually. For instance, research has shown that patients with chronic diseases, like cancer-related chronic edema, scored lower in total quality of life and made less use of coping resources, proving the significance of healthcare professionals to assess and enhance patients' coping resources rationally (Armer et al., 2017). The presence of resources also plays a significant role in determining the efficiency of coping activities among cancer patients. Healthcare professionals play a crucial role in facilitating access to a range of resources, including psychosocial support systems, educational materials, and community services. Integrating communications skills into the treatment process raises patients' awareness of available resources, thereby allowing them to access support more effectively. A qualitative patient-experience study demonstrated that effective communication between oncologists and patients was a prerequisite for establishing trust and initiating active health management. By addressing patients' cognitions and affective states, providers are then in a position to deliver improved overall quality of cancer care and equip patients with the necessary tools to cope successfully throughout their treatment process (Mestre et al., 2019). Furthermore, regular monitoring of coping efforts and available resources should be a standard component of oncologic care. This is not just about promoting formal support systems, such as therapy or support groups, but also about encouraging patients to engage with informal networks, including family and friends. The multidimensional needs of cancer care necessitate that emotional resilience be enhanced by considering a range of approaches that address both clinical and supportive needs. Therefore, nursing interventions that target facilitating strengthening coping resources should offer an amiable environment where patients are open to articulating their preferences and needs. Lastly, a general equilibrium between emotional and informational support is crucial for ensuring effective coping mechanisms, which leads to improved cancer management outcomes and patient satisfaction (Armer et al., 2017).

Test Your Knowledge

1. How may cancer diagnosis and therapy influence the emotional, social, and psychological well-being of a patient?
2. What are the approaches nurses can use to provide effective psychosocial care of patients and families with cancer?

12.6. Ethical and Legal Issues in Oncology

Learning Outcome

1. Describe the informed consent and patient autonomy
2. Define the end-of-life care and decision-making
3. Identify the ethical dilemmas in treatment

Oncology raises ethical and legal issues that are multifaceted and must be managed by the clinician through subtle situations arising when there is a diagnosis of cancer. At the heart of the ethical assumptions surrounding the issue is the obligation to tell the truth, especially when a diagnosis has a profound impact on patients' lives. For cancer patients and those with gastrointestinal disease, not just the revelation of the diagnosis but also the emotional and psychological impact that follows is necessary. A study on interaction in the treatment of cancer underscores the importance of effective communication, with doctors and nurses both playing a part in establishing a climate of trust through the imparting of accurate information about patients' states and the treatments offered. There needs to be consideration of how ethical demands can influence patients' consent to treatment and their understanding of end-of-life choices, which are particularly complex in oncology (Andreea et al., 2019). Another significant area of concern in oncology is the legal aspect of consent, particularly in clinical trials. Patient autonomy is a core principle of modern medical ethics; however, its application can become complicated when patients are faced with the need to decide on experimental therapies. Informed consent is a procedure that requires transparency, allowing patients to make informed decisions about their treatment while protecting healthcare providers from excessive legal repercussions. Despite the focus on patient rights, research shows that the majority of oncologists believe they are duty-bound to prioritize clinical outcomes over explanations, which can erode informed consent. By discussing the advantages and disadvantages of treatment versus clinical trials in detail, medical professionals can better align their ethical responsibilities with legal ones, thereby informing patients thoroughly about their options (Lampugnane et al., 2017). Lastly, physician-assisted suicide (PAS) is still an emotive cause of ethical as well as legal debate in oncology. Given the fact that the outlook for cancer is often accompanied by suffering and loss of quality of life, discussions around PAS face medical professionals with reconciling medical ethics with personal faith as well as statutory law. Legal policies for PAS vary greatly, where jurisdictions offer PAS under strict criteria, but other regions are subject to strict prohibition. Oncologists and oncology nurses must handle such laws humanely and sensitively, being mindful to provide information and support to the patients regarding this method. Ethical concerns are most appropriate when addressing the demands and wishes of dying patients, placing into perspective the vital significance of palliative care for oncology. This complexity requires ongoing education and debate within the healthcare community to address the ethics of PAS and establish a legal system that respects both patient autonomy and the sanctity of life (Andreea et al., 2019) (Figure 12.17).

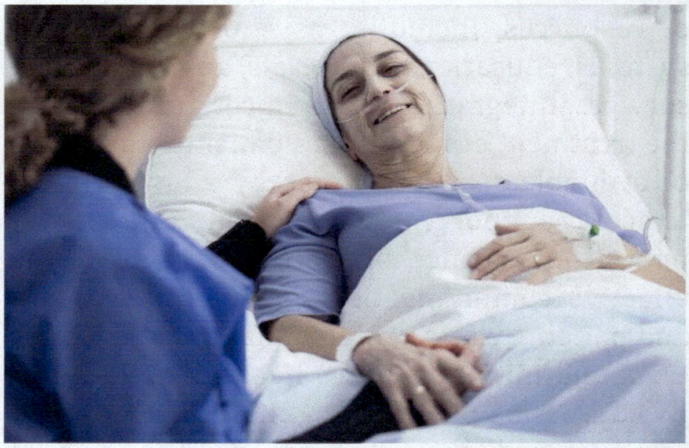

Figure 12.17. Nurse ethics in oncology.

Source: https://www.amnhealthcare.com/siteassets/candidate-blog/nursing/travel/oncology-nurse-ethics-1.jpg.

12.6.1. Informed Consent and Patient Autonomy

In cancer nursing, informed consent plays important role in promoting patient autonomy, with the intention of enabling individuals to possess the ability for decision-making with regard to their treatment options. Informed consent is not merely a procedural requirement, but instead involves the understanding of the relevant medical facts, risks, benefits, and alternatives to interventions being considered. This means that oncology nurses must be adept at explaining sophisticated medical jargon in simple, everyday terms, creating an atmosphere in which patients can ask questions and raise concerns with ease. The inherent ethical principle of respect for autonomy leads healthcare providers to approach patients as active partners in their care rather than passive recipients, thereby enhancing trust and collaboration in the healthcare setting. Thus, informed consent plays an essential role not only due to legal requirements but also as a statement of the dignity and autonomous decision-making of cancer patients. Recognizing the importance of informed consent underscores the profound implications of patient autonomy in the treatment of oncology. Patient autonomy is the capacity of individuals to make choices on their own values, beliefs, and interests. In cancer care, this can be especially important because patients are presented with decisions that can affect not just their physical health, but also their quality of life and mental state. Empowering patients to actively participate in their treatment decisions can make a significant difference. Oncology nurses are ideally suited to be the drivers of a model of shared decision making, in which patients and providers cooperatively weigh options based on informed consent. Such a model respects transparency and personal values, acknowledging that the typically challenging emotional and moral landscape of cancer care can be navigated, with patients' wishes and values given considerable consideration. Furthermore, the nuances of patient autonomy and informed consent become a crucial issue in cases wherein patients may possess diminished decision-making capacity due to the physical and psychological weight of cancer. For instance, as in the settings of oncology and palliative care, clinicians often encounter situations wherein the patient refuses food as an expression of autonomy within end-of-life care. The inclination to respect a patient's decision, even in states of partial capacity, underlines the delicate equilibrium between ethical duties and the demand for empathy in treatment protocols. Consequently, doctors who practice medicine must receive additional training to recognize and manage such occurrences effectively. Developing a sensitive definition of informed consent not only prevents accurately labeling patients' actions incorrectly but also upholds the dignity of patients in their intense autonomy of end-of-life decisions, symbolizing the intense ethical obligation to defend patients' dignity throughout the trajectory of cancer (Esteves et al., 2016; Büche et al., 2020).

12.6.2. End-of-Life Care and Decision-Making

Decision-making at the end of life and care for cancer patients is a , profound, and sensitive realm of oncologic care. When the patient reaches this phase of his/her course, integration of palliative care is paramount, with prioritization of comfort and quality of life over curative treatment. Decision-making must be multidisciplinary, involving oncologists, nurses, palliative care specialists, and social workers to ensure that all aspects of patient health—physical, emotional, and spiritual—are considered. Effective communication is essential, as healthcare practitioners must navigate patient and family wishes, cultural beliefs, and ethical dilemmas. Ensuring dialogue about goals of care occurs is paramount, as this can guide interventions and provide some degree of relief regarding impending loss. Lastly, decision-making towards the end of life should prioritize patient dignity and desires, while establishing an environment where informed choices can be made in unison. In cancer nursing, there is a critical role for professionals in advocating for effective end-of-life care, such as assessment in a profound and holistic context that captures not only the physical symptoms but also psychosocial dynamics. Nurses are typically directly involved with patients and their families, providing direct care and support, and thus placed in a position where they can assess the dynamic needs of patients and their families. The utilization of comprehensive geriatric assessments in this population can help gain a clearer insight into the specific issues faced by elderly cancer patients. Such assessments can reveal underlying issues, such as frailty or loneliness, which significantly influence treatment decisions and quality of life (Lampugnale et al., 2017). Through this identification, nurses can become active participants in conversations with patients and the healthcare team about what quality of life means to them at the end of life. Additionally, the decision-making model of end-of-life care is enhanced through an understanding of global training paradigms for surgical oncologists, which span every level of the healthcare system (Are et al., 2016). Because variations in training exist globally, possessing a foundation for understanding these variations can inform practice adaptation of end-of-life care in multicultural settings. Developing an international curriculum in surgical oncology also creates a uniform yet malleable model for oncologic care that recognizes the unique sociocultural determinants influencing patient decision and availability of care. This wide-ranging education equips healthcare professionals for the competencies required to navigate the complex emotional environment of end-of-life conversations, to provide increased and compassionate care for cancer patients and families (Figure 12.18).

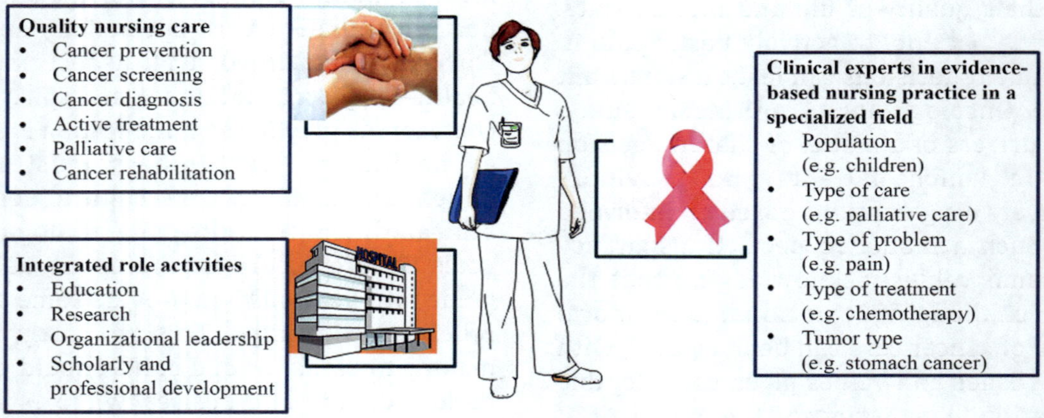

Figure 12.18. The oncology nurse's role in quality nursing care.

Source: https://www.researchgate.net/publication/370346735/figure/fig1/AS:11431281242179291@1715419885943/The-oncology-nurses-role-in-quality-nursing-care-integrated-role-activities-and.tif.

12.6.3. Navigating Ethical Dilemmas in Treatment

In oncologic practice management, navigating ethical challenges in treatment becomes an indispensable aspect of cancer nursing. With the set of ethical issues that arise in the management of patients with cancer, there are challenges of honesty of communication and psychological impacts to patients and their families. The ethical doctrine of patient autonomy provides a platform through which patients are presented with credible information regarding their condition and care, enabling them to make informed decisions concerning their care. The principle becomes particularly applicable in the context of digestive cancers, where communication complexity is further increased. Such ethical needs compel nurses and physicians to engage in open conversations that not only inform patients with clinical facts but also meet patients' emotional needs, thereby creating a facilitating environment amidst the often-overwhelming reality of diagnosis (Andreea et al., 2019). Moreover, the ethical decision in dealing with treatment becomes even more complex when treating the special needs of geriatric patients with cancer. As the demographic of the aging population is expected to grow further in the United States, oncogeriatric patients present particularly challenging issues for medical practitioners. Oncogeriatric patients tend to be at a greater risk for comorbidities that complicate treatment, so informed consent becomes even more critical. Ethical dilemmas may also arise as a result of pugnacious treatment suggestions being in opposition to worries for the quality of life in patients. This dilemma highlights the importance of geriatric assessments before surgery, as they aid in identifying the optimal treatments based on patients' varying frailty and support systems. By prioritizing these appraisals more highly, healthcare workers are better able to navigate the ethical landscape, weighing the risks and benefits of treatment in accordance with the principle of beneficence while protecting patient-directed care (Lampugnale et al., 2017). Finally, the ethical issues surrounding end-of-life care and decision-making further complicate the landscape of cancer care. Palliative care, euthanasia, and physician-assisted suicide discussions are fraught with ethical issues that need to be handled with care and sensitivity. While nurses engage in advance directives and respect the end-of-life wishes of patients, they must balance professional requirements with respect for patient autonomy and family dynamics. Providing holistic care and making sure palliative patients receive empathetic treatment in accordance with their wishes is a pillar of ethical oncology practice. Lastly, embracing a holistic approach that integrates ethical principles into treatment planning not only enhances the quality of patient care but also empowers nurses and other healthcare professionals to make ethically sound judgments as they handle the complex issues of cancer management (Lampugnane et al., 2017) (Figure 12.19).

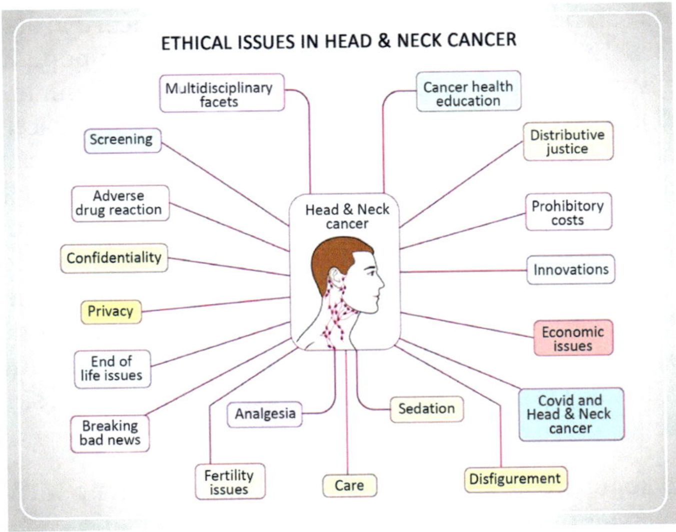

Figure 12.19. Social, ethical and treatment related problems faced by healthcare workers in the care of head and neck cancer patients.

Source: https://media.springernature.com/lw1200/springer-static/image/art%3A10.1007%2Fs12070-023-03738-w/MediaObjects/12070_2023_3738_Fig1_HTML.png.

Test Your Knowledge

1. What are the frequent ethical challenges in cancer care faced by oncology nurses, particularly in end-of-life issues?
2. How do oncology nurses promote informed consent and patient autonomy in the treatment process?

SUMMARY

From the discussion of cancer nursing and the principles of oncologic management, it is evident that an approach with multiple facets is essential for effective patient care. Cancer nurses are pivotal agents, enabling the integration of clinical expertise, patient advocacy, and psychosocial care through an integrated treatment model. Their role extends beyond the mere provision of treatment administration; it encompasses the management of patients' experiences, which involve coping with complex health decisions, particularly in terms of fertility and family planning during treatment. As seen in the findings, the majority of patients reported very minimal conversations about contraception choices with their oncology providers, which is a key shortage in the care continuum that must be addressed. The requirement for such discussions is based on patient empowerment and safeguarding of their reproductive rights and health outcomes (Lindsay et al., 2018). The necessity to address the unique healthcare needs of selected patient populations, such as oncogeriatric patients, has also emerged as a pressing concern in oncologic care. The increasing geriatric population in the United States necessitates an age-related approach to surgical interventions and care interventions for the elderly with cancer. Risk stratification is mandated by comprehensive geriatric assessments, which remain underutilized due to time constraints in clinical practice. With the incorporation of these assessments in oncologic practice, quality of life and outcomes for patients can be significantly enhanced by healthcare professionals. Complications of this practice, particularly in conducting thorough tests among the population, remain significant issues that healthcare systems should prioritize in their pursuit of enhancing the quality of care (Lampugnale et al., 2017). Lastly, the evolution of oncologic nursing practice relies on continuous evaluation and adaptation of care models to meet the evolving needs of cancer patients. Improved guidelines that guarantee enhanced contraception screening and geriatric assessments must be developed and implemented through multidisciplinary collaboration among oncologists, nurses, and other interdisciplinary teams. With the evolution of cancer treatment, ongoing education of health professionals on the principles of oncologic care will be essential. This will not only ensure compliance with best standards but also restore patient autonomy and facilitate shared decision-making, thereby improving the patient experience along their cancer journey. Integration of these premises will, in the end, promote the quality of cancer nursing care to patients and health populations alike.

In the context of oncologic medical-surgical unit care management, identifying the multifaceted challenges that define cancer nursing, particularly in acute settings, is necessary. According to evidence, nurses posted in oncologic medical-surgical units are likely to experience low patient admission rates for those requiring critical therapies, such as chemotherapy and follow-up care. This condition can result in low professional confidence among nursing staff, who pose safety concerns regarding whether or not they can handle chemotherapy or provide complete care for cancer patients (Littlepage et al., 2020). These shortcomings can be overcome through the establishment of competency validation programs dedicated explicitly to oncologic nursing. With the integration of web-based learning and simulation training, hospitals can enhance nursing capabilities and foster a deeper understanding of oncologic concepts among their staff. Further, the integration of innovative educational approaches is evident in ongoing efforts to develop nursing capacity in cancer care through comprehensive training programs. The efforts involve both theoretical foundations and practical applications, facilitating nurses in addressing oncologic concepts effectively. Initial research findings on nursing education have shown promising results. For instance, nurses participating in competency programs reported considerable gains in their self-assessed knowledge and self-perceived confidence with respect to oncologic nursing care and chemotherapy administration, the latter going from 46.4% to 78% (Littlepage et al., 2020). These findings confirm the effectiveness of these learning approaches, indicating promise in equipping nurses with the necessary skills to manage complex oncologic cases and, by extension, enhancing patient care outcomes. Aside from professional education, the emotional and psychological aspects of cancer care should not be downplayed. For patients and caregivers who have to cope with the complexity involved in life-threatening diagnoses, the importance of holistic care becomes increasingly apparent. Research has shown that patients and caregivers often experience severe emotional distress and undergo a significant decrease in quality of life upon receiving a cancer diagnosis. For these conditions to be improved, incorporating palliative care principles into oncologic treatment is essential. To effectively accomplish this, however, one should practice caution regarding the integration because the conventional interpretation of palliative care runs the risk of evoking death- and treatment-ceasing anxieties. By redefining these conversations and promoting genuine about end-of-life care, health care providers are able to give patients sensitive, holistic care that honors their individual preferences and needs and thus improves the oncologic care experience overall.

KEY TERMS FROM THIS CHAPTER

- Biopsy
- Cancer Pain Management
- Chemotherapy
- Immunotherapy
- Nausea and Vomiting (CINV)
- Nutritional Support in Cancer
- Oncology
- Psychosocial Support
- Survivorship Care Plan
- Bone Marrow Transplantation
- Carcinogenesis
- Fatigue Management
- Metastasis
- Neutropenia
- Oncologic Emergencies
- Palliative Care
- Radiation Therapy
- Targeted Therapy

CRITICAL THINKING QUESTIONS

1. **What is the primary goal of cancer screening in nursing practice?**
   a. To treat cancer aggressively
   b. To detect cancer early and improve outcomes
   c. To determine the patient's pain threshold
   d. To provide palliative care only
2. **Which of the following treatments is considered systemic cancer therapy?**
   a. Surgery
   b. Radiation therapy
   c. Chemotherapy
   d. Biopsy
3. **A major side effect of chemotherapy that nurses must monitor for is:**
   a. Hypertension
   b. Hypercalcemia
   c. Neutropenia
   d. Bradycardia
4. **What is the nurse's primary responsibility during radiation therapy?**
   a. Prescribing analgesics
   b. Instruction:
   c. Patient education on skin care and tissue damage monitoring
   d. Operation of radiation equipment
   e. IV fluids administration
5. **What is the definition of symptom relief and quality of life-focused care in late stages of cancer?**
   a. Curative care
   b. Aggressive therapy
   c. Preventive care
   d. Palliative care

Short Answer Questions

1. Define oncology nursing and its chief objectives.
2. What are two side effects of chemotherapy that must be met by nurses?
3. Define the TNM cancer staging system briefly.
4. What is the nurse's role in patient education regarding cancer treatment?
5. Detail nursing roles in administering and managing chemotherapy side effects.
6. Explain how nurses support the psychosocial needs of cancer patients and families throughout the disease progression.
7. Discuss the role of early detection in cancer and the nurse's role in screening and health promotion.
8. Compare and contrast curative, adjuvant, and palliative cancer therapies and how the nursing care differs with each.

Answers to Critical Thinking Questions

1. (b) 2. (c) 3. (c) 4. (b) 5. (d)

REFERENCES

1. Puts, M. T. E., Hsu, T., Szumacher, E., Sattar, S., Toubasi, S., Rosario, C., Brain, E., Duggleby, W., Mariano, C., Mohile, S., Muss, H., Trudeau, M., Wan-Chow-Wah, D., Wong, C., & Alibhai, S. M. H. (2017). Meeting the Needs of the Aging Population: The Canadian Network on Aging and Cancer—Report on the First Network Meeting, 27 April 2016. *Current Oncology*, *24*(2), 163-170. https://doi.org/10.3747/co.24.3455Andreea, G., Badiu, D. C., Dumitru, A., Hulea, V., et al. (2019). Ethical aspects in managing patients diagnosed with digestive cancers: A review of literature. https://core.ac.uk/download/216811031.pdf (accessed on 28th June 2025).
2. Are, C., Audisio, R. A., Berman, R. S., Cummings, C., et al. (2016). Global curriculum in surgical oncology. https://core.ac.uk/download/46580365.pdf (accessed on 28th June 2025).
3. Armer, J. M., Cohen, S., Cormier, J., Davidson, T. N., Fallowfield, L., International Lymphoedema Framework, International Society of Lymphology, et al. (2017). Psychological factors in chronic edema: A case–control study. https://core.ac.uk/download/161525056.pdf (accessed on 28th June 2025).
4. Assaf, K. (2016). Oncological and aesthetic-functional evaluations of almost 200 patients who underwent in 2014 to breast cancer surgery. https://core.ac.uk/download/79620953.pdf (accessed on 28th June 2025).
5. Barber, M., Boyd, K., Cowey, E., Kendall, M., et al. (2018). Outcomes, experiences and palliative care in major stroke: A multicenter, mixed-method, longitudinal study. https://core.ac.uk/download/159991977.pdf (accessed on 28th June 2025).
6. Beauchemin, M. P. (2019). Supporting clinical decision making in cancer care delivery. https://core.ac.uk/download/231878618.pdf (accessed on 28th June 2025).
7. Bennett-Guerrero, E., Bergamaschi, R., Gan, T. J., Gottumukkala, V., et al. (2017). American Society for Enhanced Recovery (ASER) and Perioperative Quality Initiative (POQI) joint consensus statement on measurement to maintain and improve quality of enhanced recovery pathways for elective colorectal surgery. https://core.ac.uk/download/81681180.pdf (accessed on 28th June 2025).
8. Büche, D., Fringer, A., Ott, S. C., Schnepp, W., et al. (2020). The associations of palliative care experts regarding food refusal: A cross-sectional study with an open question evaluated by triangulation analysis. https://core.ac.uk/download/304636098.pdf (accessed on 28th June 2025).
9. Carron, P. N., Dami, F., Diawara, F., Hugli, O., et al. (2014). Palliative care and prehospital emergency medicine: Analysis of a case series. https://core.ac.uk/download/77180728.pdf (accessed on 28th June 2025).
10. Cerminara, K. L. (2011). Hospice and health care reform: Improving care at the end of life. https://core.ac.uk/download/51092475.pdf (accessed on 28th June 2025).
11. Colomer, R., Ferro, T., Jiménez, M. del M., Muñoz, M., et al. (2016). Advanced breast cancer clinical nursing curriculum: Review and recommendations. https://repositorio.uam.es/bitstream/10486/680256/5/advanced_vila_cto_2017.pdf (accessed on 28th June 2025).
12. Copeland, L. I. B. T., James, D., Duinkerken, M. S. I., & Kelsey, A. (2018). Jefferson Digital Commons quarterly report: April–June 2019. https://core.ac.uk/download/220159103.pdf (accessed on 28th June 2025).

13. Esteves, F., Mega, A. C., Mesquita, J., Nóbrega, T., et al. (2016). Adaptación del modelo ABCDE de medicina humana para comunicar malas notícias a lo dueño del paciente oncologico en medicina veterinaria. https://core.ac.uk/download/80518348.pdf (accessed on 28th June 2025).

14. Fonseca, C., Lopes, M. J., Mendes, F., Parreira, P., et al. (2017). Control of pain and dyspnea in patients with oncologic disease in acute care: Non-pharmacological intervention. https://core.ac.uk/download/154812508.pdf (accessed on 28th June 2025).

15. Fuly, P. D. S. C., Oliveira, B. G. R. B. de, Padilha, K. G., Pires, D., et al. (2016). Carga de trabalho de enfermagem de pacientes oncológicos sob cuidados paliativos. https://core.ac.uk/download/268283548.pdf (accessed on 28th June 2025).

16. Lampugnale, C. A. (2017). Surgical assessment of the geriatric oncology patient. https://open.bu.edu/bitstream/2144/26707/5/Lampugnale_bu_0017N_13146.pdf (accessed on 28th June 2025).

17. Lindsay, S. (2018). Understanding facilitators and barriers to contraception screening and referral in young women with cancer. https://open.bu.edu/bitstream/2144/32681/7/Lindsay_bu_0017N_14014.pdf (accessed on 28th June 2025).

18. Littlepage, D. (2020). Using simulation for oncology nursing competency evaluation in hospitals. https://core.ac.uk/download/428348772.pdf (accessed on 28th June 2025).

19. Mestre, C. A. J. (2019). Talk and let talk: Communication is the key: Patients' perspective about oncologic consultations and its implications for quality of cancer care. https://core.ac.uk/download/542329619.pdf (accessed on 28th June 2025).

20. Rughani, R. (2022). Early integration of palliative care with curative oncology treatment for patients with advanced cancer: Implications for clinical nursing practice. https://core.ac.uk/download/559452572.pdf (accessed on 28th June 2025).

INDEX

G

H

I

K

L

M

Q

R

S

W